VENEERS

FANTASY RISK SUCCESS

MACIEJ ŻAROW

Co-authors:
WALTER DEVOTO
LOUIS HARDAN
MARGARIDA HENRIQUE
MARCO NICASTRO
DANIELE RONDONI

VENEERS

FANTASY RISK SUCCESS

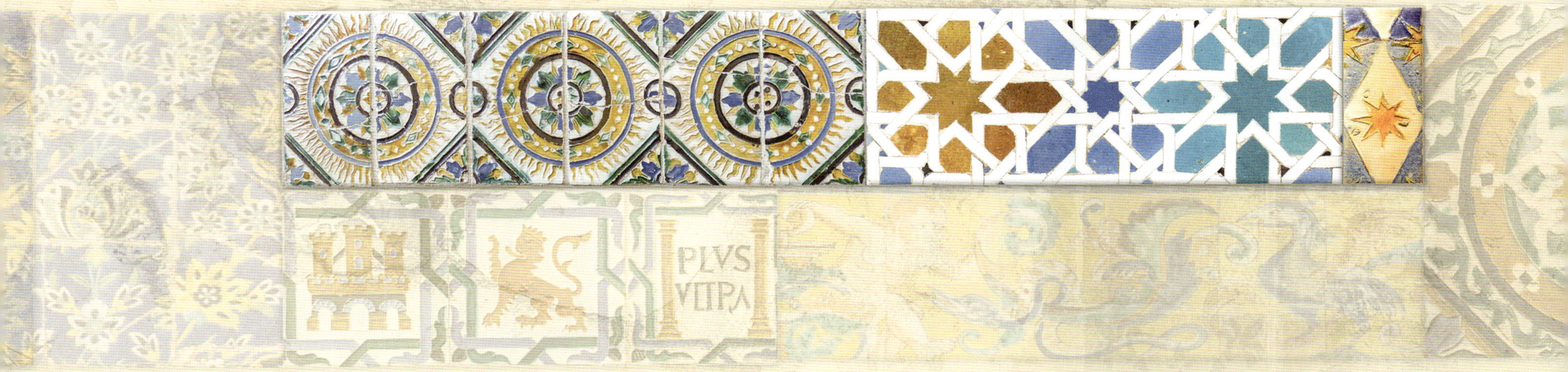

QUINTESSENCE PUBLISHING

Berlin | Chicago | Tokyo
Barcelona | London | Milan | Mexico City | Paris | Prague | Seoul | Warsaw
Beijing | Istanbul | Sao Paulo | Zagreb

One book, one tree: In support of reforestation worldwide and to address the climate crisis, for every book sold Quintessence Publishing will plant a tree (https://onetreeplanted.org/).

A CIP record for this book is available from the British Library.

QUINTESSENCE PUBLISHING DEUTSCHLAND

Quintessenz Verlags-GmbH
Ifenpfad 2–4
12107 Berlin
Germany
www.quintessence-publishing.com

Quintessence Publishing Co Ltd
Grafton Road, New Malden
Surrey KT3 3AB
United Kingdom
www.quintessence-publishing.com

Editor: Iwona Koziel, Anya Hastwell
Design: Janina Knap
Design, typesetting and layout: Janina Knap, Małgorzata Trębicka, Sabine Theuring
Drawings: Julia Gebel
Translation: Natalia Jakubowicz, Anthony Casey

ISBN 978-1-78698-116-5

Printed in Croatia

"A goal without a plan is just ... a wish"
Antoine de Saint-Exupéry

I DEDICATE THIS BOOK
TO PROFESSOR ZBIGNIEW JAŃCZUK,
OUR TIRELESS MENTOR

ABOUT THE AUTHORS

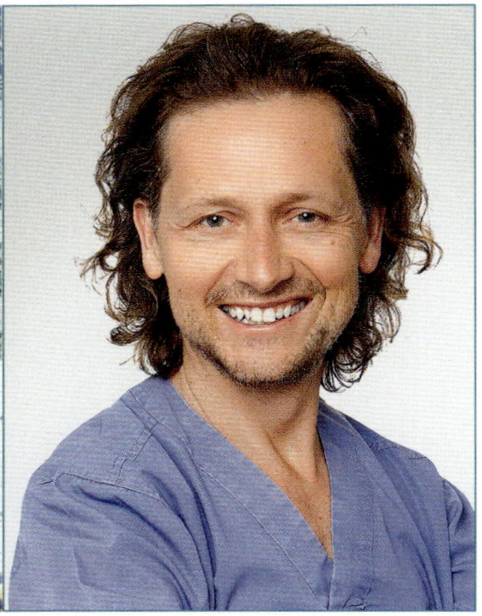

Maciej ŻAROW

Professional profile

He received his dental degree from the Faculty of Dentistry at Semmelweis University, Budapest (Hungary). Upon his graduation, Maciej pursued a Doctor of Medical Sciences title, obtained after Pass with Honors for his dissertation defense on composite inlays-onlays in the restoration of endodontically treated teeth. Maciej has been a long-time researcher and lecturer, working with dental students at the Department of Propedeutics of Conservative Dentistry of CMUJ, Krakow. During his International Association of Dental Research scholarship, he conducted research work on adhesive bridges (FDPs) as well as the restoration of endodontically treated teeth at the universities of Leeds and Manchester. He has been a visiting professor at the University of Chieti (Italy), and visiting lecturer the UIC University (Barcelona). In 2021 he became a mentor at the prestigious Kois Center in Seattle. In 1999 Maciej established his private practice "Dentist" in Krakow and maintains it with his energetic attitude and everlasting passion.

Clinical practice

Maciej is an experienced clinician working with an extensive spectrum of practical approaches to dental treatment. He is keen on promoting and implementing new restorative techniques in his everyday practice. He furthermore favors initiating modern interdisciplinary procedures that harmonize esthetics with function and minimize interference with the natural mechanisms of functioning of the whole stomatognathic system. Maciej successfully carries out this philosophy in his private dental practice "Dentist" in Krakow, as well as in his Postgraduate Courses Center.

Professional activity

Maciej takes pride in being Editor-in-Chief of the *Quintessence for Dentists* journal. His book, *EndoProsthodontics: A Guide for Clinical Practice*, has achieved success and is now published in English, Chinese, Croatian, French, and Russian. He has authored more than 80 scientific papers in both national and international journals. Maciej is also an active member in the Italian restorative dentistry research group "Style Italiano," as well as the Polish Academy of Esthetic Dentistry. In 2019 he became a certified member of European Society of Cosmetic Dentistry.

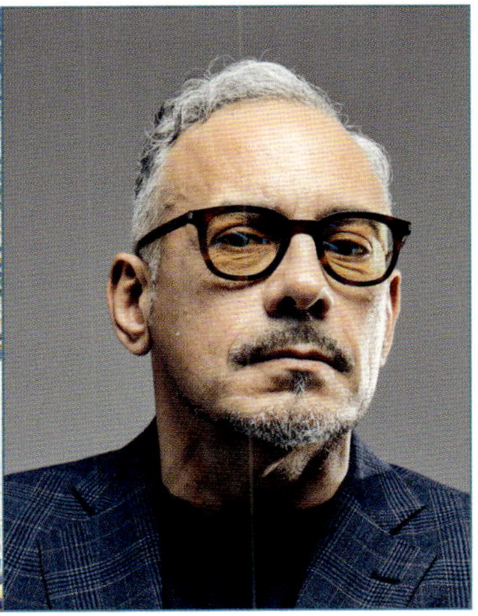

Walter DEVOTO

Professional profile
A graduate w th honors from the Faculty of Dentistry and Prosthodontics at the University of Genoa (Italy), Walter's postgraduate studies are in the field of dental prosthetics. Initiator and participant of university research programs. University lecturer at medical schools in Madrid and Siena.

Clinical practice
Runs private practices specializing in esthetic dentistry and dental surgery in Sestri Levante and Portofino (Italy). He cooperates clinically with prestigious centers of esthetic dentistry around the world. Visiting professor at the Universitè de la Méditerranée in Marseille (France).

Professional activity
Member of the European Academy of Esthetic Dentistry – a founding member of its counterpart in Italy. Founder of the Style Italiano research group. An innovator of instrument technology and methods in the field of esthetics with composite material. Renowned lecturer at national and international congresses, author and co-author of books, including *Le Guide Estetique*, *Odontoiatria Restaurativa*, *Traumatologia Oral*, and *Layers*.

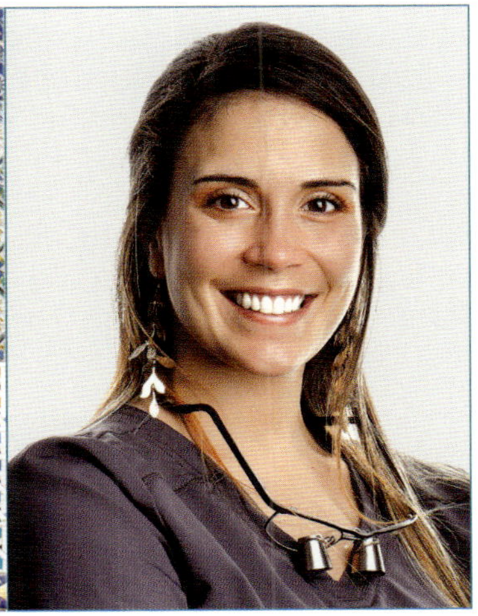

Margarida HENRIQUE

Professional profile
A dentist by choice and a graduate of the Medical University of Porto (Portugal), a few years later becoming a Master of Implantology at the University of Seville (Spain). There, she completed postgraduate studies in the field of esthetic dentistry.

Clinical practice
Runs a private dental clinic specializing in surgical and prosthetic treatment. She improves her knowledge and gains new experiences as a participant of renowned courses and congresses in prestigious dental training centers. She has unique knowledge in the field of tooth morphology, so necessary to optimize the esthetics and function.

Professional activity
Since 2019, she has actively participated in the activities of the Style Italiano group.

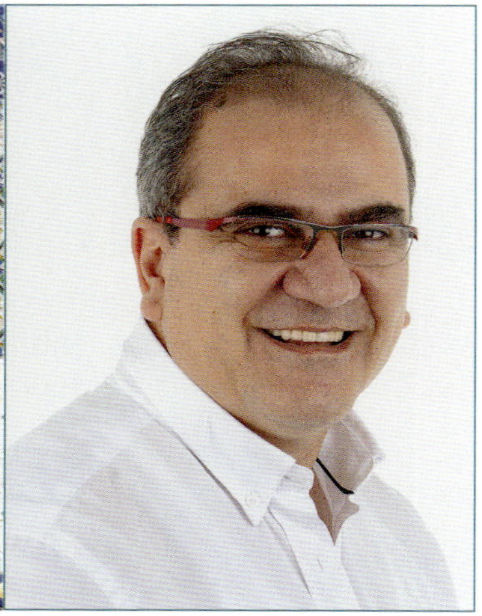

Louis HARDAN

Professional profile
A graduate of the Saint Joseph University of Beirut-Lebanon. Full Professor, DDS, CES, DEA, Ph.D. – and former head of the restorative and esthetic department and director of the Master's program. He graduated in dentistry in 1989 and was awarded his Ph.D. in oral biology and dental materials in 2009.

Clinical practice
Owns a private practice in his hometown Byblos (Lebanon), dealing with esthetic dentistry. Inventor of Mobile Dental Photography systems for anterior and posterior documentation and optimizing dentist's communication with the dental laboratory.

Professional activity
Member of the Lebanese Dental Society – former general secretary of this organization. Scientific Director and Honorary Member of Style Italiano. Renowned congress lecturer, author of numerous publications in international specialist journals and author of the book: *Protocols for Mobile Dental Photography with Auxiliary Lighting* (Quintessence Publishing, 2020).

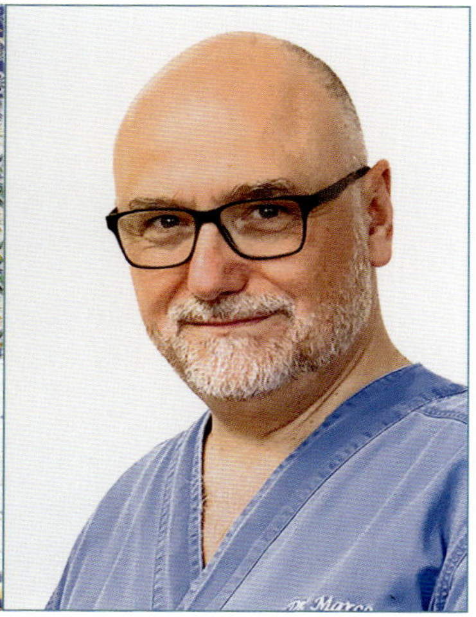

Marco NICASTRO

Professional profile
A graduate of the Faculty of Dentistry and Prosthodontics at the University of La Sapienza in Rome (Italy). He also completed studies in the field of prosthetics. He gained new experience in prosthetic procedures at Oral Design Center Roma, and in the field of new directions of esthetic dentistry by participating in courses conducted at the University of Geneva (Switzerland).

Clinical practice
His practice "Studio Dr. Nicastro" in Rome uses modern therapeutic methods. Minimally invasive procedures, shaping optimal occlusive conditions, integrating esthetics and functions, and finally, the methodology of digital dentistry set the tone for everyday practice in this therapeutic center. This renowned center is dominated by two specialties: esthetic dentistry and implantology, with a wide range of accompanying prosthetic procedures.

Professional activity
Member of the Italian Dental Society and the Italian Academy of Dental Prosthetics, and one of the founders of the Interdisciplinary CAD/CAM Study. Author of many international publications, lecturer at national and international congresses in the field of esthetic restorative dentistry.

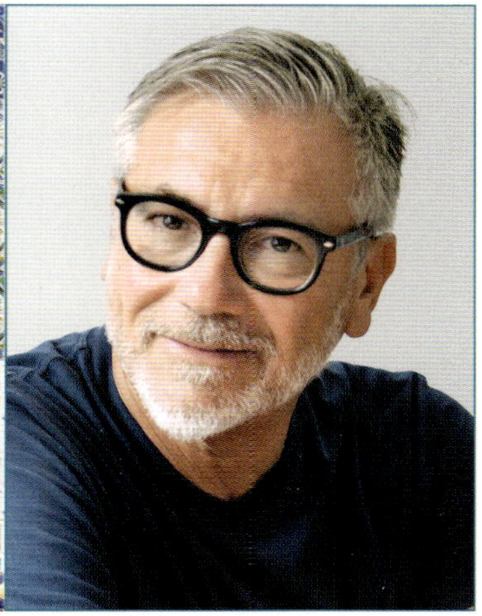

Daniele RONDONI

Professional profile

Master of Dental Technology. A graduate of the renowned P. Caslini Dental School in Genoa (Italy). Lecturer and co-founder of Dental Technician School in Savona (Italy). He gained professional experience in leading centers for dental technicians in Switzerland, Germany, and Japan. Visiting professor at the University of Chieti-Pescara.

Clinical practice

Since 1982, he has been running his own dental laboratory. By devoting himself to an in-depth analysis of dental morphology and creating optimal esthetics in restorative dentistry, he has gained a reputation as a respected authority in the world of modern dentistry. He is the creator of original protocols of performing indirect composite techniques on metal structures and restorations on implants, known as the Inverted Hardness Layering System.

Professional activity

Member of the European and Italian Academy of Esthetic Dentistry. Persistently participates in the activities of Style Italiano. Author of the book *Ceramic Multilayering Technique* and co-author of the book *Conservative Restoration of Anterior Teeth*. He lectures on numerous educational projects and as a key lecturer at international congresses.

FOREWORD

I have known Dr. Maciej Żarow as a consummate student, gifted practitioner, and provocative thinker. He also is an excellent writer who answers complex clinical questions with clarity and simplicity.

I am honored to recommend his newest book, *Veneers*. Dr. Żarow's combined teaching, research, and clinical expertise are evident in the book's content. As you read, you will be exposed to new ways of thinking about veneers. The book begins with consideration of the "why" of veneer placement. Then, he carefully describes in detail the systems and proven methodologies that will allow the reader to achieve predictable, excellent outcomes. His treatment planning process includes a functional risk assessment to better ensure the long-term survival of the veneers. He also provides in-depth selection criteria for porcelain vs composite material choices. Other chapters include dental morphology, photographic communication, tooth preparation, provisional fabrication, and cementation.

I am certain this book will help any dentist fabricate and deliver veneers with predictable outstanding outcomes using a practical workflow that can be incorporated into any dental practice.

John C. Kois DMD MSD
The Kois Center, Founder and Director
University of Washington School of Dentistry,
Affiliate Professor, Graduate Restorative Program
The Compendium of Continuing Education in Dentistry,
Co-Editor-in-Chief

PREFACE

It is a great honor to introduce a book for my good friend Maciej Żarow. Maciej is passionate about life, a passion manifested in everything he does: in personal relationships, in travel, in fun, in treating patients, in teaching ... Over the years, he has been able to forge bonds of friendship all over the world, and from humility, study, and work, he has developed a deep and solid knowledge of broad aspects of dentistry, which has made him a referent in conservative and esthetic dentistry worldwide.

In this book, he has managed to bring together a team of excellent dentists and technicians, as well as great friends, to show us a new vision of ceramic veneers, a classic treatment of renewed validity. It is not a book to impress, but a book to teach, where his deep knowledge of the foundations of dentistry is revealed. The need to carry out adequate diagnoses that consider functional aspects fundamental to achieving success in this compromised type of treatment is emphasized. Through detailed clinical cases, it shows us when they are indicated, when we have to avoid them, what risks lie in wait for us, how we have to prepare the teeth, what type of materials to use, how to proceed with cementation, and also shows us where the future of this type of treatment is going, with the incorporation of digital workflow.

This is an excellent book by an exceptional person, which should be a must for clinicians dedicated to esthetic restorative dentistry.

Miguel Roig Cayón
President
Spanish Society of Prosthodontics and Esthetic Dentistry
Professor and Head
Department of Restorative Dentistry
Universitat Internacional de Catalunya
Barcelona, Spain

INTRODUCTION

Is veneering a challenge? What do you need to have a predictable key to success in your workshop? What did I have to learn and remember well, after an era of uncertainty, trials, and material choices to treat this therapy as an ordinary but demanding clinical procedure?

For 20 years, I have been offering my patients porcelain and composite veneers, and – more precisely – comprehensive esthetic treatment, in which the beauty and harmony of the anterior teeth put life in first place. I have come across dozens of cases of varying degrees of difficulty. Do I know enough about this micropart of modern dentistry today to authoritatively face every challenge that nature can give us? Probably not – although already in the hundreds of clinical situations that I have encountered over many years of practice, I find an extensive set of experiences, regularities, and rules that allow me to search for effective treatment procedures. And that is what I wanted to share in the pages of this book.

To make the book even more comprehensive and valuable, I invited my dear friends and eminent dentists to contribute. They are: Dr. Marco Nicastro, Dr. Walter Devoto, Prof. Louis Hardan, Dr. Margarida Henrique, and dental technician Daniele Rondoni. The first has been my mentor of esthetic dentistry for 20 years; the second is a long-standing motivator in the constant search for newer and simpler treatment methods; and the third is an innovator in dental photography. Margarida, on the other hand, is an absolute "freak" when it comes to her passion for her field – which made me consider that her extraordinary knowledge about the details of teeth would be a great enrichment of the knowledge contained in this book. The artist of the sketches is Dr. Julia Gebel, whom I would like to thank for her commitment and the countless number of drawings made. I must thank Dr. John Kois from Seattle – my teacher and mentor – who had put together my knowledge about functional risk assessment in esthetic cases.

In addition, I must acknowledge two outstanding Polish professors. The first is Prof. Stanisław Suliborski, whose lecture in 1995 and passion for veneers inspired me to become involved in this field, and the second is Prof. Jerzy Krupiński, my great teacher and friend. He had endless patience in teaching me how to logically put my thoughts on paper.
I hope that all the students, novice dentists, and experienced practitioners who read this book will find many useful tips for their practice.

Maciej Żarow
Cracow, Poland 2021

Ceramic tiles "azulejos"! I have always been fascinated by the facades of Andalusian and Portuguese cities. The experts in their fabrication and "gluing" did it well enough that they could survive for hundreds of years. They have been my inspiration when planning porcelain veneers...

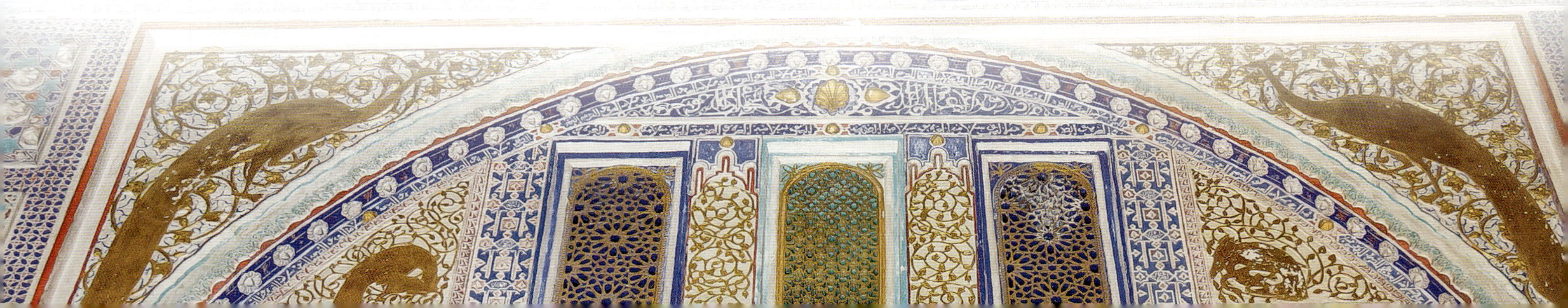

CONTENTS

CHAPTER 1

WHY VENEERS?

MACIEJ ŻAROW

Patients are interested in veneers because they consider them an excellent way to change their smile. Veneers have, after all, glamorized many famous people, including actors, politicians, and other celebrities. Patients believe that the world of veneers will open the door to a fuller and better life ...

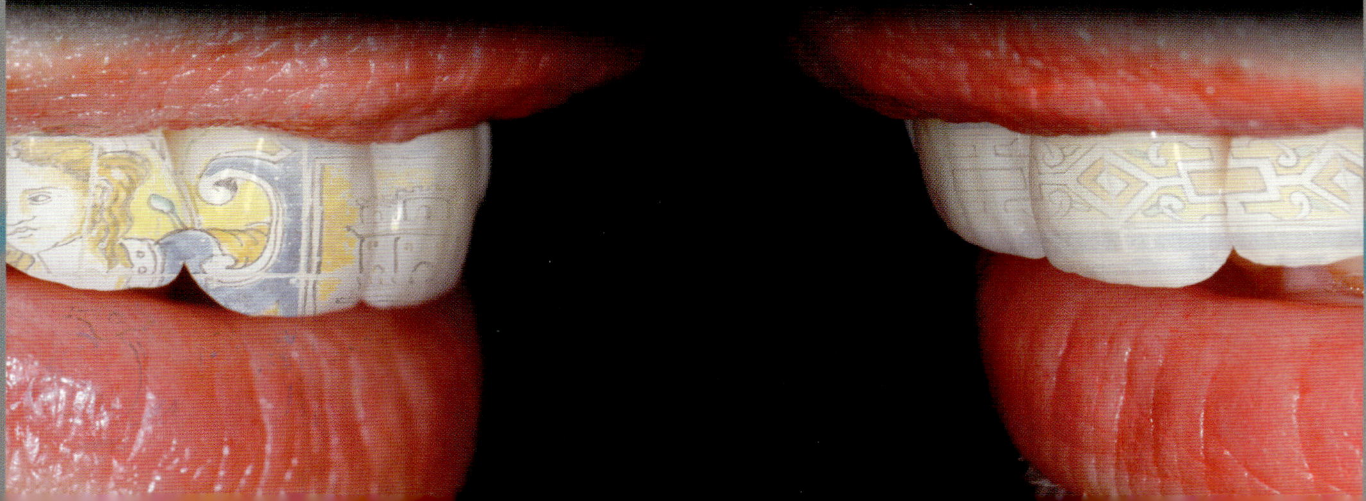

Why veneers?

Veneers start a risky game. They can improve the patient's well-being and comfort, increase their chance of professional success and social standing. On the other hand, they can also – even irreversibly – change everyday life for the worse. Do we know the answers to all the questions that a patient might ask?

THE PATIENT'S POINT OF VIEW

Patients are interested in veneers because they are an attractive treatment; they improve their smile and well-being relatively quickly. They know that veneers have glamorized many famous people, such as actors, entrepreneurs, politicians, and celebrities. They hope that entering the world of veneers will change their daily life, give them social confidence, increase their chances of professional success, and raise their social position. Therefore, it is safe to say that veneers or esthetic treatment can sometimes work in the same way as good psychological therapy.

More than once, I have hosted in the dental clinic modest and almost non-smiling patients who, after veneer treatment, have completely changed their lifestyle; they smile widely, are more talkative change their hairstyle to a new, more sophisticated cut, and alter their wardrobe for a more fashionable one often intended for young and confident people.

CLINICAL POINT OF VIEW

I write on purpose about veneer treatment, not about cosmetic change. After all, this type of therapy is, in most cases, a dental treatment. Despite all the aspects of our changing reality, the role of social media into our clinics, and the generational change in the business approach to running dental practices, we must not forget that we are dentists, and our primary goal is to treat. Veneers do not only change the shape and the color of the teeth, but they also have a therapeutic effect, which goes beyond the improvement of esthetics and the patient's comfort. Their therapeutic meaning can be outlined in ten aspects[1–10]:

1. They improve the function of anterior guidance and lateral guidance,-protecting molars and premolars from tooth wear
2. They improve the function of eating
3. They can have a positive effect on phonetics
4. With gentle preparation, they often strengthen tooth stiffness, which is compromised due to root canal treatment and structural loss
5. They are nearly non-invasive for the periodontium (with supra- or juxtagingival preparation and with an appropriate emergence profile)
6. They are less invasive than prosthetic crowns, where the preparation means a significant structural loss
7. They improve health conditions for the gingival papilla by creating carefully planned and stable contact points
8. They reduce plaque accumulation by covering the composite fillings
9. They protect thin and chipped incisal edges, thanks to their appropriate material strength

QUESTIONS THE PATIENT MAY ASK:

Do veneers require significant tooth damage?

We can plan and minimize the range of the tooth preparation. Using appropriate methods, it is possible to perform veneers with a preparation depth of 0.2–0.4 mm or less into the hard tissues (Fig 1-1). What is important is that we try to prepare the tooth so as not to remove the entire thickness of the enamel or expose the dentin (exposing the dentin may reduce the durability of the veneers).[1,11–12]

How long do veneers last?

Under optimal conditions (a significant amount of enamel ensures good adhesion of the veneer to the tooth), we can expect durability up to 15 years and more (Fig 1-2).[13–15] However, with age, physiological atrophy of the gums may progress and, after many years, the veneer–tooth transition can be visible. That is why professional oral hygiene and plaque control are important, contributing to slowing down the periodontal aging process.

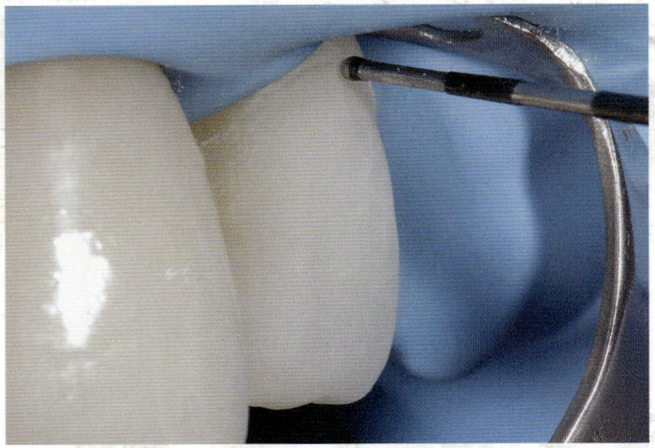

Fig 1-1
It is possible to perform veneers with reduced tooth preparation using appropriate methods. (The photograph shows tooth 22 before veneer cementation.)

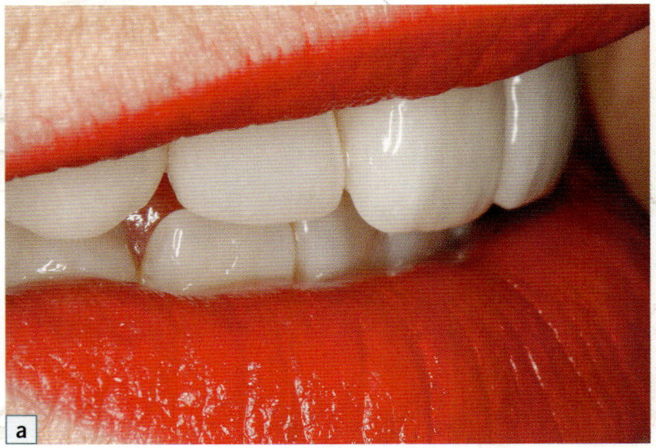

a

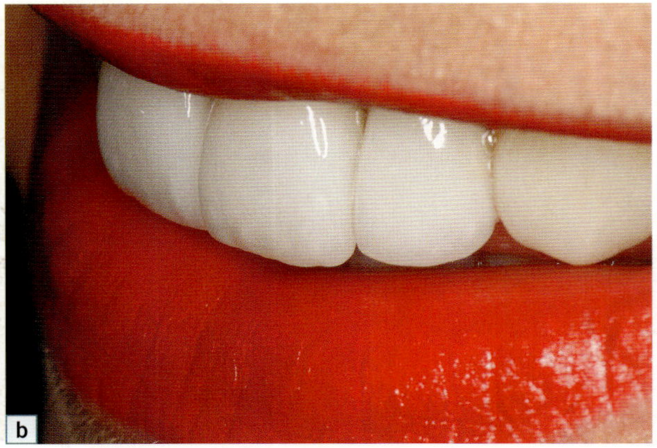

b

Fig 1-2
Under optimal conditions, we can expect the durability of these restorations to be up to 15 years or even more. These veneers have been successfully functioning in the mouth for over 12 years.

Can veneers be placed over teeth with composite restorations?

Of course, veneers are recommended wherever it would be too difficult to perform direct composite restorations, especially in the case of multiple restorations. In such complex situations, it is much easier to improve the smile with the indirect veneers (Fig 1-3).[16]

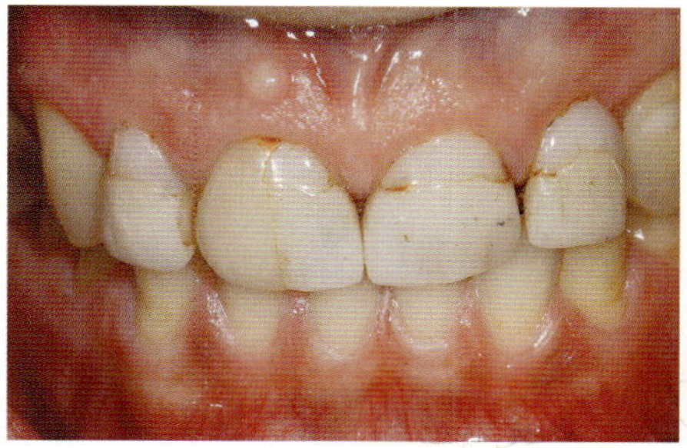

Fig 1-3a
A patient presented to the dental office to improve the smile esthetics in the maxillary anterior sextant. The patient was unsatisfied with unesthetic tooth reconstructions.

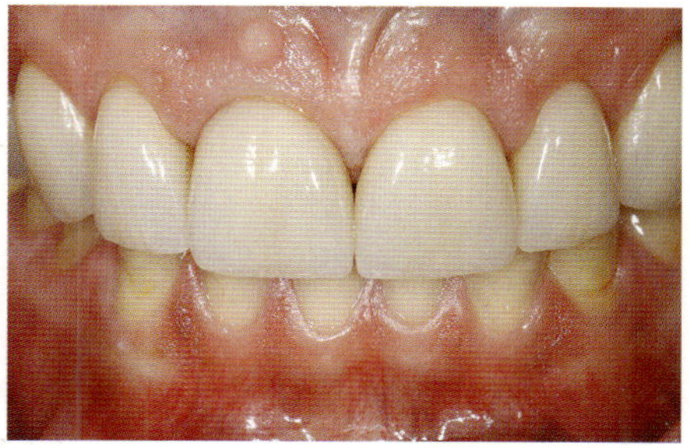

Fig 1-3b
Six feldspathic porcelain veneers were performed.

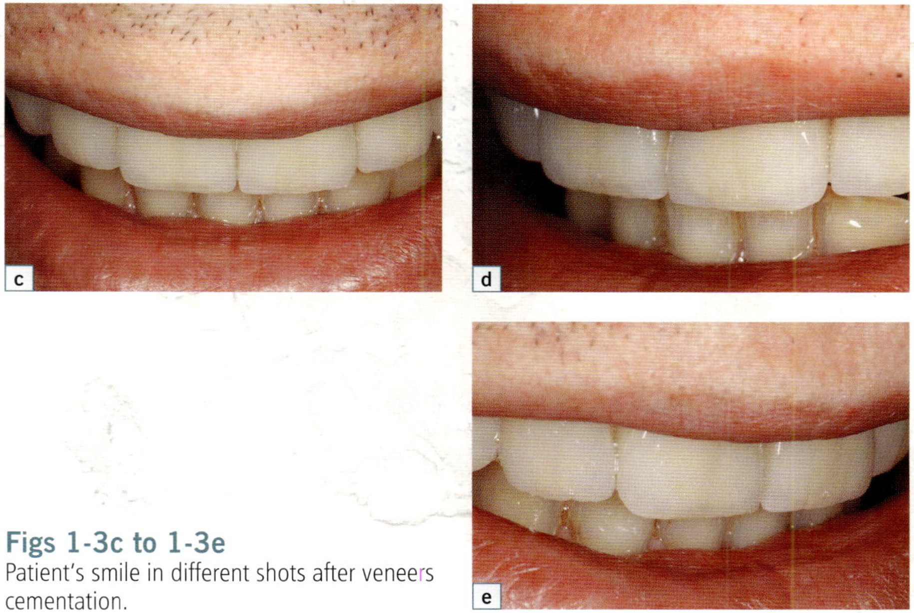

Figs 1-3c to 1-3e
Patient's smile in different shots after veneers cementation.

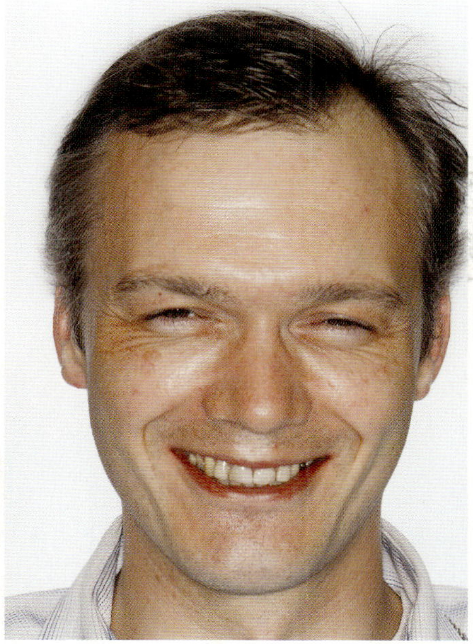

Fig 1-3f
The initial situation, before veneer treatment.

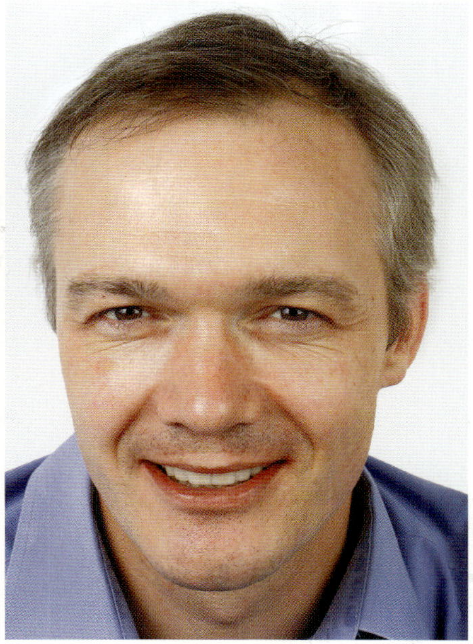

Fig 1-3g
Clinical situation after veneers cementation.

Is it true that veneers often fall off or break?

Veneers fall off due to incorrect indications (occlusal overload or structural compromise) or an error during the cementation procedure. If the teeth are overloaded, the risk of failure increases significantly. Sometimes, additional procedures should be performed in advance. Such procedures can include the functional risk assessment, removal of the premature occlusal contacts, and in certain cases, increasing the vertical dimension of occlusion (Fig 1-4).[17,18] There are also clinical cases where the tooth may not have enough of its own healthy structures, and veneer adhesion to the tooth will not be predictable.[3]

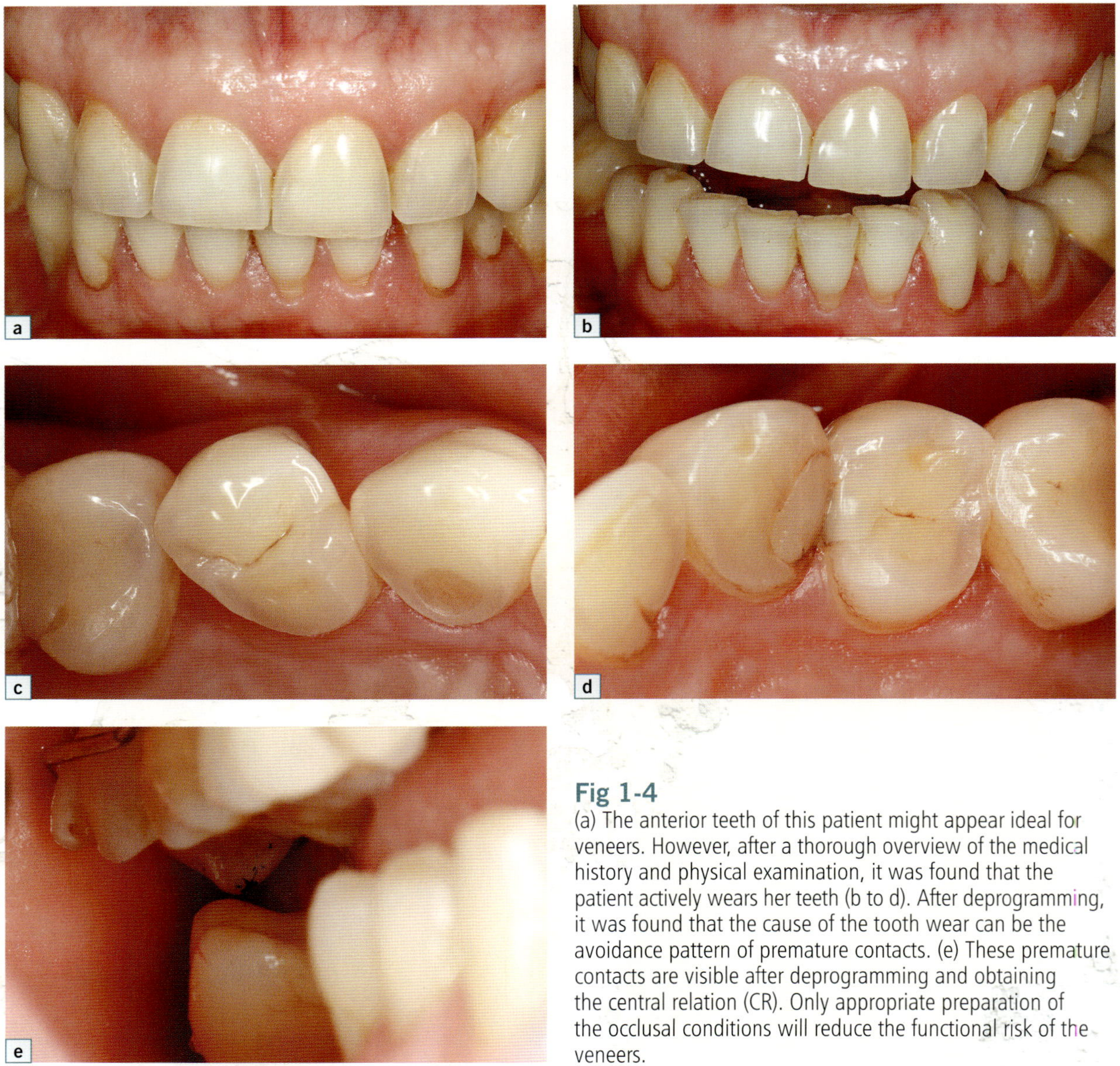

Fig 1-4
(a) The anterior teeth of this patient might appear ideal for veneers. However, after a thorough overview of the medical history and physical examination, it was found that the patient actively wears her teeth (b to d). After deprogramming, it was found that the cause of the tooth wear can be the avoidance pattern of premature contacts. (e) These premature contacts are visible after deprogramming and obtaining the central relation (CR). Only appropriate preparation of the occlusal conditions will reduce the functional risk of the veneers.

What does it mean: altering the vertical dimension?

Altering the vertical dimension means increasing the clinical height of the posterior restorations that will provide the front teeth with more necessary space for chewing, swallowing, breathing, and talking. The principle is as follows: reconstruction of the teeth in the mandibular arch, in the maxillary arch, or reconstruction in both, which will relieve the front teeth (Fig 1-5).[17,18]

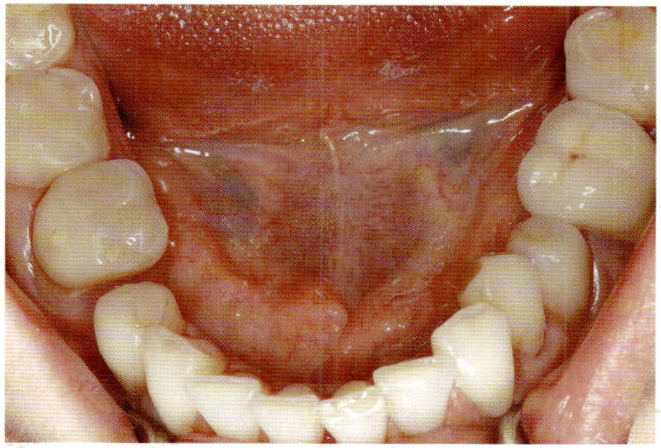

Fig 1-5a
The female patient shown in Fig 1-4 was qualified for altering the vertical dimension – initial situation.

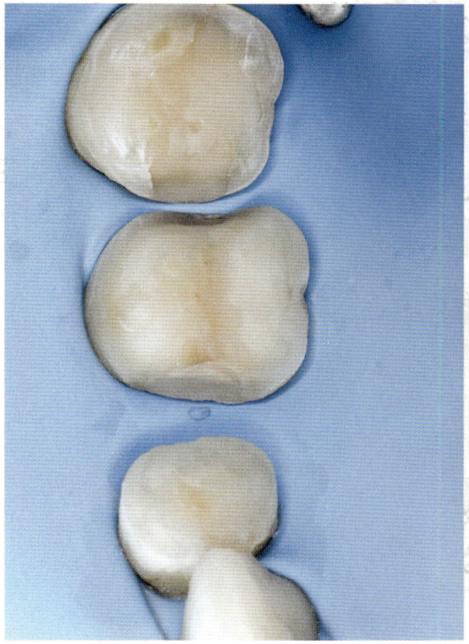

Fig 1-5b
Tooth preparation for indirect restorations in the fourth quadrant.

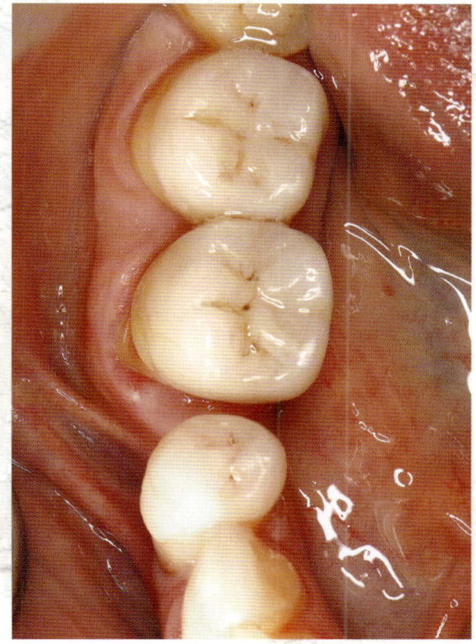

Fig 1-5c
Indirect restorations after cementation in the fourth quadrant.

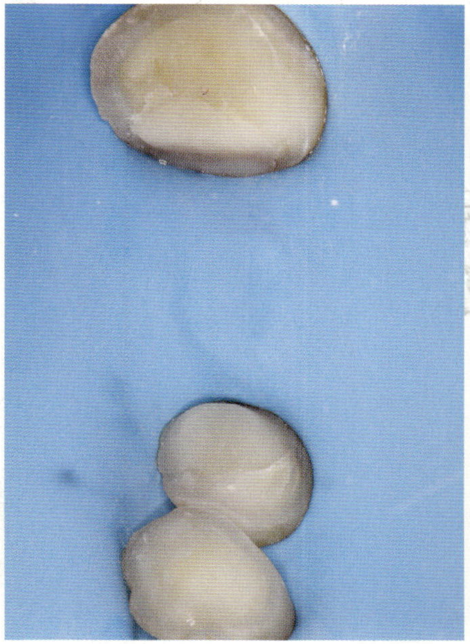

Fig 1-5d
Tooth preparation for indirect restorations in the third quadrant.

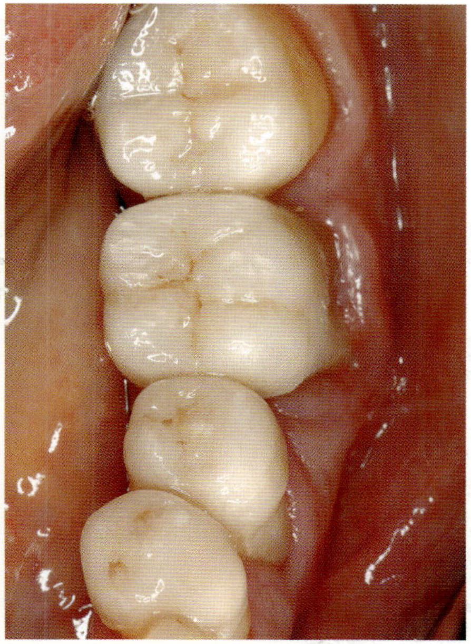

Fig 1-5e
Indirect restorations after cementation in the third quadrant.

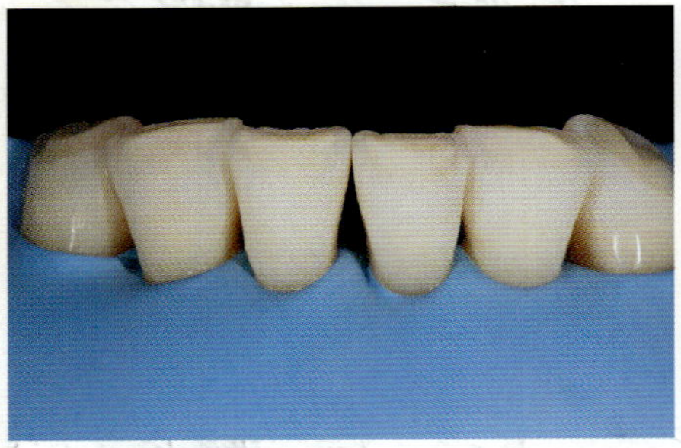

Fig 1-5f
Anterior teeth isolated with a rubber dam, ready for direct composite restorations.

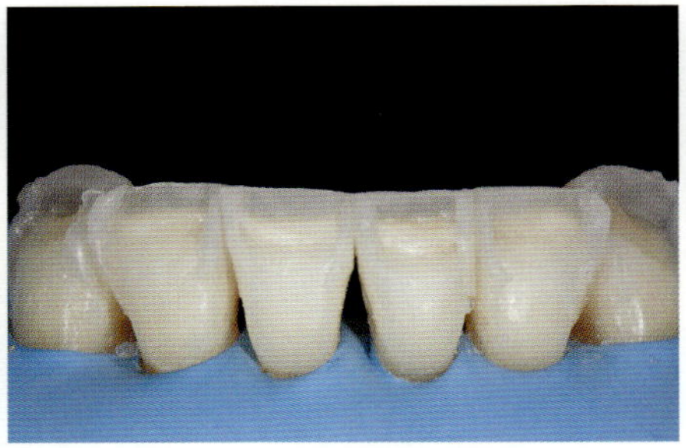

Fig 1-5g
"Palatal frames" of composite restorations were made with silicone index obtained for the diagnostic wax-up.

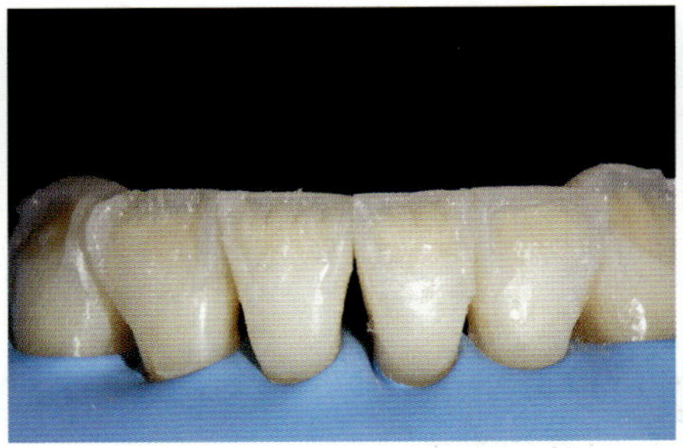

Fig 1-5h
Mamelons were created with the dentin composite resin layer.

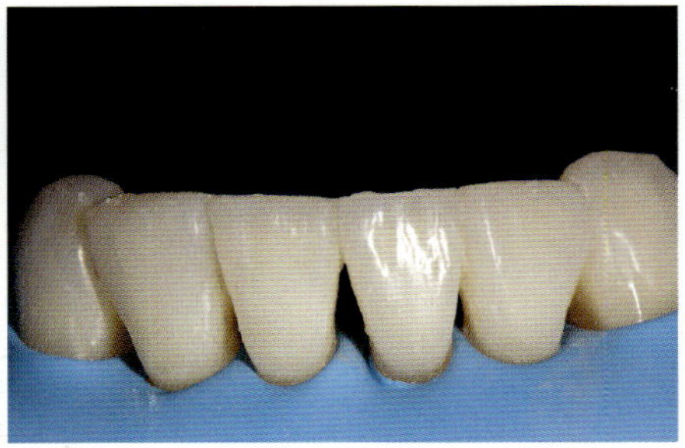

Fig 1-5i
Situation after restoration with final enamel composite and initial characterization.

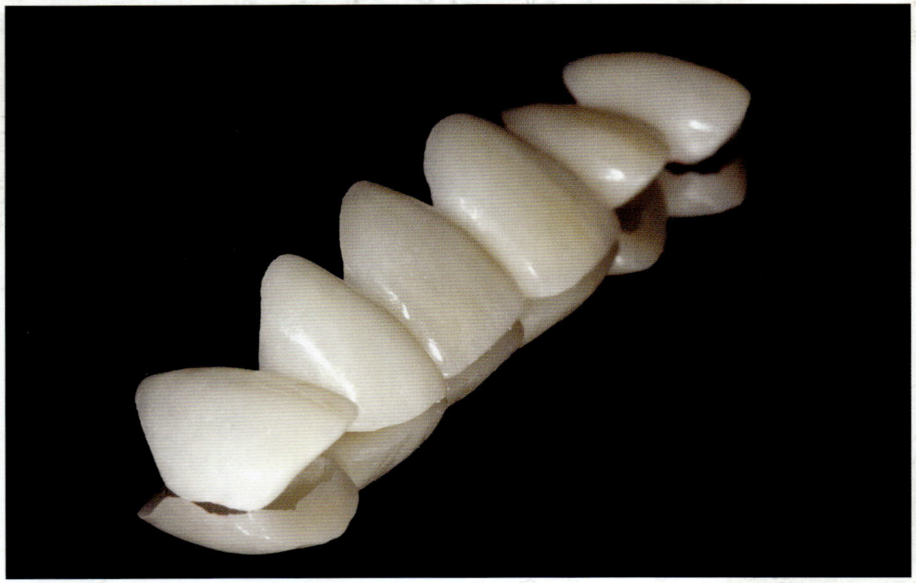

Fig 1-5j
Altering the vertical dimension of the occlusion provided appropriate space for the porcelain veneers.

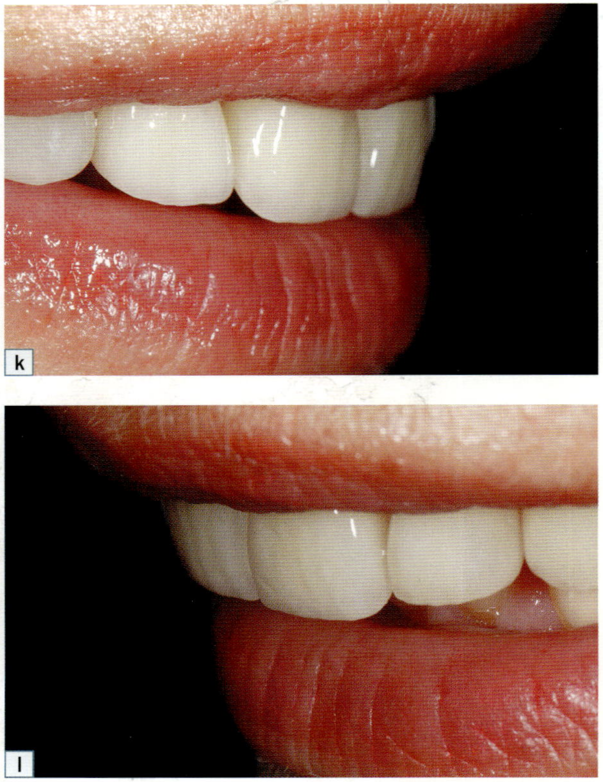

Figs 1-5k and 1-5l
Patient's smile from (k) the right and (l) the left semi-profile after veneers cementation.

Can a veneer be performed on one discolored tooth in the anterior region?

Making a single veneer is risky. If we want to achieve a predictable, satisfactory appearance of the front teeth, it is better to perform the veneers in pairs – symmetrically, so they will look natural (Fig 1-6).[19]

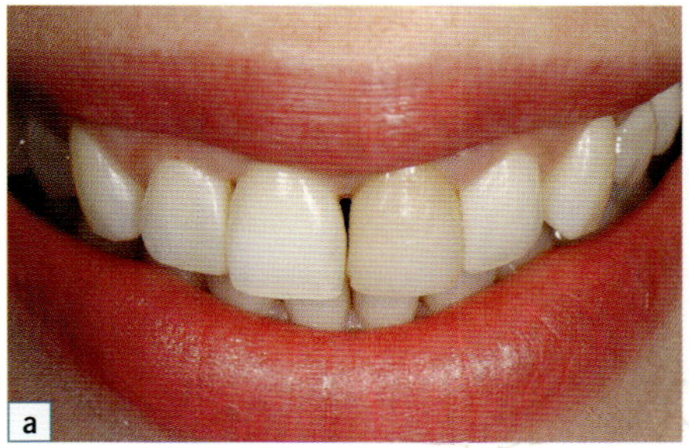

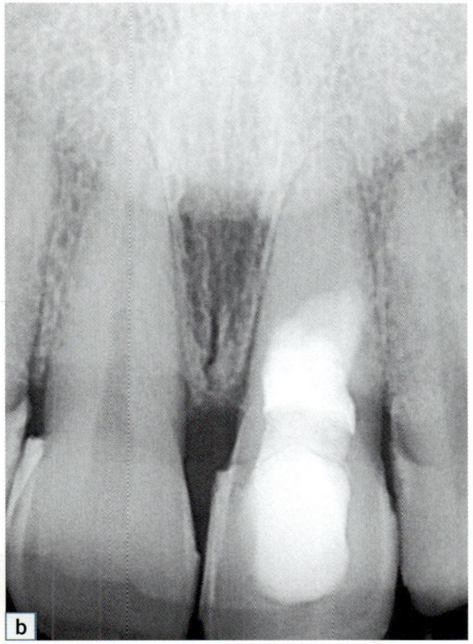

Figs 1-6a and 1-6b
(a) A 37-year-old female patient presented to the dental clinic seeking a better esthetic outcome for tooth 21. (b) Discoloration of the tooth was related to root canal treatment performed in childhood.

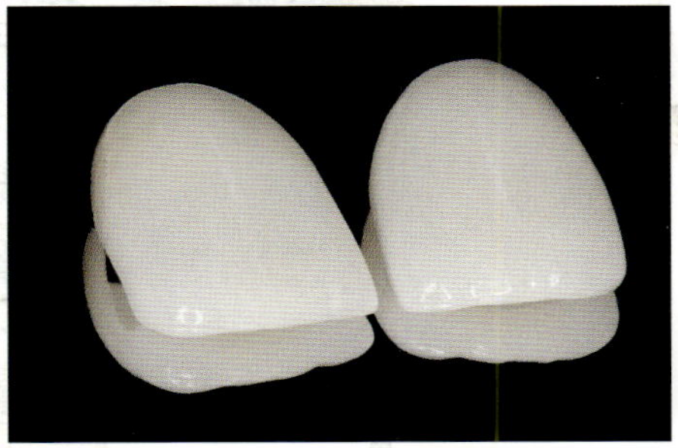

Fig 1-6c
The decision was taken to perform two feldspathic porcelain veneers on teeth 11 and 21, which will not only increase the predictability of color matching but also improve the symmetry and the incisal line of the central incisors.

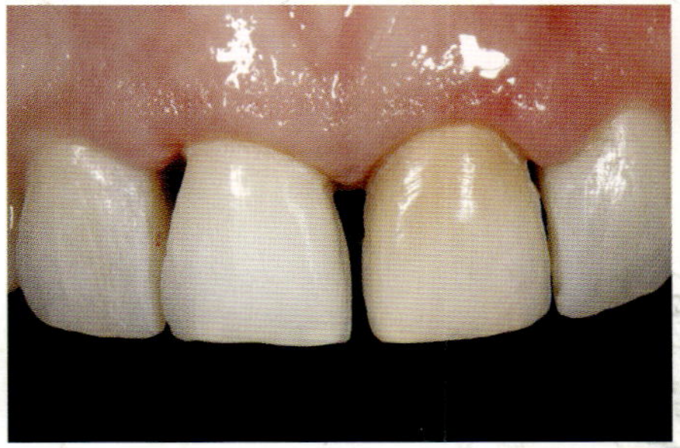

Fig 1-6d
Teeth 11 and 21 were prepared for veneers.

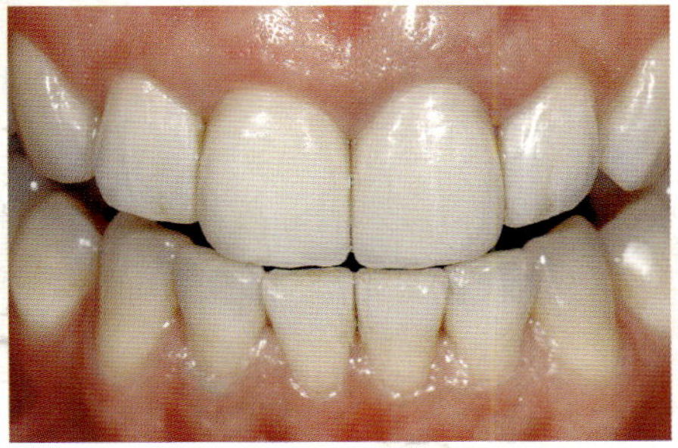

Fig 1-6e
Clinical situation 3 months after cementing veneers on teeth 11 and 21.

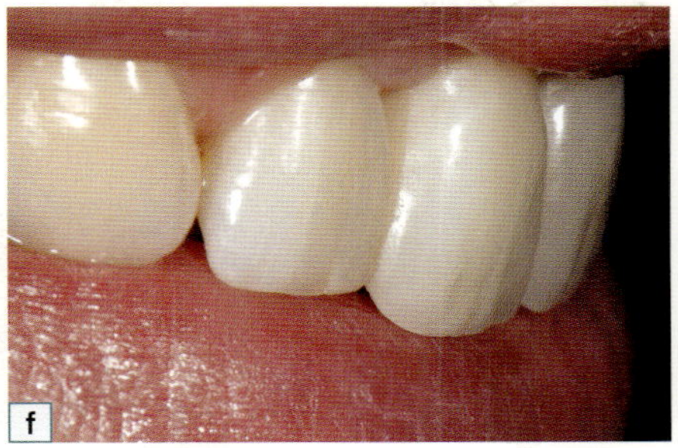

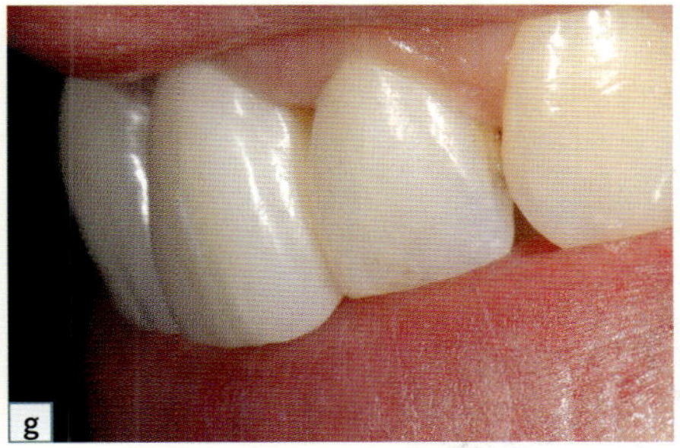

Figs 1-6f and 1-6g
Patient's smile with (f) the right and (g) the left semi-profiles after treatment is completed.

Can an old crown be replaced and a veneer performed on an adjacent tooth?

Yes. Using the same porcelain, it is possible to make an all-ceramic crown with a veneer on an adjacent tooth. Such a procedure with the central incisors will allow the same symmetrical restorations in terms of shape, color, and characterization (Fig 1-7).

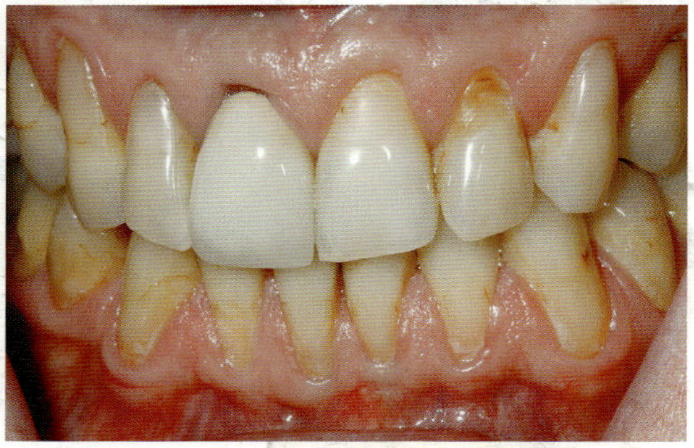

Fig 1-7a
A 52-year-old patient presented to the clinic to replace the old ceramic crown on tooth 11. It was recommended to perform a porcelain veneer on tooth 21 at the same time to achieve symmetry between the maxillary central incisors.

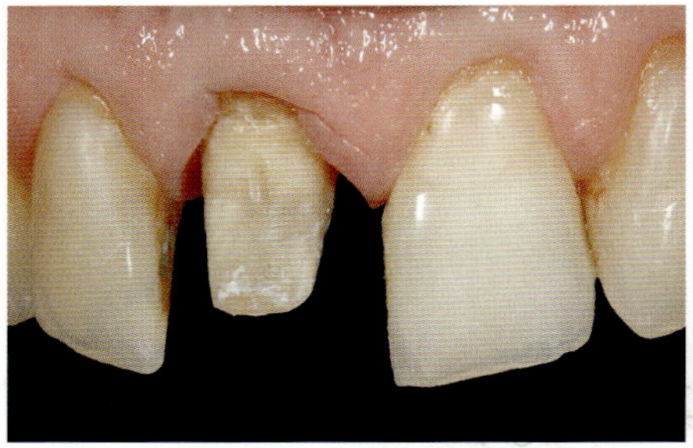

Fig 1-7b
Clinical situation after removing the old crown 11.

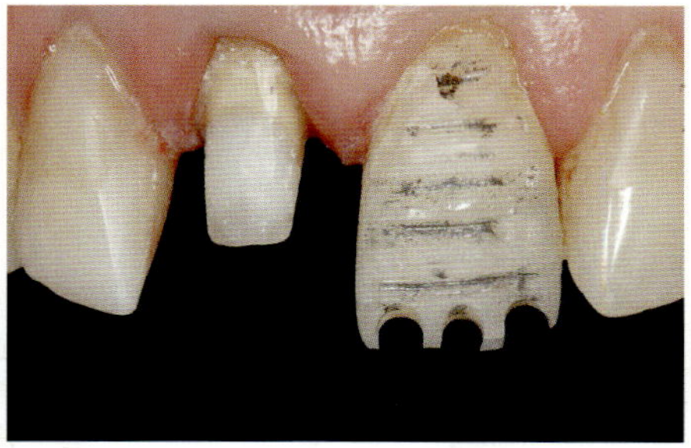

Fig 1-7c
Preparation depth grooves obtained from mock-up position on tooth 21.

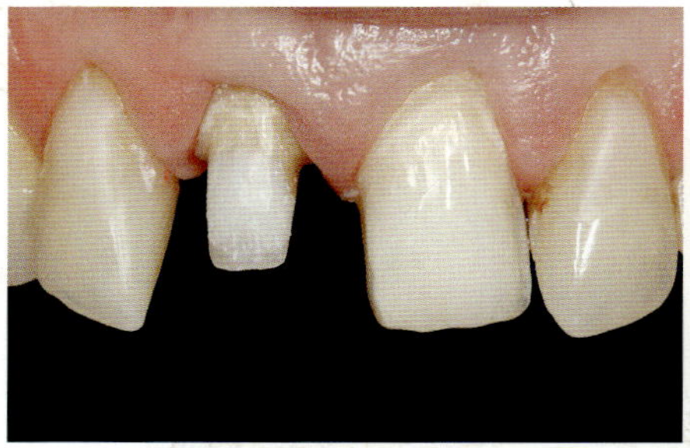

Fig 1-7d
Situation after the final preparation for the crown 11 and porcelain veneer 21.

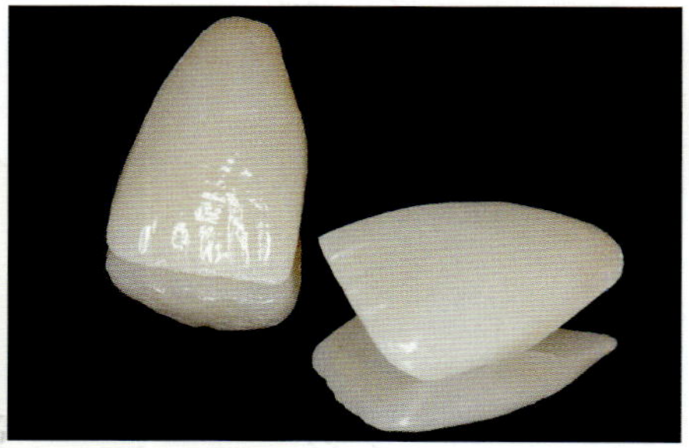

Fig 1-7e
Prosthetic crown and veneer made of lithium disilicate – ready for cementation.

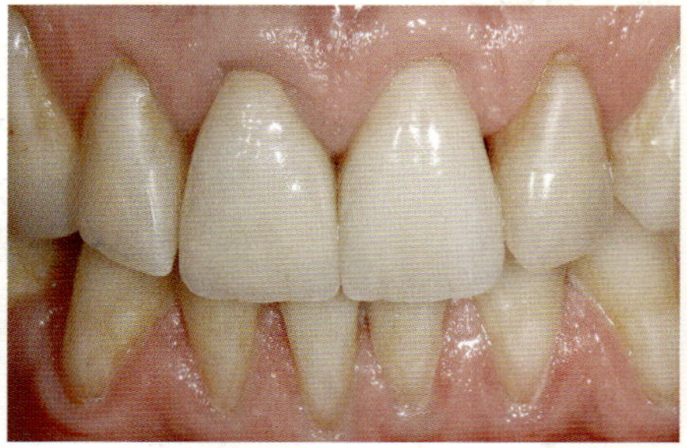

Fig 1-7f
Clinical situation after cementation of all-ceramic crown 11 and veneer 21.

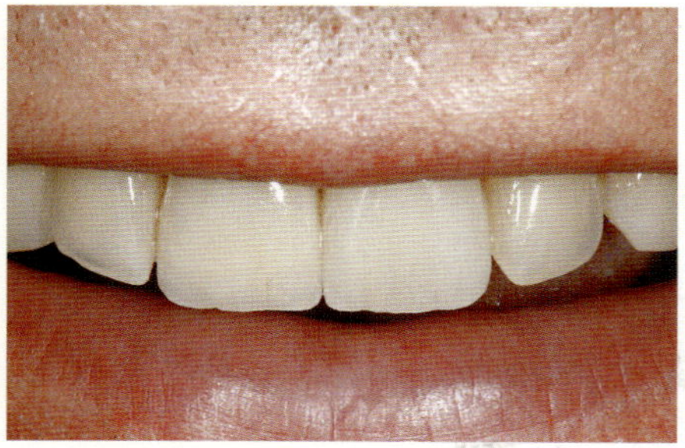

Fig 1-7g
Patient's smile after treatment is completed.

Can veneers be bleached?

Unfortunately, no. Therefore, it is strongly recommended to whiten the teeth before starting the treatment. For esthetic reasons, it is easier and better to match the veneer color to bleached teeth.[20] Moreover, the patient's appetite usually grows with what it is fed, and after cementing the veneers (if whitening has not been performed), the patient will say: "Doctor, the veneers are nice, but now I would like to whiten them, one or two tones." Remember, whitening veneers will never be possible. However, it will be possible to refresh the whitening of adjacent teeth, which can become slightly discolored over time due to the dye absorption (Fig 1-8).

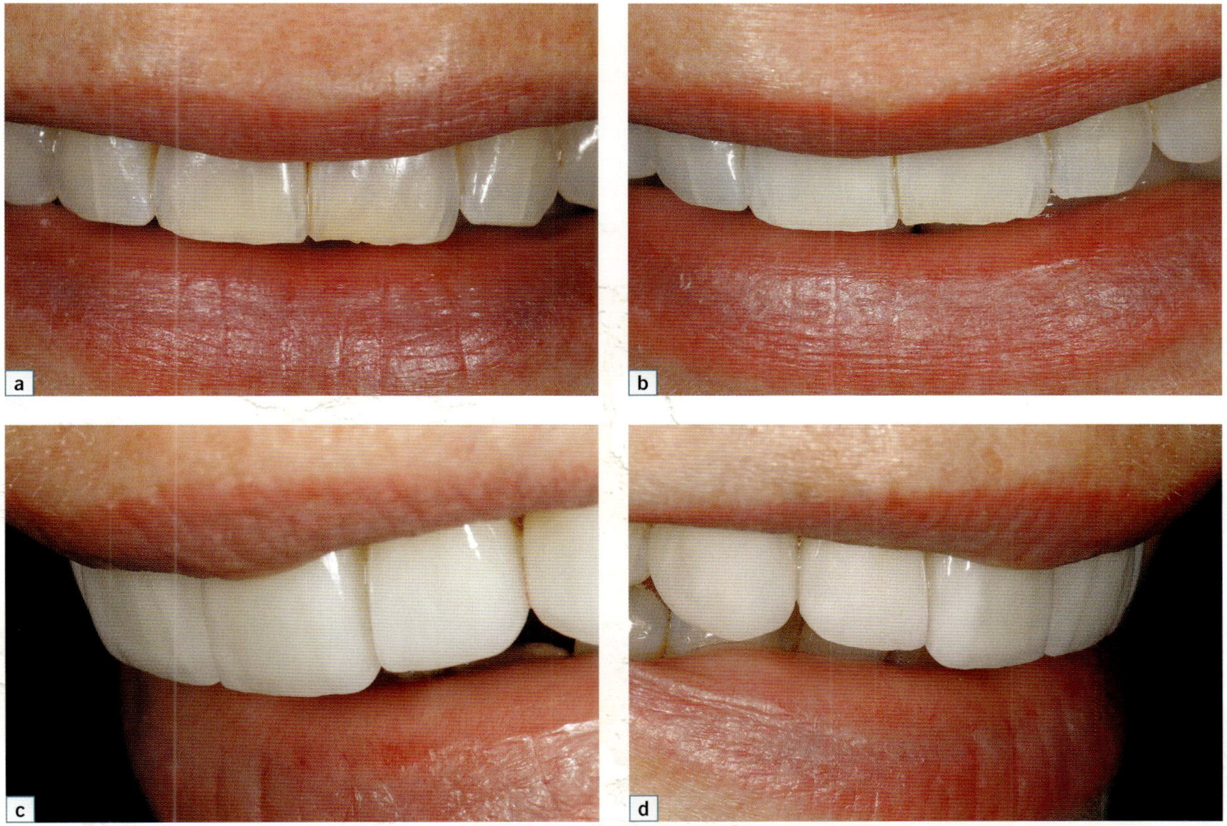

Fig 1-8
When planning porcelain veneers, teeth whitening should always be considered. After completing orthodontic therapy, the female patient presented to the dental office seeking esthetic treatment. With the help of veneers in the maxillary arch, it was planned to lighten the color of the teeth and lengthen the maxillary incisors to improve the smile line. Thanks to the whitening, the dental technician had an easier task to match the veneer color to the brighter teeth, which harmonized them with the adjacent teeth: (a) clinical situation before whitening; (b) clinical situation after whitening; (c, d) clinical situation after porcelain veneers cementation.

How should one deal with a gingival recession, making the tooth-veneer transitions or cervical tooth discoloration visible?

With proper prophylaxis (regular visits to a dental hygienist, bilaterally balanced occlusion, relaxation mouthguard, and appropriate tooth-brushing), the patient should not be exposed to rapid gingival recession (Fig 1-9). If such a situation occurs many years later, the veneers can always be redone.[21]

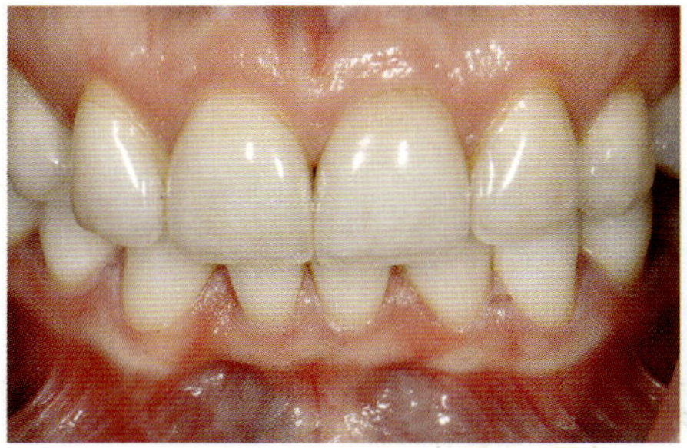

Fig 1-9a
A 40-year-old female patient presented to the dental office wishing to replace the old veneers done several years ago. She complained that the junction between the tooth and the veneer has become particularly visible over the years.

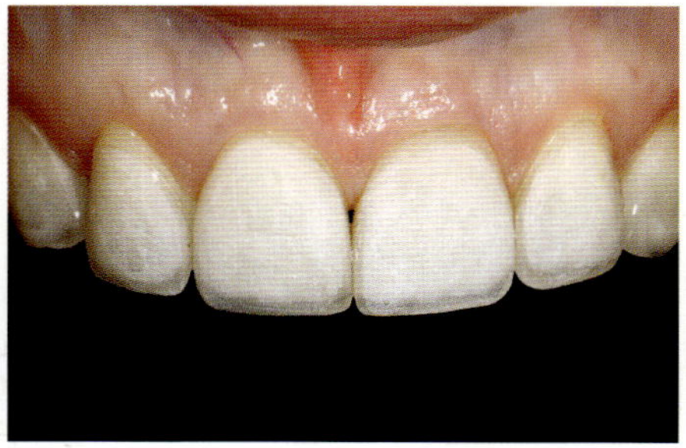

Fig 1-9b
Preparation was obtained based on existing veneers, which were used as a mock-up (preparation through mock-up), and photographs were taken during the procedure.

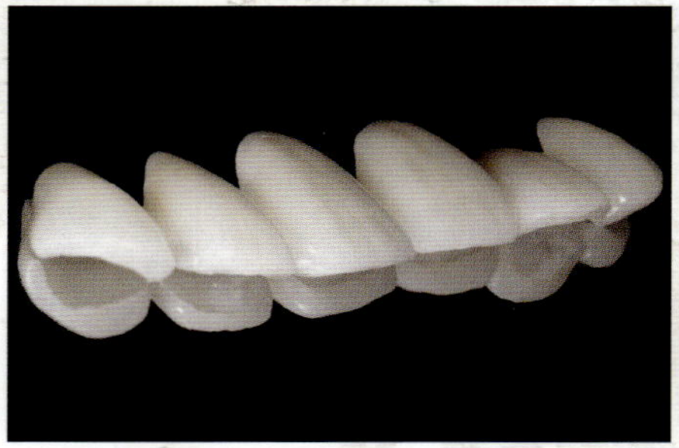

Fig 1-9c
Feldspathic porcelain veneers performed in the laboratory – ready for cementation.

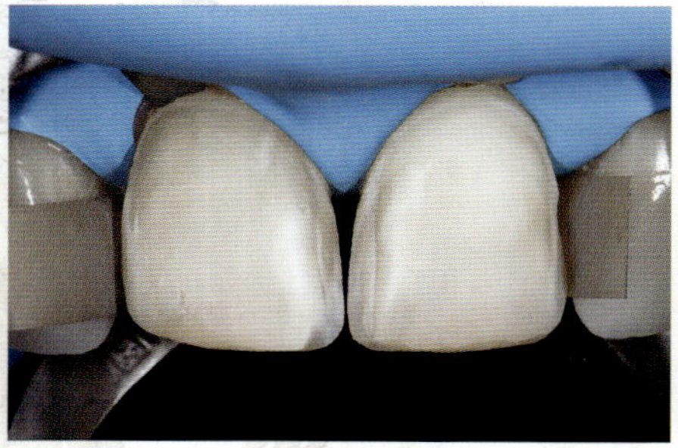

Fig 1-9d
Rubber dam isolation ensures predictable adhesive cementation.

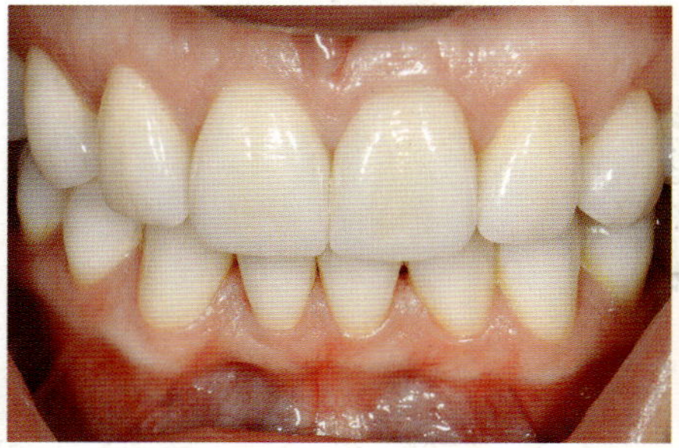

Fig 1-9e
Clinical situation after performing the veneers.

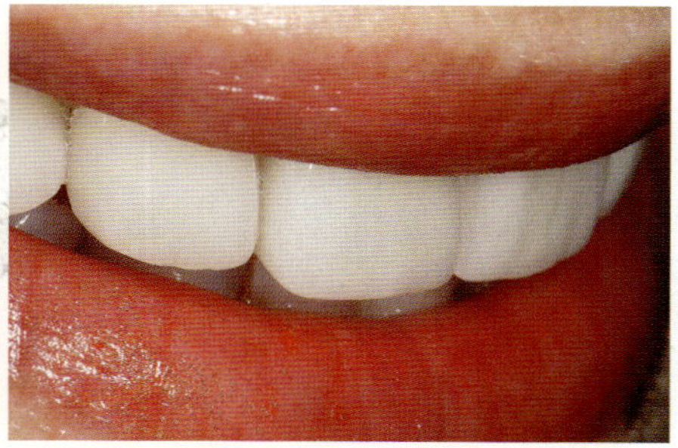

Fig 1-9f
The patient's smile after treatment.

Which porcelain should be chosen for veneers?

Currently, two main types of ceramic materials are used: feldspathic porcelain and lithium disilicate porcelain (pressed or milled). A dentist should choose based on clinical indication and cooperation with an experienced dental technician (Fig 1-10).[22]

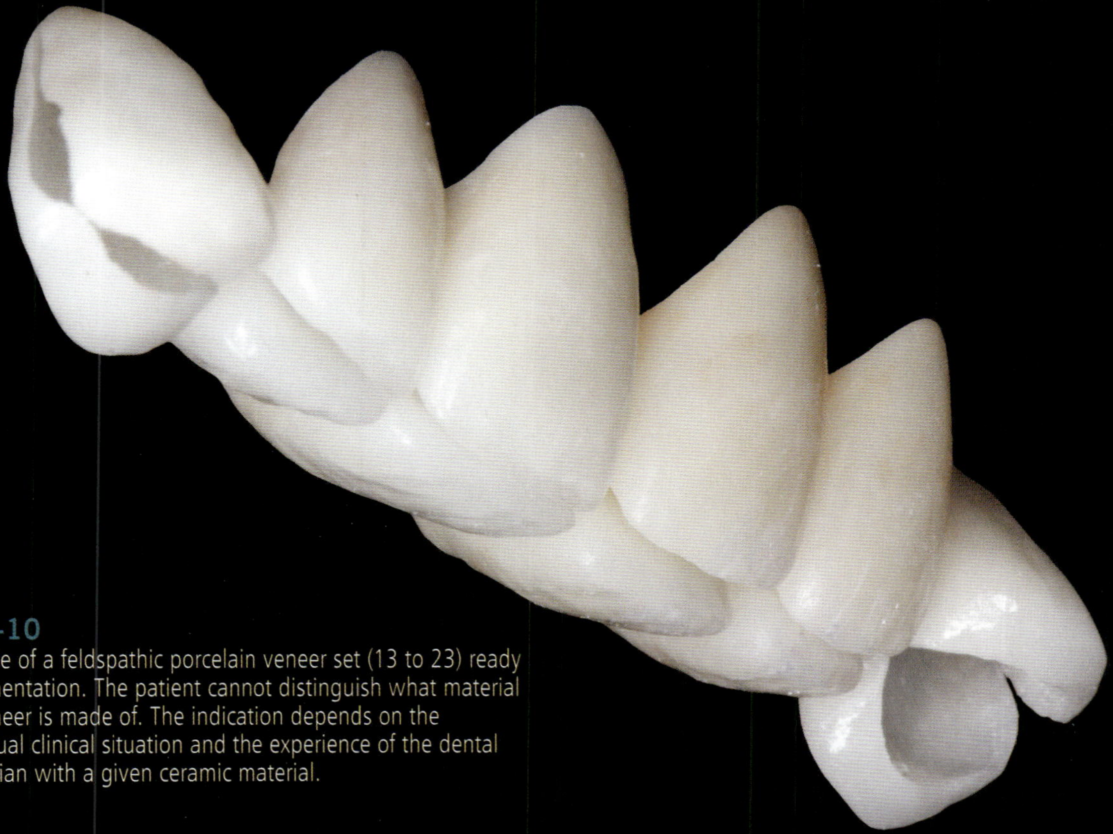

Fig 1-10
Example of a feldspathic porcelain veneer set (13 to 23) ready for cementation. The patient cannot distinguish what material the veneer is made of. The indication depends on the individual clinical situation and the experience of the dental technician with a given ceramic material.

Can veneers replace orthodontic treatment?

In some limited clinical cases, it is possible; for example, in case of slight rotation of the teeth or in case of retrusion of the maxillary incisors and the retroposition (here, the position of the teeth allows for esthetic tooth additive reconstruction). However, in the case of protrusion, when maxillary incisors extend beyond the normal contour of the dental arch, their correction with veneers requires extensive tooth preparation (Fig 1-11).[23]

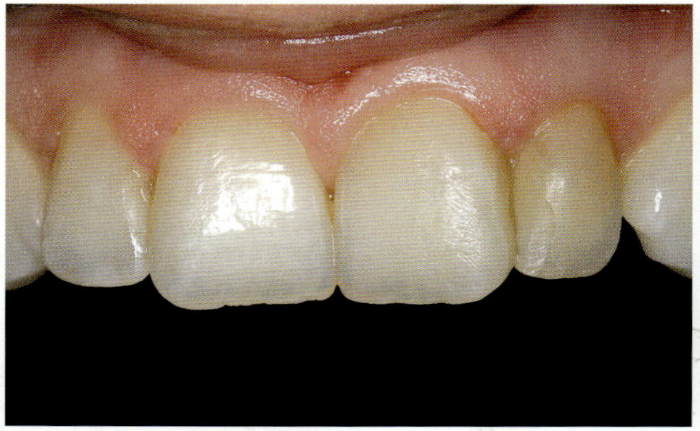

Fig 1-11a
This female patient presented with an esthetic problem of rotated central incisors.

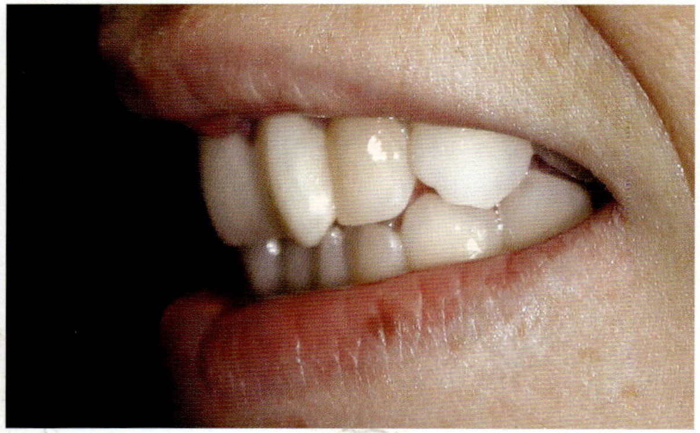

Fig 1-11b
The patient was performing on stage, and she was concerned by a shadow appearing on her teeth in some camera shots and pictures.

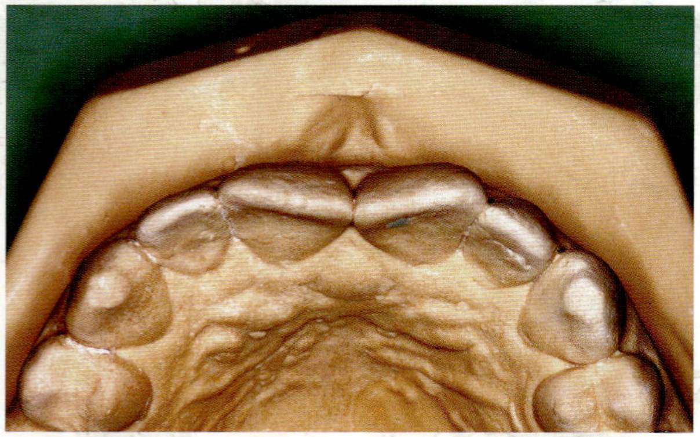

Fig 1-11c
Study cast with visible rotation of the central incisors.

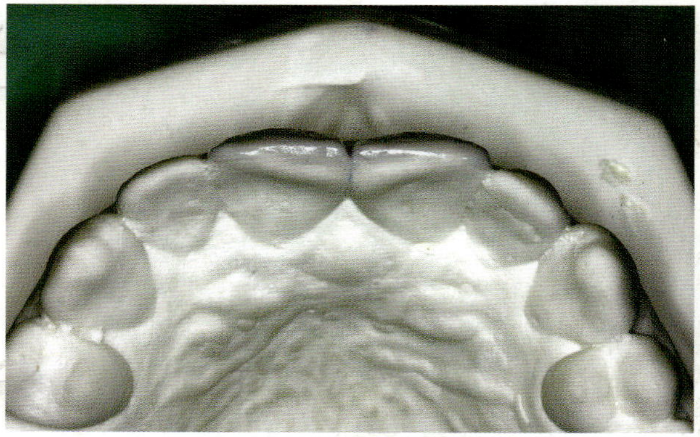

Fig 1-11d
Diagnostic wax-up shows rotated teeth correction possibility with minimally invasive porcelain veneers.

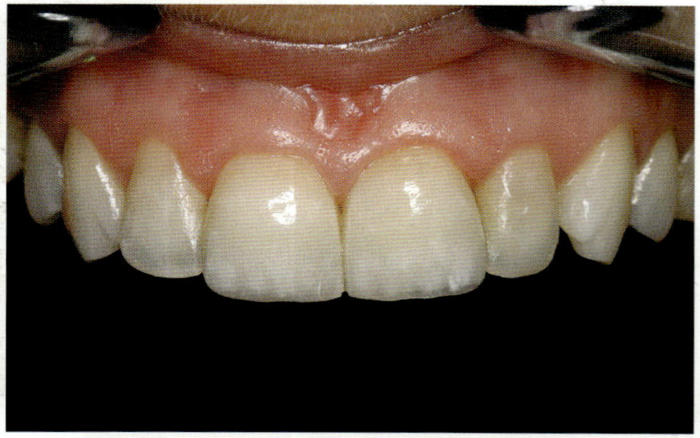

Fig 1-11e
Clinical situation after cementing porcelain veneers.

Will veneers fail on the canines?

The canines indeed fulfill a special functional aim by performing canine guidance, which creates disclusion of the posterior teeth in the lateral movement of the mandible and protects the teeth from excessive abrasion/wear.
On the other hand, the convex shape of the canine on the palatal side (more convex than the maxillary incisors) makes the stress distribution on the porcelain veneers more favorable.[24,25] So, do not be afraid to make veneers on the maxillary canines if you wisely plan them. Look at the extreme case where a veneer was made after unsuccessful orthodontic treatment (ankylosis of the maxillary canine) (Fig 1-12). However, special attention should be paid not to overdo the inclination of the canine guidance (steep guidance may result in overloading and breaking the veneers).

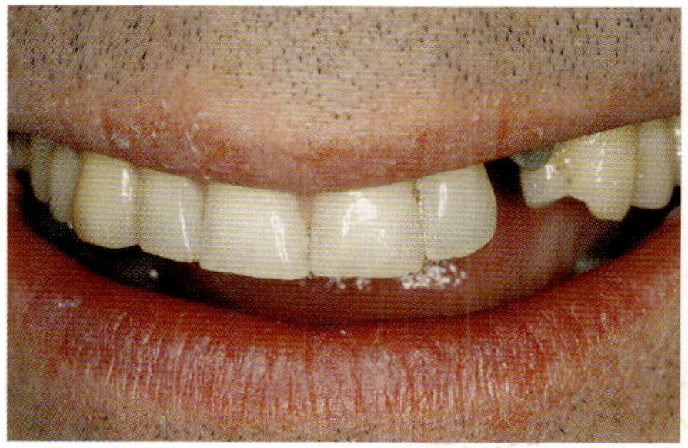

Fig 1-12a
A patient was referred to improve esthetics after unsuccessful orthodontic treatment, which involved extrusion of the retained canine 23.

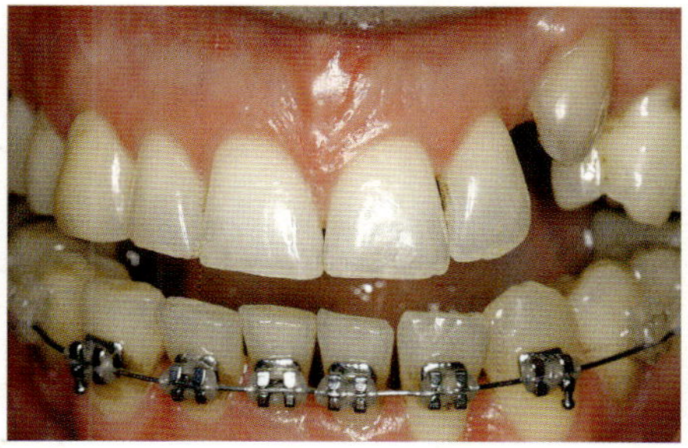

Fig 1-12b
Due to ankylosis of tooth 23, orthodontic treatment was completed at this stage.

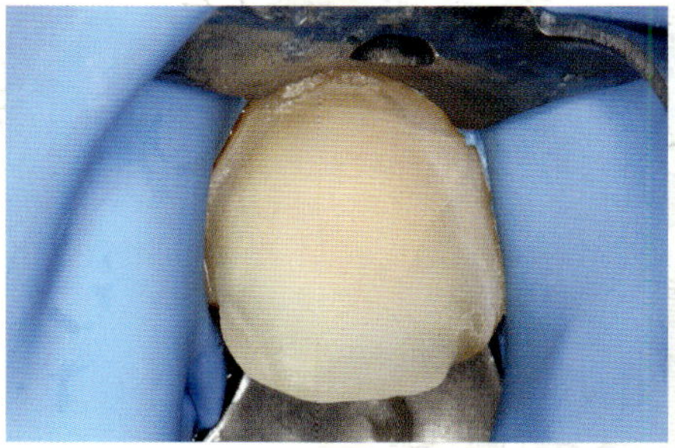

Fig 1-12c
Veneer preparation was done only in the enamel. Adhesive steps of the tooth structure were obtained in rubber dam isolation ...

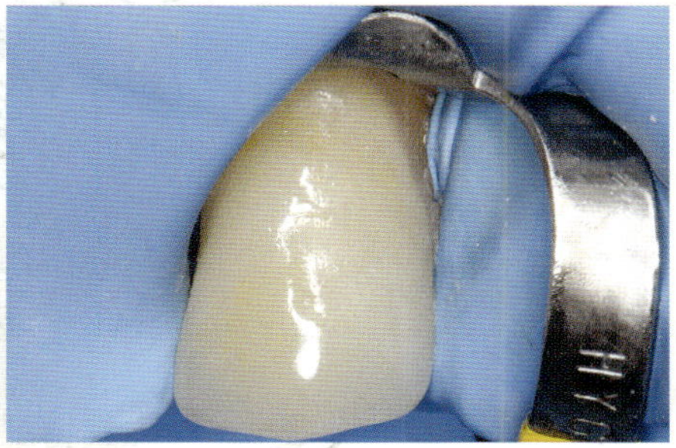

Fig 1-12d
... and the porcelain veneer was cemented.

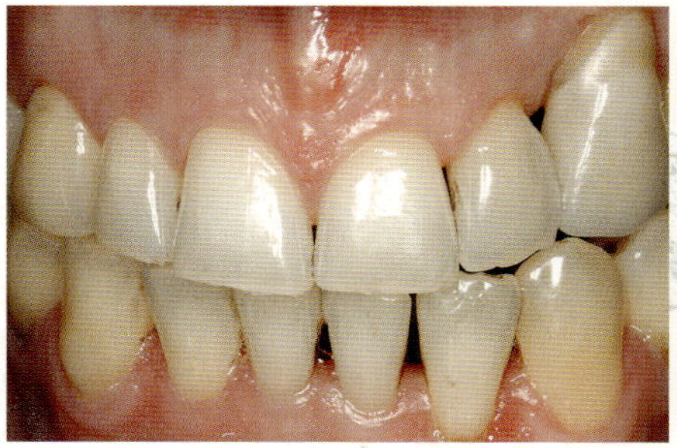

Fig 1-12e
Clinical situation after veneer cementation on the tooth 23.

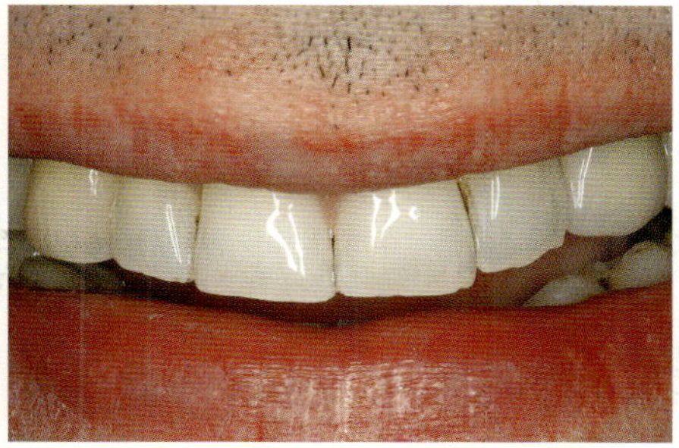

Fig 1-12f
A satisfied patient's smile after improving the esthetics of tooth 23 (it should be mentioned that the veneer has been functioning successfully for more than 14 years now).

REFERENCES

1. Burke FJ. Survival rates for porcelain laminate veneers with special reference to the effect of preparation in dentin: a literature review. J Esthet Restor Dent 2012;24:257–265.
2. Radz GM. Minimum thickness anterior porcelain restorations. Dent Clin North Am 2011;55:353–370.
3. Gürel G, Sesma N, Calamita MA, Coachman C, Morimoto S. Influence of enamel preservation on failure rates of porcelain laminate veneers. Int J Periodontics Restorative Dent 2013;33:31–39.
4. Gürel G, Morimoto S, Calamita MA, Coachman C, Sesma N. Clinical performance of porcelain laminate veneers: outcomes of the aesthetic pre-evaluative temporary (APT) technique. Int J Periodontics Restorative Dent 2012;32:625–635.
5. Gürel G, Bichacho N. Permanent diagnostic provisional restorations for predictable results when redesigning the smile. Pract Proced Aesthet Dent 2006;18:281–286; quiz 288, 316–317.
6. Magne P, Magne M. Use of additive wax-up and direct intraoral mock-up for enamel preservation with porcelain laminate veneers. Eur J Esthet Dent 2006;1:10–19.
7. Kinderknecht KE, Kupp LI. Aesthetic solution for large maxillary anterior diastema and frenum attachment. Pract Periodontics Aesthet Dent 1996;8:95–102; quiz 104.
8. da Cunha LF, Gonzaga CC, Saab R, Mushashe AM, Correr GM. Rehabilitation of the dominance of maxillary central incisors with refractory porcelain veneers requiring minimal tooth preparation. Quintessence Int 2015;46:837–841.
9. da Cunha LF, Pedroche LO, Gonzaga CC, Furuse AY. Esthetic, occlusal, and periodontal rehabilitation of anterior teeth with minimum thickness porcelain laminate veneers. J Prosthet Dent 2014;112:1315–1318.
10. Dietschi D, Argente A. A comprehensive and conservative approach for the restoration of abrasion and erosion. Part II: clinical procedures and case report. Eur J Esthet Dent 2011;6:142–159.
11. Farias-Neto A, de Medeiros FCD, Vilanova L, Simonetti Chaves M, Freire Batista de Araújo JJ. Tooth preparation for ceramic veneers: when less is more. Int J Esthet Dent 2019;14:156–164.
12. Burke F, Lucarotti P. Ten-year outcome of porcelain laminate veneers placed within the general dental services in England and Wales. J Dent 2009;37:31–38.
13. Beier US, Kapferer I, Burtscher D, Dumfahrt H. Clinical performance of porcelain laminate veneers for up to 20 years. Int J Prosthodont 2011;25:79–85.
14. Layton DM, Walton TR. The up to 21-year clinical outcome and survival of feldspathic porcelain veneers: accounting for clustering. Int J Prosthodont 2012;25:604–612.
15. Dumfahrt H, Schäffer H. Porcelain laminate veneers. A retrospective evaluation after 1 to 10 years of service: part II – clinical results. Int J Prosthodont 2000;13:9.
16. Gresnigt MM, Kalk W, Özcan M. Clinical longevity of ceramic laminate veneers bonded to teeth with and without existing composite restorations up to 40 months. Clin Oral Investig 2013;17:823–832.
17. Kois JC, Phillips KM. Occlusal vertical dimension: alteration concerns. Compend Contin Educ Dent 1997;18:1169–1180.
18. Kois DE, Kois JC. Comprehensive risk-based diagnostically driven treatment planning: developing sequentially generated treatment. Dent Clin North Am 2015;59:593–608.
19. Zarow M. Contraindicated internal bleaching: what to do? Styleitaliano; 4/2017. Dostępne. Available at: www.styleitaliano.org/contraindicated-internal-bleaching-what-to-do/
20. Berland L. Bleaching and porcelain veneers: consider the combination. Dent Today 1994;13:78–81.
21. Calamia J, Calamia Ch. Porcelain laminate veneers: reasons for 25 years of success. Dent Clin N Am 2007;51:399–417.
22. Edelhoff D, Prandtner O, Saeidi Pour R, Liebermann A, Stimmelmayr M, Güth JF. Anterior restorations: the performance of ceramic veneers. Quintessence Int 2018;49:89–101.
23. Curry FT. Porcelain veneers: adjunct or alternative to orthodontic therapy. J Esthet Dent 1998;10:67–74.
24. Magne P, Douglas WH. Design optimization and evolution of bonded ceramics for the anterior dentition: a finite-element analysis. Quintessence Int 1999;30:661–672.
25. Peumans M, De Munck J, Fieuws S, Lambrechts P, Vanherle G, van Meerbeek B. A prospective ten-year clinical trial of porcelain veneers. J Adhes Dent 2004;6:65–76.

CHAPTER 2

PORCELAIN VENEERS: YES OR NO?

MACIEJ ŻAROW

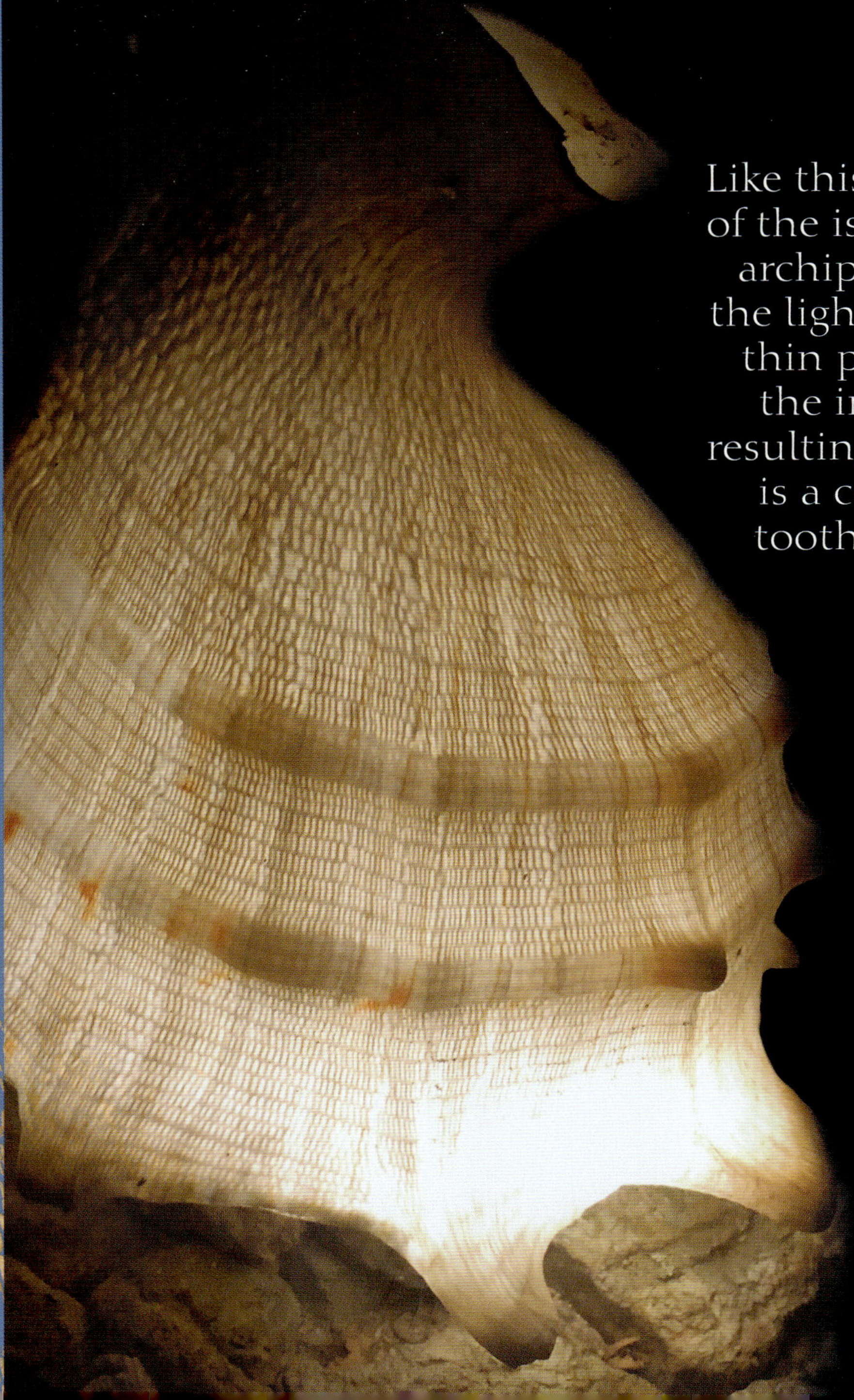

Like this shell, found on one of the islands of the Palawan archipelago (Philippines), the light penetrates through thin porcelain veneers to the inside of the tooth, resulting in a final color that is a combination of the tooth and the veneer ...

Porcelain veneers – why yes?

Are porcelain veneers a good choice? The answer is yes because they have many advantages: they are highly esthetic and look like natural teeth, and they are thin enough to let the light penetrate inside the tooth, just like alabaster or shells. In addition, preparation time is minimized, and the enamel is maintained as much as possible.

ADVANTAGES OF VENEERS FROM A CLINICAL PERSPECTIVE

- They are less invasive than prosthetic crowns[1,2]
- There is no risk of losing pulp vitality when performing a slight preparation (enamel) (Fig 2-1)[3]
- Assuming that we are preparing the tooth within the enamel, the risk of hypersensitivity is minimized (Fig 2-1)[4]
- By definition, they do not interfere with periodontal tissues (juxtagingival preparation) (Fig 2-2)[5]

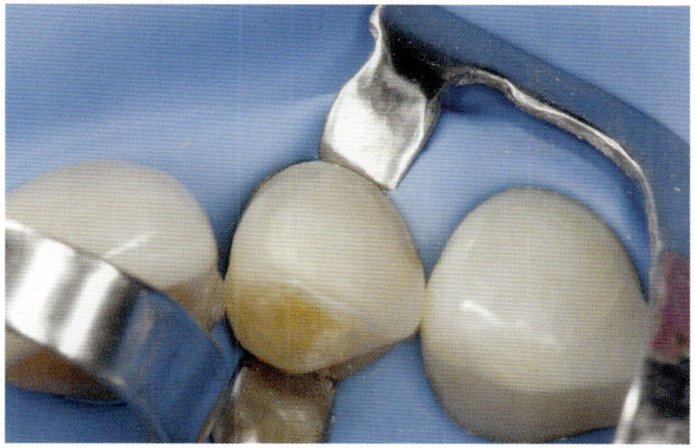

Fig 2-1
Example of a standard preparation made under the control of a silicone index to minimize the enamel.

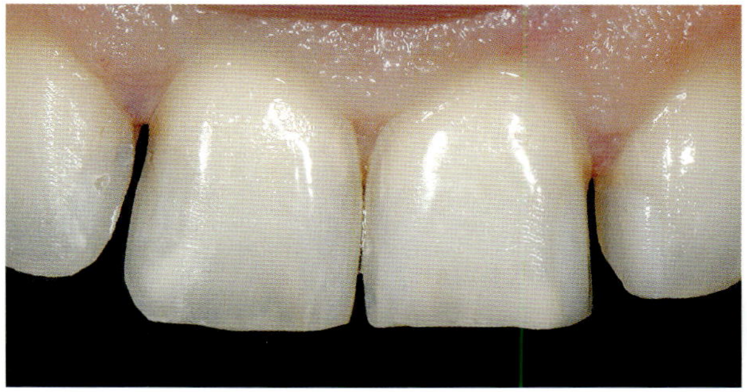

Fig 2-2a
Veneer preparation on teeth 11 and 21 with respect for the gingival margin – the juxtagingival preparation did not violate the integrity of the soft tissues.

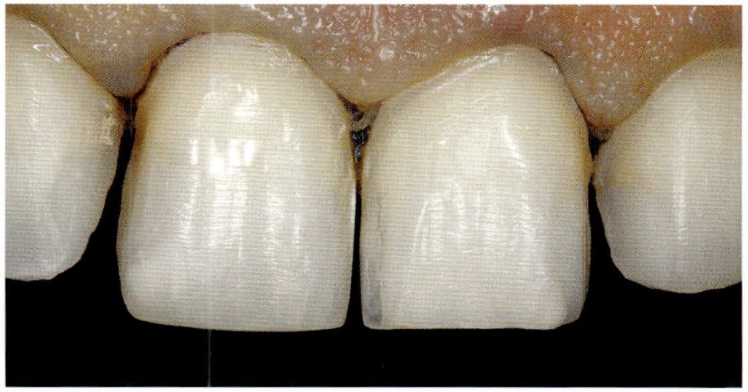

Fig 2-2b
The preparation margin becomes visible only after inserting the first and then the second retraction cord.

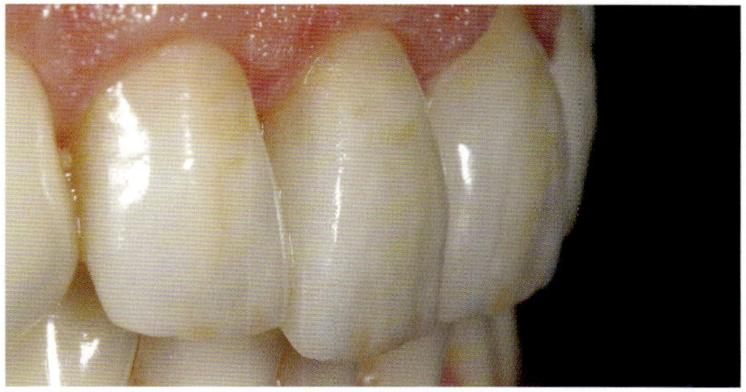

Fig 2-2c
Clinical situation after veneers cementation.

- They are biocompatible and well tolerated by the gingiva, even when a minimal subgingival preparation is performed (subgingival preparation for veneers is generally not recommended. However, in some cases, it is required to cover intense discoloration or to close the black triangles in the interdental space – the veneer gently interferes with the subgingival area)[5]
- They successfully improve function: symmetrical anterior guidance and lateral guidance (Fig 2-3)[6]
- They can be redone in the future[7]
- They restore the tooth stiffness due to the physical properties of porcelain, which is important for the functional aspects of the anterior teeth[8,9]
- They can mask tooth discoloration, which is unpredictable and extremely difficult when working with composites (Fig 2-4)[10–13]

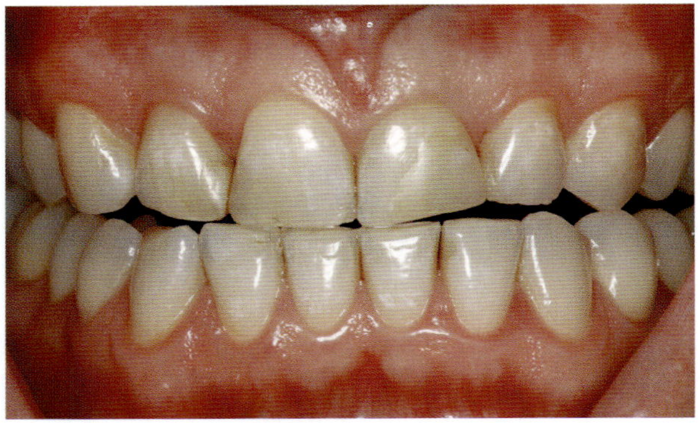

Fig 2-3a
A 41-year-old female patient was offered four porcelain veneers in the maxillary arch, not only for esthetic reasons but also to improve anterior guidance – shown here is the clinical situation in anterior guidance before treatment.

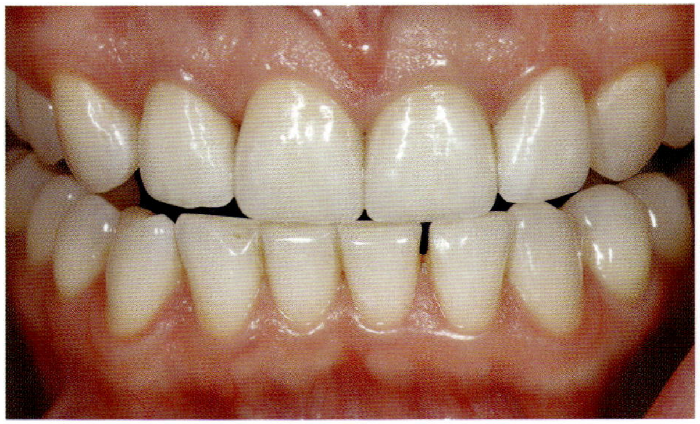

Fig 2-3b
Four porcelain veneers were obtained.

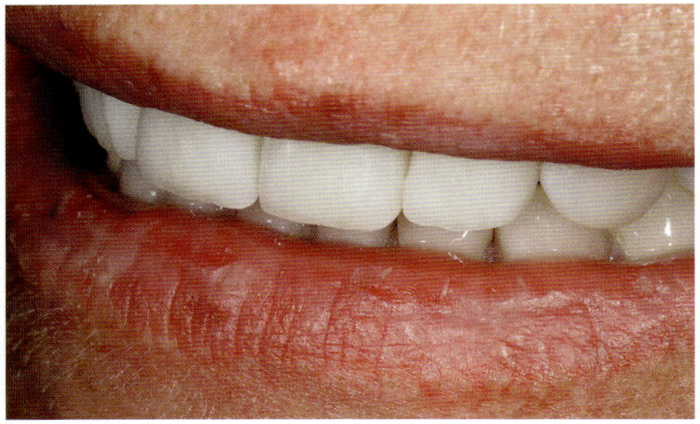

Fig 2-3c
The patient's smile from the semi-profile after cementation of the veneers.

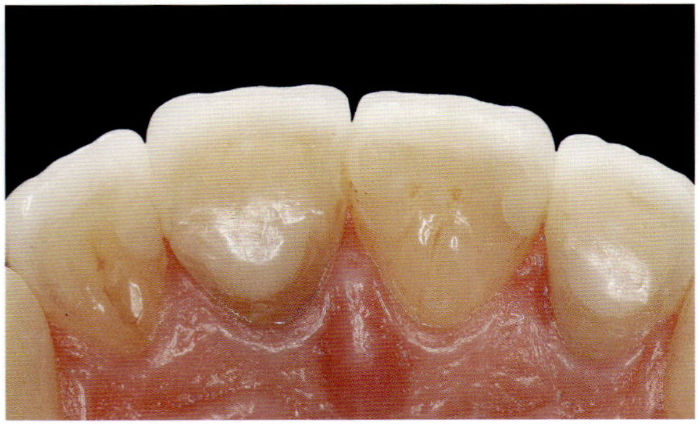

Fig 2-3d
Cemented veneers from the palatal view.

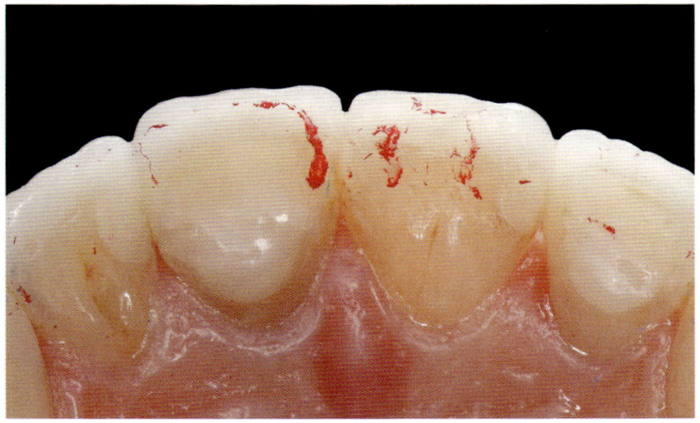

Fig 2-3e
Marking the front guidance after tooth lengthening with the veneers.

Fig 2-4a
Many years ago, a female patient presented to the dental office requesting to cover her teeth with veneers because multiple attempts at teeth whitening had not brought any results. The cause of the discoloration was taking tetracycline in early childhood.

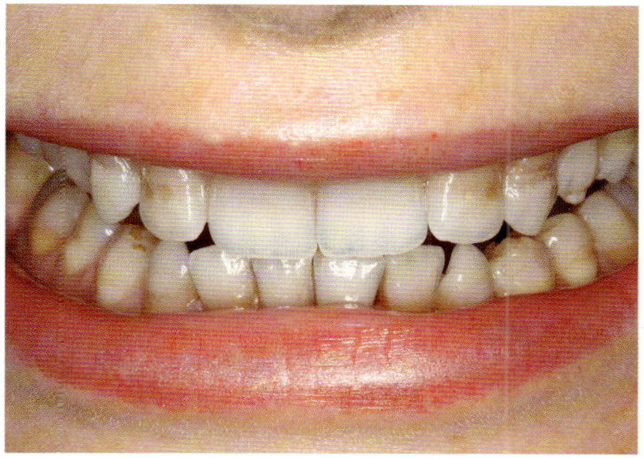

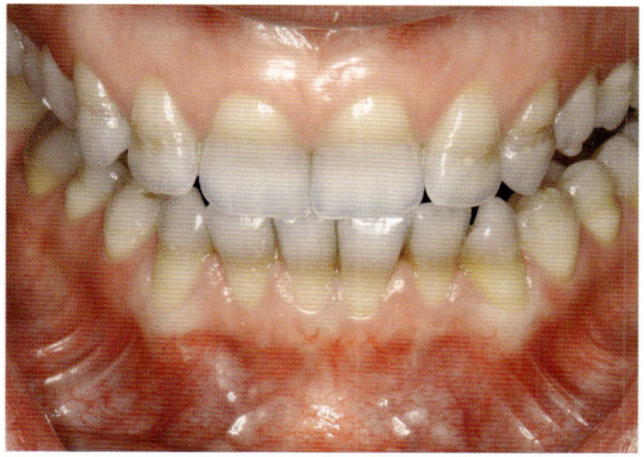

Fig 2-4b
The clinical situation in the maxillary and mandibular arches.

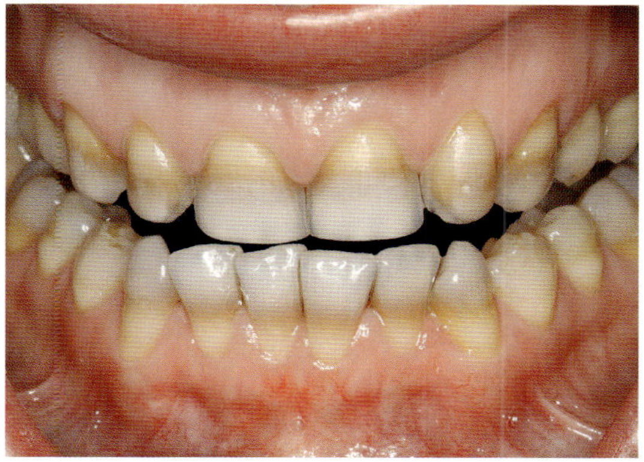

Fig 2-4c
Ten maxillary porcelain veneers were proposed as a treatment – the photograph shows minimal veneer preparation with preservation of enamel.

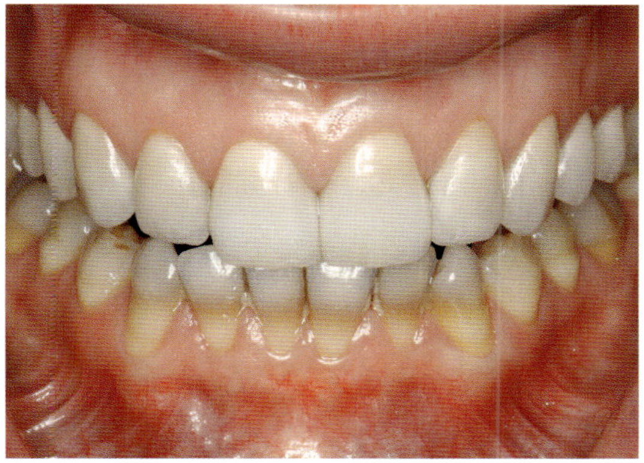

Fig 2-4d
Situation after cementing porcelain veneers (feldspathic porcelain was used, now it would be possible to use "better masking" lithium disilicate porcelain).

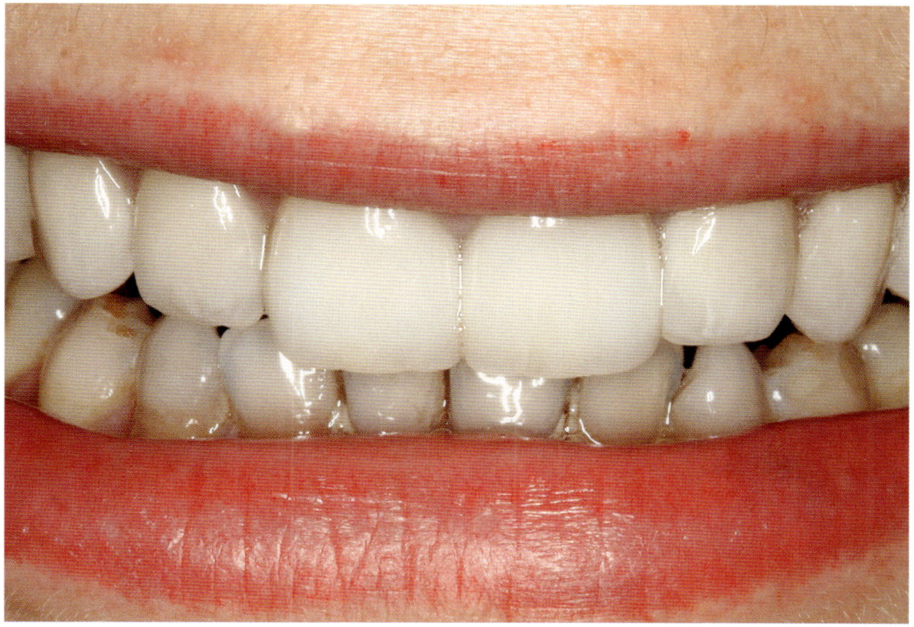

Fig 2-4e
Patient's smile after cementing 10 veneers in the maxilla.

CONSIDER PLANNING PORCELAIN VENEERS WHEN:

1. Maxillary anterior teeth have extensive, highly visible composite restorations (Fig 2-5)

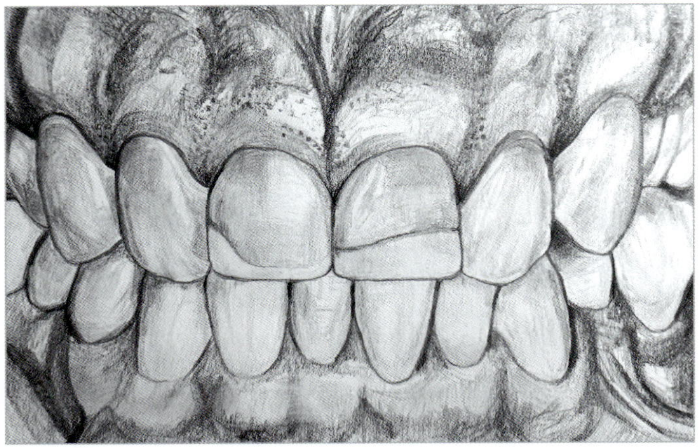

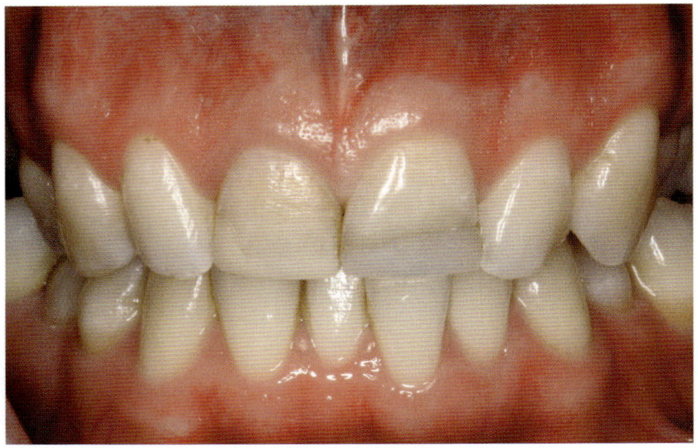

Fig 2-5
The replacement of extensive restorations can cause many difficulties, such as correct color composite matching or durability problems. In such cases, veneers can be considered.

2. Esthetic composite restorations are difficult to perform due to the need to reconstruct many teeth (Fig 2-6)

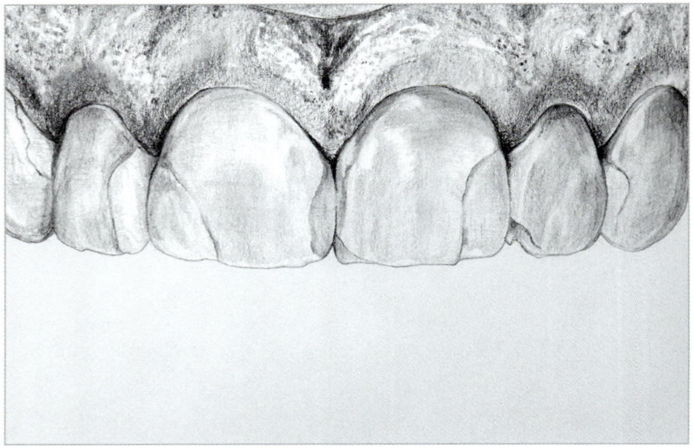

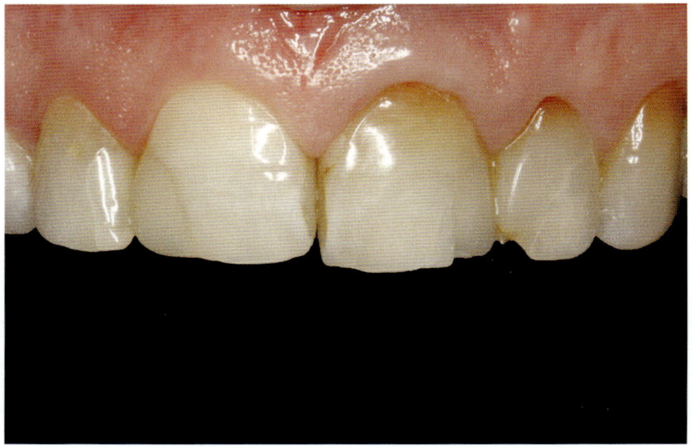

Fig 2-6
If the replacement of extensive restorations involves many teeth (for example, four or six), it is even more worth considering veneers.

Consider the advantages
of porcelain veneers when
you are planning esthetic treat-
ment ... but do not forget about
the functional risk !

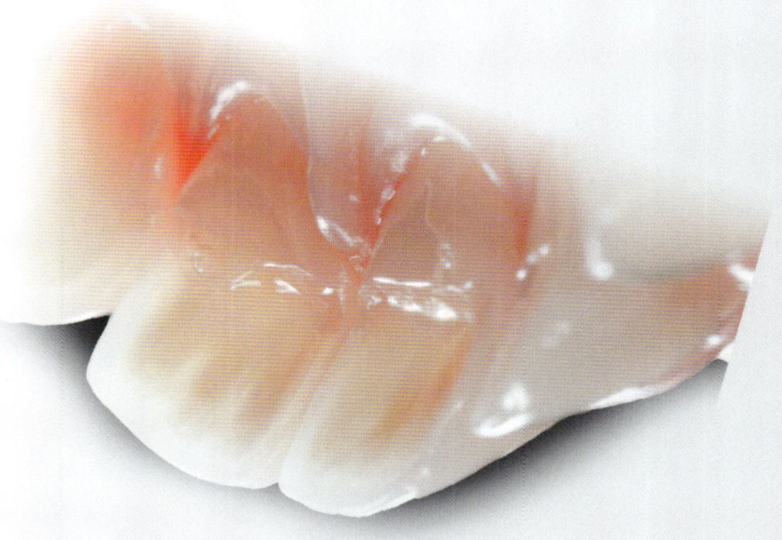

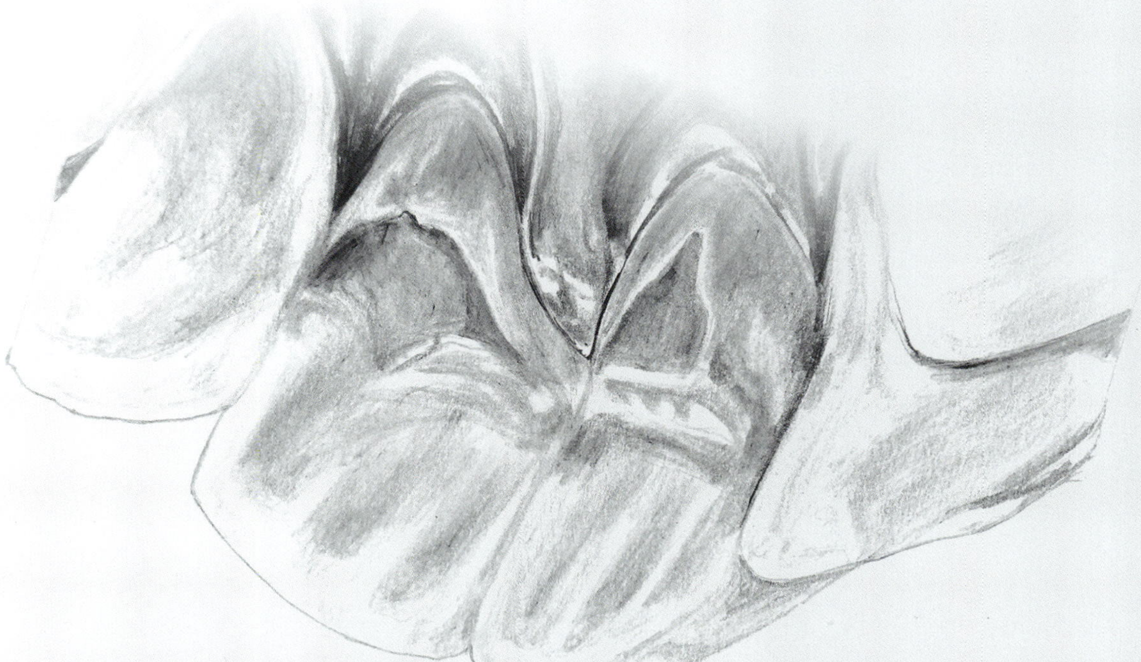

3. When a significant change of the shape or lengthening is necessary (Fig 2-7)[14–16]

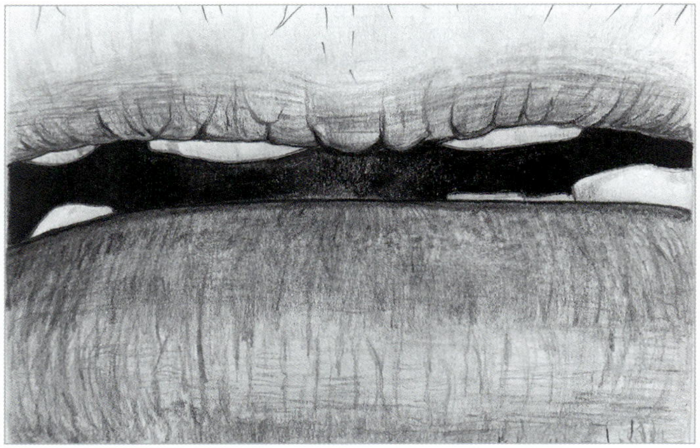

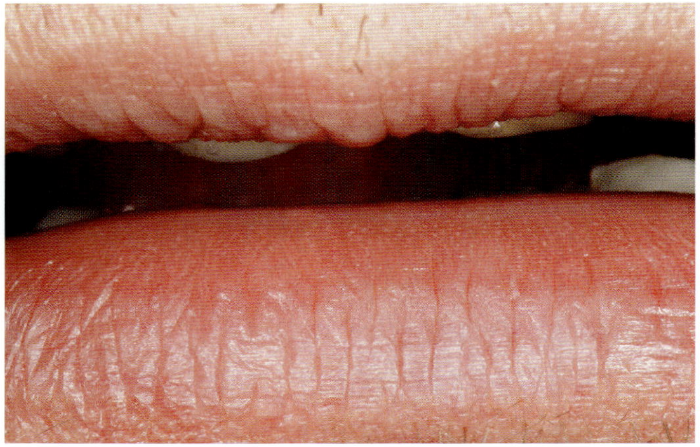

Fig 2-7a
When maxillary central incisors are not visible in the "lips at rest" position, tooth extension should be considered for esthetic improvement. In such cases, porcelain veneers are among the treatment options.

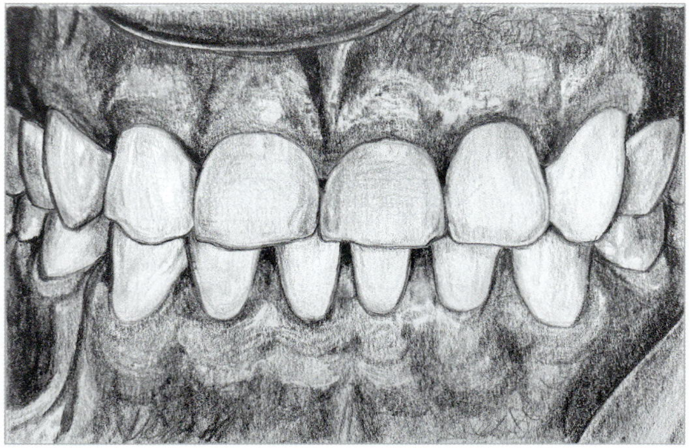

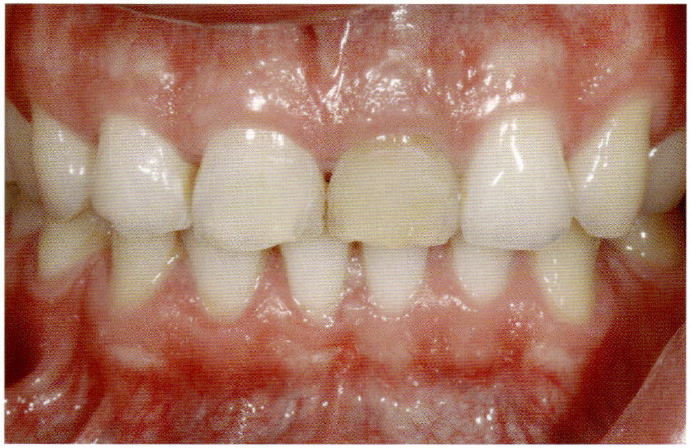

Fig 2-7b
When the maxillary central incisors have a similar length to the maxillary lateral incisors, consider changing the length or shape of the teeth to achieve dominance of the maxillary central incisors.

4. It is necessary to close the diastema (Fig 2-8)[17,18]

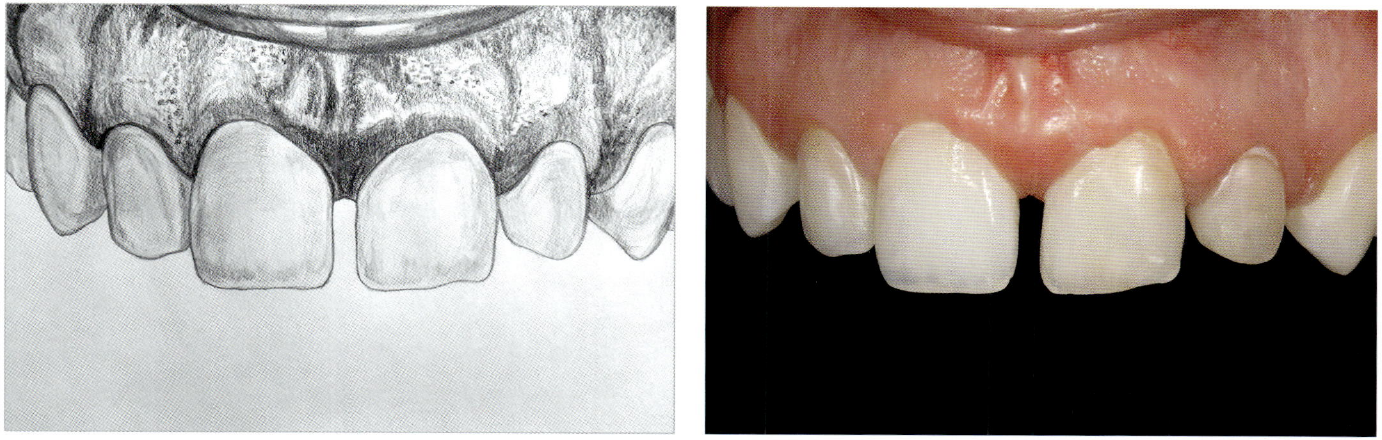

Fig 2-8
Diastema is one of the indications for porcelain veneers. However, this therapeutic option should always be analyzed individually and be visualized by mock-up before starting the treatment.

5. Reducing/closing visible black triangles (Fig 2-9)[5]

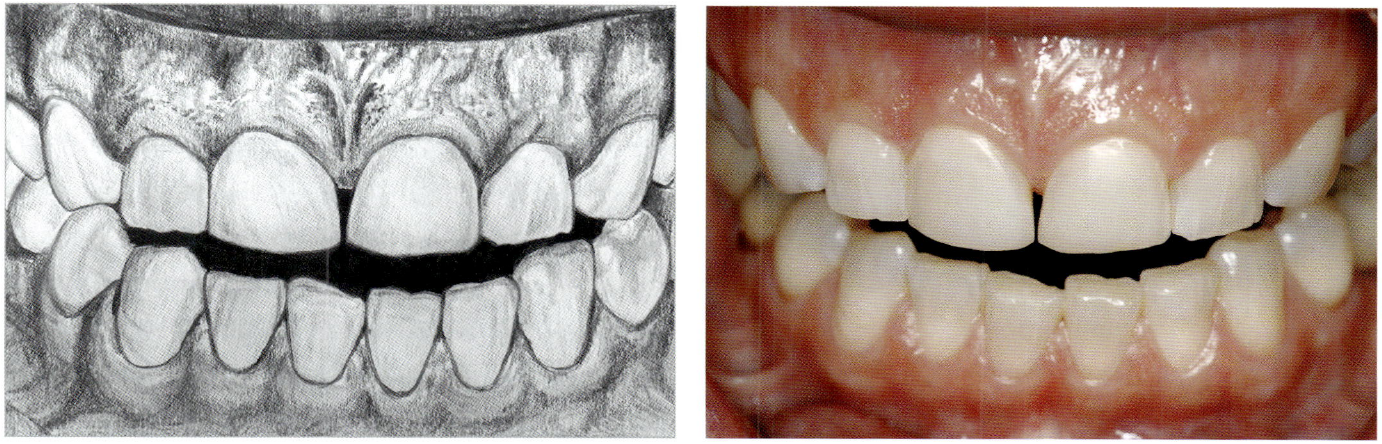

Fig 2-9
Closing black triangles is one of the indications for porcelain veneers. To achieve permanent black triangle closure, it should be done based on the knowledge of the alveolar bone position and the biological width.

6. Changing the long axis of the anterior teeth or the midline between the maxillary central incisors (Fig 2-10)[5]

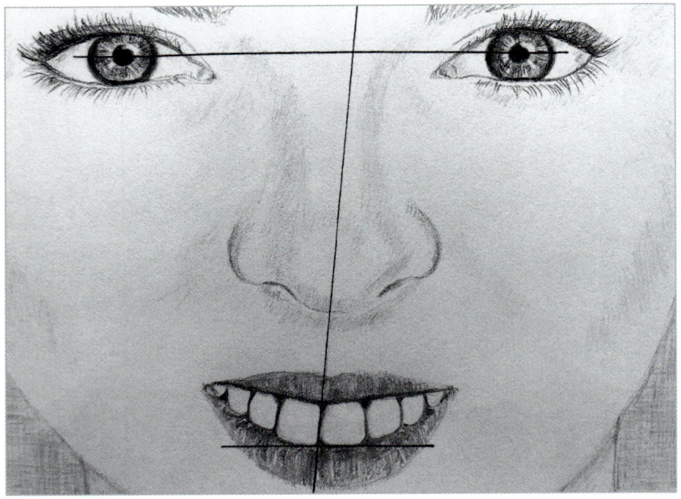

Fig 2-10
One of the indications for porcelain veneers is changing the line course between the maxillary central incisors so that it overlaps more with the facial midline and is perpendicular with the pupillary line.

> **REMEMBER**
> If you want to improve the midline course with veneers, you should plan the restoration appropriately and involve the proximal surfaces in the preparation. A photograph from the 12 o'clock position helps us understand the coincidence of a facial midline with a dental midline (see page 55, point 14).

7. Tooth is discolored and cannot be whitened or masked predictably with the composite material (Fig 2-11)[19]

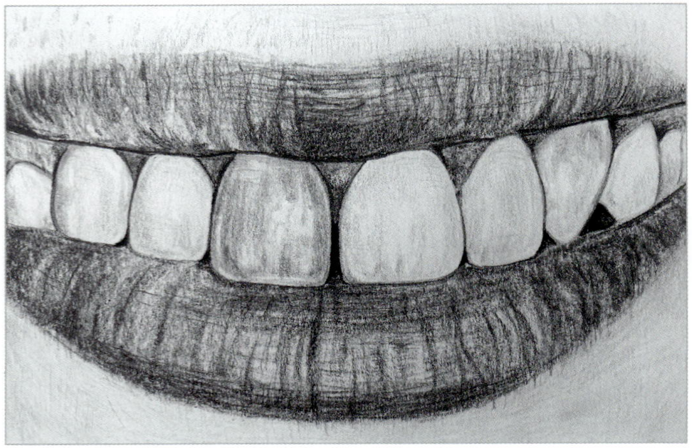

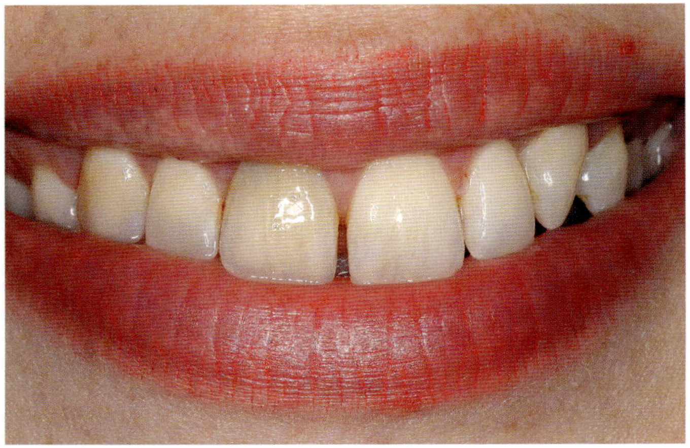

Fig 2-11
One of the indications for making two symmetrical porcelain veneers is a discolored tooth where for some reason, internal bleaching is contraindicated, so the color cannot be masked predictably with the composite.

8. We perform a single crown and want to balance the esthetics on the other side of the dental arch (Fig 2-12)[20]

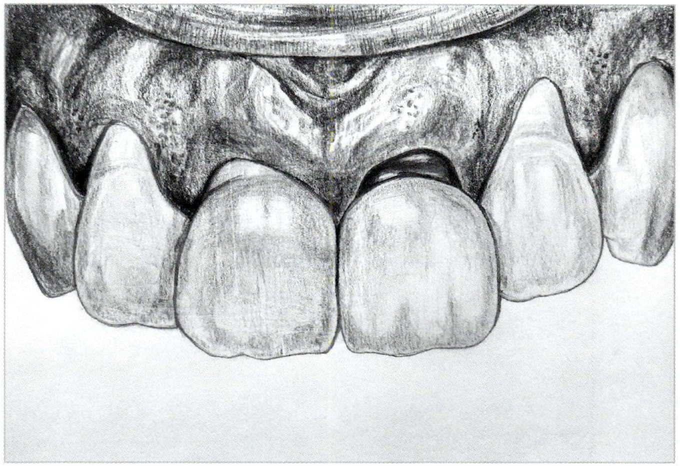

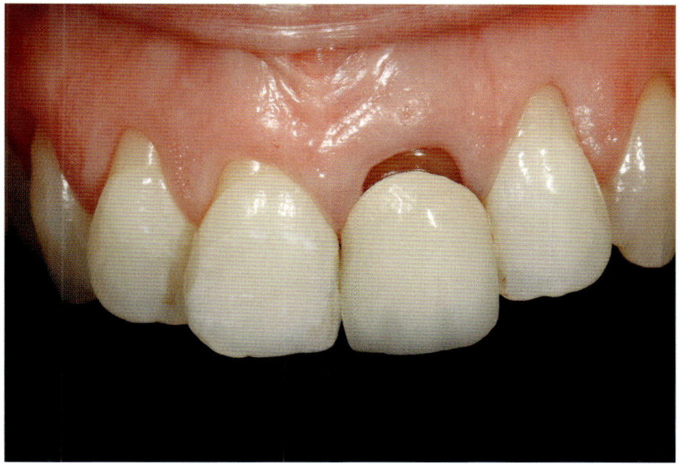

Fig 2-12
When replacing the crown on one of the maxillary central incisors, the ideal solution is to cover the symmetrically positioned incisor with a porcelain veneer made of the same porcelain as the crown.

9. When a single implant-supported crown is performed, and there is a need to balance the symmetry and to close a possible black triangle (Fig 2-13)[21]

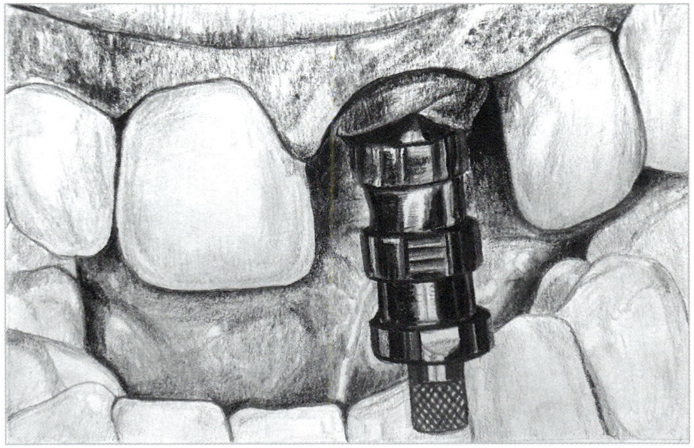

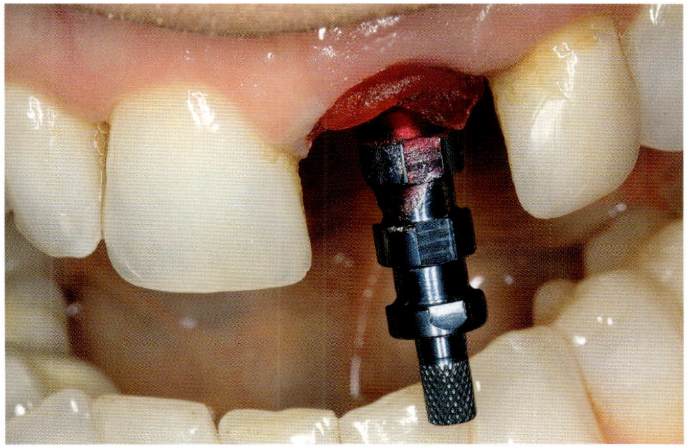

Fig 2-13
When performing the maxillary central incisor implant crown, the gingival margin can change its architecture from the baseline, requiring shape change on both teeth. For this purpose, it is often necessary to carry out a veneer on the adjacent tooth.

10. When the position of the rotated tooth needs to be corrected, and orthodontic treatment is not possible for some reason (Fig 2-14)[22]

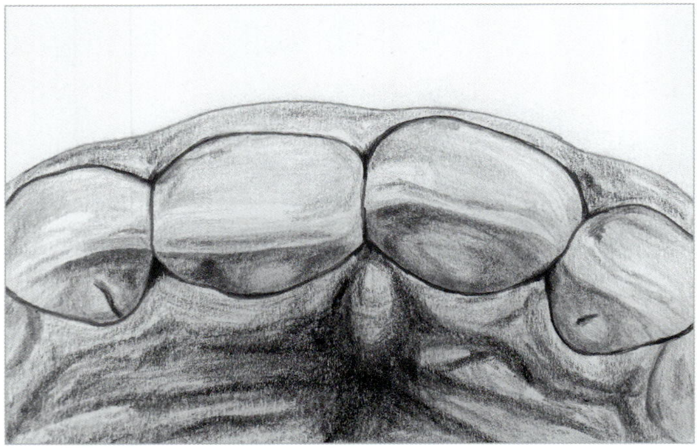

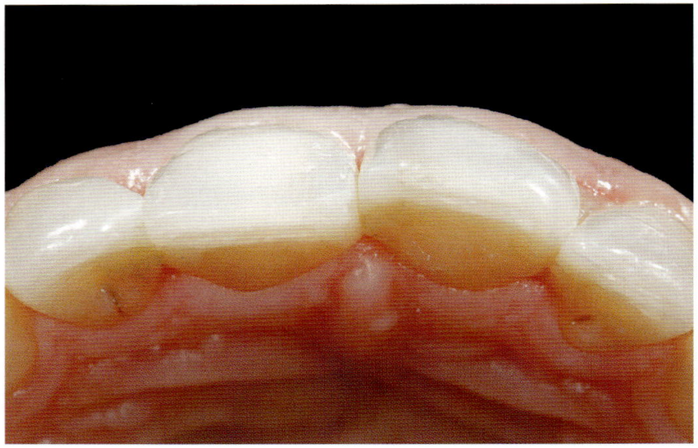

Fig 2-14
Orthodontic treatment remains the best solution for patients who require teeth aligned in the dental arch. However, it is possible to align the dental arch and improve the smile with porcelain veneers in some cases, especially when the teeth position enables us to minimize tooth preparation.

11. When complex occlusal rehabilitation is planned – as the last step of restoring the function and esthetics in the anterior segment (Fig 2-15)[23]

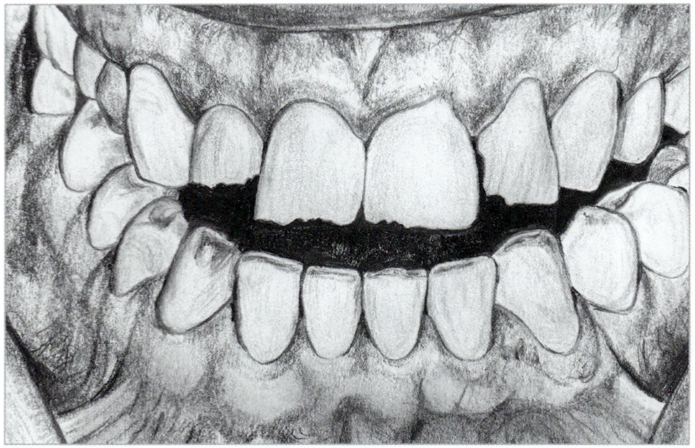

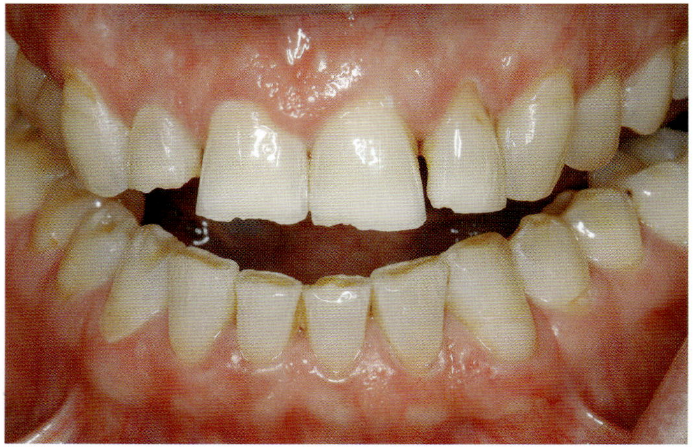

Fig 2-15
In cases like this, porcelain veneers are indicated but usually only after reconstruction of the occlusion by creating appropriate space for restorative material in the anterior teeth.

Porcelain veneers – why no?

You cannot agree to even very convincing suggestions from patients who are absolutely sure that porcelain veneers are the only possible treatment. The clinical situation and indications should be realistically assessed. Sometimes, even the greatest efforts can lead to months of disputes and resentments.

DO NOT PLAN PORCELAIN VENEERS WHEN:

1. There is a small amount of tooth structure, and less than 50% of the tooth structure would adhere to the veneer after preparation (Fig 2-16)[13]

If more than 50% of the hard tissues remain after veneer preparation, we can expect proper adhesion and durability for such reconstruction. The more enamel, especially on the margins of the preparation, the better chance for a long-lasting marginal seal. The same is true for the ratio of tooth structure to composite surface within the preparation. Although similar to tooth tissues (especially to dentin), composite behaves slightly differently over the years. It shows a tendency to water sorption and volume change, which means that the veneer may "work" differently when it is bonded to the hard tissue surface and the composite surface.

This will not matter for small composite restorations,[13] but it is difficult to predict how the veneer will behave when the base surface is a large Class 4 restoration.

Suppose we add a lack of stable occlusion and bilateral support on the lateral teeth or constricted chewing pattern. In that case, the total of the unfavorable factors becomes even greater.

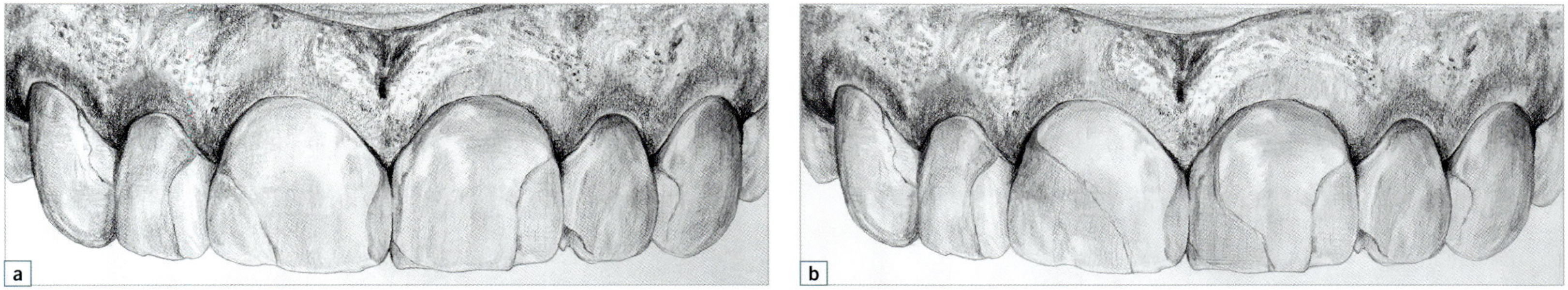

Fig 2-16
Two different clinical situations. (a) There is enough tooth structure in teeth 11 and 21. (b) After veneer preparation in tooth 11, less than 50% of the hard tissues will be left, and in tooth 21, the quantity of hard tissues will be around 50%. Therefore, the replacement of fillings or ceramic crowns should be considered. It is possible to make porcelain veneers in this case, but the risk of failure in the future (for example, cracks) increases significantly when the veneer has a composite build-up on most of its preparation surface.

2. There are subgingival cavities or Class 5 restorations reaching the cementum (Fig 2-17)[24]

When Class 5 composite restorations are placed subgingivally deep enough that placing a rubber dam to control the moisture and removing excess material during cementation is not possible, veneers are contraindicated. In addition, the cervical part of the veneer is a critical zone in terms of stress distribution. The cervical area of the tooth accumulates much stress: this is where the enamel reaches the cementum (cementoenamel junction, CEJ), and main types of non-carious cervical lesions are formed, ie, abfractions (due to occlusal overload).

If the margin of the preparation can be located in the enamel in this critical gingival zone, the durability of the veneer will increase. If a significant part of the preparation is located subgingivally in the cementum, the veneer's adhesion to the tooth will decrease critically. In addition, it will not be possible to control moisture during cementation or to remove excess material.

For these reasons, the marginal seal of the veneer and periodontal health will be unpredictable. The location of the veneer margin on the composite in the gingival zone is contraindicated in the case of an existing Class 5 restoration. The veneer may cover the entire filling, but the gingival margin should not finish on the restoration but on the tooth structure.

REMEMBER

If the gingival margin of the veneer preparation is located deep subgingivally, the long-term marginal seal of the veneer and periodontal health will not be predictable. In such a clinical situation, think about alternative solutions such as direct or indirect composite restorations. In the event of chipping or other problems, they can be repaired!

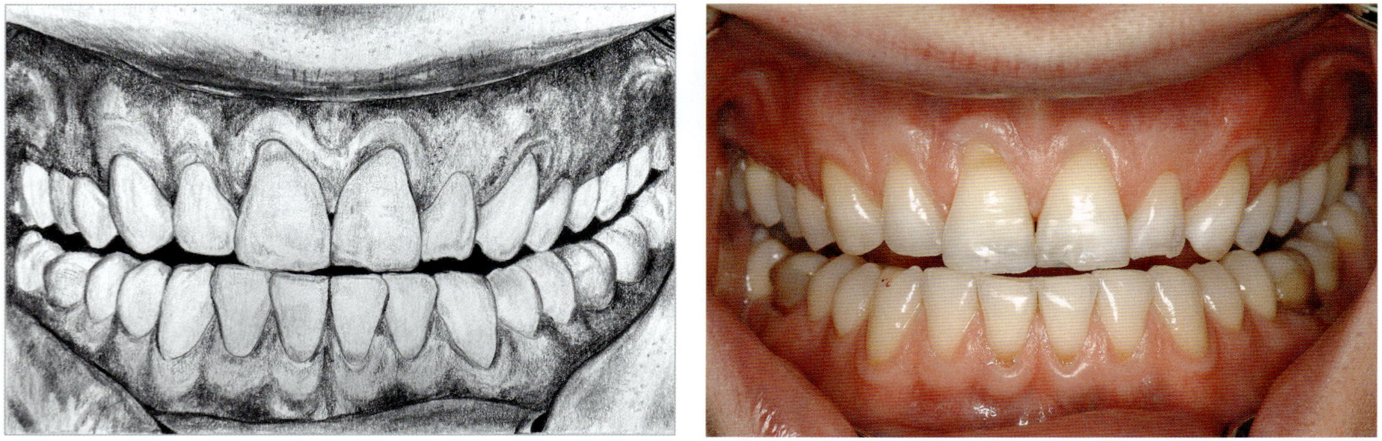

Fig 2-17
When cavities reach the cementoenamel junction and interfere in the cementum zone, the risk of the veneer entering the cementum should be taken into account (faster aging of the adhesion and risk of stress accumulation).

3. Class 3 subgingival restorations when rubber dam isolation is not possible (Fig 2-18)

As with Class 5 cavities, deep subgingival Class 3 cavities are contraindicated for porcelain veneers.[24] The veneer cannot have a margin placed juxtagingivally on the composite restoration.

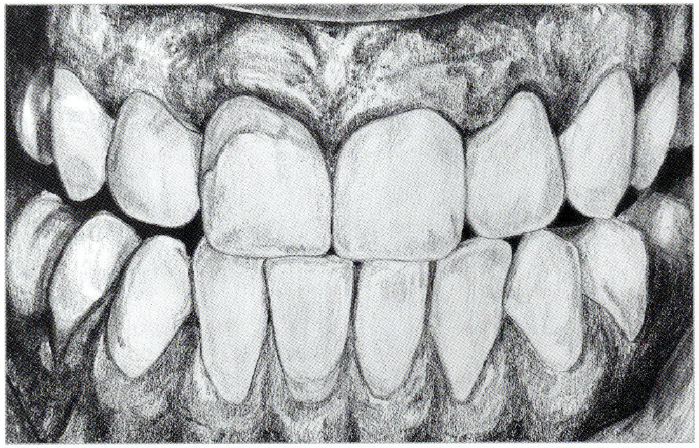

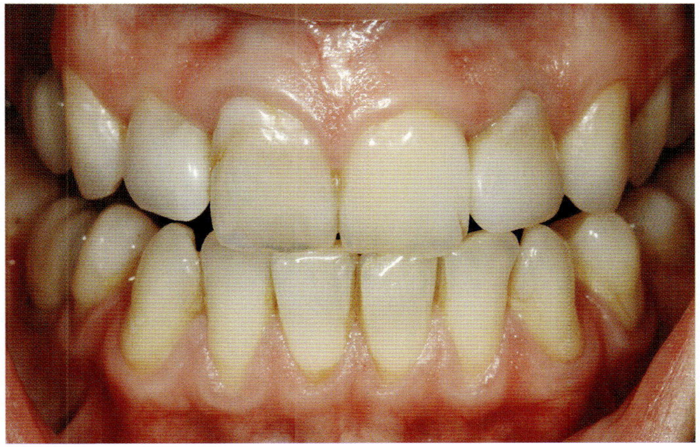

Fig 2-18
With deep subgingival Class 3 cavities, a different type of treatment than porcelain veneers should be considered.

4. The patient is an adolescent (Fig 2-19)[25]

Video: Alternative treatment of an adolescent https://books.dentist.com.pl/veneers/1

As a rule, we do not make porcelain veneers for patients under the age of 21. It used to be considered that the patient's occlusion was formed and stable by the age of 18–20; currently, it is assumed that this limit should be extended even to the age of 25. This is shown by studies related to implantation failure in patients in their early 20s. For young people, direct composite veneers will be a perfect solution.

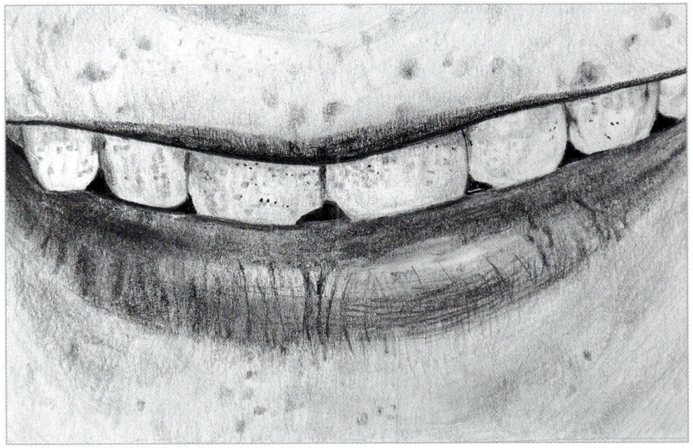

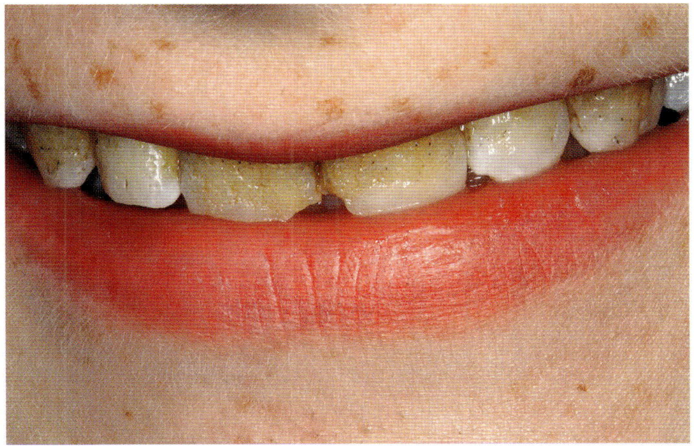

Fig 2-19
A 15-year-old female patient presented to the dental office to obtain porcelain veneers to cover the enamel hypoplasia. The patient's young age and the ongoing bone growth phase are contraindications for an indirect porcelain restoration.

5. Incorrect occlusal conditions were diagnosed[26–28]

- Lack of a stable and balanced occlusion on both sides (no lateral support) (Fig 2-20)

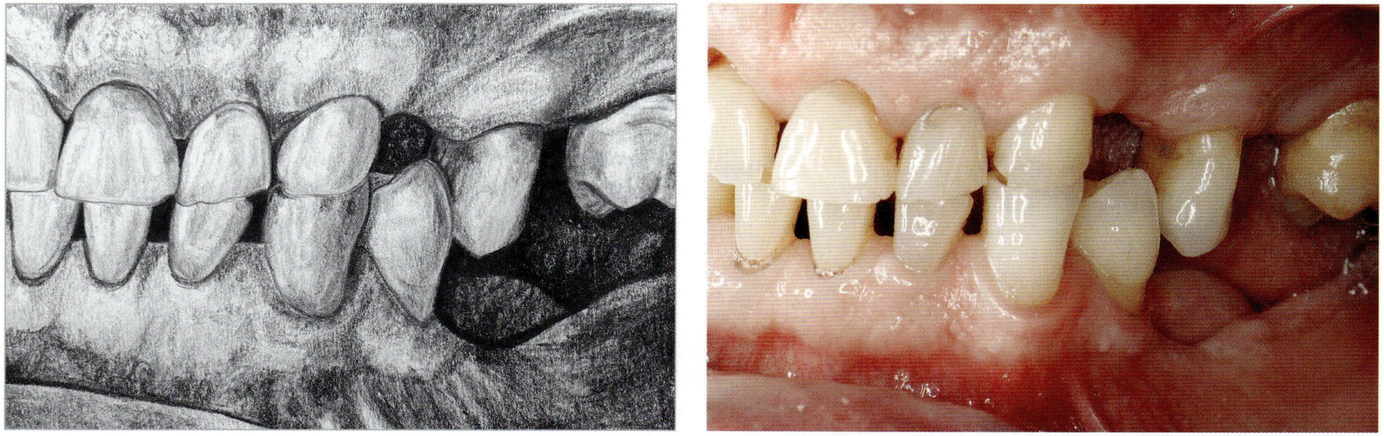

Fig 2-20
Missing teeth in the posterior segment of the dental arch is a contraindication for porcelain veneers. First, occlusion rehabilitation should be performed – only then can veneers be made according to previous planning (see Chapter 8).

- A constricted envelope of function means that there is no space between the front teeth of the maxilla and mandible when performing basic functional activities, such as chewing, talking, breathing, or swallowing. Clinically, it is common to see shelves of wear as exposed dentin on the palatal surface – Dr. John Kois calls this a vertical wear pattern (Fig 2-21).

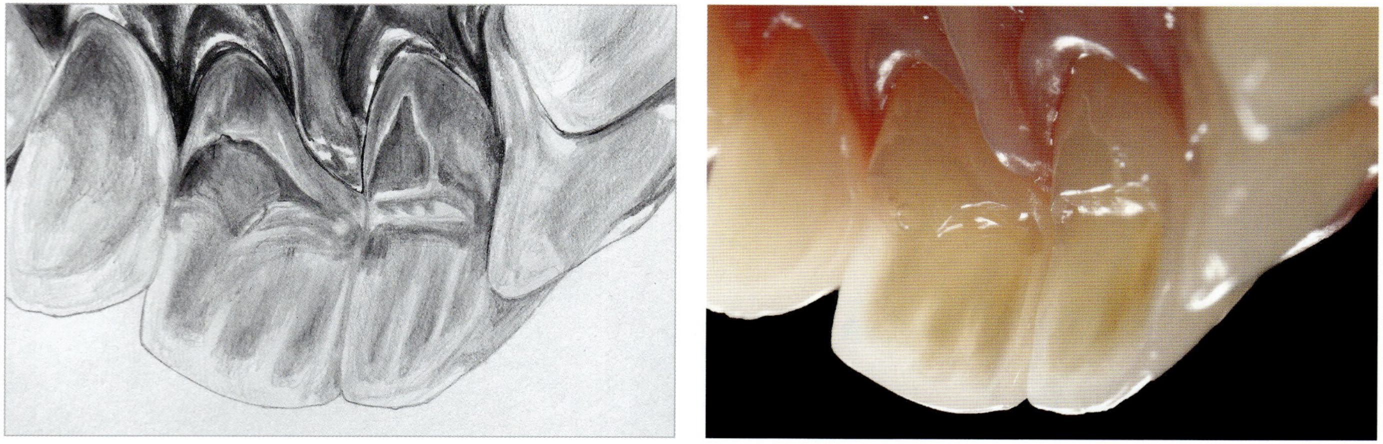

Fig 2-21
A 22-year-old female patient was diagnosed with a constricted envelope of function, which led to a vertical wear pattern on the palatal surface of the anterior maxillary teeth.

- The occurrence of premature contacts leads to bypassing with mandibular movements, which can often be destructive for the teeth by excessive abrasion. In this situation, we are usually dealing with a horizontal wear pattern (Fig 2-22).

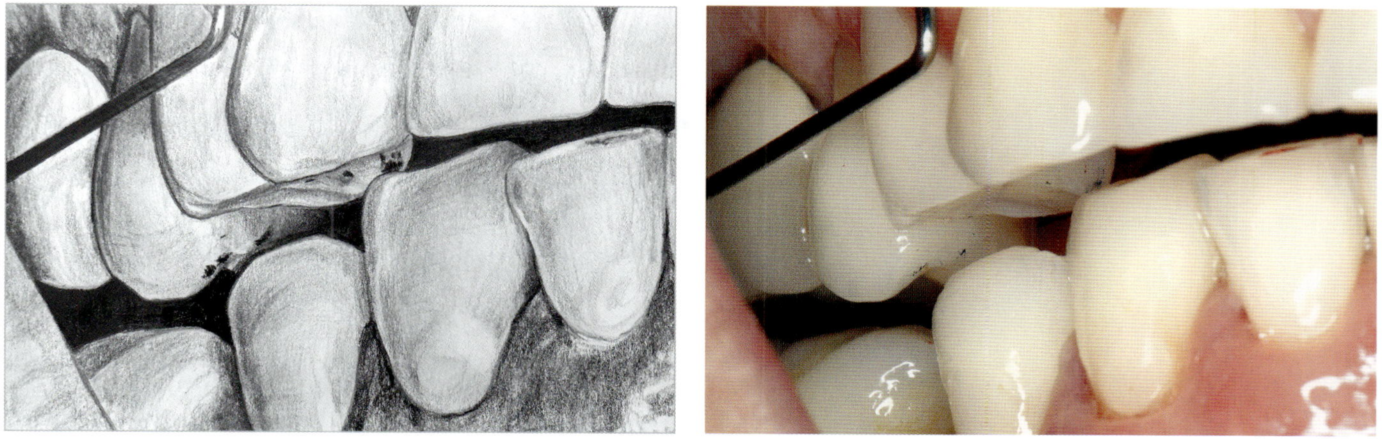

Fig 2-22
Premature contacts in the posterior segment of the dental arch were detected by a Kois Deprogrammer (KD) (horizontal wear pattern; occlusal dysfunction in Kois functional risk classification).

Video: Correction no-prep with the composite https://books.dentist.com.pl/veneers/2

6. The patient's esthetic problems can be solved in a less invasive way than performing veneers[29,30]

- Porcelain veneers, although they are minimally invasive, do in most cases require slight preparation, which can be avoided in many situations
- Teeth can be whitened and fillings can be replaced with minimally invasive composite restorations (Fig 2-23)

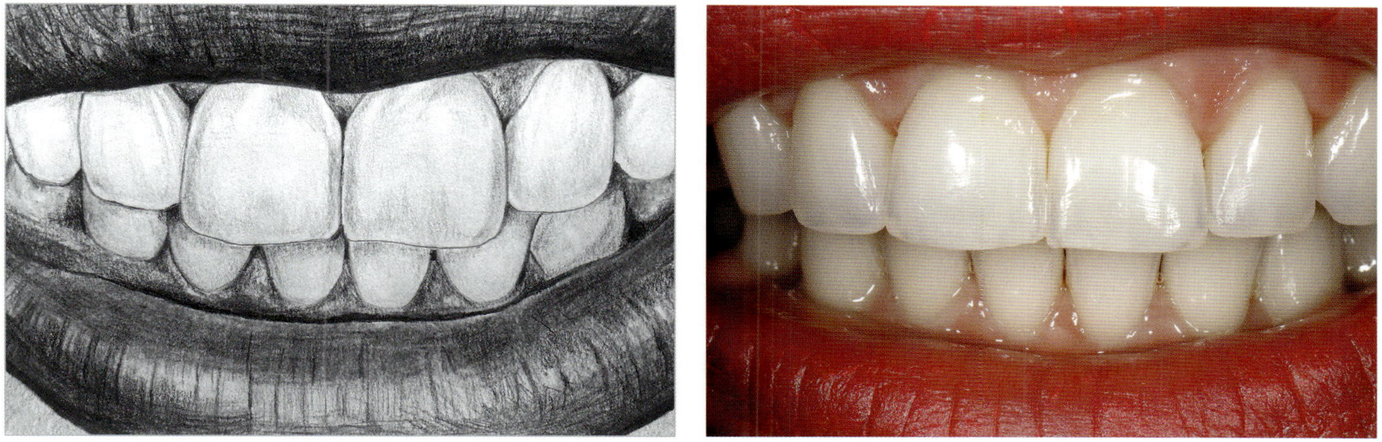

Fig 2-23
A female patient presented to the dental office seeking treatment with porcelain veneers: whitening and slight correction of the shape with composite was proposed.

- White spots (hypomineralization) that can be eliminated or removed by resin infiltration (Icon) (Fig 2-24)

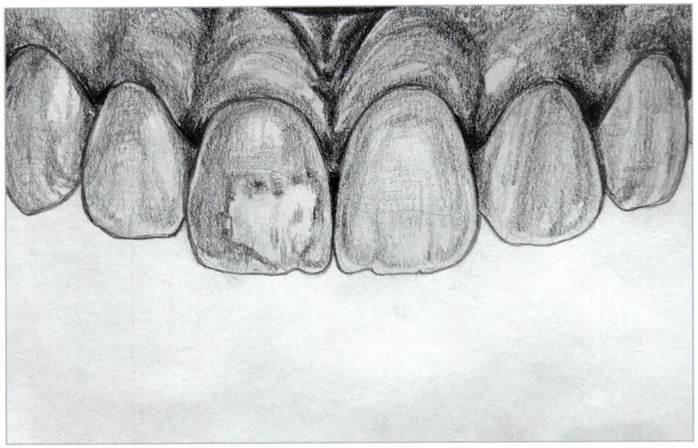

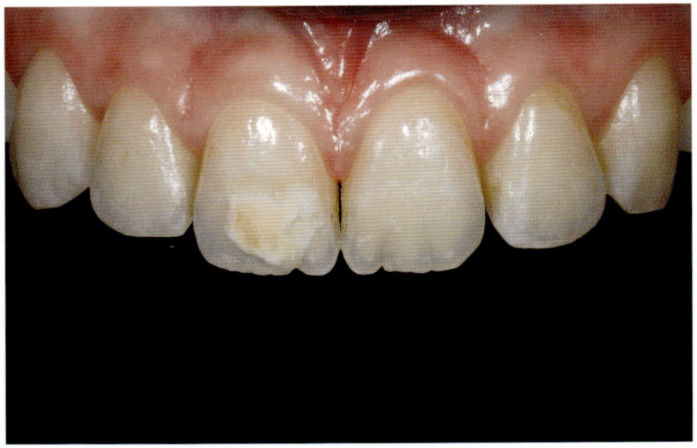

Fig 2-24
A 19-year-old female patient presented to the dental office to improve the esthetics of anterior teeth due to enamel hypoplasia occurring as white/brown spots. The solution, in this case, can be bleaching and resin infiltration (see Chapter 10).

Video: Whitening and shape correction with the composite https://books.dentist.com.pl/veneers/3

- Teeth with an unesthetic shape that can be corrected with rotary instruments (Fig 2-25)

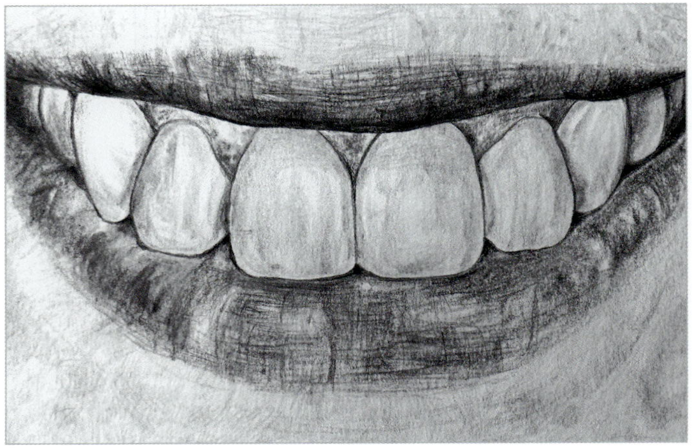

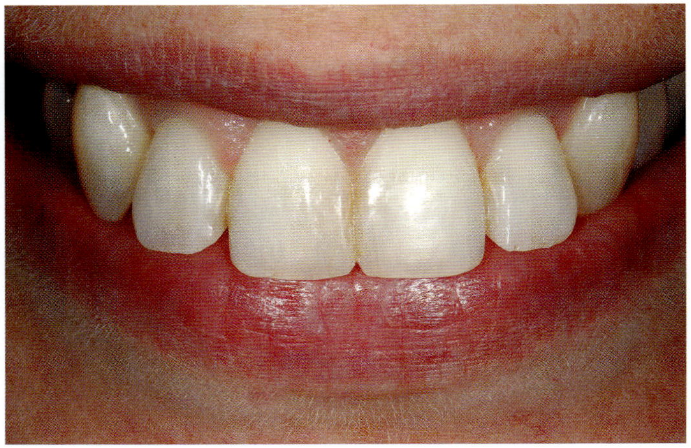

Fig 2-25
A female patient was unsatisfied with the length of the maxillary incisors, which were catching the lower lip. A minimally invasive shape correction was planned with the Sof-Lex disk (red) and the addition of composite resin, which allowed a significant improvement in the patient's smile to be achieved.

RELATIVE CONTRAINDICATIONS FOR PORCELAIN VENEERS

1. Extreme discoloration of the tooth (Fig 2-26)[31,32]

Masking very dark, discolored teeth is a difficult task and requires great skill from the dental laboratory where the restorations will be fabricated. There is a major risk that the patient will find the veneer with opaque material slightly different under different lighting, despite a positive color assessment during the try-in.

It can also happen that the dentist – often prompted by the dental technician to obtain more space for the ceramic material – prepares the hard tissues of the tooth deeply by removing the entire enamel layer – necessary for long-term adhesion and thus weakening the future bonding of the veneer with the tooth.[33] Deep preparation also means a darker base surface for the veneer.

> **REMEMBER**
>
> If the discoloration is due to pulp necrosis, we try to perform internal bleaching unless there are contraindications. By changing the tooth color, it will be possible to reduce the tissue preparation and perform a veneer without removing the entire enamel layer. Deep preparation leads to a vicious circle, as the dentin is usually darker than the enamel!

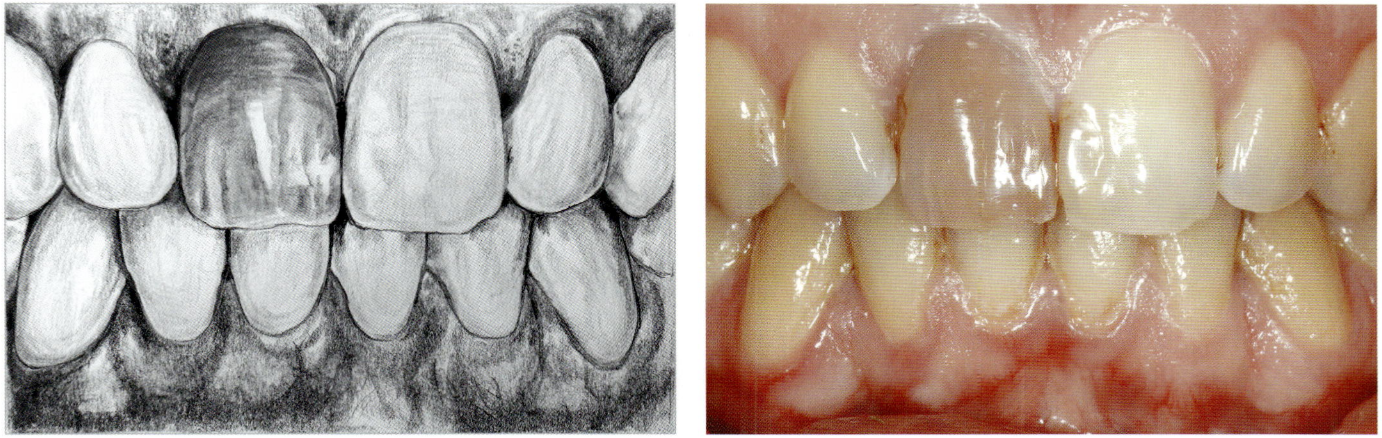

Fig 2-26
A patient presented to the dental office to improve the esthetics of the extremely discolored tooth 11. Due to the post and core, it would be too risky to perform internal bleaching. Such discoloration is not an absolute contraindication, but due to the difficulty of laboratory fabrication, it is a relative contraindication. It is easier for the dental laboratory to fabricate a ceramic crown than a thin porcelain veneer. If we can cooperate with an appropriate laboratory, an attempt should be made to perform a veneer.

2. Single porcelain veneer for central incisor (Fig 2-27)[32]

Generally, in the anterior segment, try to avoid single prosthetic restorations (veneers, crowns). This is especially true for situations where an asymmetric veneer would be planned on one maxillary central incisor. Why? Because it is extremely difficult and sometimes impossible for the laboratory to do. At the end of the treatment, a particularly demanding patient may not be satisfied because the asymmetrically placed veneer on one maxillary central incisor has slightly different optical properties (reflection, light absorption) than the natural tooth. This effect will be reduced if the veneers or crowns are made symmetrically, and even a slight difference will not be noticeable by the patient. The situation is slightly better when performing an asymmetrical veneer on the lateral incisors because a single veneer is placed laterally and is not as exposed as the central incisor.

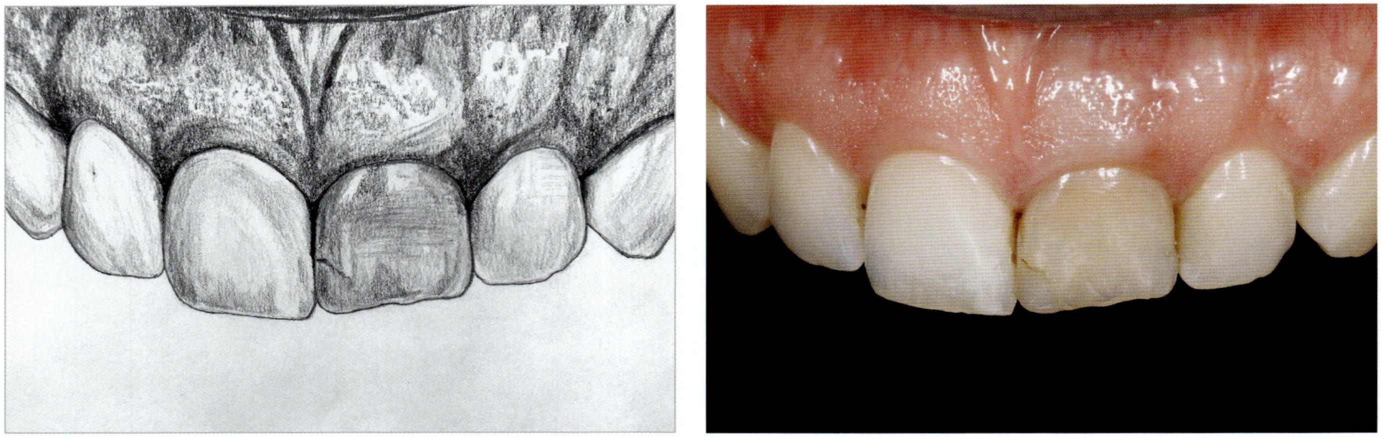

Fig 2-27
A female patient presented to the dental office to make a single porcelain veneer on tooth 21. Instead of such a solution, a direct composite veneer was proposed. Performing a single asymmetric porcelain veneer is not a good solution due to the esthetic risk (see Chapter 10).

3. Patient has relatively nice teeth and smile (Fig 2-28)

Patients sometimes ask the dentist to make porcelain veneers because they want to resemble their movie or life idols, and they do not accept their own teeth, even though they are not damaged. Sometimes, they are disturbed by the color or shape of their teeth, and sometimes by white spots on the labial surfaces. The dentist's task is to communicate properly with the patient, understand their problem, and consider the esthetic pros and cons of porcelain veneers.

> **TIP**
> A patient who has a good understanding of the treatment options will often choose a less invasive solution, such as changing the shape of the teeth by slight correction with a diamond abrasive disk or by adding a small amount of composite resin.

Fig 2-28
A female patient presented to the dental office requesting porcelain veneers. It was explained that this solution would not be best for her. Instead, deprogramming with the Kois Deprogrammer was proposed to calibrate and achieve a balanced posterior occlusal support. It was also proposed to consult a periodontist on whether it would be possible to cover the recession with a gingival graft.

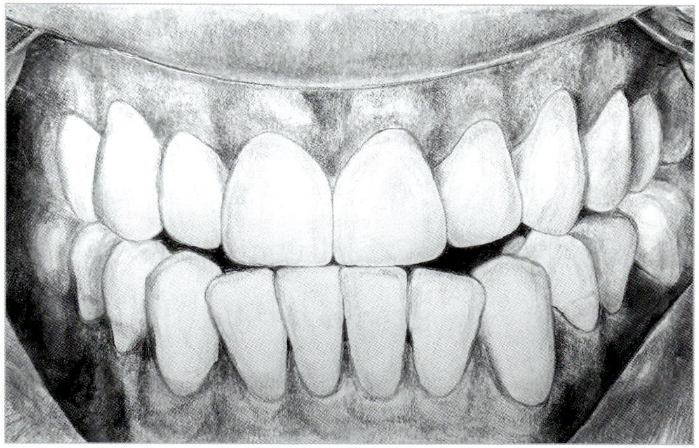

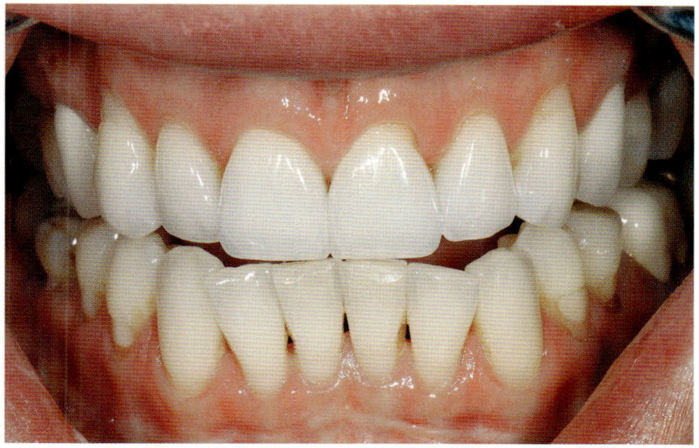

Video: How to avoid preparation – shape correction with composite https://books.dentist.com.pl/veneers/4

4. If the teeth position requires a too deep veneer preparation (Fig 2-29)[32]

In some cases, in order to obtain a satisfactory esthetic effect, preparation for the veneers will have to be very invasive and will involve dentin or pulp exposure, which represents a too high biological loss. The patient should be offered an alternative treatment, such as orthodontic therapy or reshaping the teeth with composite resin.

Fig 2-29
A female patient was referred by a periodontist to improve the esthetics of her smile. Orthodontic treatment was rejected due to periodontal problems. Performing indirect veneers would involve a very deep preparation and a significant loss of hard tissues (high biological loss). Due to the risk of possible complications, treatment with indirect veneers was not undertaken. It was decided that composite resin restorations would be the best method for changing the shape of the teeth.

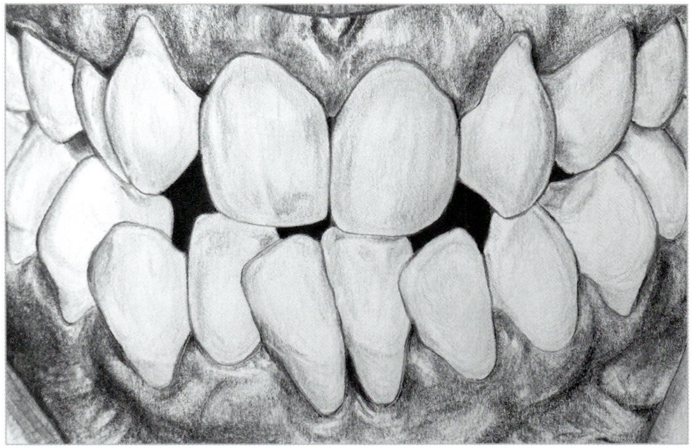

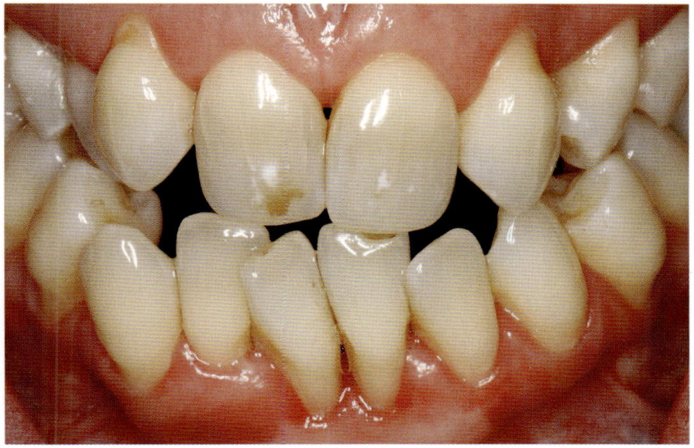

Table 2-1 Summary of indications and contraindications for porcelain veneers

Consider planning veneers when:	Do not plan veneers when:
There are extensive composite restorations in the anterior teeth	There is a small amount of tooth structure and less than 50% of the tissue would adhere to the veneer after preparation
Performing esthetic reconstructions with composite is difficult and unpredictable due to the necessity of treatment many teeth	There are deep Class 5 subgingival restorations
When a significant change of the shape is necessary	There are Class 3 subgingival restorations, which will not allow rubber dam isolation
It is indicated to lengthen the front teeth	The patient is an adolescent
The goal of the treatment is to close the diastema, and performing it with a composite will not be predictable or durable	Incorrect occlusal conditions were diagnosed, and there is no possibility to perform veneers without significant risk of failure
Changing the long axis of the anterior teeth or the midline between the maxillary central incisors	Patient's esthetic problem can be solved in a less invasive way than performing veneers
Tooth is discolored and cannot be whitened or masked predictably with the composite resin	Extreme discoloration of the tooth when we cannot predictably mask discoloration with minimally invasive veneer
As part of the complex occlusal rehabilitation, it is planned to complete the treatment of restoring the function and esthetics in the anterior segment	The patient has relatively nice teeth and smile, and the motivation to have veneers is a psychological problem
We make an asymmetrically positioned crown and want to balance the esthetics on the other side	Teeth qualified for veneers are sited asymmetrically and the patient only agrees to make one veneer on one side and has excessive esthetic expectations
We make an implant crown and there is a need to balance the symmetry and to close a possible black triangle	During the mock-up (test drive veneers) you encounter a communication problem that is impossible to solve
If, after assessing the tooth structure, direct composite restorations would be advisable but the patient's hygiene or eating habits do not allow for their predictable performing. In such cases, porcelain veneers can help to avoid discoloration and provide adequate durability	If the teeth position or their anatomy requires significant loss of tooth structure during veneer preparation

REFERENCES

1. Edelhoff D, Sorensen JA. Tooth structure removal associated with various preparation designs for anterior teeth. J Prosthet Dent 2002;87:503–509.
2. Schwindling FS, Waldecker M, Rammelsberg P, Rues S, Bömicke W. Tooth substance removal for ceramic single crown materials – an in vitro comparison. Clin Oral Investig 2019;23:3359–3366.
3. Aristidis GA. Etched porcelain veneer restoration of a primary tooth: a clinical report. J Prosthet Dent 2000;83:504–507.
4. Gresnigt MM, Cune MS, de Roos JG, Özcan M. Effect of immediate and delayed dentin sealing on the fracture strength, failure type and Weilbull characteristics of lithium disilicate laminate veneers. Dent Mater 2016;32:73–81.
5. Edelhoff D, Prandtner O, Saeidi Pour R, Liebermann A, Stimmelmayr M, Güth JF. Anterior restorations: the performance of ceramic veneers. Quintessence Int 2018;49:89–101.
6. da Cunha LF, Pedroche LO, Gonzaga CC, Furuse AY. Esthetic, occlusal, and periodontal rehabilitation of anterior teeth with minimum thickness porcelain laminate veneers. J Prosthet Dent 2014;112:1315–1318.
7. Burke FJ, Lucarotti PS. Ten-year outcome of porcelain laminate veneers placed within the general dental services in England and Wales. J Dent 2009;37:31–38.
8. Magne P, Douglas WH. Porcelain veneers: dentin bonding optimization and biomimetic recovery of the crown. Int J Prosthodont 1999;12:111–121.
9. Magne P, Douglas WH. Cumulative effects of successive restorative procedures on anterior crown flexure: intact versus veneered incisors. Quintessence Int 2000;31:5–18.
10. Igiel C, Weyhrauch M, Mayer B, Scheller H, Lehmann KM. Effects of ceramic layer thickness, cement color, and abutment tooth color on color reproduction of feldspathic veneers. Int J Esthet Dent 2018;13:110–119.
11. Sari T, Ural C, Yüzbasioglu E, Duran I, Cengiz S, Kavut I. Color match of a feldspathic ceramic CAD-CAM material for ultrathin laminate veneers as a function of substrate shade, restoration color, and thickness. J Prosthet Dent 2018;119:455–460.
12. Morimoto S, Albanesi RB, Sesma N, Agra CM, Braga MM. Main clinical outcomes of feldspathic porcelain and glass-ceramic laminate veneers: a systematic review and meta-analysis of survival and complication rates. Int J Prosthodont 2016;29:38–49.
13. Gresnigt M, Kalk W, Özcan M. Clinical longevity of ceramic laminate veneers bonded to teeth with and without existing composite restorations up to 40 months. Clin Oral Investig 2013;17:823–832.
14. da Cunha LF, Gonzaga CC, Saab R, Mushashe AM, Correr GM. Rehabilitation of the dominance of maxillary central incisors with refractory porcelain veneers requiring minimal tooth preparation. Quintessence Int 2015;46:837–841.
15. Radz GM. Minimum thickness anterior porcelain restorations. Dent Clin North Am 2011;55:353.
16. Tunkiwala A, Chitguppi R. Conservative, functional, and esthetic rehabilitation of severe palatal erosion (class IV) using modified dahl approach. Compend Contin Educ Dent 2017;38:289–296.
17. Guzmán-Armstrong S, Maia RR. Conservative treatment planning in veneer replacement. J Prosthet Dent 2016;115:393–396.
18. Chu FC, Siu AS, Newsome PR, Wei SH. Management of median diastema. Gen Dent 2001;493:282–287.
19. Albino LGB, Chaves ET, Lima VP, Lima GS. Restoration of a single darkened central incisor with a modified ceramic veneer. J Prosthet Dent 2019;121:369–372.
20. Zarrow M. Metal post and core: how to improve aesthetics. Available at: www.styleitaliano.org/metal-post-and-core-how-to-improve-aesthetics/
21. Gobbato L, Paniz G, Mazzocco F, et al. Significance of crown shape in the replacement of a central incisor with a single implant-supported crown. Quintessence Int 2013;44:407–413.
22. Curry FT. Porcelain veneers: adjunct or alternative to orthodontic therapy. J Esthet Dent 1998;10:67–74.
23. Vailati F, Belser UC. Classification and treatment of the anterior maxillary dentition affected by dental erosion: the ACE classification. Int J Periodontics Restorative Dent 2010;30:559–571.
24. Munck de J, Landuyt van K, Peumans M, Poitevin A, Lambrechts P, Braem M, van Meerbeek B. A critical review of the durability of adhesion to tooth tissue: methods and results. J Dent Res 2005;84:118–132.
25. Clark DJ. Composite versus ceramics, part I: young patients and fractures. Dent Today 2016;35:132–135.
26. Peumans M, Munck de J, Fieuws S, Lambrechts P, Vanherle G, Van Meerbeek B. A prospective ten-year clinical trial of porcelain veneers. J Adhes Dent 2004;6:65–76.
27. Kois DE, Kois JC. Comprehensive risk-based diagnostically driven treatment planning: developing sequentially generated treatment. Dent Clin North Am 2015;59:593–608.
28. Vence BS. Predictable esthetics through functional design: the role of harmonious disclusion. J Esthet Restor Dent 2007;19:185–192.
29. Borges AB, Caneppele TM, Masterson D, Maia LC. Is resin infiltration an effective esthetic treatment for enamel development defects and white spot lesions? A systematic review. J Dent 2017;56:11–18.
30. Müssig E, Lux CJ, Staehle HJ, Stellzig-Eisenhauer A, Komposch G. Applications for direct composite restorations in orthodontics. J Orofac Orthop 2004;65:164–179.
31. Zarow M. Contraindicated internal bleaching: what to do? Styleitaliano; 4/2017. Dostępne. Available at: www.styleitaliano.org/contraindicated-internal-bleaching-what-to-do/
32. Zarow M, Szczeklik K. Faccette dirette in composito come prevenzione della discolorazione dopo lo sbiancamento di denti non vitali. Case report. Il Dentista Moderno 2015;9:126–134.
33. Burke FJ. Survival rates for porcelain laminate veneers with special reference to the effect of preparation in dentin: a literature review. J Esthet Restor Dent 2012;24:257–265.

CHAPTER 3

PLANNING VENEERS

MACIEJ ŻAROW

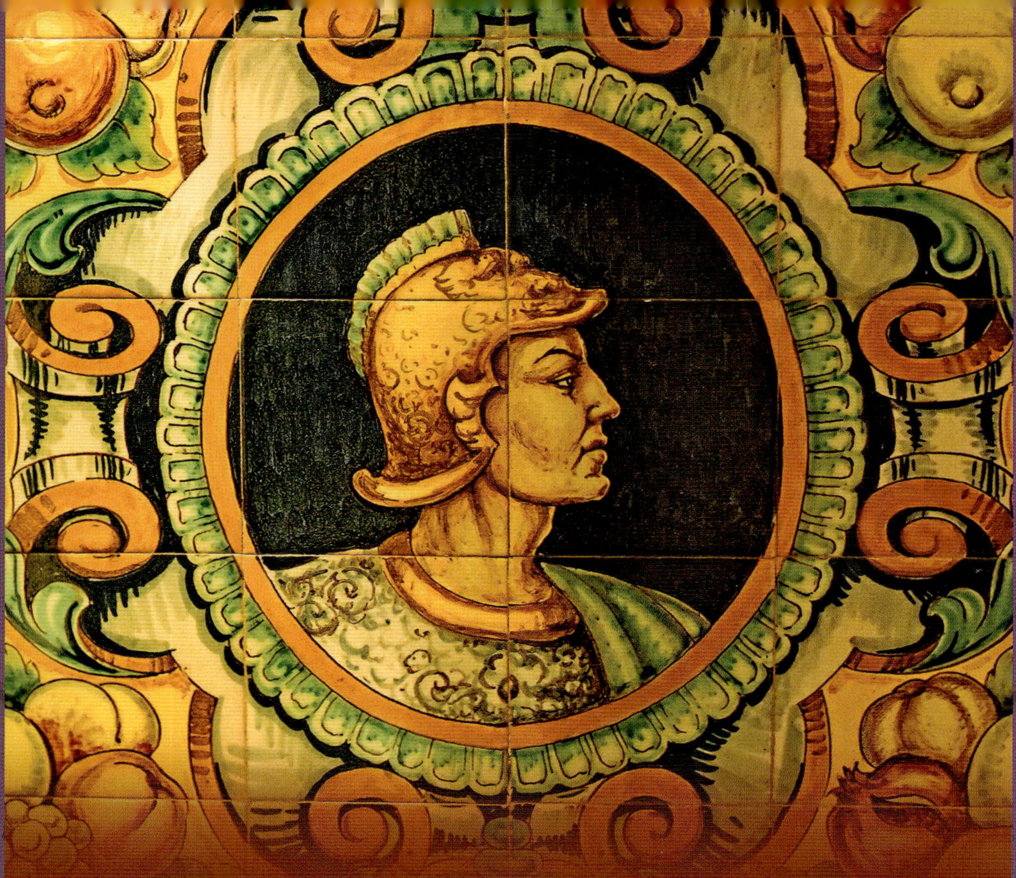

There is one main rule:
without planning we cannot interfere
with the dentition!
Of course, we can replace the restoration,
but we cannot start veneer preparation
without planning.
Preparation of the teeth carries
a lot of responsibility for the dentist.
And it is IRREVERSIBLE!

Planning veneers

When porcelain veneer preparation is performed, it is important to achieve an "equilibrium" between minimizing the preparation of the tooth structure (which will ensure maximum adhesion through the presence of enamel), achieving the necessary mechanical strength (appropriate thickness), and esthetics. This can be achieved through appropriate treatment planning.

ADHESION, MECHANICAL RESISTANCE, AND ESTHETICS

Planning the extension of veneer preparation is very important because their bonding to the tooth is purely adhesive, not retentive (Fig 3-1). If we prepare too little, the dental technicians will not have enough space for the restorative material, making them too convex, and the teeth will look like an off-road bumper or a locomotive from old times (Fig 3-2). To improve the shape, the dental technician would have to reduce the volume of the material from the labial surface, but this could also make the veneer too thin in some places and prone to cracking. However, if we prepare too much of the tooth, we will risk dentin exposure, which will weaken the veneer adhesion.[1–4]

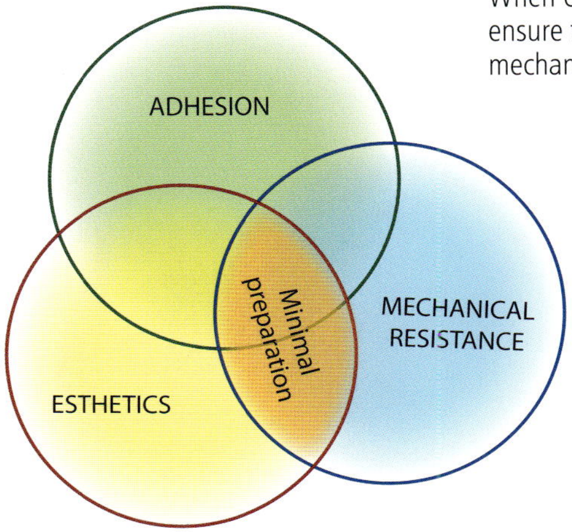

Fig 3-1
When carrying out veneer preparation, ensure the conditions for maximum adhesion, mechanical resistance, and esthetics.

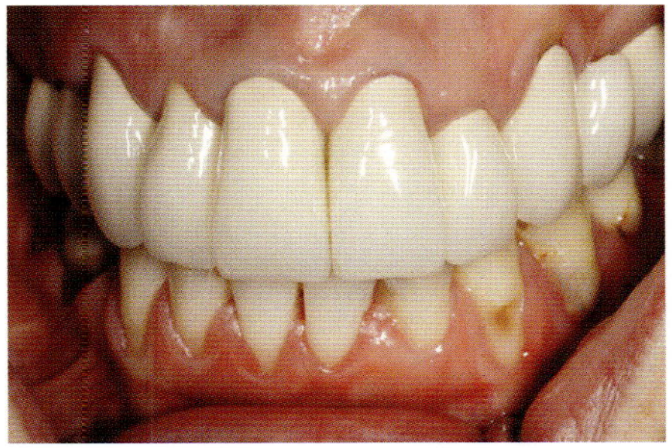

Fig 3-2
A poorly planned and disastrously performed prosthetic restoration. The teeth are too big, have an unnatural shape and resemble...

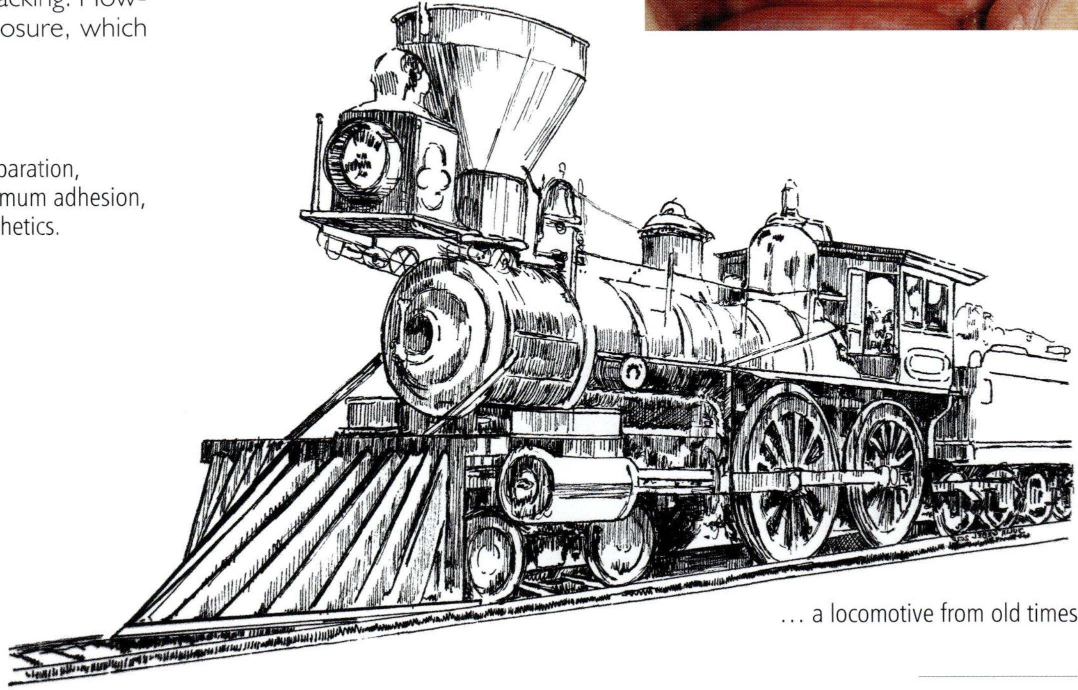

... a locomotive from old times.

CONSULTATION VISIT

The consultation visit should include:

1. Thorough medical history
2. Clinical examination
3. Photographic documentation
4. Creating diagnostic wax-up

1. Thorough medical history

Determining the needs, expectations, and risks related to the patient

First, you need to know the patient's general health. How did they find the dental office? Who (if anyone) recommended it to them? What is the patient's profession and their chief complaint? Are they satisfied with previous treatment? If not, why not? What expectations does the patient have of the initial visit? Answering these questions makes it possible to obtain information and create an initial patient profile (Fig 3-3).[5-7]

A good solution is to present the patient with a questionnaire to be filled in during the first visit. This allows an assessment of the current condition of the oral cavity. The completed questionnaire is an excellent starting point for a clinical examination and treatment plan. Thanks to the information provided, the dentist does not have to take a scattergun approach to diagnosis that may make the patient uncomfortable. Rather, the dentist's observations from the clinical examination may relate to the patient's remarks in the questionnaire, which in turn can give the patient more confidence in the diagnosis.[8]

2. Clinical examination

Structural risk related to the loss of hard tooth tissue

It is important to analyze the loss of tooth structure because the consequence of an unrecognized cause and lack of implementation of the prophylaxis/treatment may be a continuation of further hard tissues loss. This may have a negative impact on the long-term durability of restorative therapy, including veneers. The dentist/dental hygienist performing the dental examination should note any symptoms of tooth structure loss and ascertain their origin (Fig 3-4):

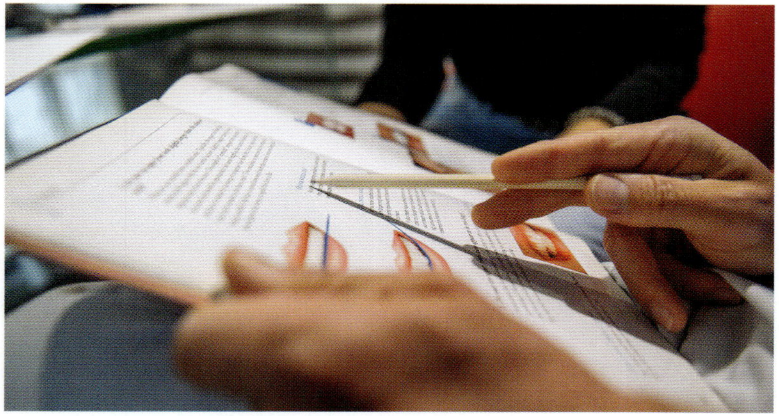

Fig 3-3
Favorable conditions for the first consultation: the right amount of time, a calm and quiet place allowing mutual trust to be established ... this seems crucial in the extremely intimate path toward creating a patient's smile. A short, hurried visit, the patient or dentist being late, disturbances, or unprofessional clinical staff members can ruin the first visit irreversibly.

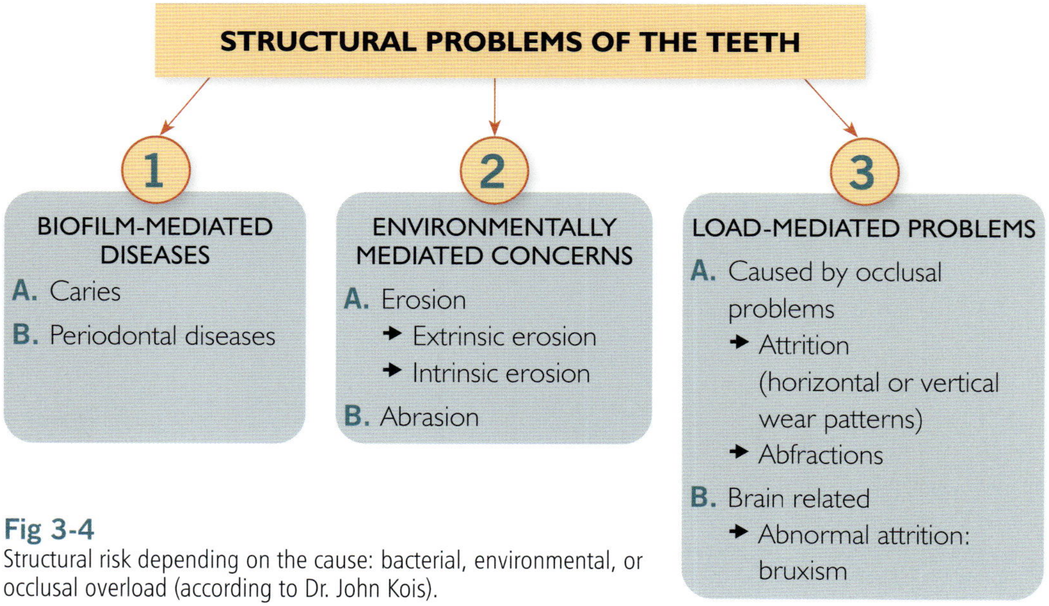

Fig 3-4
Structural risk depending on the cause: bacterial, environmental, or occlusal overload (according to Dr. John Kois).

- Structural loss related to biofilm-mediated diseases: caries result from a complex process of demineralization and remineralization of the enamel due to the exposure of organic acids produced by microorganisms living in the bacterial plaque.[9]
- Structural loss related to environmentally mediated concerns: erosion (hard tissue lesions caused by chemical processes, without cariogenic bacteria) (Fig 3-5) and abrasion (hard tissue lesions caused by physical wear by extraneous objects, such as hard bristle toothbrushes or excessively abrasive toothpaste; Fig 3-6).[10–12]

If the patient is diagnosed with erosion, the origin must be determined: intrinsic erosion (gastroesophageal reflux disease, bulimia) or extrinsic erosion (diet including lemons, grapefruits, fruit juices, energy drinks, etc.).

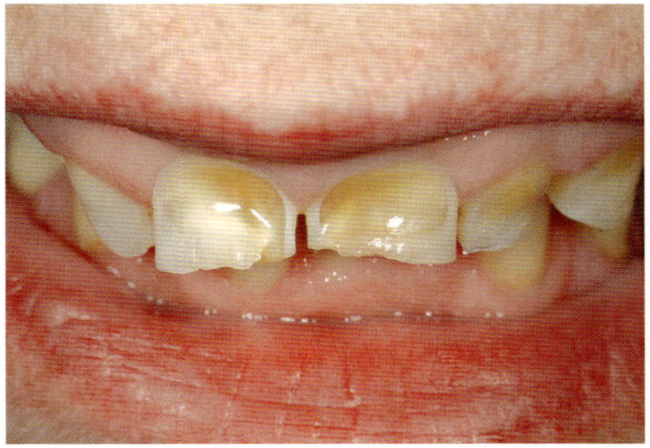

Fig 3-5a
Extrinsic erosion: a patient had a habit of consuming sauerkraut and pickled cucumbers every day. She was also fond of grapefruits and lemons. With a pH of around 2, these fruits represent a very high erosion risk factor.

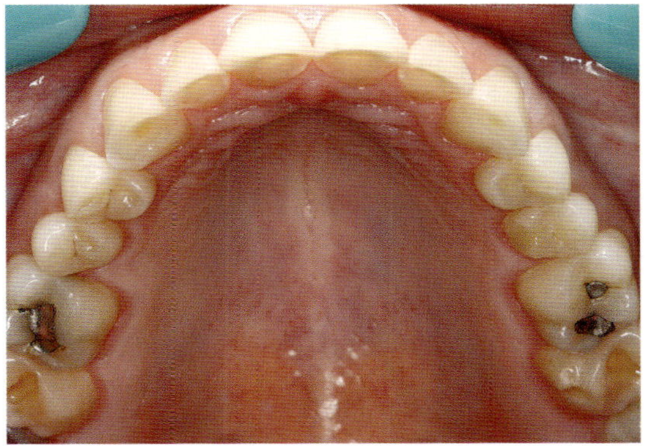

Fig 3-5b
Intrinsic erosion: a patient suffered from an eating disorder (bulimia), which caused erosion on the palatal side of the maxillary incisors (typical for intrinsic erosions) and resulted in rapid tooth wear of the incisal edges.

REMEMBER

The dental hygienist has a specific scope of procedures, such as recording and documenting (with photographs) the presence of cavities and identifying their origin – bacterial, chemical, or mechanical. The desire for white teeth makes patients buy toothpaste recommended in supermarkets or TV advertisements. These often have unfavorable abrasive properties, especially when the dentin is already exposed. The dental hygienist should monitor what kind of toothpaste is used by each patient.[13,14]
The toothpaste abrasiveness ranked by recommended daily allowance (RDA) value:
- Low abrasive: RDA below 70
- Medium abrasive: RDA 70–100
- Highly abrasive: RDA 100–150

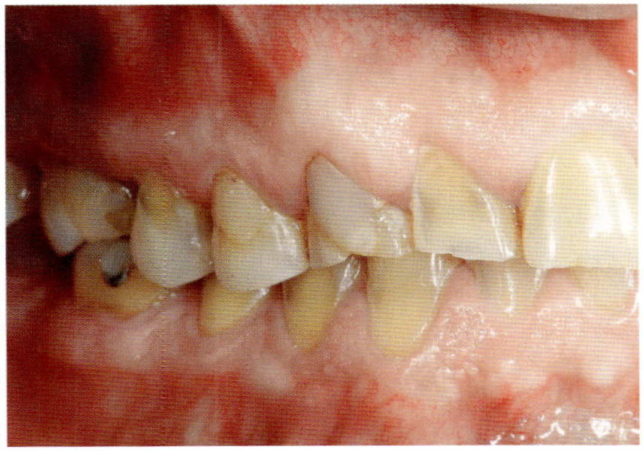

Fig 3-6
Abrasion lesions on the buccal and cervical surfaces are related to many factors, such as hard-bristle toothbrushes, abrasive toothpaste, and a diet high in acids.

Table 3-1 Acidity of common beverages and foods

Beverage	pH range
Gatorade Orange	2.99
Clear American Tropical Fruit	3.07
Vitamin Water Zero Mega-C	3.05
S. Pellegrino Sparkling Natural Mineral Water	4.96
Perrier Carbonated Mineral Water	5.25
24:7 Energy Cherry Berry	2.61
180 Blue with Acai	2.82
Red Bull	3.43
Wine	2.3–3.8
Vinegar	2.4–3.4
Apples	2.9–3.5
Plums	2.8–4.6
Orange juice	2.8–4
Lemon juice	1.8–2.4
Raspberries	2.9–3.7
Mayonnaise	3.8–4
Coca-Cola	2.48
Pepsi-Cola	2.60

Source: Kois Center (Seattle, USA)

When extrinsic erosion is diagnosed, the focus should be on raising the patient's awareness of their diet and its impact on the loss of tooth substance (Tables 3-1 to 3-4).[15]

When intrinsic erosion is diagnosed, we usually refer the patient for gastro-enterological consultation or multi-specialized behavioral therapy (in the case of bulimia nervosa).

When diagnosing abrasion, we think about the harmful effect of hard bristle toothbrushes or abrasive toothpastes, which wear away the tooth substance, especially exposed dentin (see Table 3-2), and we recommend those that are appropriate for this clinical situation.

Table 3-2 RDA value of certain products and toothpastes

Toothpaste	RDA value
Water	4
Sodium bicarbonate	7
Carifree CTx3 Gel	18.5
Enamel Plus	25
Rembrandt	53
Colgate Cavity Protection	65
Sensodyne Extra Whitening	104
Aquafresh Triple Protection	105
Amway Glister	110
Aquafresh All Tartar Control	110
Crest Pro-Health Whitening	168
Colgate 2-in-1 Whitening	200

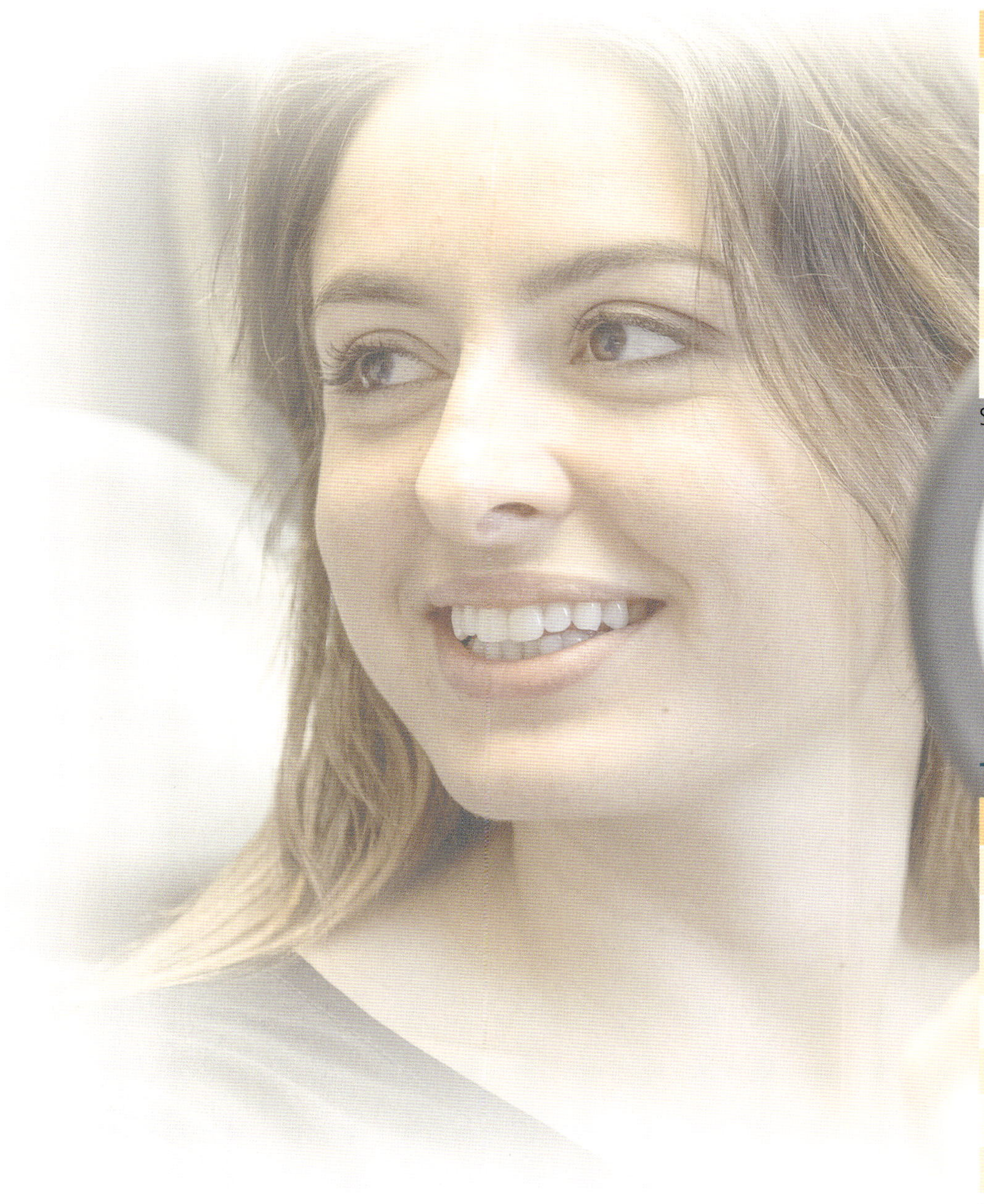

Table 3-3 Enamel dissolution in mg/cm^2

Beverage	pH	14-day weight loss (mg/cm^2)
Coca-Cola	2.48	2.78
Pepsi-Cola	2.60	3.07
Sprite	3.27	8.60
Canada Dry Ginger Ale	2.94	6.31
Mountain Dew	3.14	14.31
Diet Mountain Dew	3.17	14.82

Source: Kois Center (Seattle, USA)

Table 3-4 Main acids in common food products and beverages and their source

Acid	Food product and beverages
Acetic acid	Products containing wine vinegar, pickled cucumbers
Ascorbic acid	Vitamin C lozenges, some beverages
Carbonic acid	Fizzy drinks
Citric acid	Lemon and fruit juices
Malic acid	Apples and apple juices
Tartaric acid	Grapes, grape juices, wine
Phosphoric acid	Soft drinks (such as Coca-Cola)

Source: Kois Center (Seattle, USA)

- **Structural loss due to load-based mediated problems:** It is important to diagnose and record symptoms caused by occlusal loading, such as:

– **Attrition:** Mechanical wear resulting from mastication limited to contacting surfaces of opposing teeth (Fig 3-7).

In the patient's record, note the type of wear: whether it is horizontal or more vertical (typical "shelves of wear" are visible on the palatal surface of the maxillary incisors) and draw appropriate conclusions about this type of wear.[16,17] It is also crucial to diagnose whether tooth wear is due to occlusal or neurological problems (such as bruxism; Fig 3-8). Suppose the patient has used an occlusal splint. In that case, it can be a useful tool to diagnose bruxism (patients diagnosed with bruxism usually leave characteristic transverse scratches on the splint, indicating nocturnal activity of the masticatory system).

– **Abfractions:** The pathologic loss of tooth substance in the cervical area can indicate premature contact on given teeth or other types of biomechanical loading forces, leading to cavities at the cementoenamel junction (Fig 3-9). An acidic diet, incorrect toothbrush movement while brushing teeth, too hard bristle toothbrushes, or abrasive toothpaste may deepen the abfraction.

– **Cracked tooth syndrome:** The lines of the fracture in the posterior teeth usually run between the marginal ridges of the contact surfaces, with pain while biting down or temperature change; this may indicate pathological occlusal activity that led to the cracked tooth (Fig 3-10). The remaining teeth should be inspected, the cause should be found, and a plan for preventive (occlusal splint) or therapeutic measures developed (for example, physiotherapy or changing occlusal conditions – analysis of premature contacts, etc.).

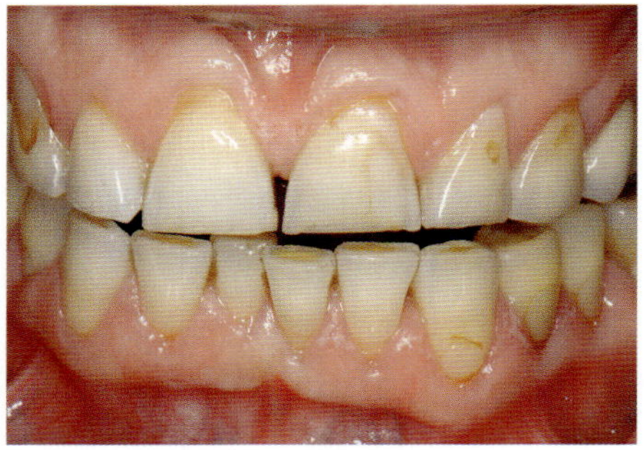

Fig 3-7
Attrition: clear horizontal wear pattern is characteristic of occlusal dysfunction. The cause is usually the lack of bilateral simultaneous posterior occlusal support and a widened envelope of function leading to horizontal wear of the incisors. In this case, factors accelerating wear can include diet, too abrasive toothpaste with abrasive agents, or a hard-bristle toothbrush.

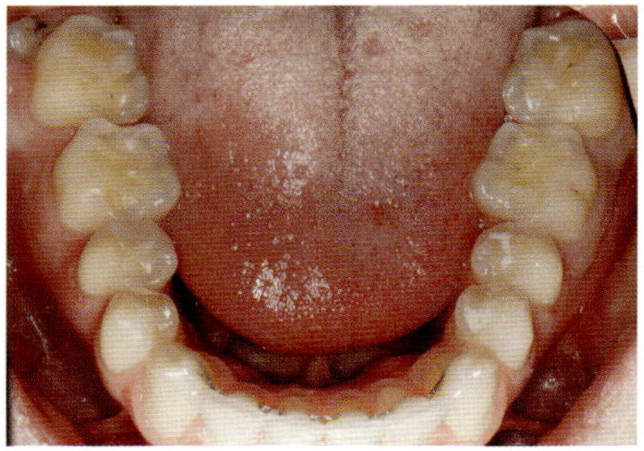

Fig 3-8
Bruxism: a 22-year-old patient, despite his young age, has worn out a large part of the enamel of the posterior teeth. This was caused by clenching his teeth at night combined with an acidic diet.

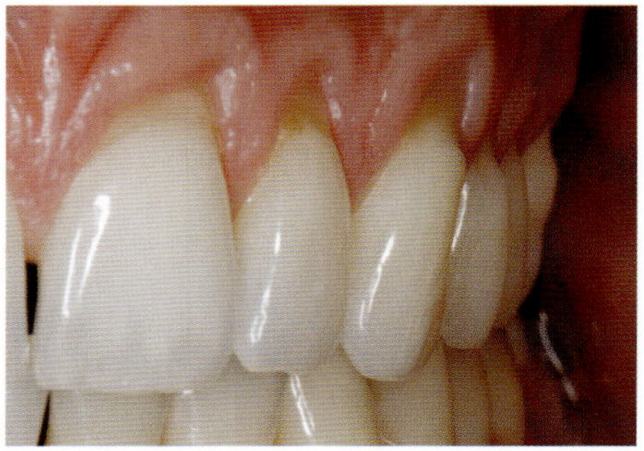

Fig 3-9
Abfractions: a 21-year-old patient, predisposed to clenching his teeth during the day, presented to the dental office with numerous non-carious cervical lesions in the premolars and anterior teeth. Many abfractions were rapidly deepened due to an acidic diet and improper tooth brushing.

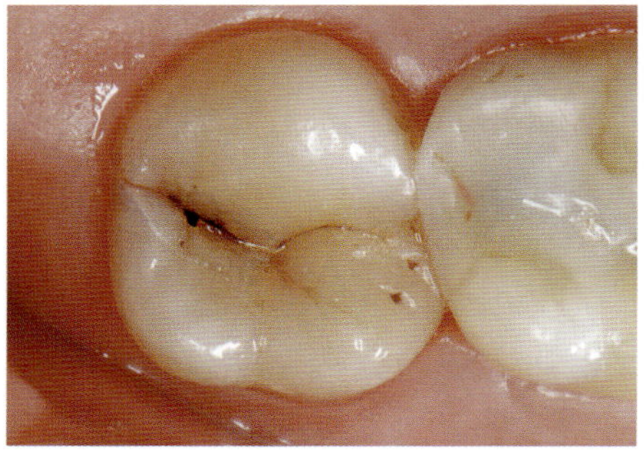

Fig 3-10
Cracked tooth syndrome: a patient who worked in a highly stressful profession (stockbroker) ground his teeth during the day and night. The results are numerous initial cracks in the enamel of the posterior teeth. Cracked tooth syndrome was detected in tooth 17. The patient presented with pain upon temperature change and while biting down. A lithium disilicate overlay and an occlusal splint therapy were proposed.

TIP

Recent studies define the following risk groups for non-carious cervical lesions:[18,19]

- Group 1: Post-orthodontic patients (65% of patients under the age of 30)
- Group 2: Clenching habits – psychological effects of anxiety
- Group 3: Athletes – amateurs and professionals attending fitness clubs, gyms
- Group 4: GERD – gastroesophageal reflux disease and post-bariatric surgery patients
- Group 5: Drug users and/or illicit substances

The risk of periodontal disease

The examination of the current periodontal condition, measurement of the depth of the sulcus or the periodontal pocket, and radiological evaluation of the alveolar ridge level are crucial for maintaining the teeth.[20,21]

If there is periodontal disease, we start periodontal treatment or refer the patient to a periodontist. Even the presence of one gingival pocket with a depth greater than 5.5 mm places the patient in a high-risk group.[22]

Regular visits combined with removal and plaque control and the patient's motivation are mandatory to prevent gum disease.[21] Scientific research has confirmed that regular periodontal debridement carried out on patients between 20 and 30 years old reduces tooth loss after the age of 40.[21]

Functional risk

Functional risk assessment is an important step in the patient diagnosis before qualification for veneers, and inaccurate qualification may cause the rapid destruction of new reconstructions.[23–28]

Porcelain veneers can be planned when:

- **There is no occlusal overload in the anterior teeth** (when the palpation test is done, the fingertips placed on the anterior teeth do not detect vibration, symptomatic of fremitus) (Fig 3-11)
- **There are no symptoms of tooth wear, or wear symptoms do not indicate an active, progressive process:** according to Dr. John Kois, significant progress has been made in this respect in the last five years, unlike the situation that once led to tooth wear but has now stopped – ie, adapted patient
- **There are no clear premature contacts** that would change the path of closure of mandible, leading to destruction/overloading/tooth wear
- **The patient does not report any pain or discomfort in the temporomandibular joints (TMJs). Basic examination of the joints includes:**
  - Examination of the vertical movement of the mandible – maximum opening (range of 35–60 mm)
  - Examination of the horizontal movement of the mandible (average range of motion 8–10 mm, ie, slightly more than the width of the maxillary central incisor)
  - Deviation during mandibular closure. The path of closure should be in a straight line. Use the facial midline as a reference to observe the course of deviation; the direction of the deviation goes toward the joint with the disorder
  - Muscle pain during palpation
  - Immobilization test: with the teeth held together, the patient tries to move the mandible in the horizontal direction (Fig 3-12a)

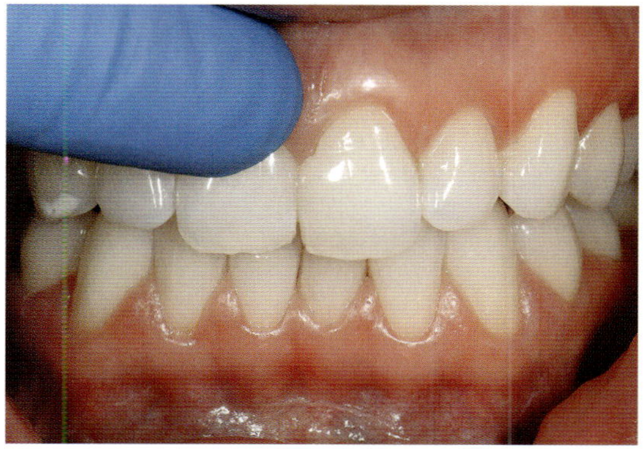

Fig 3-11
Fremitus is a symptom of occlusal overloading of a given tooth or group of teeth while closing in the centric relation or maximum intercuspation. The tooth vibration is felt when the index finger touches the tooth while closing the teeth.

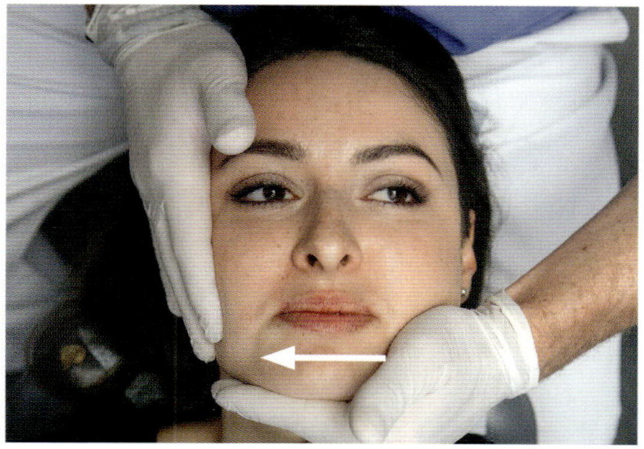

Fig 3-12a
Mandibular immobilization test: with the teeth held together, the patient tries to move the mandible in the horizontal direction against the hand of the dentist.

– TMJ sounds evaluation during mandibular opening
– TMJ loading test in centric and eccentric relation (Figs 3-12b and 3-12c)

Tenderness and pain during the test may also indicate disc displacement. The feeling of tension may suggest that the muscle contraction is persisting, which prevents the correct position of the condylar process in the mandibular fossa.[27–29] In the case of a negative test, the pain symptoms are probably related to muscle problems – a Kois Deprogrammer is a good diagnostic and therapeutic tool.[30] When the tests are positive, the appropriate initial treatment is occlusal splint therapy with support on all teeth (Michigan splint), and the patient's TMJ should be monitored. If the symptoms persist, another therapeutic solution is a consultation with a physiotherapist or gnathologist. In the case of high functional risk, we will discuss the diagnosed problem with the patient and create a treatment plan that would allow veneers to be performed with reduced functional risk (Fig 3-13).

TIP

The TMJs should be capable of transferring heavy loads without tenderness, tension, or pain in centric relation.
If the reaction in this case is positive, it means that the disc and complex process are not correctly aligned in the centric relation, and the joint should be examined more closely.

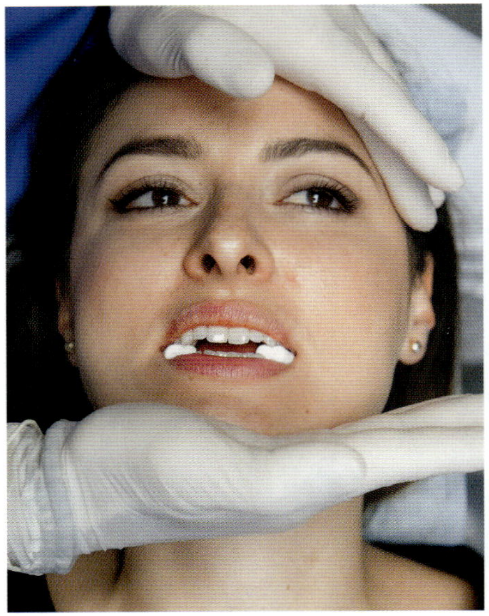

Fig 3-12b
The temporomandibular joint load test with lateral direction of force: the load force is directed on one of the TMJs, first the right and then the left (eccentric load test).

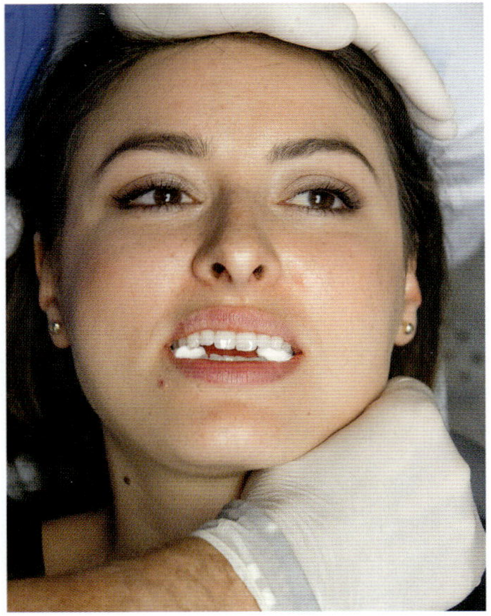

Fig 3-12c
The temporomandibular joint loading test is used to identify if we are dealing with a healthy TMJ. Place cotton rolls between the teeth in the posterior region, and then press the chin toward the TMJs (centric load test).

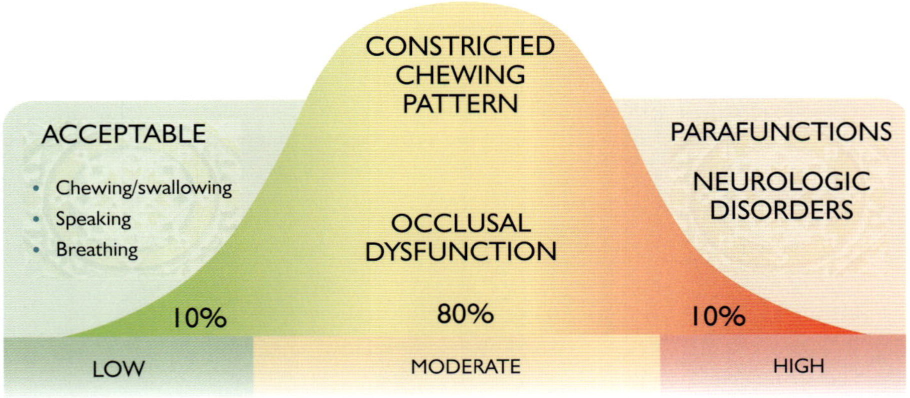

Fig 3-13
Functional risk assessment according to Dr. John Kois.

Esthetic risk

Esthetic risk assessment involves many factors that should be considered before deciding whether to cover anterior teeth with veneers.

- **Smile line:** Depending on the dynamics of the upper lip, the following can be distinguished:
  – High smile line (11% of the studied population)
  – Medium smile line (69% of the studied population)
  – Low smile line (20% of the studied population)[31–33]

A high smile line reveals the gingiva and makes the border between the porcelain veneer and the tooth structure visible. The same problem exists in high smile line patients if the veneer does not cover any tooth discoloration (high esthetic risk).

- **Upper lip dynamic range when smiling** (Fig 3-14)[34–35]:
  - Medium: 8 mm (from rest position)
  - Minimum: <6 mm
  - Normal: 6–8 mm
  - Hypermobile: >10 mm

- The course of the midline: The course of the midline should be carefully analyzed before starting veneer treatment. The midline in the esthetic canons should run perpendicularly to the pupillary line and not deviate significantly from the facial midline (Fig 3-15a).[36] In the case of an oblique midline (Fig 3-15b), planning should include preparing the mesial proximal surfaces of the central incisors to enable the dental technician to correct them. If the biological loss of the tissues will be too great to correct the midline, orthodontic treatment should be considered. Therefore, the dentist should always evaluate the scope of the planned preparation.

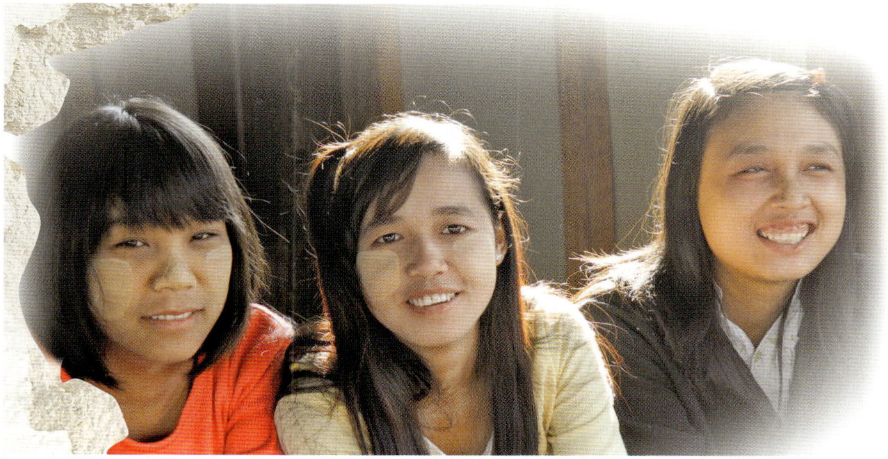

Fig 3-14
Different range of the upper lip dynamic when smiling: from left – minimal, normal, and hypermobile (assuming that all subjects smiled maximally).

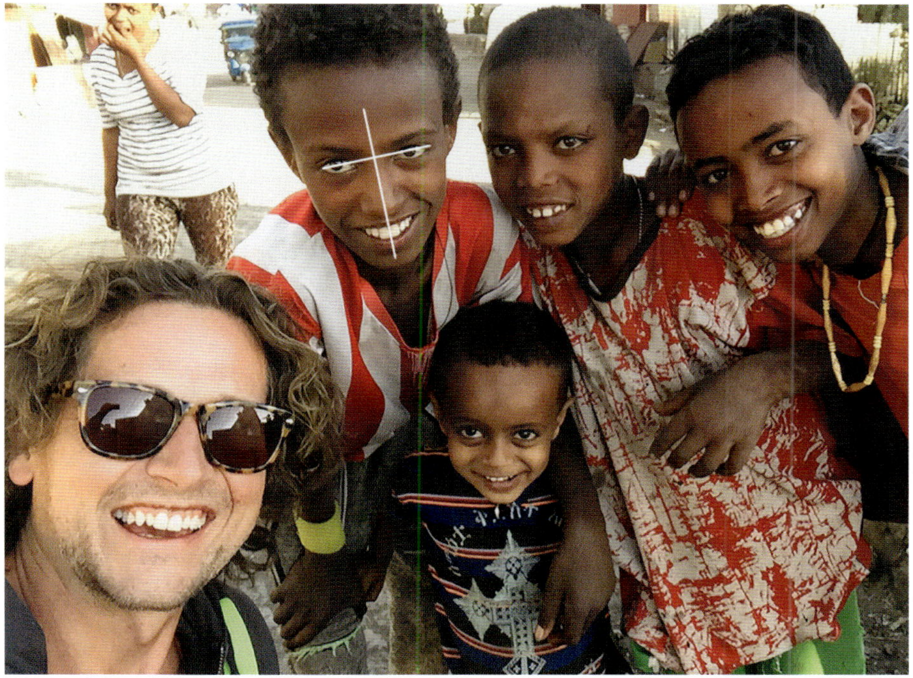

Fig 3-15a
The course of the midline is symmetrical and perpendicular to the pupillary line (face with drawn lines).

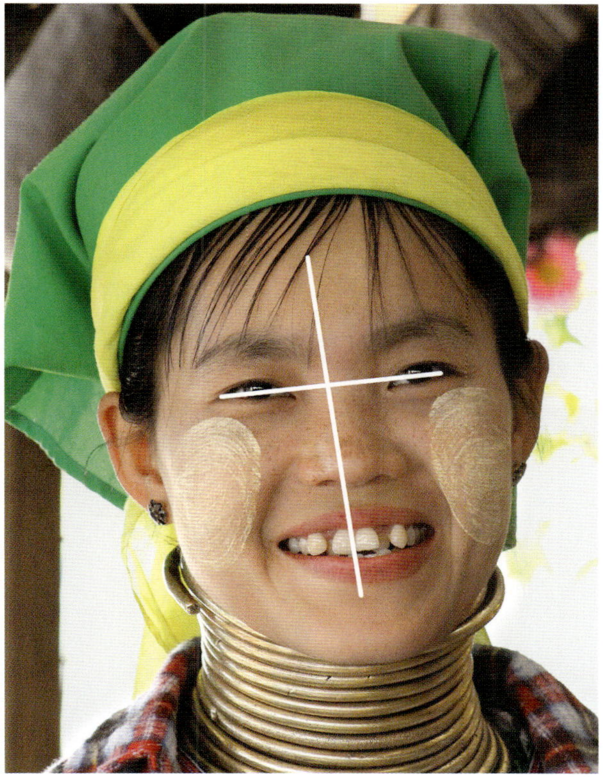

Fig 3-15b
Midline course: oblique to the pupillary line.

When the preparation could be too aggressive (significant exposure of the dentin, risk of losing pulp vitality), the dentist should think about an alternative plan (orthodontic treatment). It should be emphasized that porcelain veneers should not be an alternative treatment for teeth alignment if orthodontic therapy is required.

- **The shade of the tooth after veneer preparation:** Before the veneer preparation, it is necessary to (Fig 3-16):
  - Discuss any discoloration with the dental technician (is it possible to hide it?)
  - Consider the possibility of internal bleaching, which would avoid the use of an opaque material blocking the light transmission into the tooth
  - Whiten the neighboring teeth (it will make the work easier, as it is always simpler to make slightly brighter veneers)
  - Avoid dentin exposure during veneer preparation; in discolored teeth, the exposed dentin is even darker and more difficult to mask.

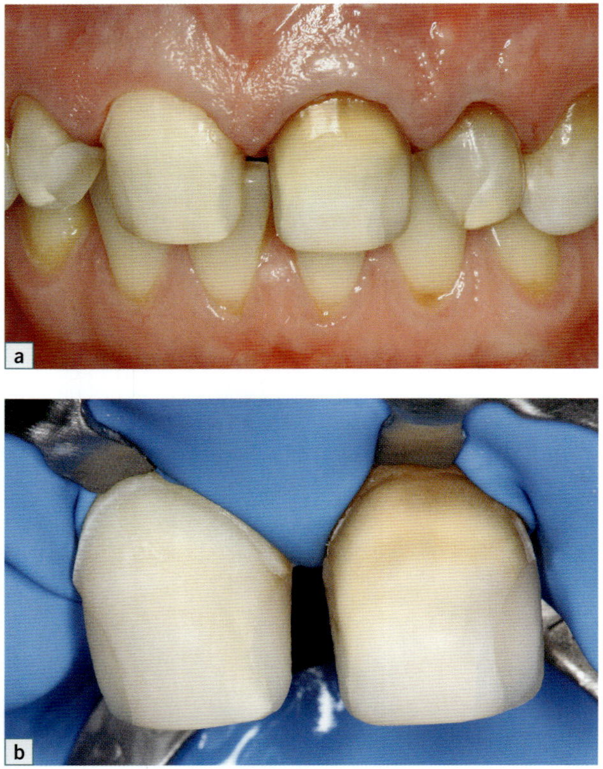

Fig 3-16
Discolored tooth vs veneer: when planning veneers on discolored teeth, the additional aspect of the dark dentin must be taken into account. If the dentin is exposed during the preparation, the discoloration will be even more difficult to mask. Discolored teeth 21 and 22 (a and b) with exposed dentin after preparation. We do not qualify this as a mistake, but we intend to avoid dentin exposure as much as possible.

3. Photographic documentation

Photographic documentation is an important stage of treatment planning, including porcelain veneers. It is the foundation for considering many treatment aspects and comparing the photographs with the diagnostic casts, even when the patient is no longer present in the dental office.

Such documentation is a starting point for treatment, which should also be included in medical history for legal reasons. The photographs provide a visual presentation of the problem to patients who may not be fully aware of their actual oral health condition.[37–40]

Photographs and communication with the patient and the dental laboratory. Photography is an excellent tool in dentist–patient–laboratory communication. Providing the technician with a set of well-made photographs of the patient gives them a greater opportunity to select the perfect restoration color and give individual characteristics (fracture lines, discoloration, etc.), which will result in highly esthetic restorations, similar to natural dentition.

Thanks to digital photographs, the dental technician's work is not based only on casts, but they also gain important information about the symmetry of the face, the midline, the smile line, and the position of the teeth in relation to the lips in their rest position.

> **TIP**
>
> With digital photographs, communication with the patient also becomes easier. Discussing the clinical situation with the patient based on photographic documentation allows not only for identification of the main oral cavity problems but also involves the patient actively in the entire treatment process.

There are several recognized protocols for performing circumferential supracrestal fiberotomy (CFS), including the American Academy of Cosmetic Dentistry (AACD), such as Dr. Coachman's, used routinely in Digital Smile Design, and Dr. Kois', used at the Seattle Kois Center. These protocols are used in everyday practice depending on each dental clinic's need and profile. Aside from the main purpose of making digital documentation, each protocol has a distinguishing element.[41,42]

The sequence of photographs suggested by the AACD is used to obtain accreditation. It includes 12 extraoral and intraoral photographs taken before and after treatment to show the results. Photographs are taken according to strictly defined parameters determined by the AACD.

The protocol proposed by Dr. Coachman allows detailed analysis of the teeth position in relation to the pupillary line and the symmetry of the face. Therefore, the most important photograph in this protocol is this one of the teeth with the use of buccal retractors, including the entire face of the patient. A characteristic element of this protocol is the photograph of the face from the 12 o'clock position, which is done while standing behind the patient with their head lying on the dentist's chair. Based on multiple photographs in this sequence, dental reconstruction is planned with a computer simulation, called Digital Smile Design (DSD).

Dr. John Kois, in his original sequence, pays special attention to the photograph of the lips in repose and the position of the canines in relation to the upper lip. The photograph that distinguishes this protocol is the shot of the profile showing the position of the anterior teeth in order to determine their position in relation to the lips (upper and lower).

As can be seen, the scope of work performed in a given dental practice is significant when choosing an effective method of photographic documentation. The sequence of photographs – proposed in the Dentist Educational Centre in Cracow/Poland for esthetic treatment planning – is shown in Table 3-5.

Photographic documentation and planning of porcelain veneers

While taking the photographs, the composition of the maxillary teeth is analyzed. A photograph of the patient's lips in repose is a key element in planning[41,42]: Whether to elongate the teeth? How much to elongate the teeth? Whether to elongate toward the incisal edge or the gingival margin?

Several of these photographs allow an assessment of the current length of the teeth in relation to the upper lip. How do the central incisors look? If they are hidden under the lip in the rest position, I would like to slightly elongate them to be more exposed from under the upper lip in repose. The younger the patient is, the greater the exposure of the maxillary incisors should be; the older the patient is, the less visible the exposure of the maxillary incisors should be.

The sex of the patient also matters because women tend to expose their teeth slightly more than men (Fig 3-17), and their central incisors are more dominant than their lateral incisors.

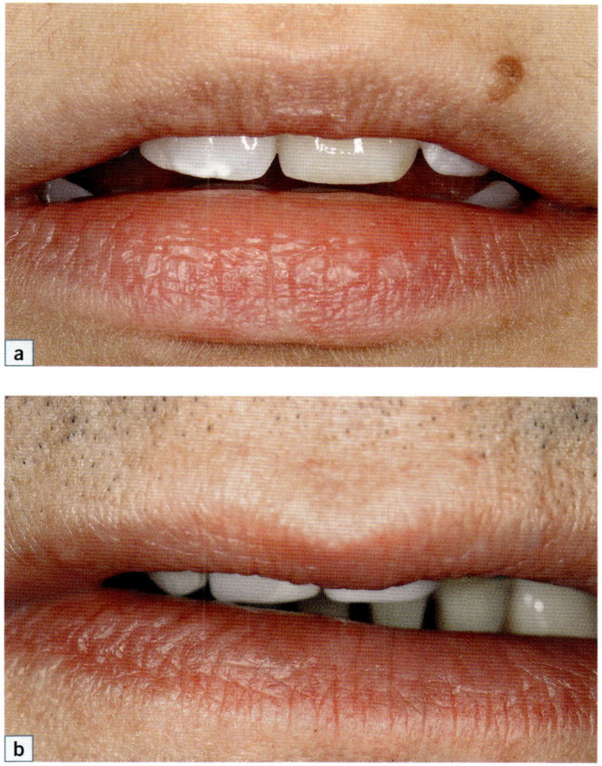

Fig 3-17
The exposure of the maxillary central incisors from under the upper lip in a rest position may vary depending on the patient's sex or age. Example of (a) major and (b) minor exposure of the central incisors from under the upper lip.

REMEMBER

Performing the proper sequence of photographs and mock-up simulation, and then presenting these simulations to the patient in the form of a PowerPoint/Keynote presentation, provides:

- Motivation for the dentist and confirmation of whether the planned esthetics are a reasonable motivation for the dental assistant and other members of the dental team to include them in the "spiral of adrenaline" necessary in a modern, motivated dental office
- Motivation for the patient, who would like to see the final result of treatment

Table 3-5 Sequence of photographs taken during the patient's first visit[37]

A. Extraoral photographs, the so-called portrait photography (f/8, 1:15, autofocus)				
	Projection	Description	Purpose of the photograph	Photograph
1	Minimal smile	• Lips in repose; pupillary line parallel to the horizontal plane • Plain background (for example, white, gray) • Camera lens in the same plane as the patient's face • Focus point: patient's eyes	Determining the symmetry, shape, and proportions of the face	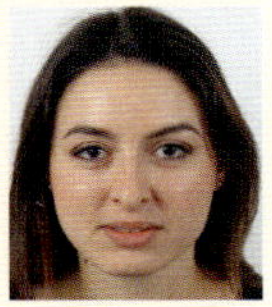
2	Maximum smile	• Patient's wide, natural smile	Esthetic analysis of the smile	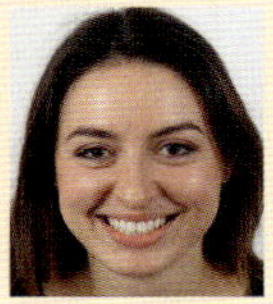
3	Profile	• Frankfurt (horizontal) plane, parallel to the floor • Focus point: the patient's eyebrows	Analysis of the Ricketts esthetic plane course and the nasolabial angle	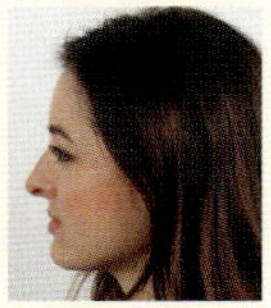
4	Face with retractors	• Pupillary line symmetrical to the floor • Midline perpendicular to the horizontal line	Planning of the esthetics DSD analysis Communication with the dental technician (the dental technician analyzes the position of the teeth in relation to the face symmetry)	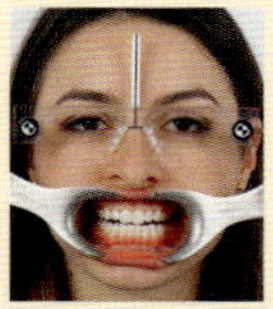
B. Intraoral photographs and close-ups (f/20, 1: 3, M-focus)				
5	Lips in repose	• "En face" projection • The patient says, for example, the word "Emma"	Analysis of the exposure of maxillary incisors from under the upper lip in repose (the norm of exposure of the maxillary incisors is 1–3 mm; may vary depending on sex, age, and individual factors)	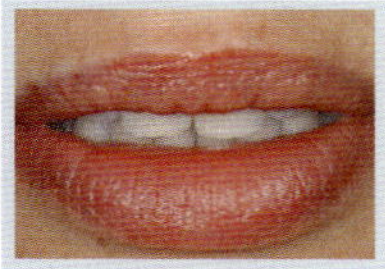
6	Maximum smile	• "En face" projection • Focus point: central incisors • We try to take the patient's most natural smile	Esthetic analysis of the smile – vertical and horizontal symmetry, the smile line course, assessment of the presence of anterior and lateral negative space, analysis of red esthetics (analysis of the esthetic risk)	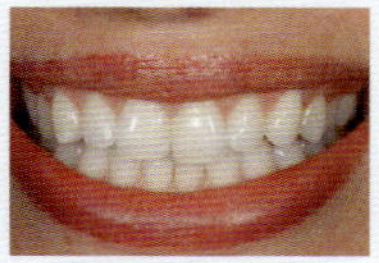
7	Position of maximum intercuspation	• "En face" projection • Use buccal/labial retractors • Center point of the photography: proximal contact point of the central incisors • Focus point: canines or first premolars	Documentation of current occlusal conditions (in MIP)	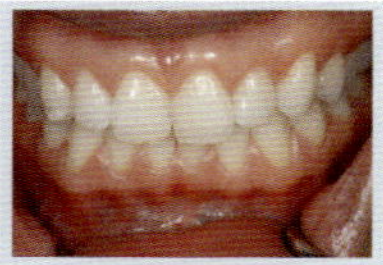

8	Edge to edge position	• Protrusive position of the patient's mandible • Contact is only on the incisal edges of the maxillary and mandibular central incisors	Assessment of the anterior guidance and exposure of mandibular incisors	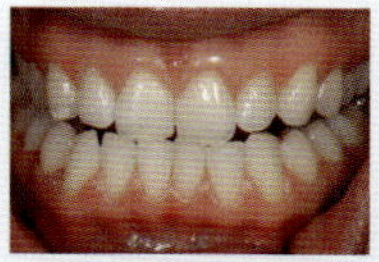
9	Maxillary anteriors on a black background	• Use an anterior black contrastor	Exposing the characteristics of the anterior maxillary teeth	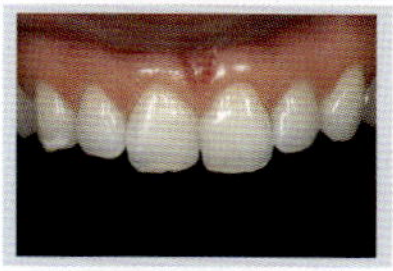
10/11	Buccal lateral right/left	• Use a buccal mirror and a buccal retractor at the opposite side to be photographed • Focus point: canines or first premolars	Analysis of occlusal contacts in the lateral region, analysis of non-carious cervical lesions, for example, abfractions, abrasions, erosions	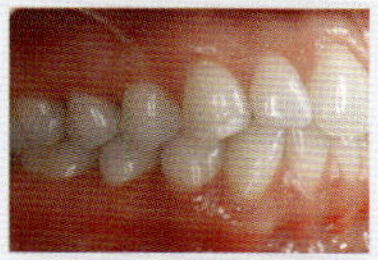 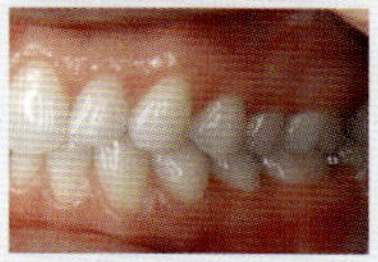
12	Occlusal-upper arch	• Use an occlusal mirror and labial retractors • Mirror is resting on the lower arch • Photography is taken at an angle of 45° to the mirror surface • Dentist takes a photograph while standing behind the prone patient in the supine position • Focus point: first premolars	Documentation of the maxillary arch	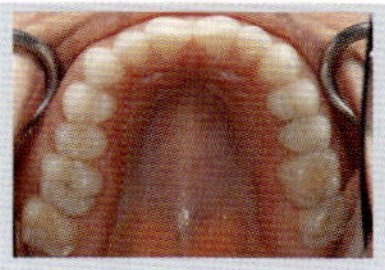
13	Occlusal-lower arch	• Use an occlusal mirror and labial retractors • Mirror is resting on the mandibular arch and retromolar trigone • Tongue lies freely on the floor of the mouth or rests on the palate 45° angle between the camera lens and the occlusal mirror surface • Dentist takes the photograph while standing in front of the prone patient in the supine position • Focus point: first premolars	Documentation of the mandibular arch	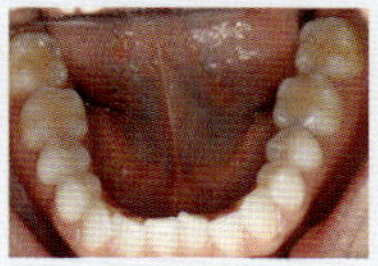
C. Additional photographs (f/10, 1: 3, M-focus)				
14	12 o'clock position	• Dentist takes a photograph while standing behind a prone patient • Photograph of a patient's natural smile	Analysis of the maxillary incisors line in relation to the lower lip line, analysis of the midline course	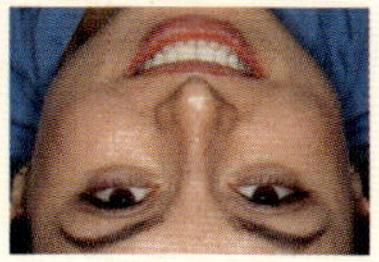

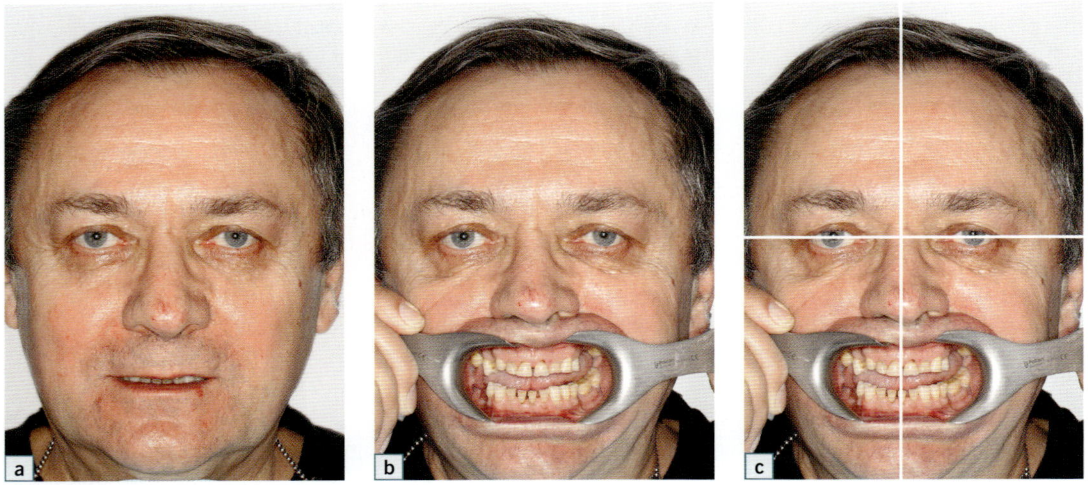

Figs 3-18a to 3-18c
Screenshots from a PowerPoint presentation showing DSD planning according to Dr. Coachman's protocol. (a) An "en face" photograph of the patient's face and (b) the face with the retractors. (c) Basic lines are drawn for esthetic planning: the pupillary line and the midline perpendicular to it.

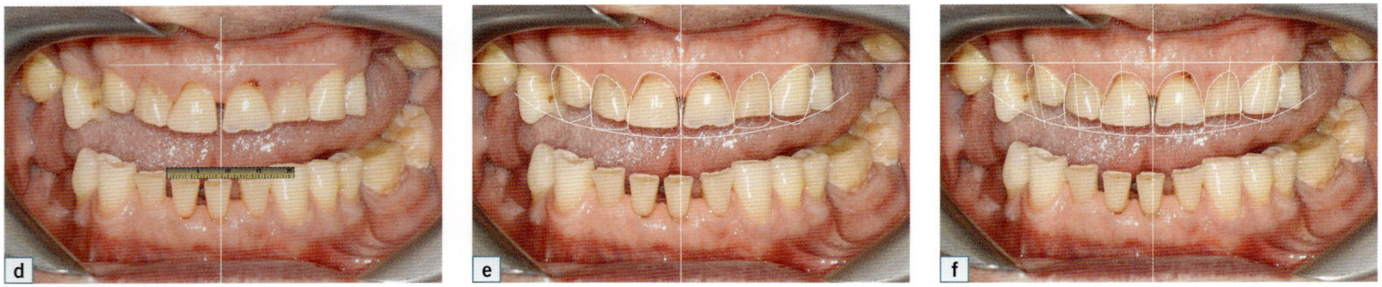

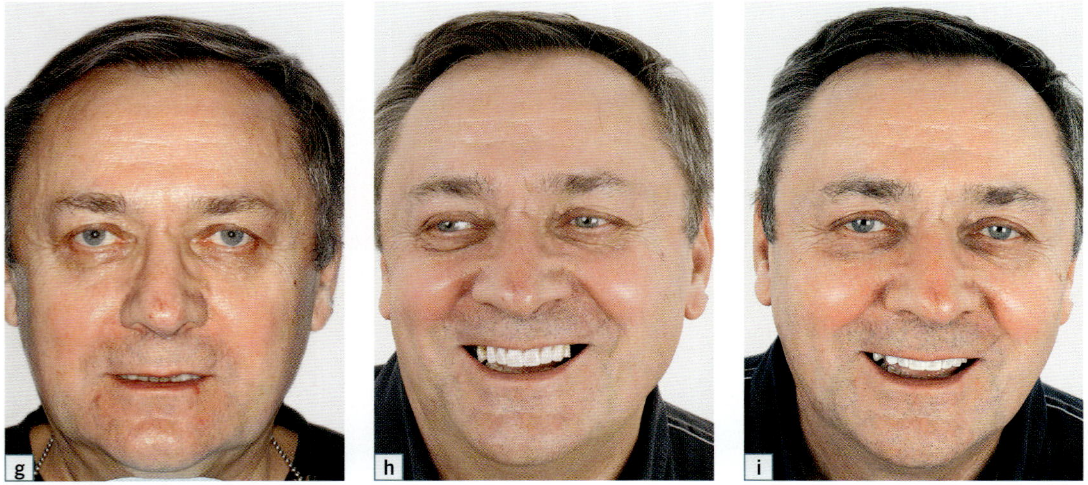

Figs 3-18d to 3-18i
Screenshots from a PowerPoint presentation showing DSD planning according to Dr. Coachman's protocol. (d) The close-up of the teeth was "cut out" from the photograph with the retractors, thanks to which we can be sure that the horizontal line is aligned with the pupillary line. (e, f) Now, we draw up the planned new teeth outlines, which will be the basis of communication with the dental laboratory in order to prepare the initial esthetic wax-up. (h to i) Wax-up was transferred into the mouth using the silicone index and Protemp (mock-up). Thanks to the photographs obtained during the mock-up (ie, with provisional restorations), we can improve communication with the patient and the dental technician. We are also able to start functional planning of the case.

4. Creating a diagnostic wax-up

To create a proper diagnostic wax-up, it is essential to provide the dental laboratory with relevant information, such as:

- Length of the maxillary central incisors (in millimeters, average length: 10–10.5 mm)
- Description of the line course along the incisal edges of the maxillary incisors (dominance of the maxillary central incisors): Major dominance? Minor dominance?
- The proposition of the tooth shape: Rectangular? Oval? Triangular?
- General information about the patient: sex, age, profession, character traits

Transferring this information may take the form of a card, PowerPoint/Keynote presentation, ie, DSD by Dr. Coachman (Fig 3-18) or simple drawings, photographs, or printouts (see dental office – dental laboratory communication card).

Taking impressions and facebow registration

Take an alginate impression of the mandibular and maxillary arches and a facebow registration to inform the dental technician about the horizontal plane based on the pupillary line (Fig 3-19).[43,44] Also, take a bite registration in the maximum intercuspation. If major occlusal changes are planned, the central relation should also be registered (see Chapter 8).

Creating an esthetic wax-up

The technician mounts the casts in the articulator according to the facebow registration. Then, using all the information provided by the dentist in the form of photographs, notes, or DSD presentation, they start the esthetic waxing. The esthetic wax-up aims to create an initial esthetic treatment plan and test it with the patient (transferred to a mock-up). We do not analyze the function at this stage. Rather, it is about verifying the patient's expectations and confirming that the planned work makes esthetic and therapeutic sense.

The Kois Platform (Panadent Occlusal Platform) attached to the articulator can help the dental technician control the symmetry and the course of the horizontal plane, making the waxing process predictable. After creating the diagnostic wax-up, the dentist evaluates the esthetics on the casts (Fig 3-20). Only after the dentist's initial approval of the wax-up can the patient be invited for a "test drive," ie, transferring the wax-up to the oral cavity.[45–48]

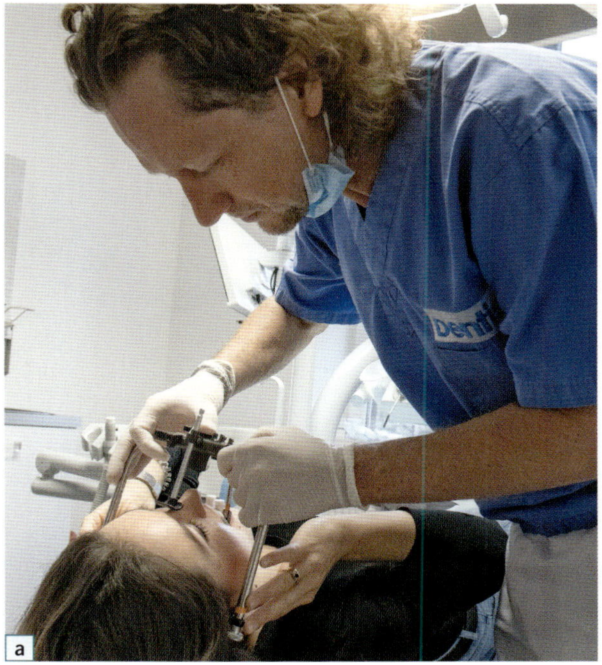

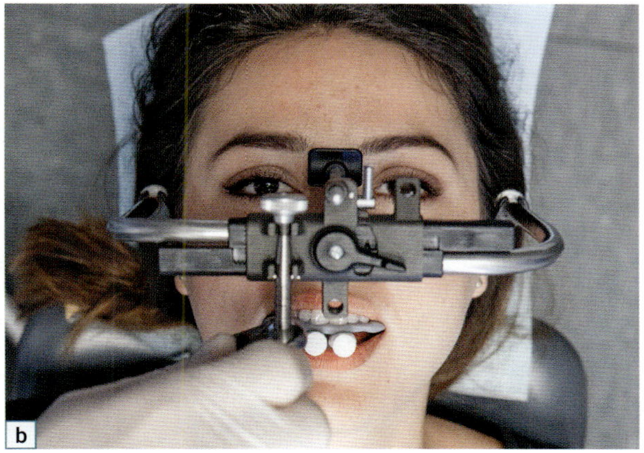

Figs 3-19a and 3-19b
Facebow registration.

Fig 3-20
The dentist should approve the diagnostic wax-up, assessing whether it has been prepared as recommended. The midline, symmetry, tooth shape, and inclination of the long axis of each tooth are all checked.

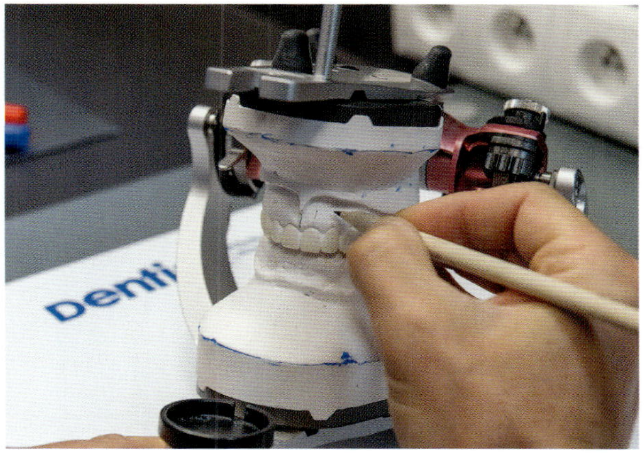

Dental office – dental laboratory communication card

(DT Janos Mako, DDS, PhD Maciej Zarow, MD)

1. Date of request: . . . .
2. Patient's name and surname: . . . .
3. Patient's age: . . . .
4. Patient's sex: . . . .
5. Patient wishes: . . . .
   . . . .
   . . . .
   . . . .

6. **Supplementary materials available for the dental laboratory:**
   - **a.** Diagnostic wax-up? ☐
   - **b.** Alginate impression reflecting the treatment plan (of mock-up or initial situation)? ☐
   - **c.** Photographs of the initial situation? ☐
   - **d.** Mock-up photographs? ☐
   - **e.** "Historical" patient's photographs? ☐

7. **Description of the planned restoration:**

8 - 7 - 6 - 5 - 4 - 3 - 2 - 1	1 - 2 - 3 - 4 - 5 - 6 - 7 - 8
8 - 7 - 6 - 5 - 4 - 3 - 2 - 1	1 - 2 - 3 - 4 - 5 - 6 - 7 - 8

8. **Shade of the performed restorations/color map:**

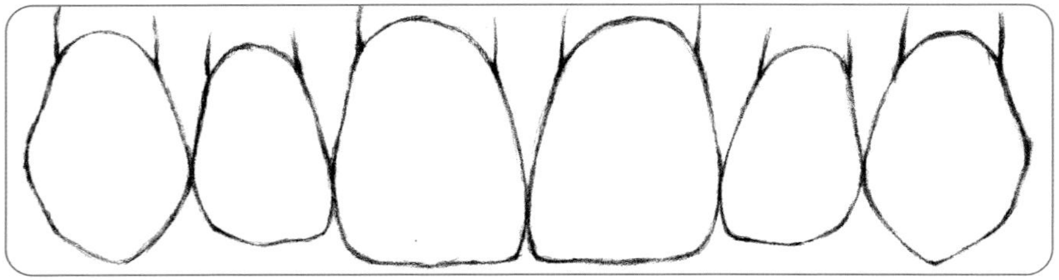

9. **Shade of the tooth after preparation (please draw):**

10. **Primary tooth shape:**

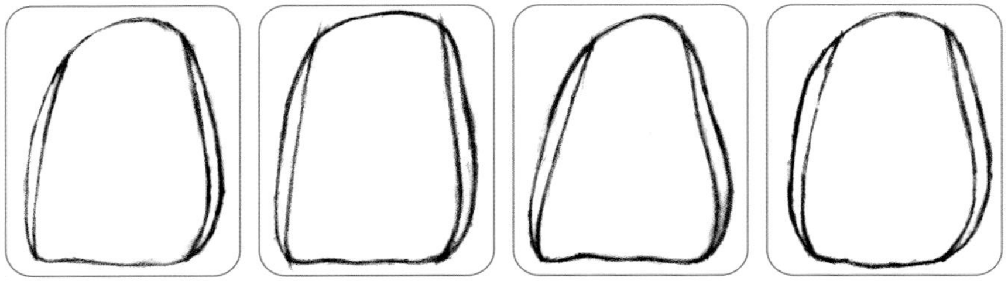

Standard ☐ Squared ☐ Triangular ☐ Oval ☐

11. **Degree of incisal edge tooth wear:**

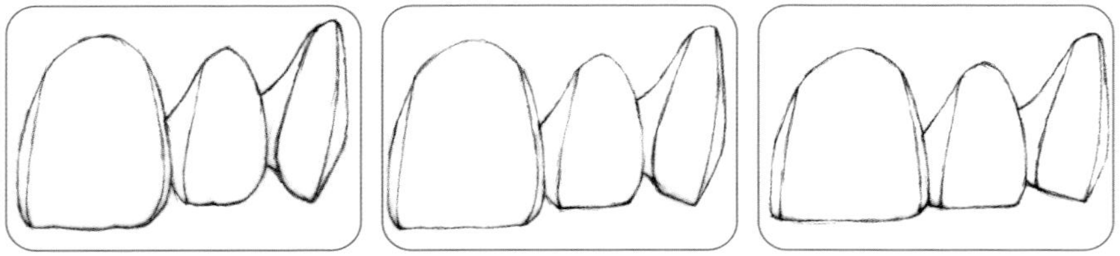

Youthful ☐ Slightly worn ☐ Very worn ☐

12. **Incisal edge characteristics:**
   a. Wrinkled? ☐ **b.** Straight? ☐

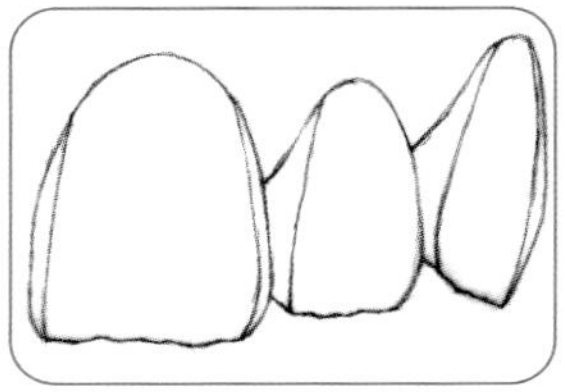

13. Characteristics of the tooth surface:

- **a.** Smooth? ☐
- **b.** Medium marked? ☐
- **c.** Clearly marked? ☐
- **d.** Other? (please describe) ☐

. . . .

. . . .

. . . .

14. Symmetry:

Are we trying to achieve symmetry on both sides:

Yes: ☐

No: ☐

Freely: ☐

If the symmetry deviates, how to make the restoration? . . . .

. . . .

. . . .

. . . .

15. Other information:

a. Length of the incisors (mark or write down the planned length of the teeth)

- Maxillary central incisors (mm):

  . . . . 8.0 8.5 9.0 9.5 10.0 10.5 –11.0 11.5 . . . .

- Maxillary lateral incisors (mm):

  . . . . 7.0 7.5 8.0 8.5 9.0 9.5 10.0 . . . .

b. Level of domination of central incisors:

- Clearly dominant: ☐
- Moderately dominant: ☐
- Barely dominant: ☐

c. Level of dominance/exposure of canines:

- Clearly dominant: ☐
- Moderately dominant: ☐
- Barely dominant: ☐

d. Strongly arched incisor edges of the lateral incisors: ☐

e. Color of the gingiva . . . .

. . . .

. . . .

f. Method of closing the interdental spaces/black triangles (determine the distance of the proximal contact point from the preparation margin in the interdental spaces)

- **a.** Gentle proximal contact point ☐
- **b.** Medium-length proximal contact area ☐
- **c.** Long proximal contact area ☐

g. Other: . . . .

. . . .

. . . .

h. Other supplementary drawings (please draw):

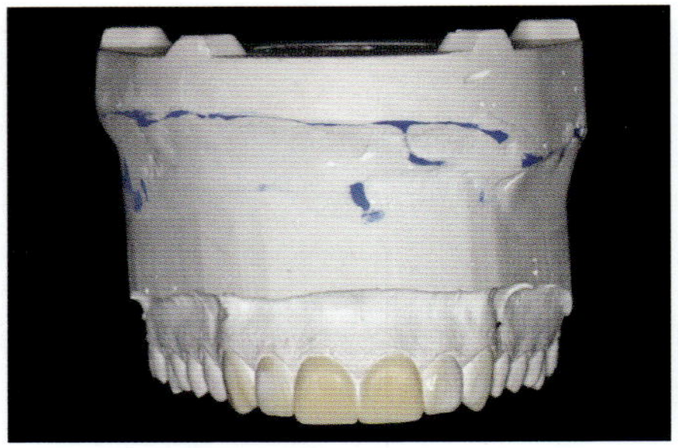

Fig 3-21a
The silicone index is taken from an approved diagnostic wax-up.

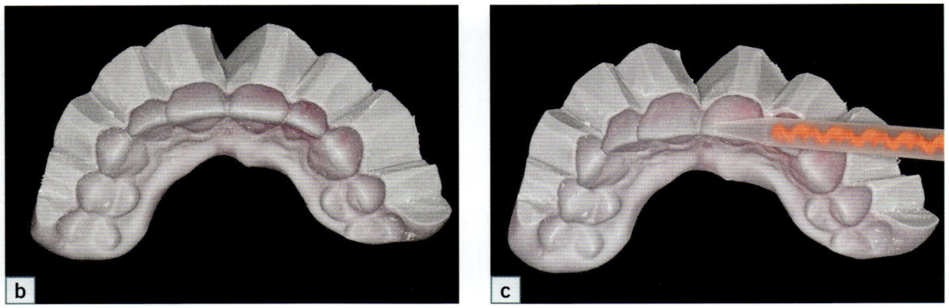

Figs 3-21b and 3-21c
(b) Cut away the silicone excess with a straight handpiece carbide bur or with a surgical scalpel, which will facilitate the removal of resin excess during the mock-up. (c) Composite temporization material is applied to the silicone index.

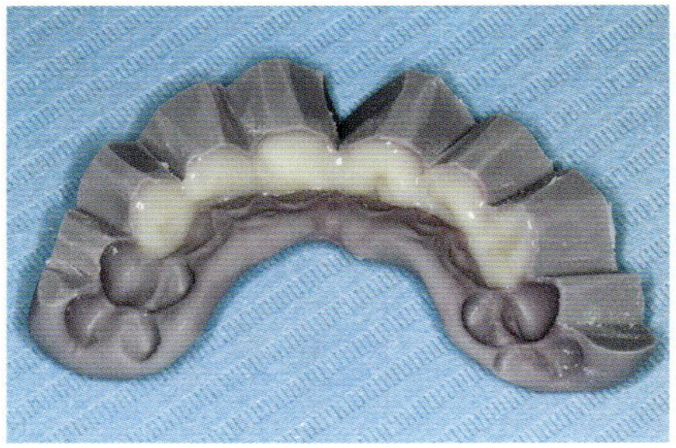

Fig 3-21d
Silicone index filled with the temporization material is transferred to the mouth …

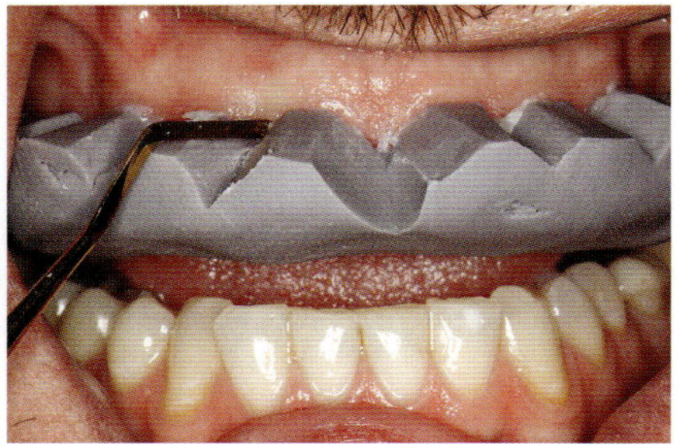

Fig 3-21e
… and after its initial setting, resin excess is removed from the adjusted proximal surfaces of the silicone index with the aid of a dental spatula.

MOCK-UP OR TEST-DRIVE VENEERS

Spending enough time to perform the test veneers is a critical step in communicating with the patient, understanding their expectations, and achieving mutual trust at the beginning of treatment planning.

Transferring the shape of the teeth from the wax-up is performed by means of a silicone index (Fig 3-21a). The silicone excess is cut away with a surgical scalpel or a straight handpiece carbide bur (Fig 3-21b), then a composite temporization material (Fig 3-21c) (for example, Protemp) is applied to the index, which is transferred to the mouth (Fig 3-21d). Next, wait for the initial setting of the resin and start removing excess material with a dental spatula.

After the composite resin has fully set (about 5 minutes), gently remove the silicone index and proceed with the removal of the excess material from the palatal side and the proximal surfaces (Fig 3-21e).

At this stage, the author would give the patient a mirror and ask whether they liked the work. This is a mistake! The patient immediately brings the mirror closer and searches for inaccuracies that will certainly be visible at close range. While looking at the mock-up, the patient also asks many questions, such as: Will the veneers be connected as in the case of the mock-up? Will they have bumps near the gums? Will they be rough?

TIP

Instead of looking for the right answers to unfavorable questions, we take a series of photographs in an improvised photographic studio (with appropriate face lighting).
Photographs must be taken in a relaxed atmosphere.

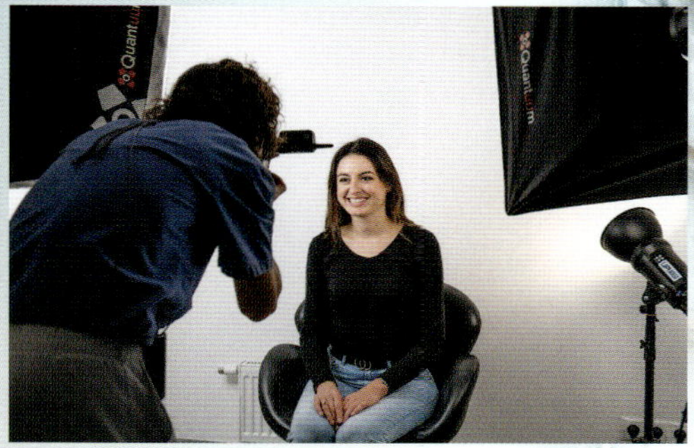

Fig 3-22
A photographic studio allows us not only to take professional photographs of the patient's face and smile, which helps to plan proper treatment, but is also a part of building a relationship with the patients and recognizing their expectations.

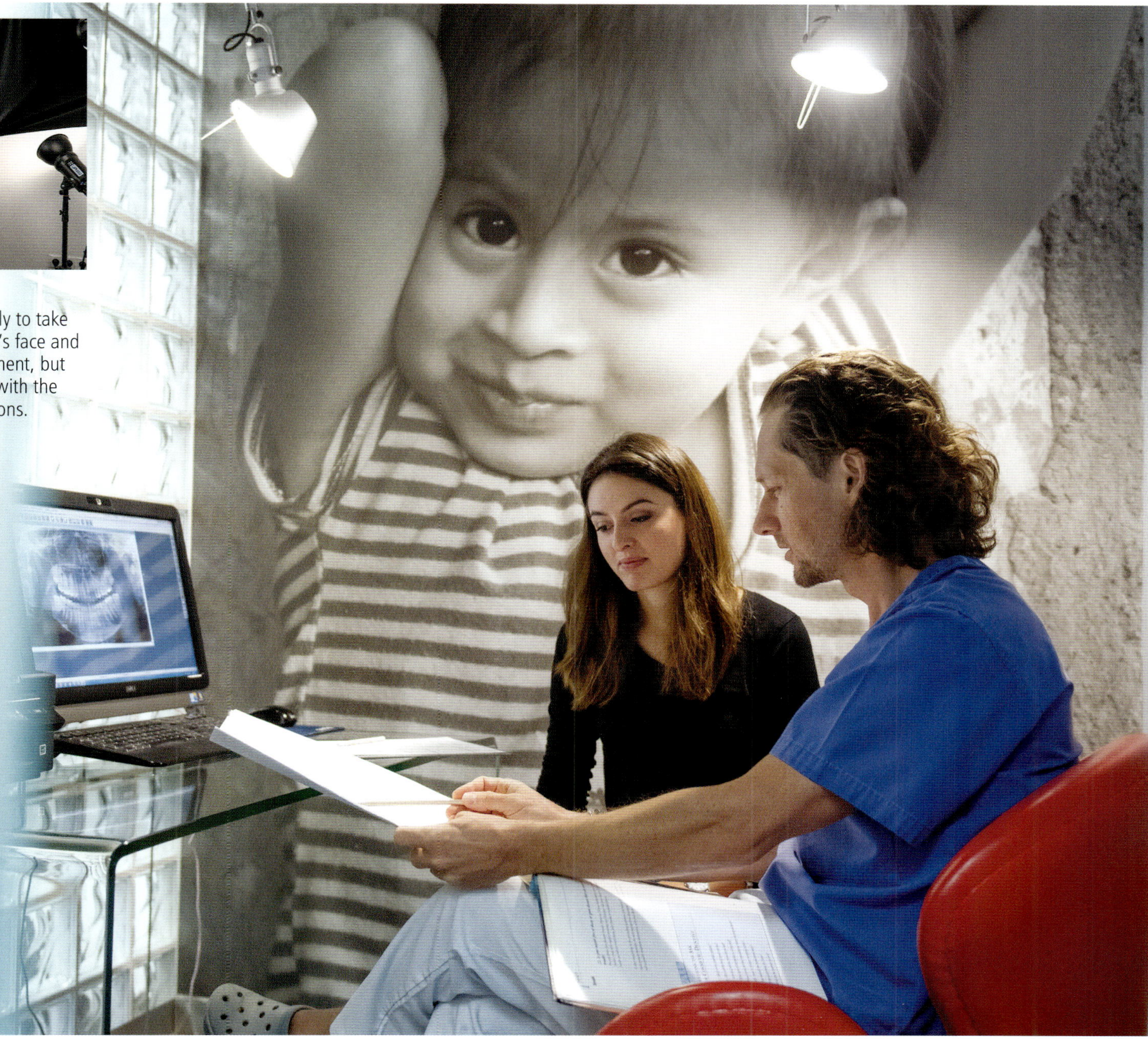

Fig 3-23
Conversation in a quiet room and presentation of photographs and drawings illustrating the concept of planned treatment is a basic element of communication with the patient. Without communication skills, one may be an excellent professional but will not be a good dentist. These skills should be improved throughout life, for the benefit of the clinic and the patients.

The photography session can be a pleasure with some patients, while with others it can be a much more difficult task, depending on the nature and attitude of the person, and on the dentist's empathy (Fig 3-22).

The atmosphere created during the photography session is very important. A patient intimidated by a tense situation will look scared and not show their teeth with relaxed lips. On the contrary, a patient who is naturally smiling or even laughing will fully reveal the created mock-up, which will allow a rational assessment of the planned esthetic treatment.[49]

Everyone probably has their own method of talking to the patient and relaxing the atmosphere; the method preferred by the author is to ask the patient to recall their most "cheerful" friend from college or high school and ask what their name was, or to recall a funny situation from the school times. Now, when a natural smile appears on the patient's face, you can start taking photographs. Then they are transferred to a computer and put into slides to be compared with the initial photographs. It is reasonable to sit down with the patient in a place where no one will disturb you, and spend 15–20 minutes to unhurriedly discuss the esthetic plan and show the photographs before and after the mock-up (Fig 3-23).

The conversation with the use of photographic documentation and the result of this discussion, and the patient's response are decisive in undertaking the treatment by the dental team and for the patient's acceptance (Fig 3-24). Sometimes it is better to withdraw from the planned treatment if it is clear that there is no agreement, if the patient's expectations may not be met, or are not in line with our medical ethics (for example, if tooth preparation would not have a medical indication in a given case).

On the other hand, the patient must feel comfortable, convinced of the planned treatment, and confident that their dental team will perform this treatment in the proper way.[50]

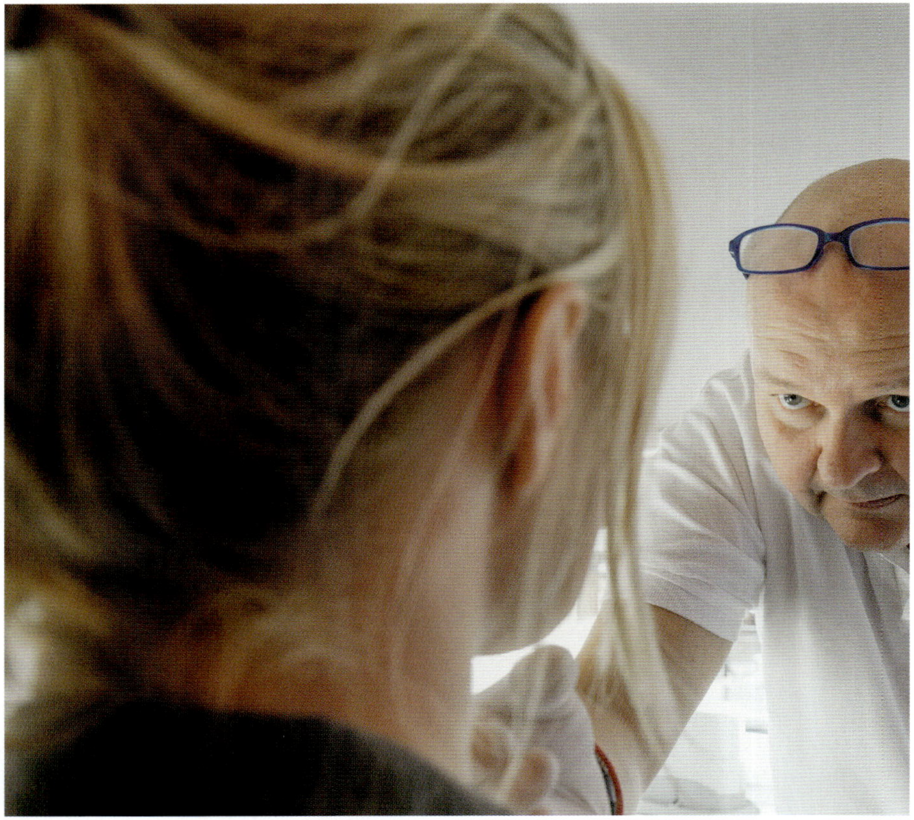

REMEMBER

Not every person who expects esthetic improvement has to become your patient. Sometimes, a dentist would give a lot to go back in time and decline to undertake treatment.

The decision on a common path in the form of comprehensive treatment requires responsibility from the dentist and should only be made if they can meet the patient's expectations. When the dentist sees that the patient's expectations are not in line with the treatment plan, the therapy should not be started.

Fig 3-24
The dental technician's ability to get to know the patient before the treatment begins is important in building trust and understanding the patient's full expectations. Planning with wax-up and mock-up provides key information before starting laboratory work.

REFERENCES

1. Hui K, Williams B, Davis EH, Holt RD. A comparative assessment of the strengths of porcelain veneers for incisor teeth dependent on their design characteristics. British Dent J 1991;17:51–55.
2. Sheets CG, Taniguchi T. Advantages and limitations in the use of porcelain veneer restorations. J Prosthet Dent 1990;64:406–411.
3. Peumans M, Van Meerbeek B, Lambrechts P, Vanherle G. Porcelain veneers: a review of the literature. J Dent 2000;28:163–177.
4. Burke FJ. Survival rates for porcelain laminate veneers with special reference to the effect of preparation in dentin: a literature review. J Esthet Restor Dent 2012;24:257–265.
5. Davis LG, Ashworth PD, Spriggs LS. Psychological effects of aesthetic dental treatment. J Dent 1998;26:547–554.
6. Mizrahi B. Visualization before finalization: a predictable procedure for porcelain laminate veneers. Pract Proced Aesthet Dent 2005;17:513–566.
7. Small BW. How communication can affect aesthetic outcome. Pract Periodontics Aesthet Dent 1992;4:11–15.
8. Kois DE, Kois JC. Comprehensive risk-based diagnostically driven treatment planning: developing sequentially generated treatment. Dent Clin North Am 2015;59:593–608.
9. Rechmann P, Kinsel R, Featherstone JDB. Integrating Caries Management by Risk Assessment (CAMBRA) and prevention strategies into the contemporary dental practice. Compend Contin Educ Dent 2018;39:226–234.
10. O'Toole S, Bartlett D. The relationship between dentine hypersensitivity, dietary acid intake and erosive tooth wear. J Dent 2017;67:84–87.
11. O'Toole S, Bernabé E, Moazzez R, Bartlett D. Timing of dietary acid intake and erosive tooth wear: a case-control study. J Dent 2017;56:99–104.
12. Wiegand A, Schwerzmann M, Sener B, et al. Impact of toothpaste slurry abrasivity and toothbrush filament stiffness on abrasion of eroded enamel – an in vitro study. Acta Odontol Scand 2008;66:231–235.
13. Schemehorn BR, Moore MH, Putt MS. Abrasion, polishing, and stain removal characteristics of various commercial dentifrices in vitro. J Clin Dent 2011;22:11–18.
14. González-Cabezas C, Hara AT, Hefferren J, Lippert F. Abrasivity testing of dentifrices – challenges and current state of the art. Monogr Oral Sci 2013;23:100–107.
15. Reddy A, Norris DF, Momeni SS, Waldo B, Ruby JD. The pH of beverages in the United States. J Am Dent Assoc 2016;147:255–263.
16. Mesko ME, Sarkis-Onofre R, Cenci MS, Opdam NJ, Loomans B, Pereira-Cenci T. Rehabilitation of severely worn teeth: a systematic review. J Dent 2016;48:9–15.
17. Loomans B, Opdam N, Attin T, et al. Severe tooth wear: European Consensus Statement on Management Guidelines. J Adhes Dent 2017;19:111–119.
18. Soares PV, Machado AC, Zeola LF, et al. Loading and composite restoration assessment of various non-carious cervical lesions morphologies – 3D finite element analysis. Aust Dent J 2015;60:309–316.
19. Teixeira DNR, Zeola LF, Machado AC, et al. Relationship between noncarious cervical lesions, cervical dentin hypersensitivity, gingival recession, and associated risk factors: a cross-sectional study. J Dent 2018;76:93–97.
20. Page RC, Kornman KS. The pathogenesis of human periodontitis: an introduction. Periodontol 2000 1997;14:9–11.
21. Joshi S, Suominen AL, Knuuttila M, Bernabé E. Toothbrushing behaviour and periodontal pocketing: an 11-year longitudinal study. J Clin Periodontol 2018;45:196–203.
22. McGowan T, McGowan K, Ivanovski S. A novel evidence-based periodontal prognosis model. J Evid Based Dent Pract 2017;17:350–360.
23. Ramseier CA, Anerud A, Dulac M, et al. Natural history of periodontitis: disease progression and tooth loss over 40 years. J Clin Periodontol 2017;44:1182–1191.
24. Dawson PE. Centric relation. Its effect on occluso-muscle harmony. Dent Clin North Am 1979;23:169–180.
25. Lundeen HC, Shryock EF, Gibbs CH. An evaluation of mandibular border movements: their character and significance. J Prosthet Dent 1978;40:442–452.
26. Ekfeldt A, Karlsson S. Changes of masticatory movement characteristics after prosthodontic rehabilitation of individuals with extensive tooth wear. Int J Prosthodont 1996;9:539–546.
27. Dawson PE, Cranham JC. Aesthetics and function: conflict or complement? Dent Today 2007;26:80–83.
28. Dawson PE. A classification system for occlusions that relates maximal intercuspation to the position and condition of the temporomandibular joints. J Prosthet Dent 1996;75: 60–66
29. Wang MQ, He JJ, Li G, Widmalm SE. The effect of physiological nonbalanced occlusion on the thickness of the temporomandibular joint disc: a pilot autopsy study. J Prosthet Dent 2008;99:148–152.
30. Zarow M. Finding the Centric Relation – The Kois Deprogrammer. Available at: www.styleitaliano.org/finding-centric-relation-kois-deprogrammer/
31. Tjan AH, Miller GD, The JG. Some esthetic factors in a smile. J Prosthet Dent 1984;51: 24–28.
32. Nold SL, Horvath SD, Stampf S, Blatz MB. Analysis of select facial and dental esthetic parameters. Int J Periodontics Restorative Dent 2014;34:623–629.
33. Hochman MN, Chu SJ, Tarnow DP. Maxillary anterior papilla display during smiling: a clinical study of the interdental smile line. Int J Periodontics Restorative Dent 2012;32:375–383.
34. Andijani RI, Tatakis DN. Hypermobile upper lip is highly prevalent among patients seeking treatment for gummy smile. J Periodontol 2019;90:256–262.
35. Van Der Geld P, Oosterveld P, Berge SJ, Kuijpers-Jagtman AM. Tooth display and lip position during spontaneous and posed smiling in adults. Acta Odontol Scand 2008;66: 207–213.
36. Silva BP, Jiménez-Castellanos E, Stanley K, Mahn E, Coachman C, Finkel S. Layperson's perception of axial midline angulation in asymmetric faces. J Esthet Restor Dent 2018; 30:119–125.
37. Bunk S, Żarow M. Fotografia cyfrowa jako składnik nowoczesnej dokumentacji medycznej. Med Prakt Stomatol 2016;2:85–91.
38. Coachman C, Calamita MA, Coachman FG, Coachman RG, Sesma N. Facially generated and cephalometric guided 3D digital design for complete mouth implant rehabilitation: a clinical report. J Prosthet Dent 2017;117:577–586.

REFERENCES

39. Coachman C, Calamita MA, Sesma N. Dynamic documentation of the smile and the 2D/3D Digital Smile Design process. Int J Periodontics Restorative Dent 2017;37: 183–193.
40. Zimmermann M, Mehl A. Virtual smile design systems: a current review. Int J Comput Dent 2015;18:303–317.
41. Dindaroğlu F, Duran GS, Görgülü S. Reproducibility of the lip position at rest: a 3-dimensional perspective. Am J Orthod Dentofacial Orthop 2016;149:757–765.
42. Dong JK, Jin TH, Cho HW, Oh SC. The esthetics of the smile: a review of some recent studies. Int J Prosthodont 1999;12:9–19.
43. Samet N, Smidt A, Samet N, Weiss EI. A clinical and cost-benefit evaluation of five face-bows. Quintessence Int 2002;33:511–515.
44. Squier RS. Jaw relation records for fixed prosthodontics. Dent Clin North A 2004;48:vii, 471–486.
45. Gurrea J, Bruguera A. Wax-up and mock-up. A guide for anterior periodontal and restorative treatments. Int J Esthet Dent 2014;9:146–162.
46. Vailati F, Carciofo S. Treatment planning of adhesive additive rehabilitations: the progressive wax-up of the three-step technique. Int J Esthet Dent 2016;11:356–377.
47. Fabbri G, Cannistraro G, Pulcini C, Sorrentino R. The full-mouth mock-up: a Dynamic Diagnostic Approach (DDA) to test function and esthetics in complex rehabilitations with increased vertical dimension of occlusion. Int J Esthet Dent 2018;13:460–474.
48. Coachman C, Gürel G, Calamita M, Morimoto S, Paolucci B, Sesma N. The influence of tooth color on preparation design for laminate veneers from a minimally invasive perspective: case report. Int J Periodontics Restorative Dent 2014;34:453–459.
49. Khalifah AM, Celenza A. Teaching and assessment of dentist–patient communication skills: a systematic review to identify best-evidence methods. J Dent Educ 2019;83:16–31.
50. Ayn C, Robinson L, Nason A, Lovas J. Determining recommendations for improvement of communication skills training in dental education: a scoping review. J Dent Educ 2017;81:479–488.

CHAPTER 4

DENTAL MORPHOLOGY

MARGARIDA HENRIQUE

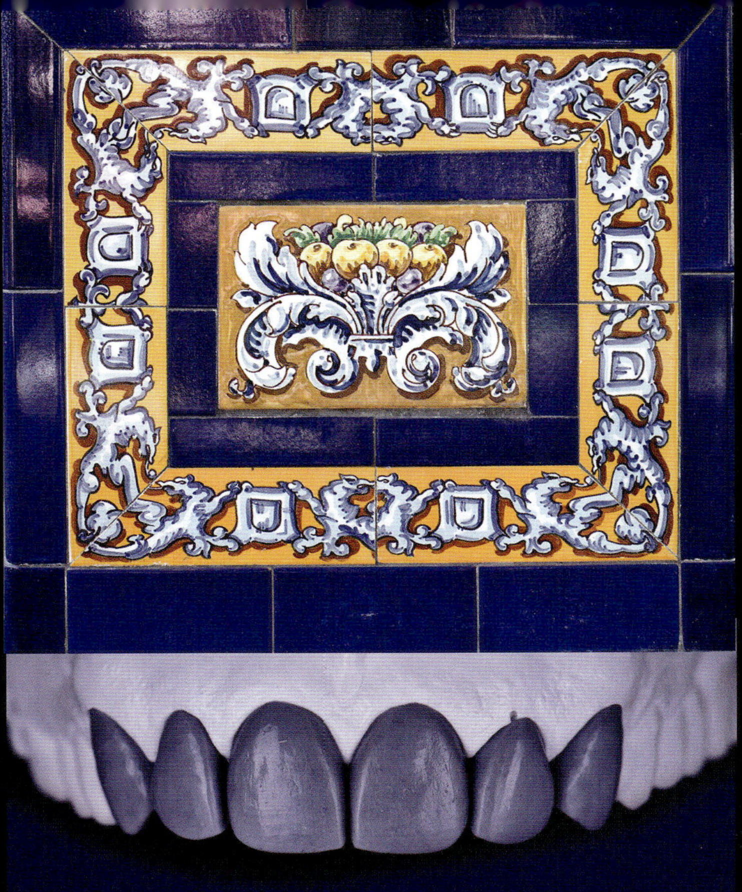

Dental morphology is unique for each person, like a fingerprint. Thus, there is a huge variation of tooth shapes in nature. Although this huge variation of dental anatomy, there has been much research to discover common features in esthetically pleasant teeth arrangements and shapes...

Dental morphology

A restorative treatment, the assumption of which is to perform a reconstruction of the patient biology, function, structure, and consequently also esthetics, cannot be done without the knowledge of tooth morphology. A dentist who understands the morphology of hard tissues can rebuild the missing tissues in a way that meets the appropriate criteria.

NATURAL ESTHETIC RESULTS

A knowledge of dental morphology is fundamental in the practice of dentistry. We want to replicate nature and give biological, functional, structural and, consequently, esthetic restorations to our patients. Nature is so well designed that each morphological characteristic of a tooth has a certain function, so if you have developed knowledge about morphology, you will know how to restore a tooth fulfilling all these premises. That is why dental professionals should search for this knowledge in a cognitive, visual and, most importantly, practical way.[1–4]

Dental morphology is so complex and variable that there are no absolute truths. However, every tooth has some basic characteristic features, and when integrated into a smile according to some established esthetic parameters, it produces an esthetically pleasant result, a beautiful smile.

It is important to note that esthetics, although not well defined, is a universal language, and frequently people of the same society or culture agree about the beauty of a person or not. Indeed, this high concordance in judging beauty in the same culture can simply reflect the media, which is today highly competitive and a dictator of trends. However, research from diverse cultures suggests that the shared beauty ideals do not depend on a preformed image.[5]

In dentistry, esthetic treatments enhance a patient's natural beauty, restore and reproduce the natural characteristics of teeth and smile.[6] There is always the need to search for more beautiful restorations, and many esthetic criteria that should be present in a beautiful smile can be proposed.

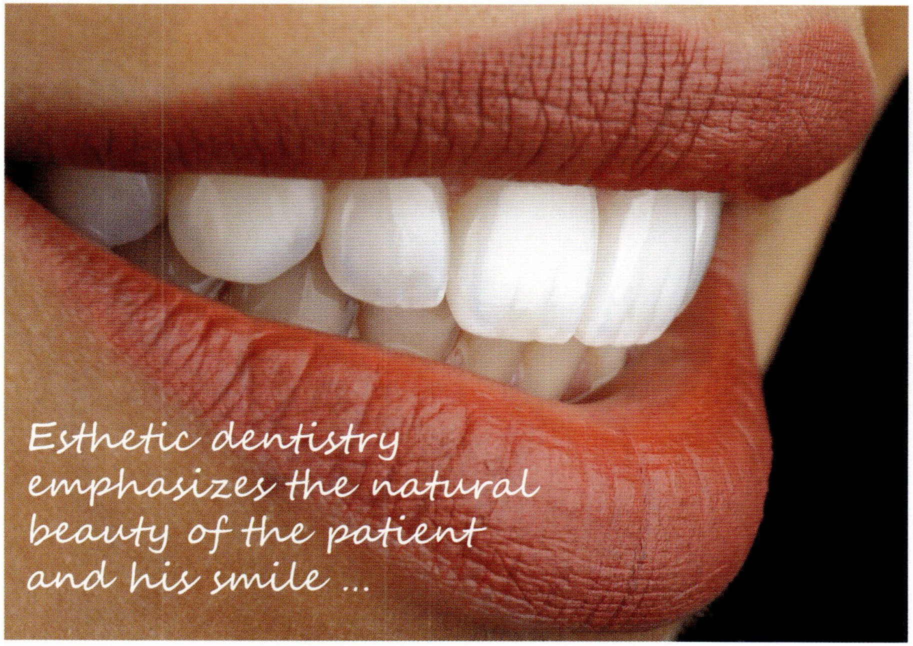

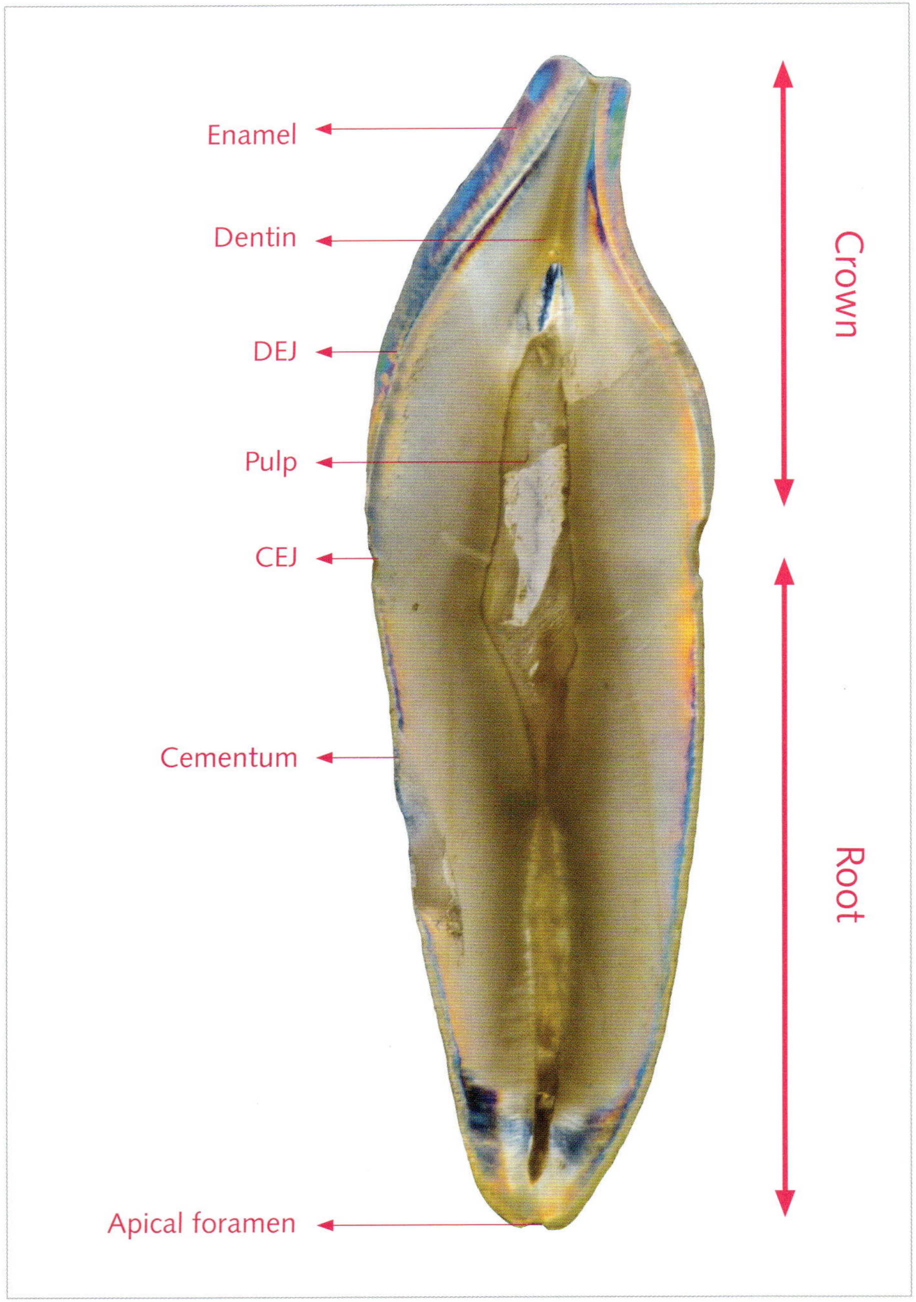

TOOTH STRUCTURE

When we think about dental morphology is important to have knowledge about the tooth structure per se. In Fig 4-1, we have a polarized photograph of a tooth cut of approximately 1 mm, in which we can appreciate the various components of a tooth.

We know that a tooth is composed of several tissues: enamel, cementum, dentin, and pulp. And that it is divided into two parts: the crown that is exposed in the oral cavity, and the root that is covered by the cementum and submerged and anchored to the bone tissue through the periodontal ligament. To better understand this structure, we will briefly describe the basic characteristics of each of its components (Fig 4-2).

Cementum (Fig 4-3)

Very thin (50–100 μm) mineralized connective tissue covers all the root area dentin, from the cervical anatomical line to the apex. Its principal function is the connection of the fibers of the periodontal ligament.

We can compare it with bone since its hardness and chemical composition are similar. It is not vascularized, and it lacks proper innervation. It also has no ability to be remodeled and is generally more resistant to resorption than the bone.

It presents a pearly white color, is darker and more opaque than enamel but less yellow than dentin.

Composition:

- Cellular components: cementoblasts and cementocytes
- Calcified extracellular matrix (46–50% inorganic matter, 22% organic matter, and 32% water)[7]

REMEMBER

The natural tooth is polychromatic, which means that it has a large variety of colors and nuances that can be observed and perceived by the human brain. To reproduce all the internal characteristics of a tooth is not an easy task, and the dentist should have the knowledge and artistic sense to identify all the details and define the different characteristics of each one.

Fig 4-1
Tooth structure and its components.

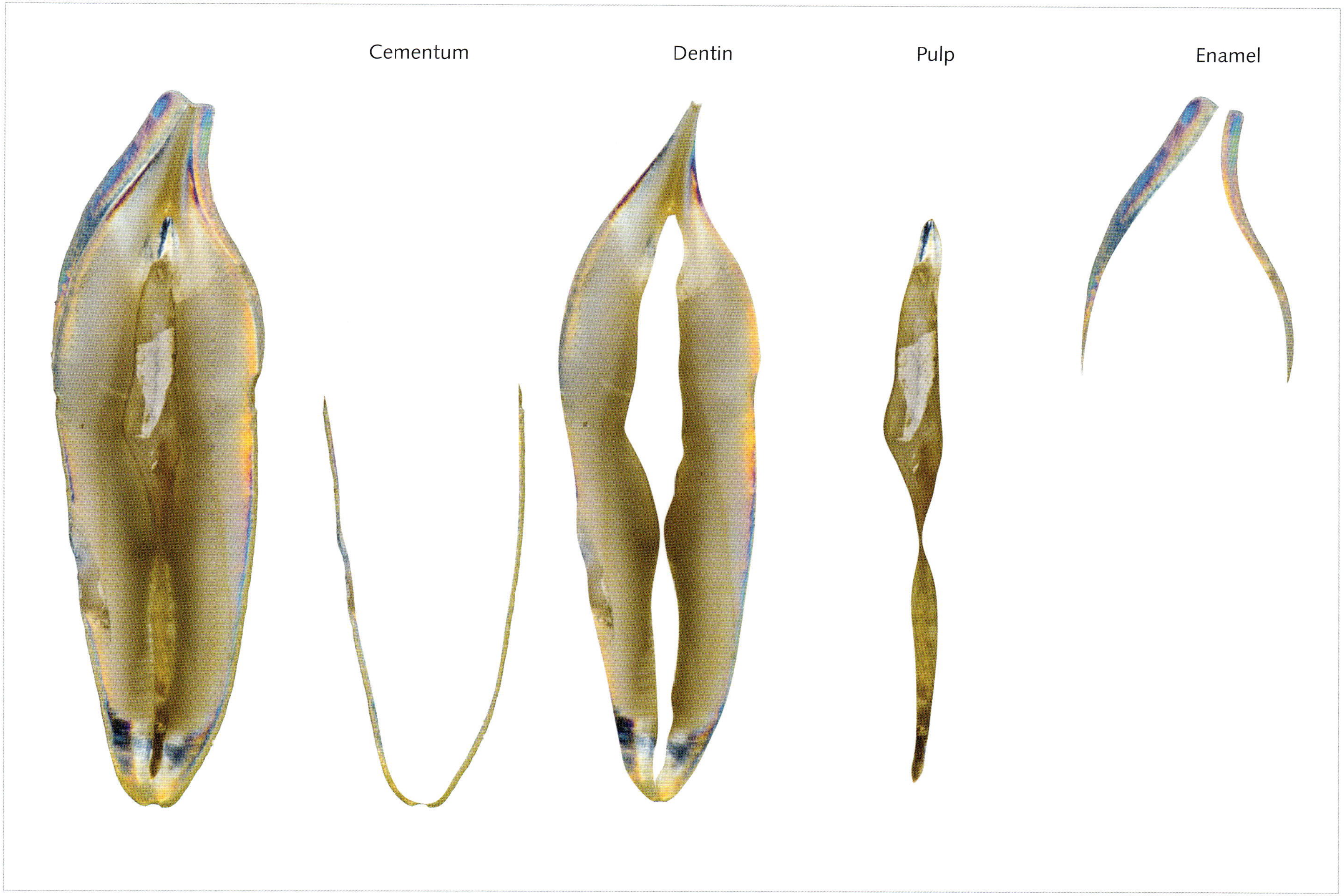

Fig 4-2
Tooth components.

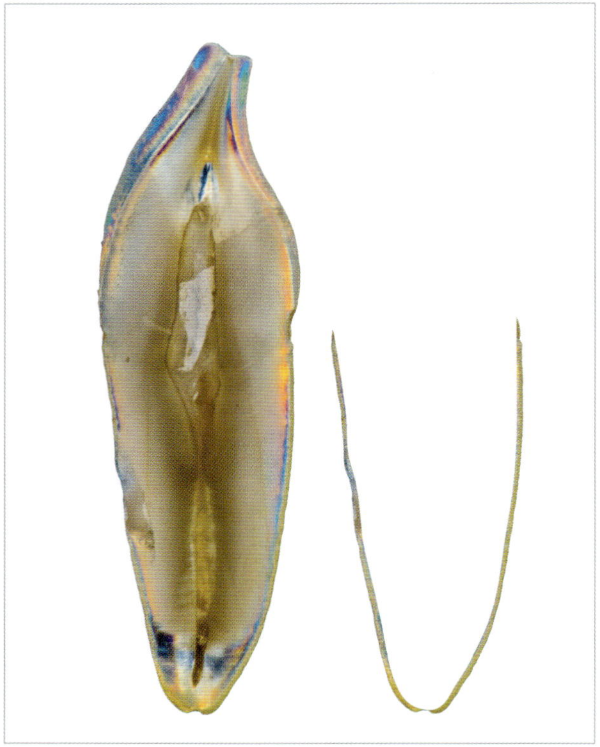

Fig 4-3
Schematic division of the cementum.

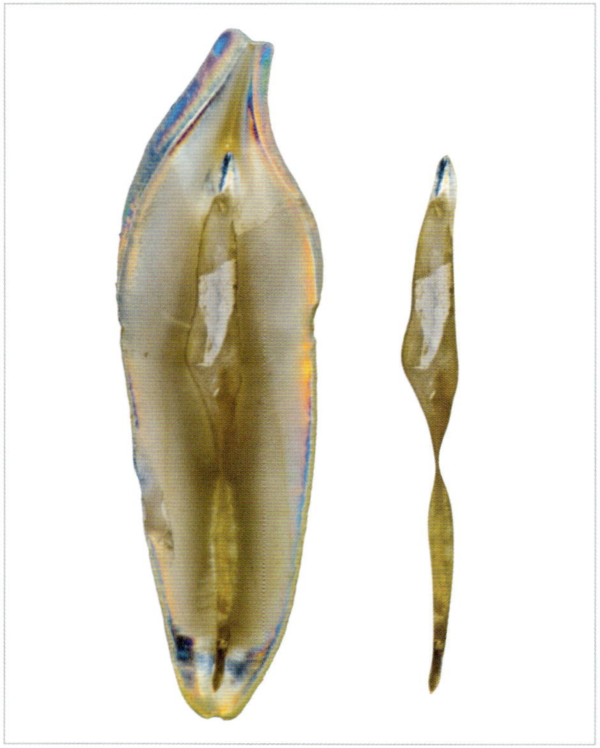

Fig 4-4
Schematic division of the pulp.

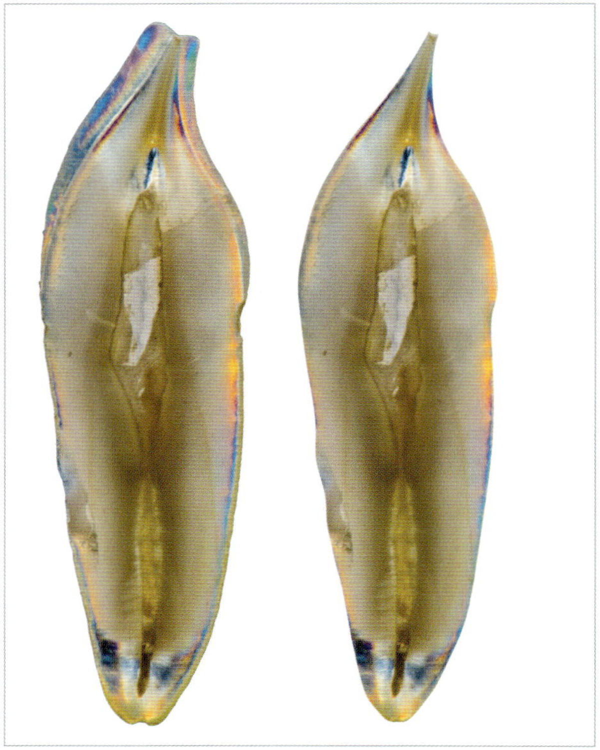

Fig 4-5
Schematic division of the dentin–pulp complex.

Pulp (Fig 4-4)
Conjunctive tissue organ is located in the center of each tooth, constituted by numerous structures like arteries, veins, lymphatic system, and nerves. Its principal function is to form the dentin.

In newly erupted teeth, the pulp is big, and it progressively reduces as the tooth is completed.

Pulp maintains its tissue-forming activity (secondary dentin), especially when caries advances into the pulp. Sometimes the pulp chamber can be totally obliterated by the secondary dentin to protect the pulp.

It has a coronal portion (pulp chamber) and a root portion (pulp or root canal). The opening of the pulp in the apex is constricted, and it is called apical foramen. The pulp connects directly with the periodontal ligament in this area through the periapex. The blood vessels and nerve fibers enter and exit the pulp through it.[7,8]

Approximated composition:

- 75% water
- 25% organic matter (cells and extracellular matrix)
- Dentin–pulp complex (Fig 4-5)
- Structural unit – odontoblasts prolongations are included on the dentin
- Functional unit – the pulp maintains the vitality of the dentin, and the dentin protects the pulp
- Their embrionary origin is common

Dentin (Fig 4-6)

This is mineralized tissue that forms the largest volume of a tooth. We can distinguish two basic components: mineralized matrix and dentinal tubules that cross all its thickness and lodge the odontoblastic processes, which are prolongations of the odontoblasts, responsible for the production of the collagen matrix and calcification of the dentin.

The odontoblasts are located in the most peripheral region of the pulp, and their prolongations are included in the dentin; that is why dentin and pulp are considered a unit: a dentin–pulp complex (see Fig 4-5).

It presents with yellowish-white color, but it may vary from one individual to another, and also throughout life. It is less translucent than the enamel due to its lower degree of mineralization.

Approximate composition:

- 70% inorganic matter (hydroxyapatite crystals)
- 18% organic matter (collagen fibers)
- 12% water

This composition is variable between the different regions of the dentin:

- Microhardness = 0.57 to 1.13 GPa
- Young elasticity modulus = 17.6 to 22.9 GPa; Vickers hardness = 60–70 HV; Compressive strength = 200–350 MPa

The natural tooth is polychromatic, which means that it has a large variety of colors and nuances that can be observed and perceived by the human brain. To reproduce all the internal characteristics of a tooth is not an easy task, and the dentist should have the knowledge and artistic sense to identify all the details and define the different characteristics of each one. Dentin and enamel have a rich composition and detail of optical characteristics.

> **TIP**
>
> Dentin anatomy is a way to understand internal teeth characteristics.

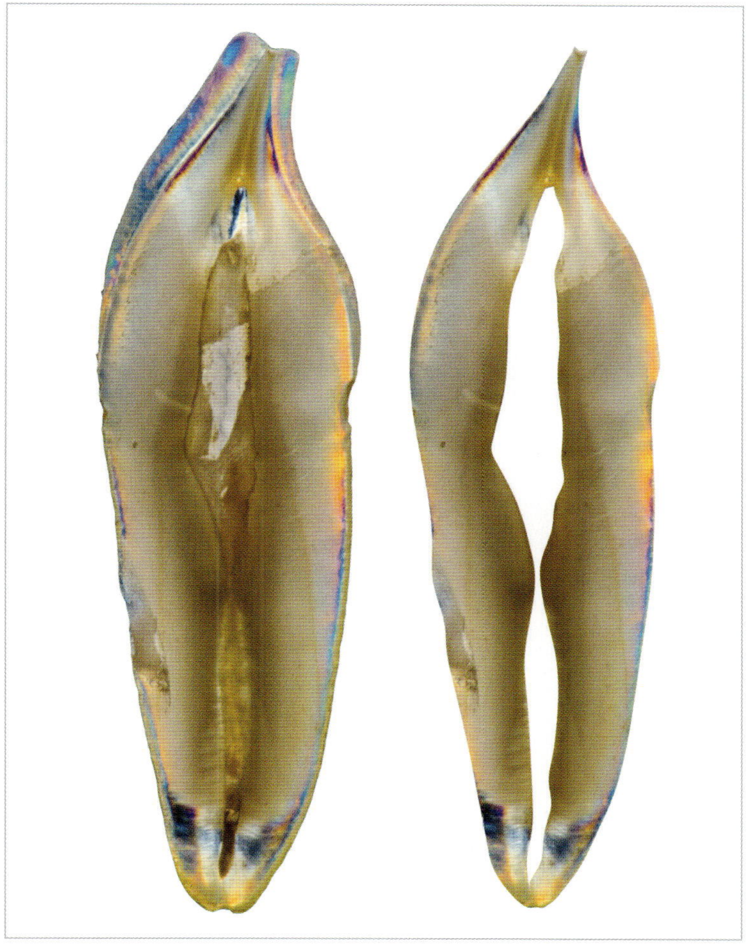

Fig 4-6
Schematic division of the dentin.

Dentin is responsible for the basic color of the tooth (hue), and enamel modulates the chroma and the value of the hue according to its thickness. Comprehension of the thickness, both of the enamel and dentin necessary to emulate the natural tooth, is fundamental to achieving a great esthetic result. To better understand it, I did the removal of the enamel layer of several teeth following the protocol suggested by Bazos and Magne, submerging the natural teeth in 10% hydrochloric acid (HCL) under ultrasonic vibration for 20 minutes, and I have obtained the structures shown in Fig 4-7. We can observe the dentoenamel junction (DEJ) surface, and understand that its morphology has a crucial role on the enamel surface morphology.[9,10]

To better understand and train the morphology of the dentin surface, I have tried to reproduce it with a characterized wax-up of each of the anterior teeth (13-12-11-41-42-43) as shown in Figs 4-8 and 4-9.

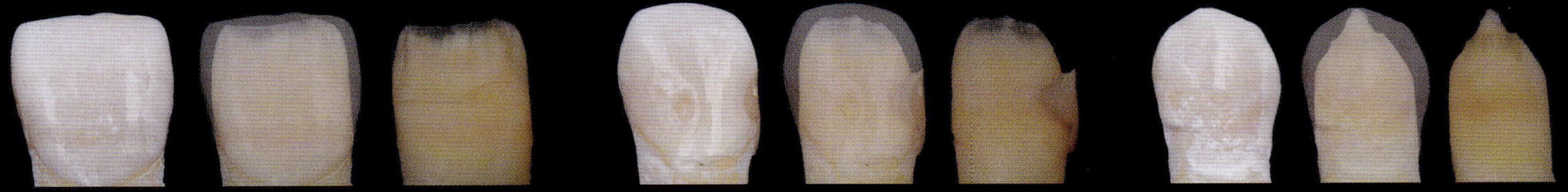

Fig 4-7
Natural teeth treated with hydrochloric acid (HCL) at 10% to remove all the enamel layer and have a better comprehension of the dentin morphology.

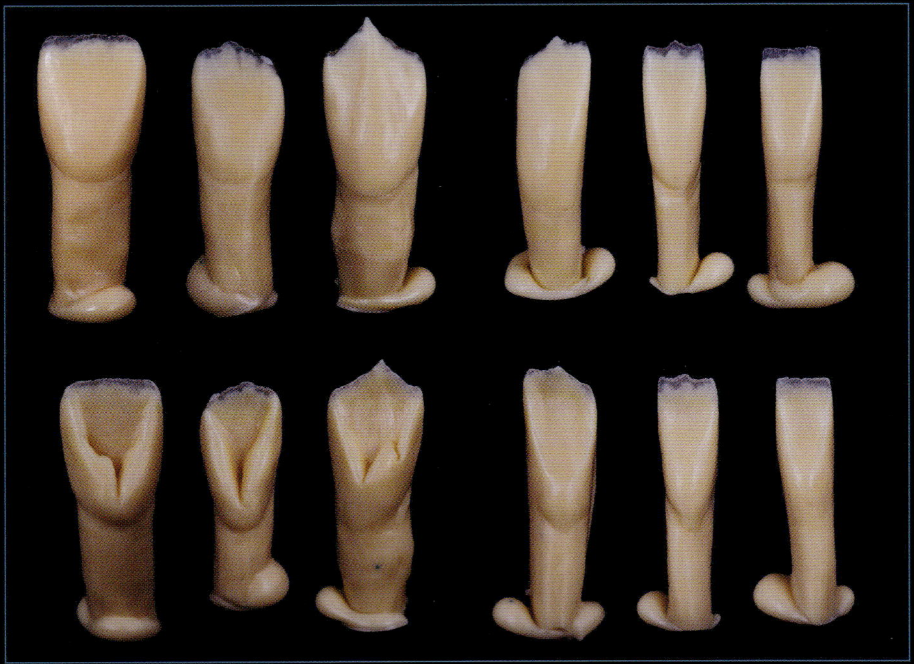

Fig 4-8
Total wax dentin cores to simulate dentin morphology, facial and lingual view (note the simulation of the mantle of dentin).

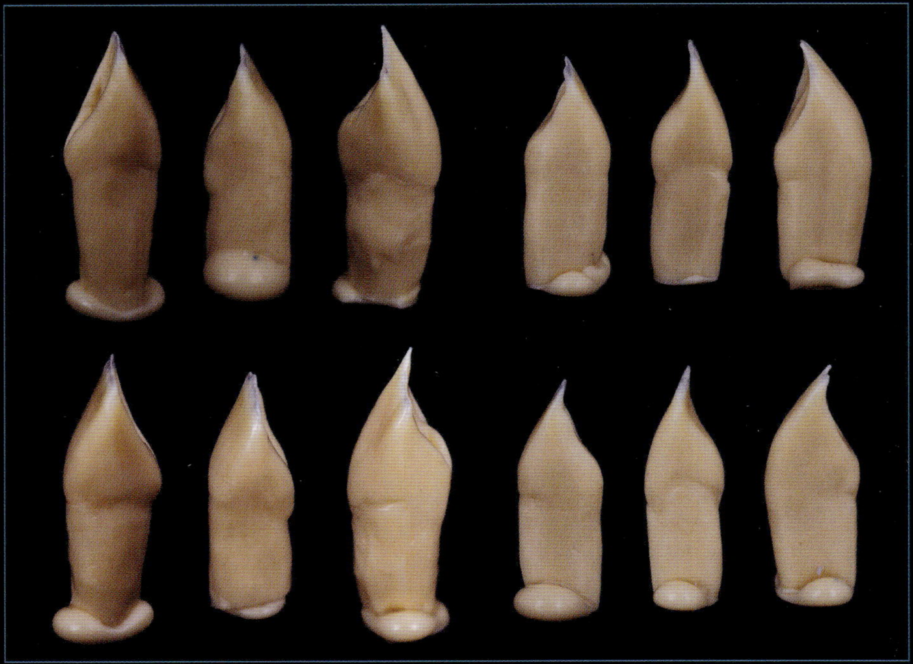

Fig 4-9
Total wax dentin cores to simulate dentin morphology, mesial and distal view (note the simulation of the mantle of dentin).

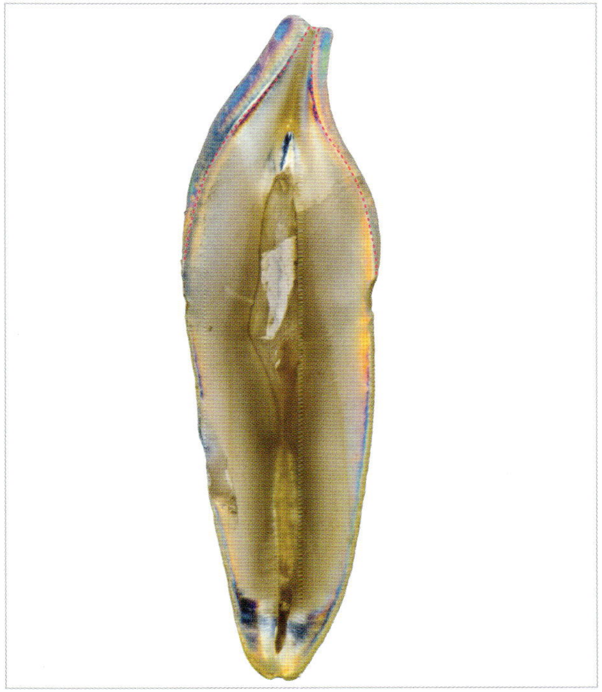

Fig 4-10
Scheme indicating the dentinoenamel junction (DEJ) position.

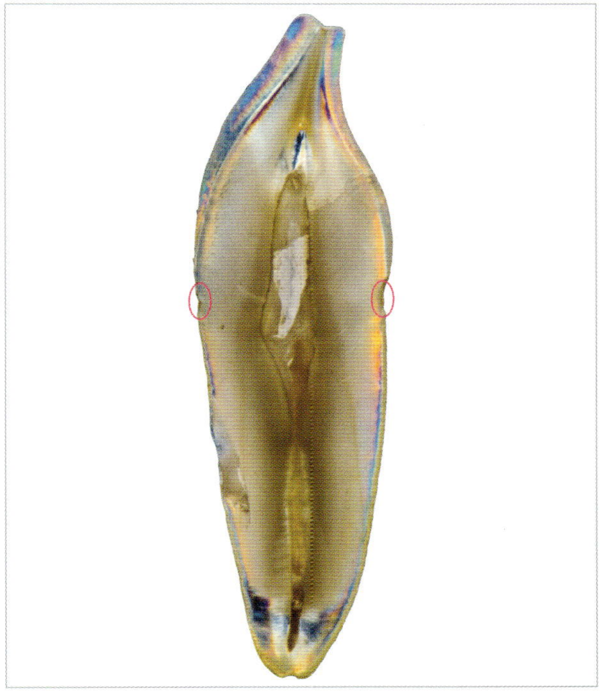

Fig 4-11
Scheme indicating the amelocementary junction (JAC) position.

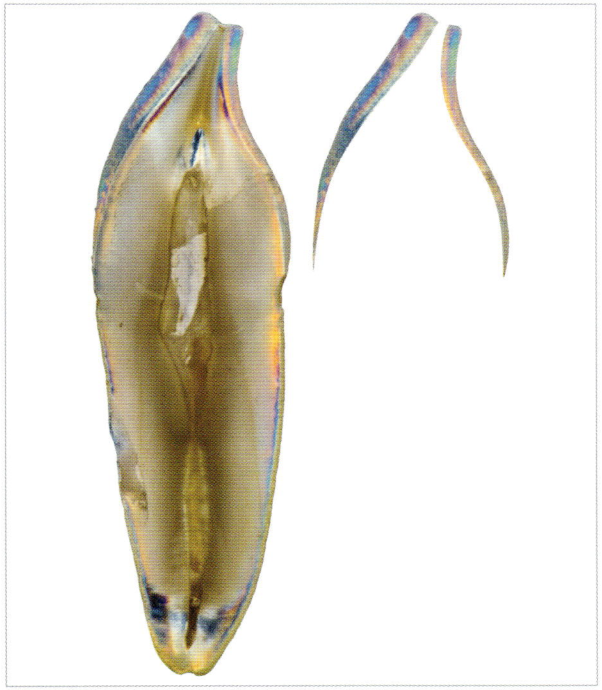

Fig 4-12
Schematic division of the enamel.

DEJ – dentinoenamel junction (Fig 4-10)

Well delimitated line resultant of the union of the enamel with the dentin.[7] A less simplistic view suggests that the DEJ complex should also include the inner aprismatic enamel and the mantle dentin.[11] The DEJ and the outer enamel surface are essential features of the tooth's three-dimensional structures and significantly affect its visual appearance. It is known that the shape of the DEJ is very similar to the shape of the outer surface enamel.[9,12,13]

JAC – amelocementary junction (Fig 4-11)

Also known as the cervical anatomic line. There are four possibilities for its presentation (the Choquet cases)[8]:

1. The cement covers the enamel (60% of cases)
2. The enamel covers the cement (less frequent)
3. Enamel and cement are in contact, and there is no exposed dentin (30% of cases)
4. There is a lack of connection between the enamel and the cement

Enamel (Fig 4-12)

Also known as an adamantine substance, it covers the dentin, offering protection to the dentin–pulp complex. It is the hardest tissue on the human body and is constituted by millions of mineralized prisms – hydroxyapatite crystals. It is acellular, avascular, and has no innervation, so it cannot self-repair. Its thickness varies in the different regions of the tooth.

Its major thickness is located at the incisal edge and the minimum in the cervical, where it ends in a sharp edge. It is translucent, and its color is dependent on the subjacent dentin. In areas of greater thickness, it has a white-grayish color, and where it is thinner, it presents a yellowish-white color.

Approximate composition:

- 95% inorganic matter (hydroxyapatite crystals)
- 1–2% organic matter (protein origin with no collagen)
- 3–5% water

DENTAL MORPHOLOGY

It is essential tohave a basic notion about the structure of a tooth to understand its morphology. As we have seen before, dentin plays a major role in defining the final shape and color. Now, we are ready to go for the study of the basic morphological characteristics of each one of the anterior human teeth. To facilitate the comprehension of a tooth, the crown and root are normally divided into thirds to precisely define the location of its characteristics[14] (Fig 4-13).

BASIC CHARACTERISTICS OF ANTERIOR TEETH MORPHOLOGY

- **Anatomical cervical line:** Continuous and sinuous line that divides the tooth into crown and root. It is concave in vestibular and palatal and convex in mesial and distal.
- **Surface:** Each anterior tooth presents five surfaces: facial, lingual or palatal, mesial, distal, and incisal.
- **Border/Edge:** These delimitate the transition between two surfaces, taking note of the ones that they're in, forming a dihedral angle.
- **Angle:** When the different surfaces of a tooth meet, there is a formation of angles between them.
- **Bulges:** They are enamel elevations that protrude on dental surfaces. Four humps are common in every anterior tooth, and their location is:
  - Cervical third in the buccal surface.
  - Incisal third in the mesial surface.

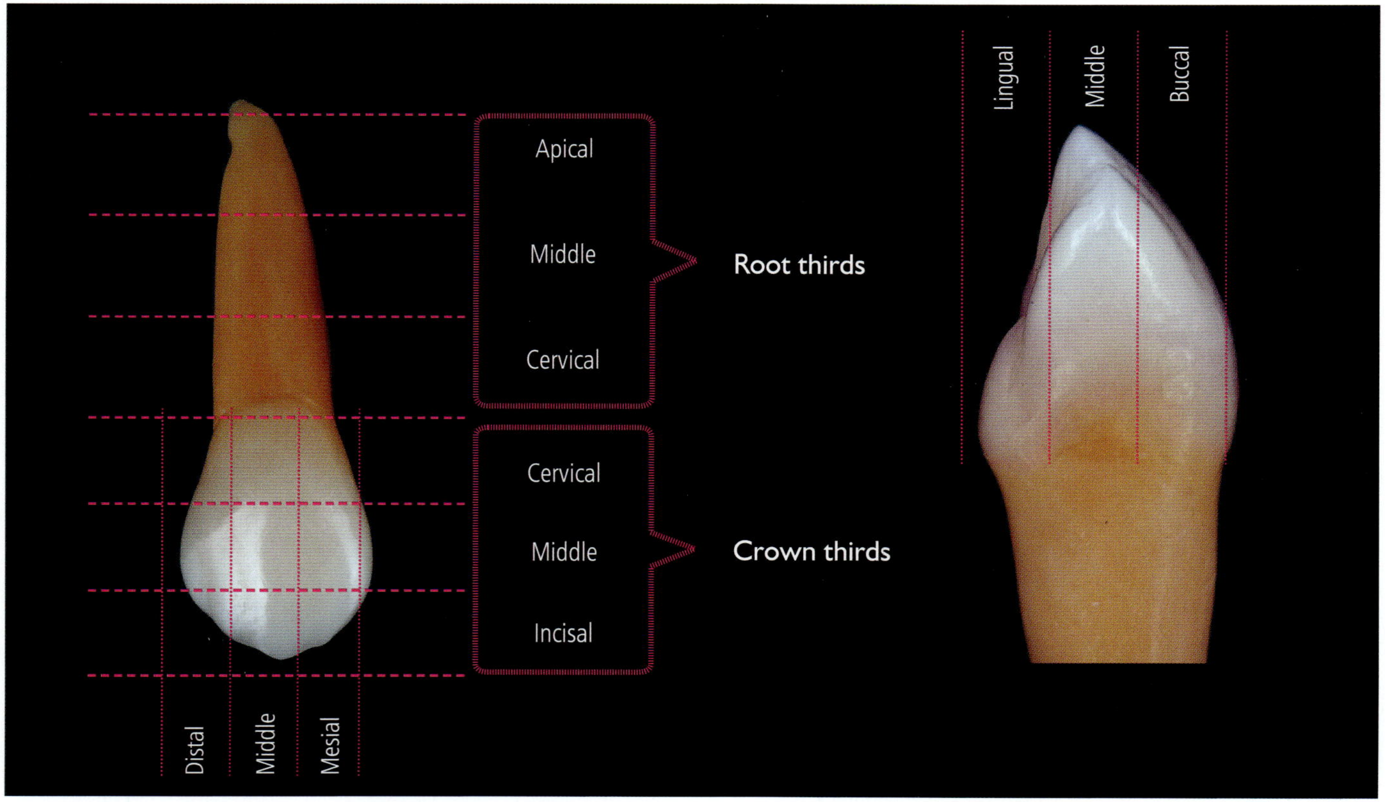

Fig 4-13
Total wax-up in a 1:1 ratio of a superior canine vestibular and proximal views. (left) Division in thirds of the tooth crown and root viewed from vestibular, in horizontal and vertical directions. (right) Division in thirds of the tooth crown viewed from proximal, in a vertical direction.

- Incisal third, slightly going to the medium third on the distal surface.
- Cervical third, in the ingual surface.

❖ **Marginal crest:** Cylindrical enamel projections located on the proximal portions of the lingual surface, going from the incisal edge to the cingulum on the anterior teeth. They act as a reinforcement pilar and allow the maintenance of the vertical occlusion dimension of the anterior sector

❖ **Cingulum:** Lingual lobe of anterior teeth, which determines the width of the cervical third of the lingual surface. It is important in the masticatory process to protect the soft tissue from the friction produced.

❖ **Lingual fossa:** A concavity or irregular depression delimited by the incisal edge, marginal ridges, and the cingulum. It is located on the palatal/lingual surface of the anterior teeth. It is less evident on the mandibular canines and incisors.

❖ **Scape groove:** A small sulcus located between the coronal portion of the termination of the marginal crests and the incisal edge. It runs from the lingual fossa into the proximal surface and provides the function of escape for food during the masticatory process.

❖ **Pit:** A sharp, pointed depression point between the cingulum and the lingual fossa. It can be found in both superior incisors but is more frequent in the lateral one.

❖ **Development grooves**: Two linear depressions (mesiovestibular and distovestibular), parallel to the major axis of the tooth, located on the vestibular surface of anterior teeth. They have variable development and are more frequent in younger teeth. They go from the cervical third (where they are less evident) to the incisal edge.

❖ **Development lobes:** Three lobes that are formed by the development grooves: mesial, medial, and distal. They can divide the incisal edge and form the incisal mamelons.

❖ **Equatorial line:** The line of the major contour of the tooth crown, resulting from the union of all the humps. It passes through the areas of bigger convexity of the dental surfaces. It divides the crown into two parts: one retentive located cervically to the equatorial line, and one expulsive located occlusally to it.

With the aim of a schematic description of each of the already mentioned characteristics, I have tried to replicate one of each tooth of two anterior sectors, three superior and three inferior. They were made in wax, applying a stratification technique, and then photographed. The morphological characteristics allow the teeth to have a correct function. The primordial function of teeth is to accomplish a good masticatory process; they are formed for cutting, tearing and crushing food, but they also have other functions.

THE FUNCTIONS OF INCISORS AND CANINES

The functions of incisors, situated anteriorly, are to cut the food, enable articulated speech, support the lip, maintain an esthetic appearance, and aid mandible guidance during the final closing phase. They all have some common characteristics that can help us identify them: a relatively straight incisal edge with a curvature in distal, a relatively rectangular crown, three labial lobes (form the vestibular surface) and one palatal/lingual (form the cingulum), a crown outline more convex on the distal surface (except the inferior central incisors, which are symmetrical), the mesioincisal angles are more acute than the distal ones (except on the inferior central incisors) and the mesial contact areas located on the incisal third, while the distal ones are in between the incisal third and the middle third. They all have a wedge shape when viewed from proximal and an S-shaped lingual outline.

Canines have the function of cutting, piercing, or shearing food, supporting the lip and facial muscles, and functional protection due to their occlusal lateral guidance. They also have some common characteristics, which are: the presence of two incisal cusp ridges, being the mesial shorter than the distal one; the presence of a vertical labial ridge; they are the only teeth with just one cusp; the mesial contact areas are also located on the incisal third while the distal ones are in between the third and middle third; the crown outline is also more convex in distal than in mesial.

When viewed from proximal, they also have a wedge shape and an S-shaped lingual outline.[14]

TIP

The morphological characteristics allow the teeth to have a correct function. The primordial function of teeth is to accomplish a good masticatory process; they are formed for cutting, tearing, and crushing food, but they also have other functions. Anatomy is a way to understand internal teeth characteristics.

ANTEROSUPERIOR TEETH (FIG 4-14)

- **Superior central incisor** (Figs 4-15 to 4-17)

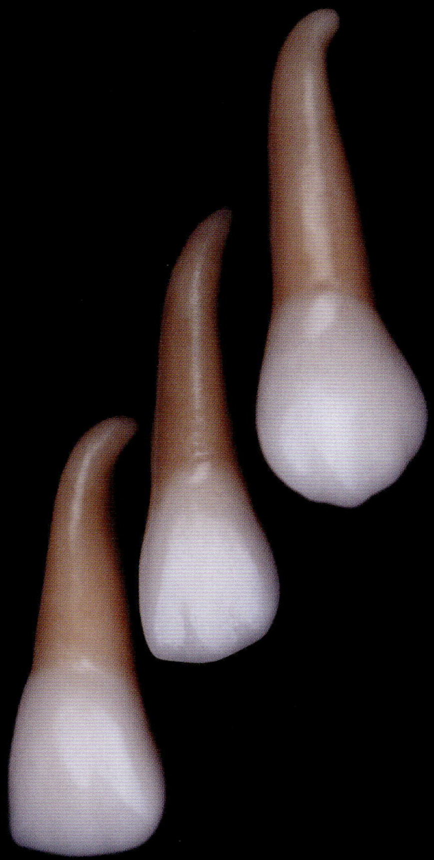

Fig 4-14
Photographs of anterosuperior teeth (11, 12, and 13) made of wax, applying a stratification technique.

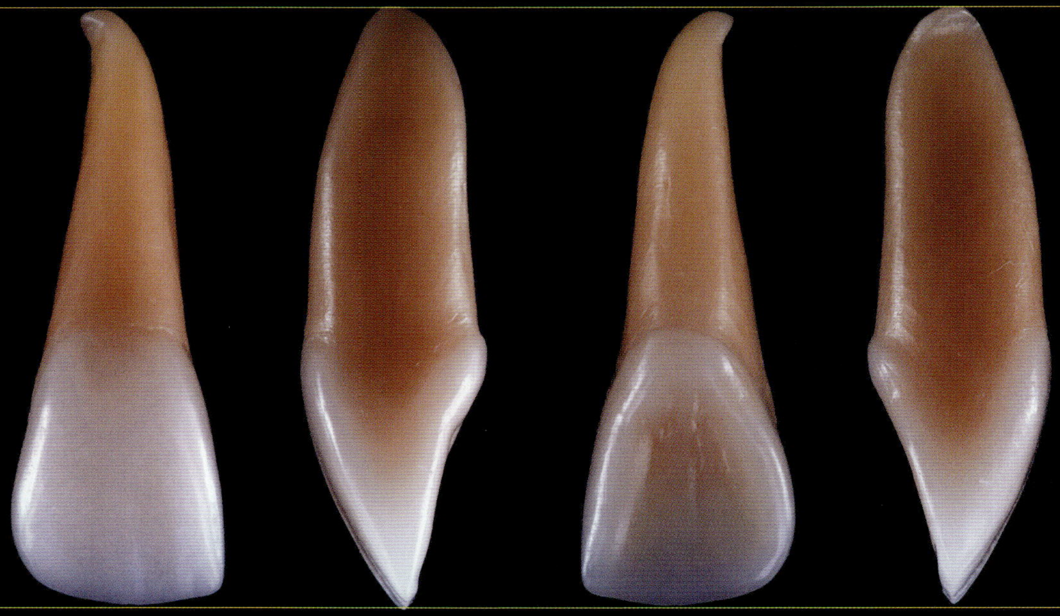

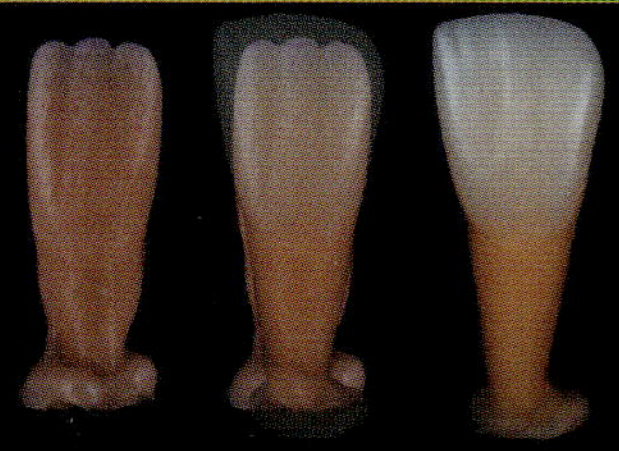

Fig 4-15
Photographs of tooth 11 (vestibular, mesial, palatal, and distal views). Stratification technique.

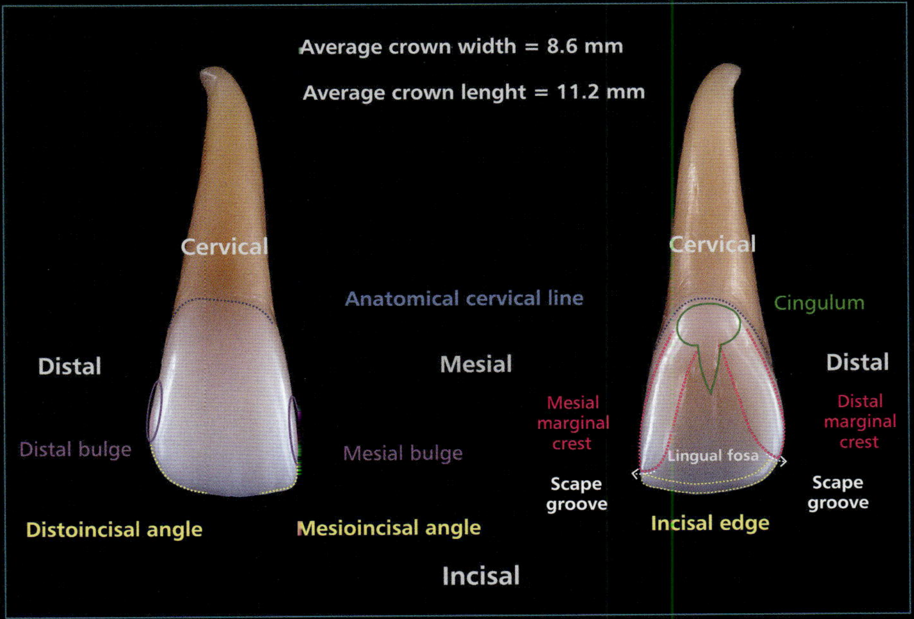

Fig 4-16
Tooth 11 (vestibular and palatal views). Scheme with basic tooth characteristics.

Tooth characteristics:

- Mesioincisal angle is a right angle
- Incisal edge closer to horizontal
- Mesial outline is flat
- Distal outline is more rounded
- Distal contact is more cervical than mesial one
- Larger shallow lingual fossa
- Distal marginal ridge more curved than mesial one

Fig 4-17
Tooth 11 (mesial and distal views). Scheme with basic tooth characteristics.

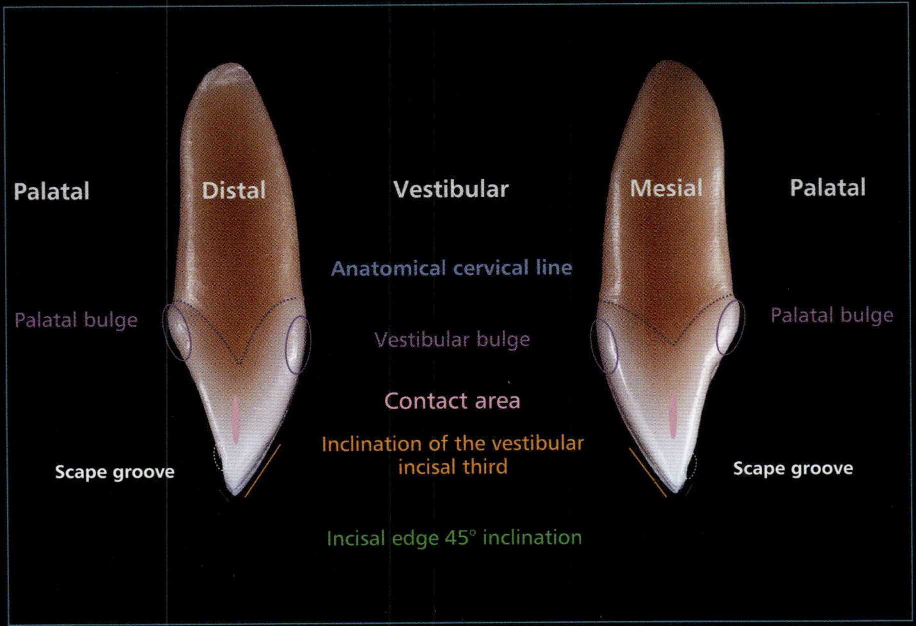

Superior lateral incisor (Figs 4-18 to 4-20)

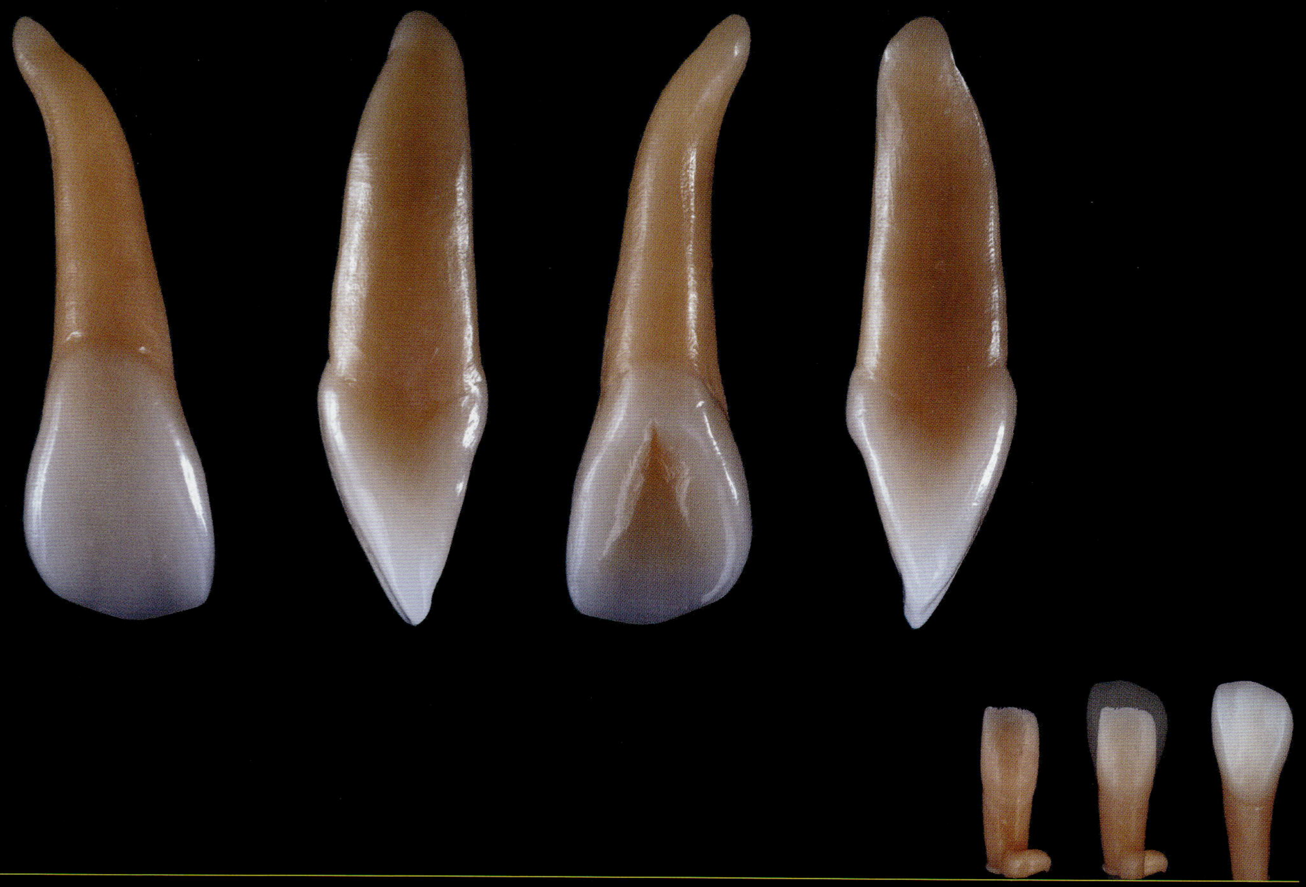

Fig 4-18
Tooth 12 (vestibular, mesial, palatal, and distal views). Stratification technique.

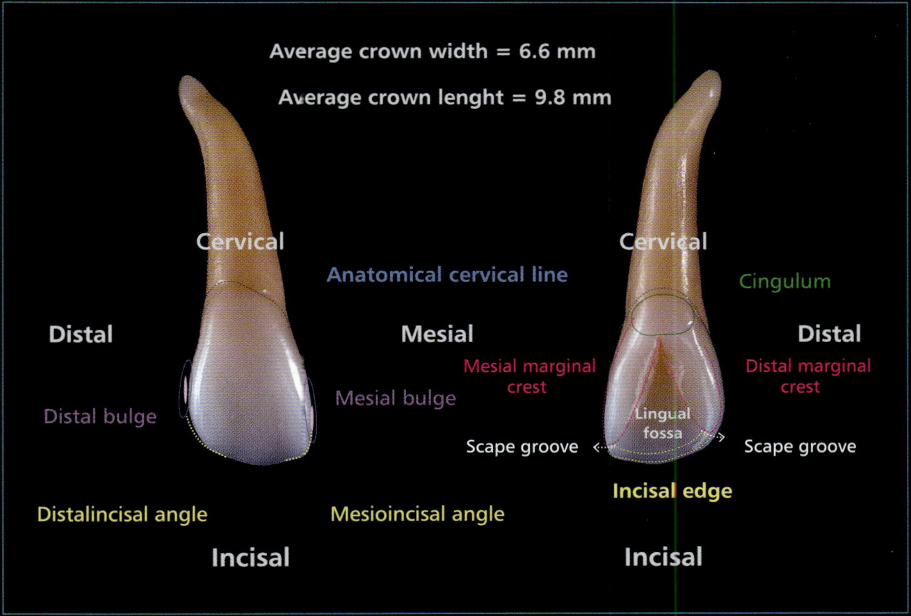

Fig 4-19
Tooth 12 (vestibular and palatal views). Scheme with basic tooth characteristics.

Tooth characteristics:

- Smaller crown, narrower cervically
- Mesioincisal angle is rounder than in the central incisor, but still straighter than the distal angle
- Distal outline is round
- Distal contact is near the middle third incisal edge toward cervical in distal
- Deep but small fossa

Fig 4-20
Tooth 12 (mesial and distal views). Scheme with basic tooth characteristics.

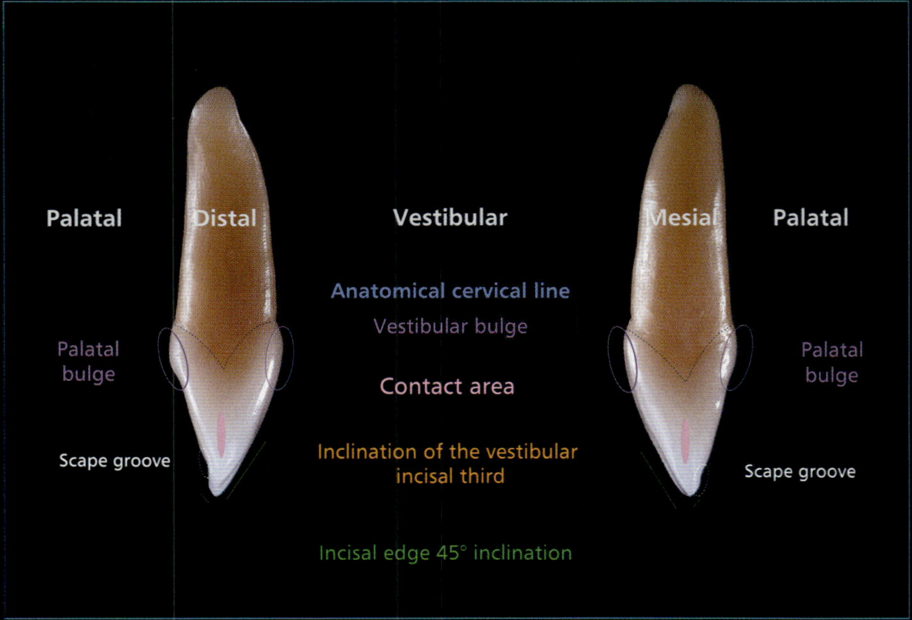

◆ **Superior canine** (Figs 4-21 to 4-23)

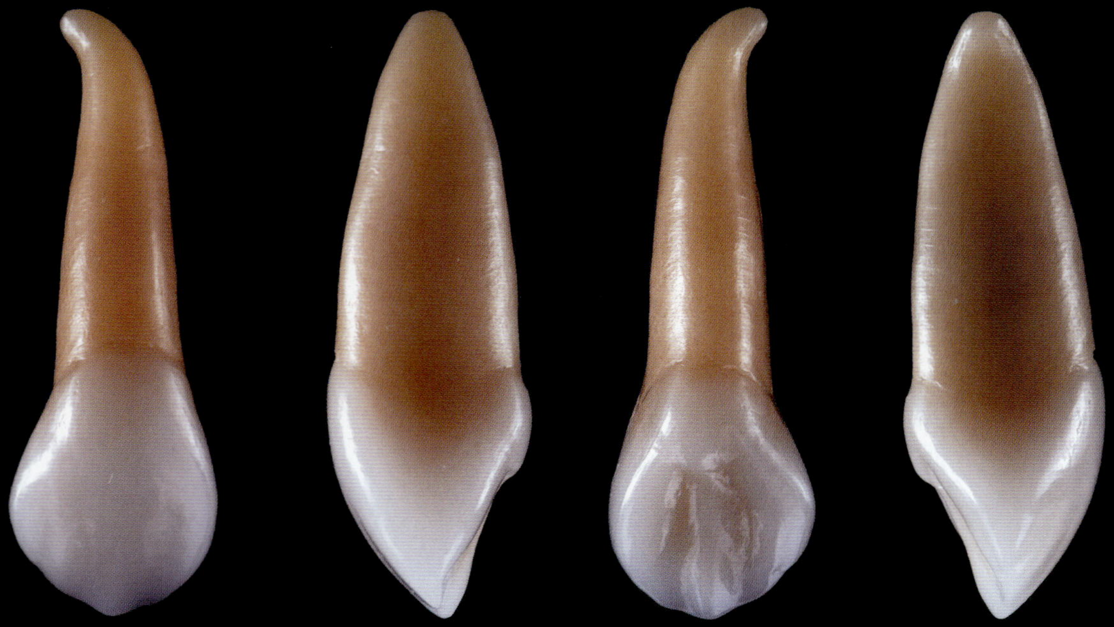

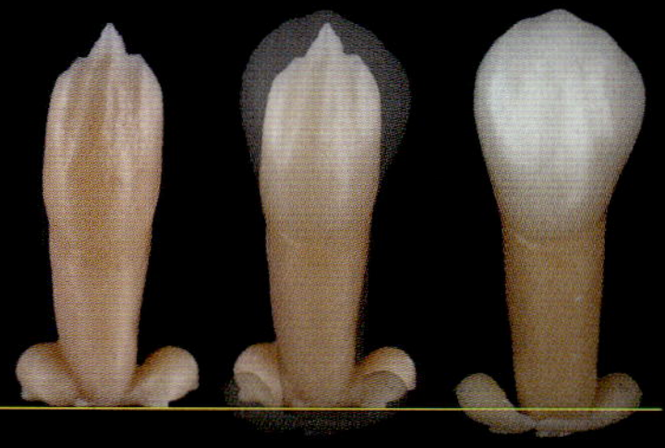

Fig 4-21
Tooth 13 (vestibular, mesial, palatal, and distal views). Stratification technique.

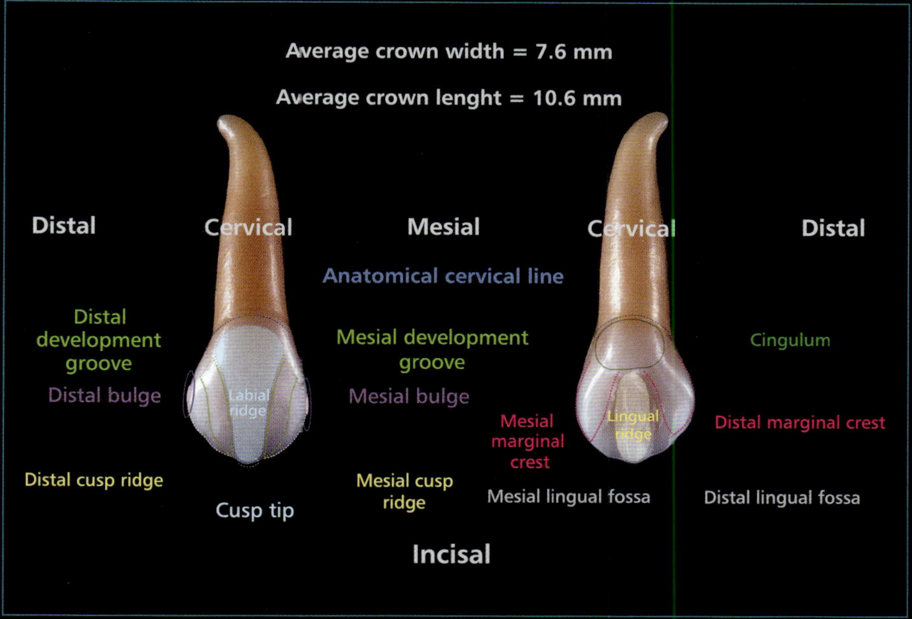

Fig 4-22
Tooth 13 (vestibular and palatal views). Scheme with basic tooth characteristics.

Tooth characteristics:

- They do not have mamelons, but they can have a notch on either cusp ridge
- The labial ridge is always vertical
- The distal contact area is more cervically positioned than the mesial one
- The crown outline is more convex on the distal than on the mesial
- The anatomy is more prominent in lingual (marginal crests and lingual ridge)

Fig 4-23
Tooth 13 (mesial and distal views). Scheme with basic tooth characteristics.

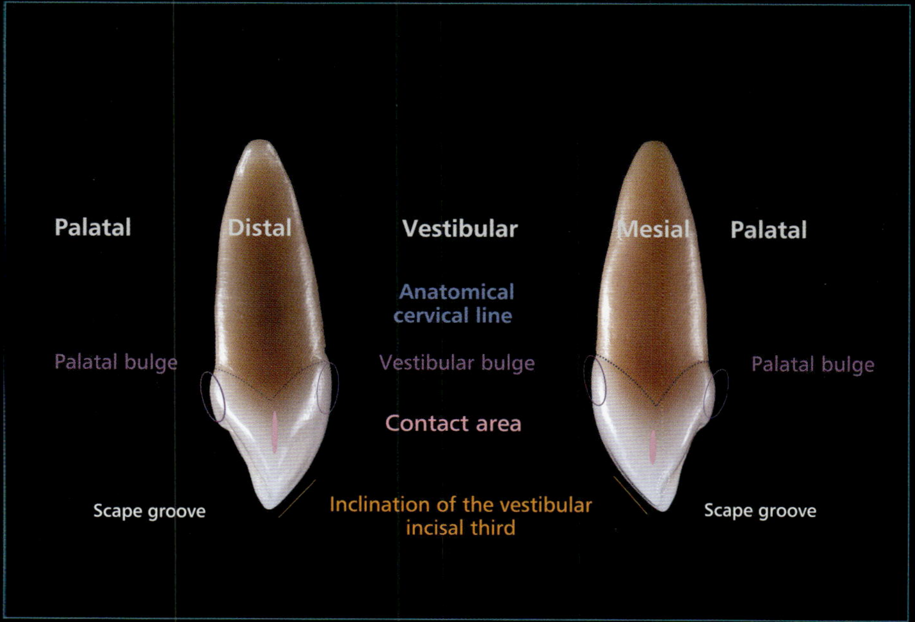

ANTERIO-INFERIOR TEETH (FIG 4-24)

◆ **Inferior central incisor** (Figs 4-25 to 4-27)

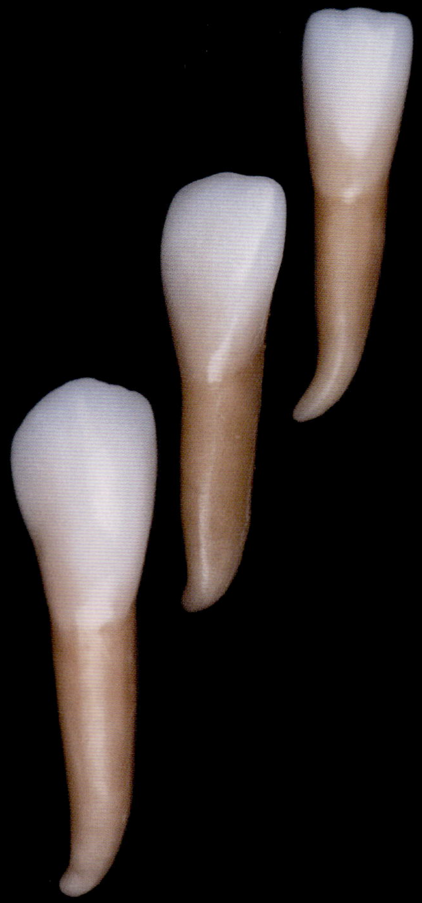

Fig 4-24
Teeth 41, 42, and 43 wax-ups, applying a stratification technique.

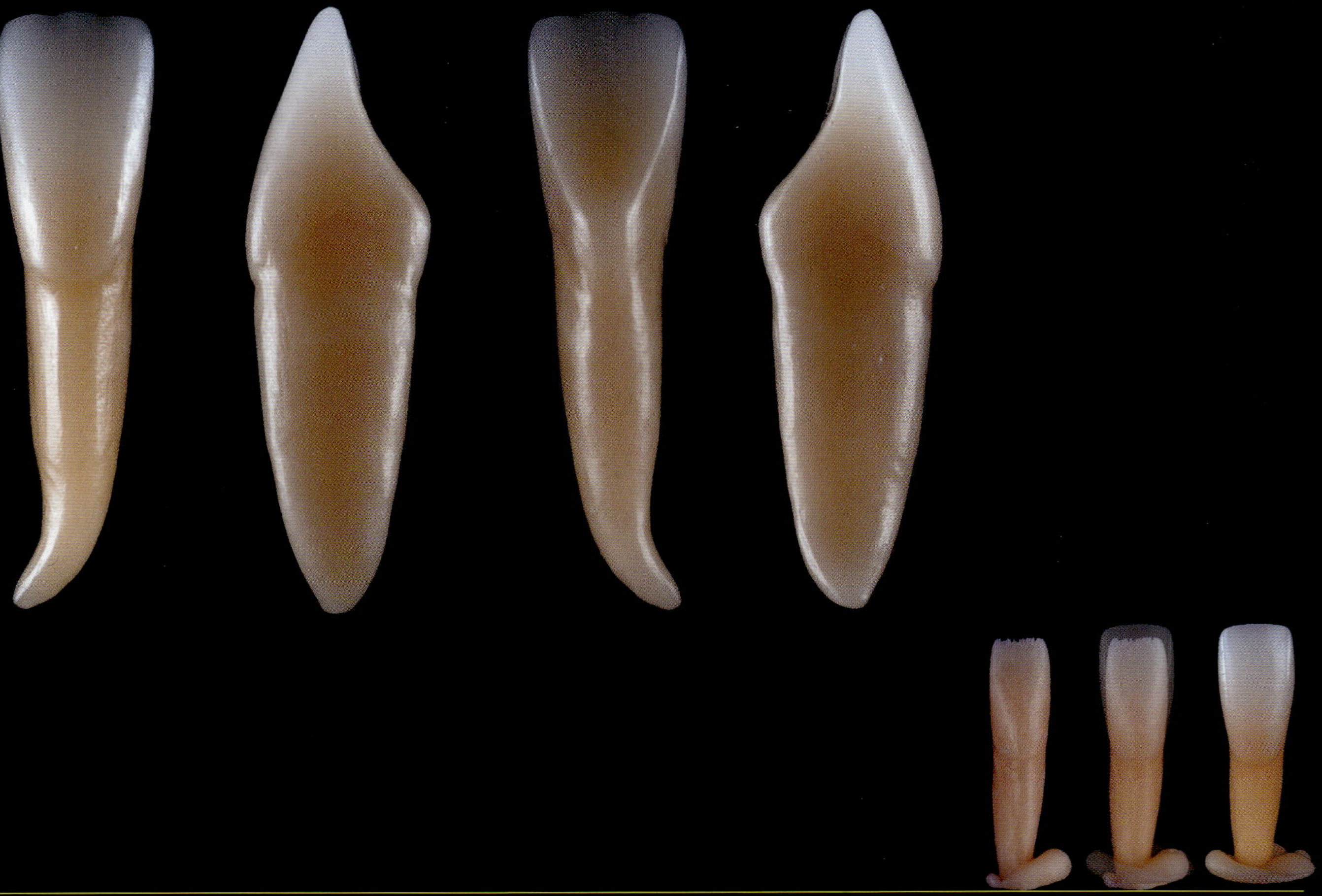

Fig 4-25
Tooth 41 (vestibular, mesial, palatal, and distal views). Stratification technique.

Fig 4-26
Tooth 41 (vestibular and palatal views). Scheme with basic tooth characteristics.

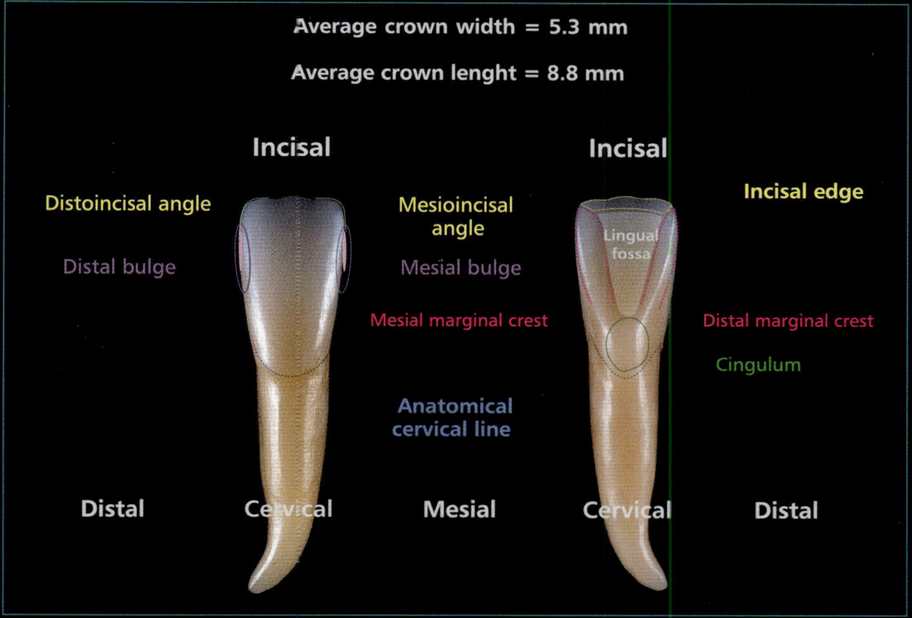

Tooth characteristics:

- It is the narrowest crown in the mouth
- It is the only symmetrical tooth in the mouth
- Mesial and distal contacts are at the same level (incisal third)
- Mesioincisal and distoincisal angles are right angles
- Straight mesial and distal outlines, becoming narrower toward cervical
- Facial surface is smooth but can have two shallow development depressions
- The lingual fossa is barely visible, smooth, without grooves, and shallow, slightly concave in the middle and incisal thirds

Fig 4-27
Tooth 41 (mesial and distal views). Scheme with basic tooth characteristics.

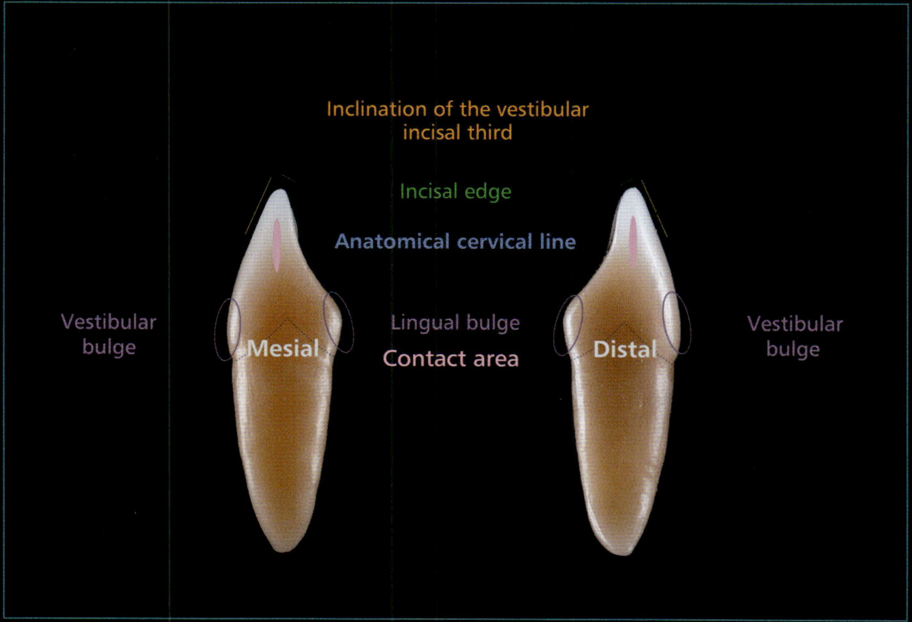

◆ **Inferior lateral incisor** (Figs 4-28 to 4-30)

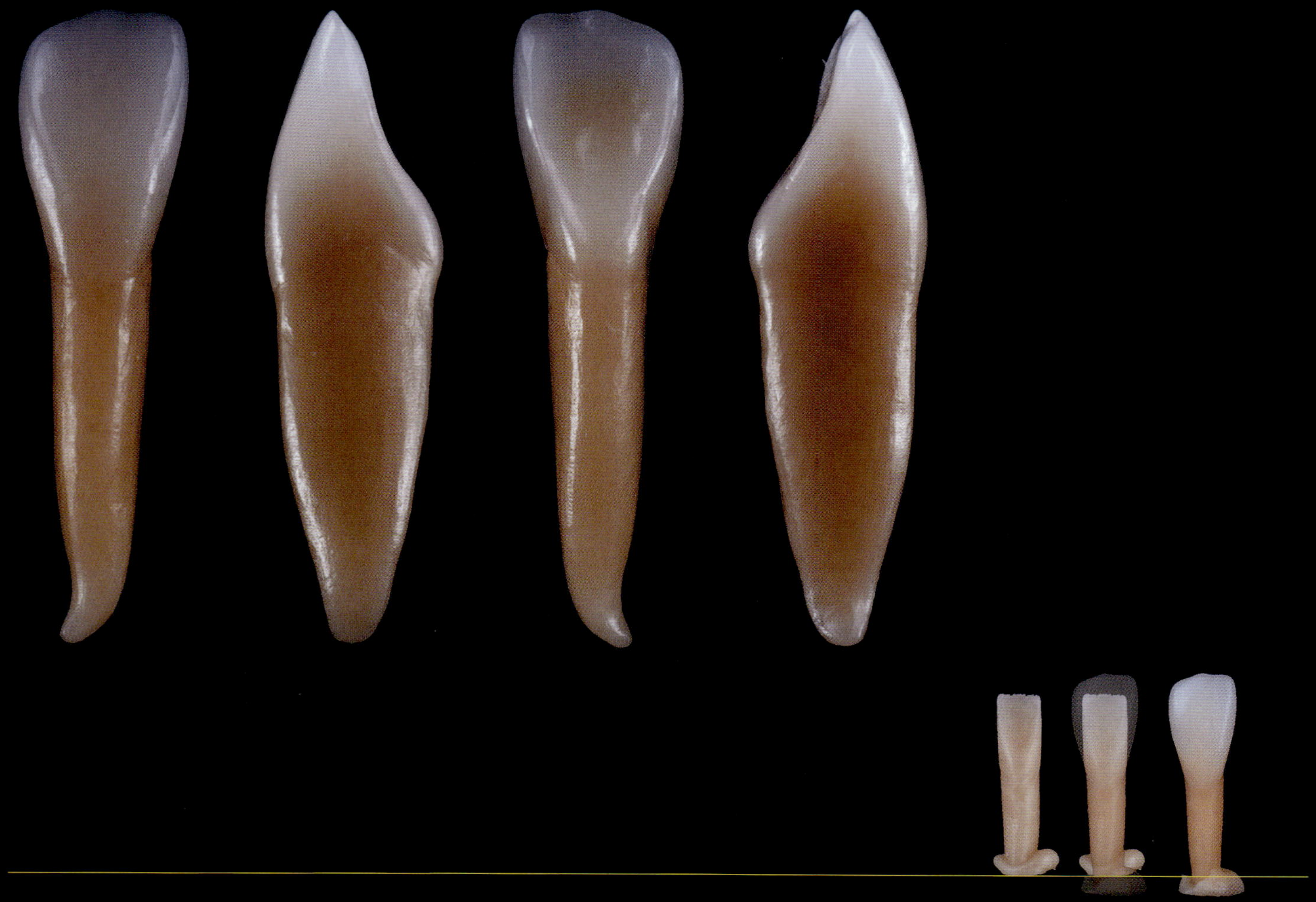

Fig 4-28
Tooth 42 (vestibular, mesial, palatal, and distal views). Stratification technique.

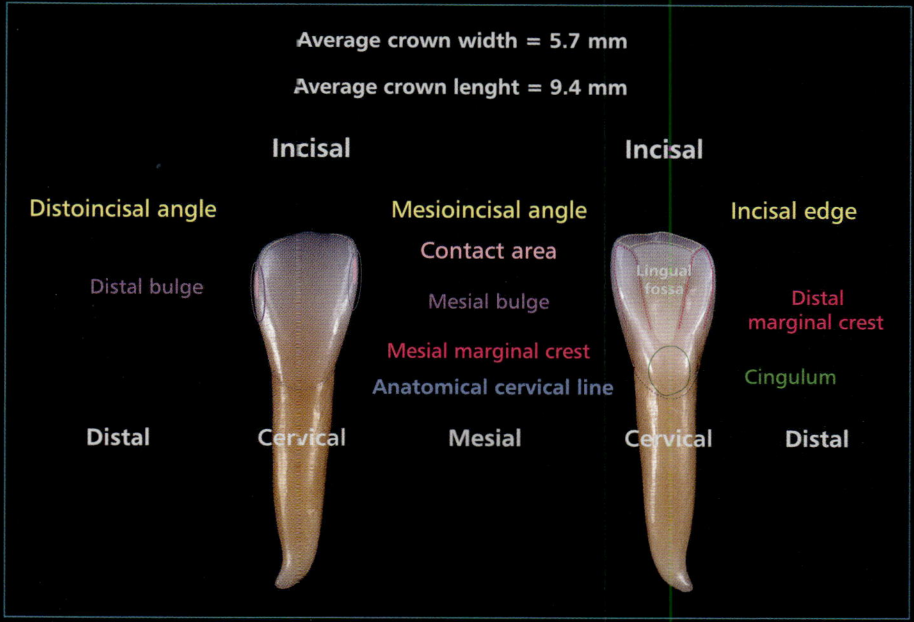

Fig 4-29
Tooth 42 (vestibular and palatal views). Scheme with basic tooth characteristics.

Fig 4-30
Tooth 42 (mesial and distal views). Scheme with basic tooth characteristics.

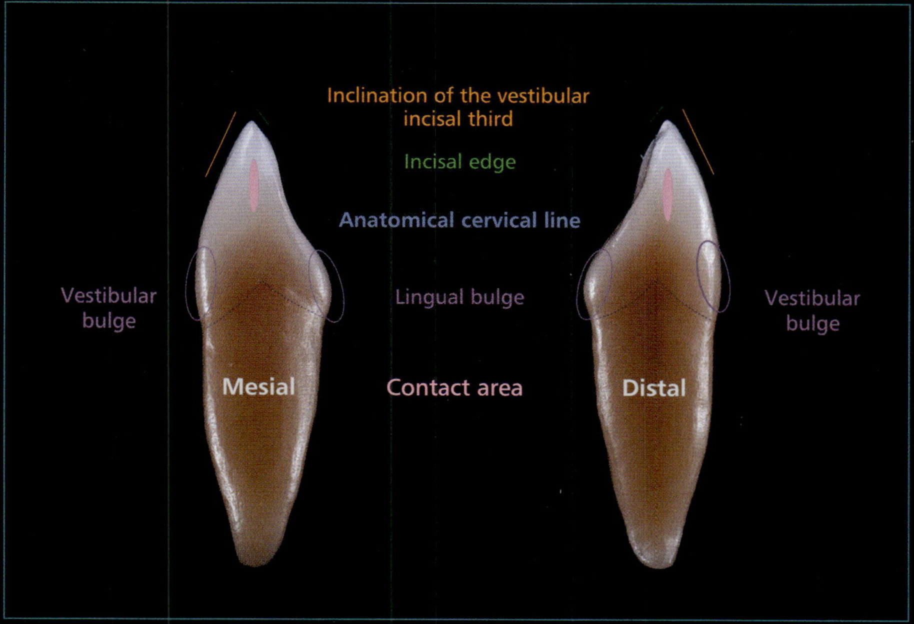

Tooth characteristics:

- The crown is slightly wider than the mandibular central incisor
- Distal crown outline is rounded, and the mesial one is straight
- Mesial proximal contact is more incisal
- Distal proximal contact is in a more cervical position
- Larger than mandibular central incisor
- Facial surface is smooth but can have two shallow development depressions in the incisal third
- The lingual fossa is barely visible, smooth, without grooves, and shallow, slightly concave in the middle and incisal thirds

◆ Inferior canine (Figs 4-31 to 4-33)

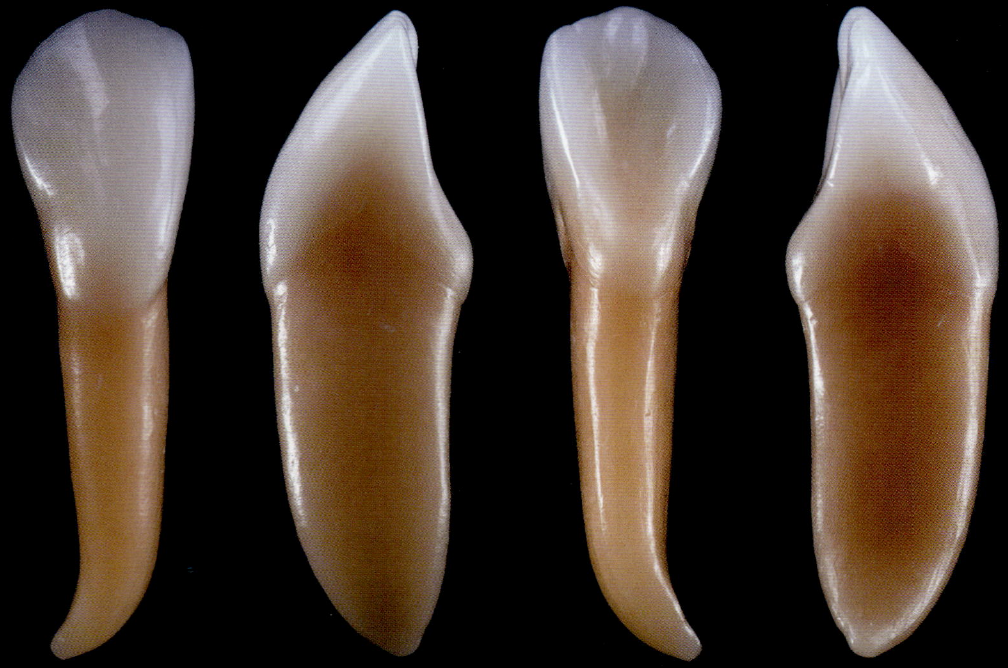

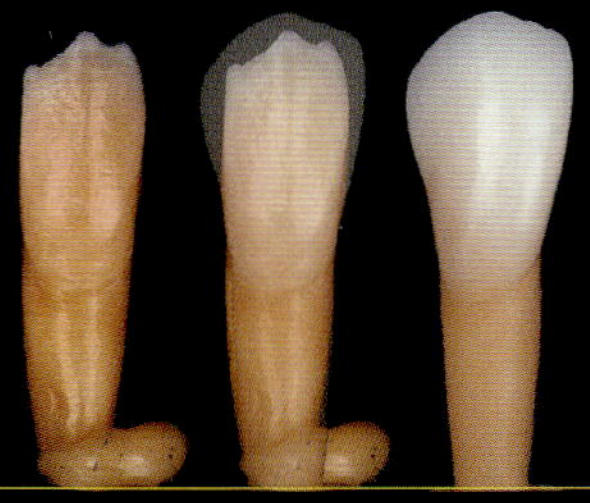

Fig 4-31
Tooth 43 (vestibular, mesial, palatal, and distal views). Stratification technique.

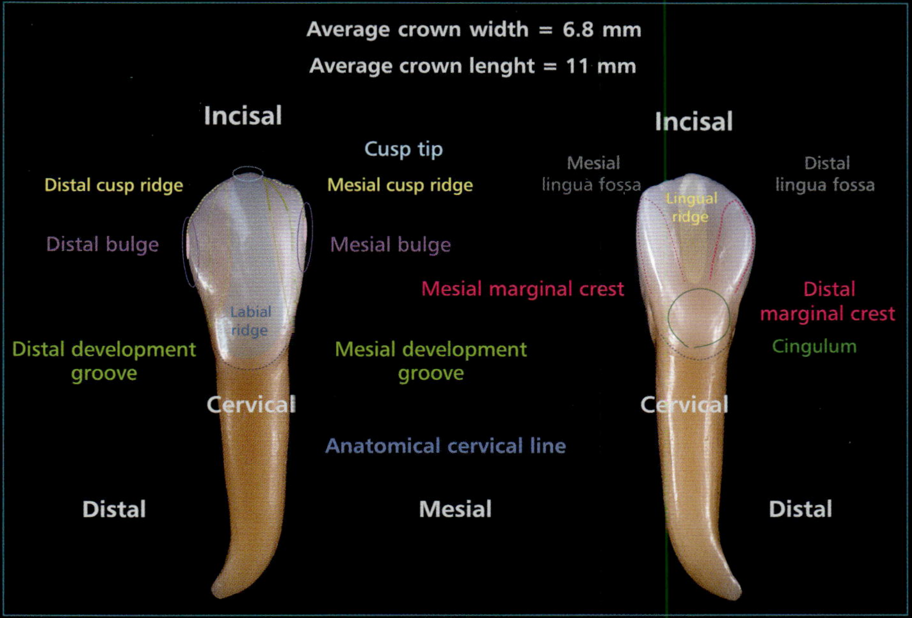

Fig 4-32
Tooth 43 (vestibular and palatal views). Scheme with basic tooth characteristics.

Tooth characteristics:

- Crown appears narrower mesiodistally and longer than the maxillary canine
- Cusp angle is obtuse, so less pronounced
- Distal outline is more convex on the distal than on the mesial surface, where it is almost flat
- Mesial cusp ridge is shorter than the distal one and is almost horizontal
- The mesial proximal contact is more incisal than the distal one
- Less pronounced labial ridge than the maxillary canine
- Lingual ridge, marginal ridges, and fossa are less prominent than in the maxillary canine

Fig 4-33
Tooth 43 (mesial and distal views). Scheme with basic tooth characteristics.

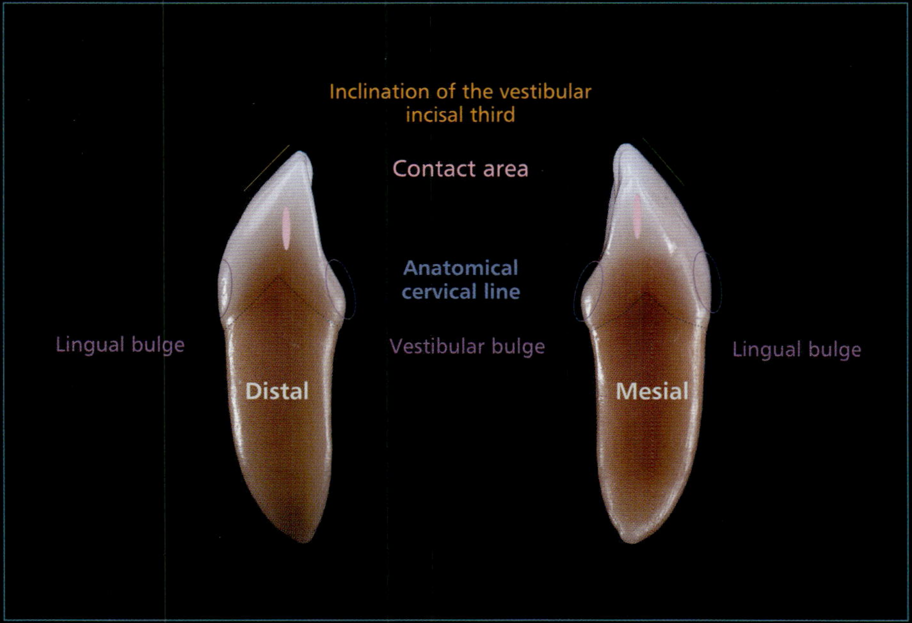

PRIMARY ANATOMY

Teeth shape: oval/triangular/squared (Fig 4-34)

Dental esthetics is a science based on the general taste of society or culture, and both dentist and patient must discuss which kind of esthetic is the most adequate for the case.

Dental morphology is unique for each person, like a fingerprint. Thus, there is a huge variation of tooth shapes in nature. Throughout this huge variation of dental anatomy, there has been much research to discover common features in esthetically pleasant teeth arrangements and shapes.[15]

In 1914 Williams concluded that human teeth could be grouped and classified into three principal shapes: oval, triangular, and square, and according to the author, the shape of the maxillary central incisor is more esthetically integrated when related to the patient facial shape.[16] It has also been stated that the different tooth shapes can be related to the patient's gender, personality, and age.[17–19]

Philip Hallawell developed a concept named "Visagism," which involves the creation of a customized personal image that expresses a person's sense of identity. It makes it possible to determine which emotions and personality traits patients wish to express through their appearance. The smile is a crucial esthetic parameter that influences appearance. The author stated that with the visagism concept, the dentist could design a smile that blends the patient's emotions, physical aspects, and personality.[20]

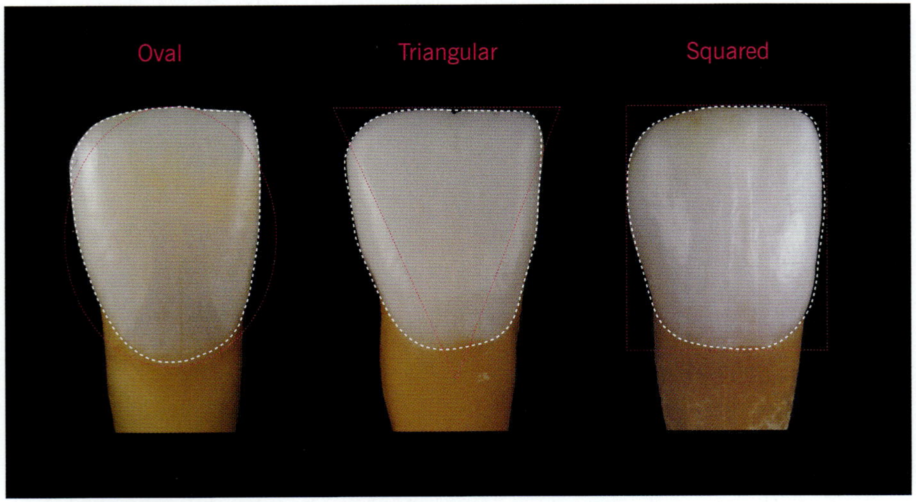

Fig 4-34
Three major groups of tooth shapes: oval, triangular, and squared.

REMEMBER

When restoring one tooth, it is easy to find which shape to follow because we will always replicate the opposite tooth present in the arch. But when restoring several teeth, we can find ourselves in a situation where we do not have any natural morphological reference. In these cases, we should use old photographs and old cast models of the patient to determine the natural morphology.

When we want to reproduce the natural shape of the patient's teeth, it is crucial to observe the remaining untouched teeth and make an exhaustive planification of the future restorations. The first anatomic characteristic that we should consider is the basic tooth shape. As said before, there are three basic tooth shapes: oval, triangular, and sqaure, and they can have innumerable variations.
Vertical, horizontal, inclined, straight, and curved lines can interact in infinite ways to create the diversity of natural tooth shapes. The shape of the maxillary central incisors plays a major role in dental esthetics because of their prominent position in the mouth. The maxillary lateral incisors are associated with intellectual and emotional aspects of the personality, while canines normally express aggressiveness, ambition, and dynamism.

Besides all of this information, this cannot serve in any way as a specific determinant for the definition of the final tooth shape, and the communication with the patient is of major importance. We should always listen to their desires and tastes.[21]

SECONDARY ANATOMY

Macrotexture

The convexities and concavities of the teeth surfaces greatly affect how they are visually perceived. The macrotexture refers to their presence, dividing the vestibular surface through these different concavities and convexities. We can modify these characteristics to create the illusion of larger or narrower teeth, which can greatly help restore esthetics.

When we do it, we will create optical illusions of size and shape that are different from reality, affecting the light reflection on the teeth surface, thus altering how the tooth is visually perceived. It is important to note that shadows create depth, light creates prominences, vertical lines accent length, and horizontal lines accent width.[22–25]

VERTICAL MACROTEXTURE

Line angles (Fig 4-35)

These represent the edges of two dental surfaces and divide a tooth crown. They show the transition of the vestibular surface to the interproximal surface and are the reflection area of light in the tooth surface. We can modify the perception of tooth size by changing its position.[22] When more separated, they create the optical illusion of a wider tooth because the reflection area of light is bigger. If they are closer, the tooth will appear narrower because the reflection area of light will be smaller.

When we need to alter the tooth size, we can alter these lines, using a pencil to mark them, and then facilitate the visual perception of the needed alteration to achieve a better esthetic result. It would help to make these alterations with a medium grain disk or with fine-grained burs at low speed.

Lobes and development grooves (Fig 4-36)

All the tooth crowns develop from lobes. In incisors and canines, crowns develop from four lobes: three vestibular lobes (mesial, central, and distal, forming three incisal mamelons) and one lingual lobe forming the cingulum area.

The development grooves are formed during tooth development, and they are located between the three lobes. There are two per tooth and are named according to their location (mesial or distal). They are wider in incisal narrowing toward the cervical third, giving a V-shape to these grooves.

The macrotexture refers to this division of the tooth in lobes and development grooves on the buccal surface of teeth, which divide the surface with concavities and convexities that can be more or less pronounced or even inexistent. They are normally more prominent in younger teeth and disappear with time for mechanical or chemical reasons.[21]

The distal development groove is usually the longest.

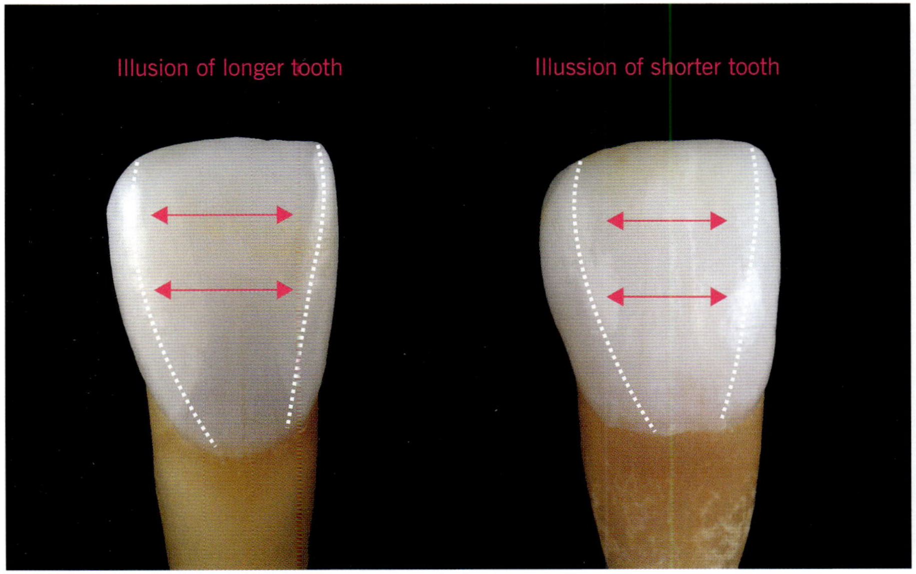

Fig 4-35
Schematic representation of the line angles. On the left, we can see that the closer the lines, the narrower the tooth appears. On the right, the opposite occurs, as the more separated the lines, the wider the tooth appears.

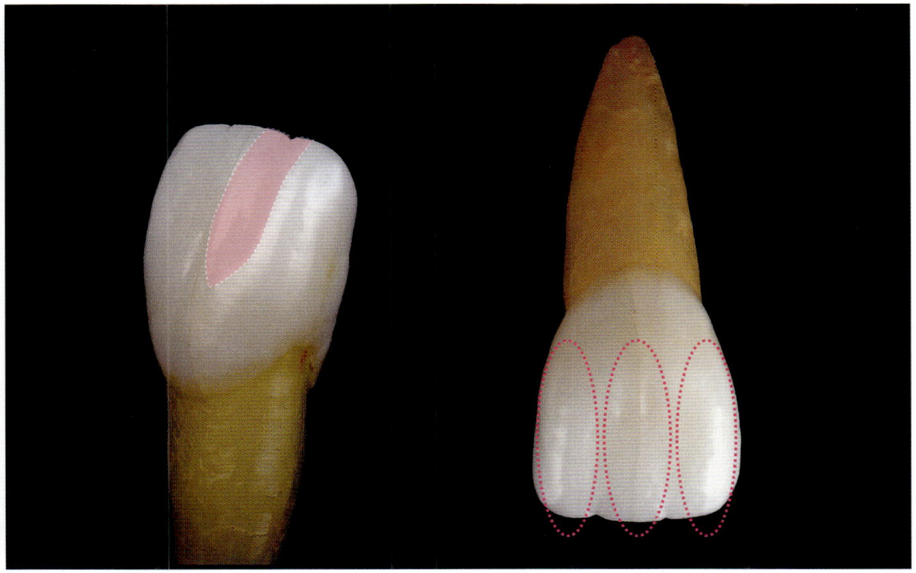

Fig 4-36
Schematic representation of the lobes and development grooves on the vestibular surface of anterior teeth.

HORIZONTAL MACROTEXTURE

This is more evident in the cervical third and in its transition to the middle third. It consists of two or three small, very smooth grooves between the transitional angular lines (Fig 4-37).

TERTIARY ANATOMY

Microtexture

The enamel surface is characterized by the presence of numerous discrete irregularities, which are the horizontal and vertical texture of the teeth, known as the microtexture.

We can map their presence with the help of silver or graphite powder; it can also be helpful to refer to black and white pictures for its correct determination. Its presence can be more pronounced (normally in younger teeth) or not (Fig 4-38); there are even cases where it is totally absent. Normally it diminishes its pronunciation or even disappears with the aging process of the patient due to mechanical or chemical causes (brushing, masticatory process, acid presence).[22]

It is very important to reproduce them in case its presence in adjacent teeth is evident; otherwise, we can completely compromise the esthetical outcome of our restoration. A natural result will always be our goal, and we have to plan accordingly, considering the tooth that we are reproducing, the adjacent tooth, the homologous tooth, and the patient's age.[6,21,22]

REMEMBER

As a horizontal texture, we have the perikymata characterized by numerous minute horizontal ridges on the enamel surface. They are formed by overlapping layers of enamel during tooth formation and are closer in the cervical third of the crown than in the incisal third. The horizontal texture is more discrete and consists of very small horizontal ridges, irregularly distributed on the enamel surface.

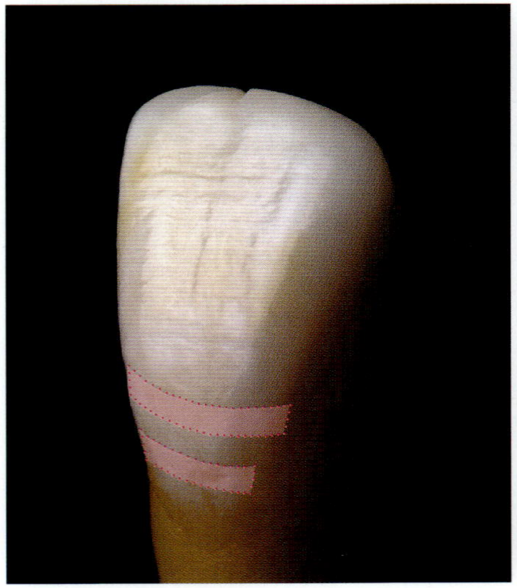

Fig 4-37
Schematic representation of the horizontal cervical grooves that exist between the transitional angular lines (horizontal macrotexture).

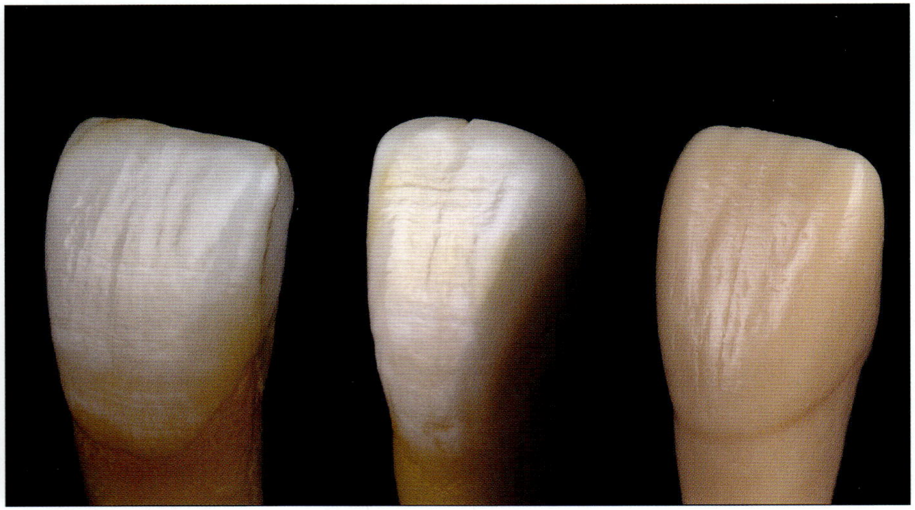

Fig 4-38
Microtexture. In this picture we can see on the left and center two natural teeth with a very rich microtexture. The tooth on the right is a wax-up attempting to reproduce the microtexture.

TEETH POSITION AND GINGIVAL ARCHITECTURE – ESTHETIC CONSIDERATIONS

It is important to mention that we must not think of teeth as separated entities. Although each has its own characteristics, they are part of the dental arch, and they must be aligned and positioned properly to achieve an esthetic and functional smile.

In the past, esthetics and function were thought of as two separate entities; in fact, the esthetic optimization usually created a functional compromise, as when we idealize the functional aspect, we sacrifice the esthetic one. Nowadays, functional prosthetic rehabilitation must represent the initial point to achieve optimal esthetics. To give a natural appearance to our restorations is for them not only to be indistinguishable from the natural dentition, but also to accomplish their correct function, which can only be accomplished with exhaustive planning. We must always think about which ideal definitive treatment we want to achieve and start planning what treatments we need to achieve it.[21]

From another point of view, esthetics is the science of beauty and harmony, and its meaning is extremely subjective and relative. There is nothing quite as personal as each patient's own perception of esthetics. It is conditioned by several factors, ie, social, psychological, and cultural parameters, besides being connected with age, which determines that it can vary from person to person.

However, we know that basic dental esthetics depend on various esthetically relevant criteria and their interactions. This means that the esthetic rehabilitation of a smile must be strictly planned, considering those several parameters. In this chapter, we will describe some of the most important intraoral ones that the dentist and dental technician should always consider.

It is very important to refer that, besides that the ideal dental composition is based on valid universal criteria, the esthetic optimization of each case must be personalized and defined accordingly with the preferences of each patient

Midline (Fig 4-39)

This is the imaginary vertical line separating the two central incisors that is perpendicular to the patient's horizon, which is normally the interpupillary line.[26–30] It should be placed in the facial midline whenever possible (70% of patients) or, in cases of asymmetrical patients, right in the middle of the smile using as reference the papilla or the labial frenum, to coincide with the symmetry of the dental composition.

It is known that the inferior midline does not coincide with the superior one in 75% of the cases; this means that we should never take the inferior midline as a reference for the establishment of the superior one.[26] Any slanting of it will disturb the dental symmetry and composition. It will result in a very unpleasant esthetic result, so it is important to make sure that it is strictly perpendicular to the patient's horizon.[6,24,29 30–33]

Smile line (Fig 4-40)

This is is an imaginary line running from the incisal edges of the anterior maxillary teeth and the buccal cusp tips of the posterior teeth that should follow the curvature of the lower lip.[31,34] It gives us the curve of Spee and should be perpendicular to the facial midline and anteroposteriorly curved to give the appearance of a younger smile. It must be parallel to the pupillary line, and it is more pronounced in women than in men.

Sometimes, due to abrasion, erosion, attrition, periodontitis, altered patterns of eruption, or poor-quality dentistry, the canines and posterior teeth present themselves longer than central incisors. This can result in a reverse smile line, which will not be esthetically harmonic and is associated with occlusal malfunction, loss of vertical dimension, and the aging process.[24]

Incisor proportion (Fig 4-41)

When treating patients with missing or badly damaged maxillary incisors, it is crucial to determine their shape, size, and position to achieve a functional and esthetical result.[27,35] The relative dimensions of teeth seem to be among the most objective dental esthetic criteria because they can be easily and physically controlled.

However, the ideal tooth dimensions remain difficult to obtain due to individual variations and incisal tooth wear.[36] Normally the width of the teeth is a measure that remains constant, while the length can vary considerably with the aging process (abrasion of the incisal edges). Then it is easy for us to find the ideal dental proportion for the teeth.

The proportion of the central incisor is achieved by calculating the width-to-length ratio of each central incisor. Harmonic proportions are essential when clinicians want to achieve an esthetic smile. Although almost every study about dental proportion concluded that the ideal width of the central incisor is between 75% and 80% of its length, it is confirmed that it can vary according to sex and race.[35,37–40]

> **TIP**
>
> The measurement of the width of the tooth must be made mesiodistally and perpendicular to the long axis of the central incisor.

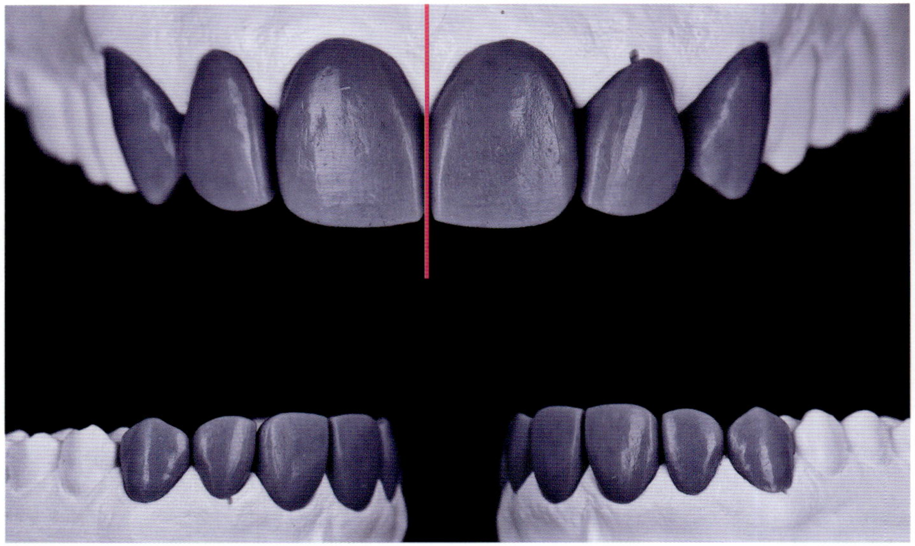

Fig 4-39
Schematic representation of the midline position.

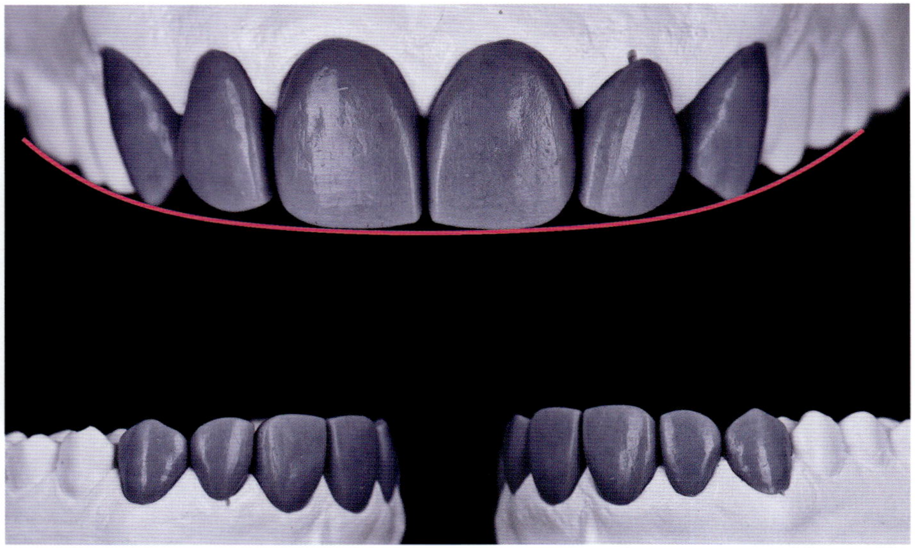

Fig 4-40
Schematic representation of the smile line position.

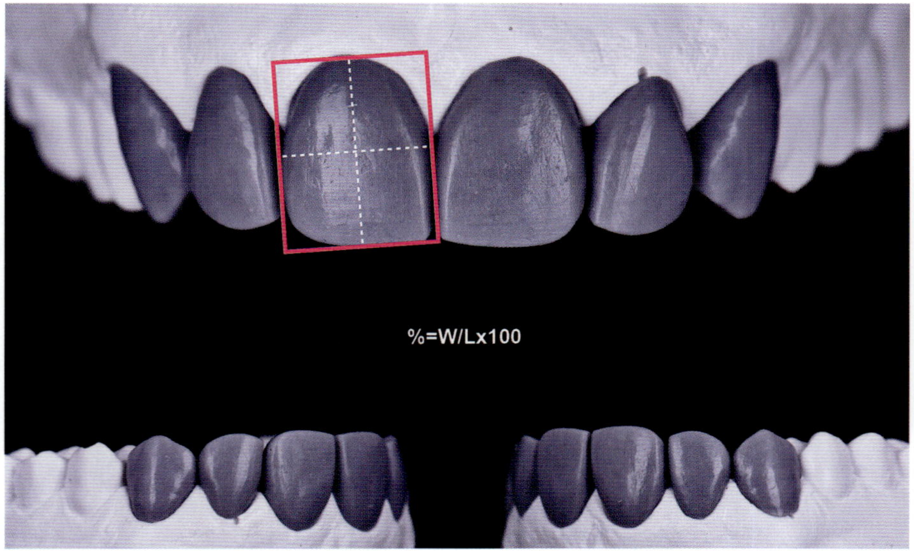

Fig 4-41
Schematic representation of how to calculate the incisor position. The mathematical formula to calculate is: length/width ×100.

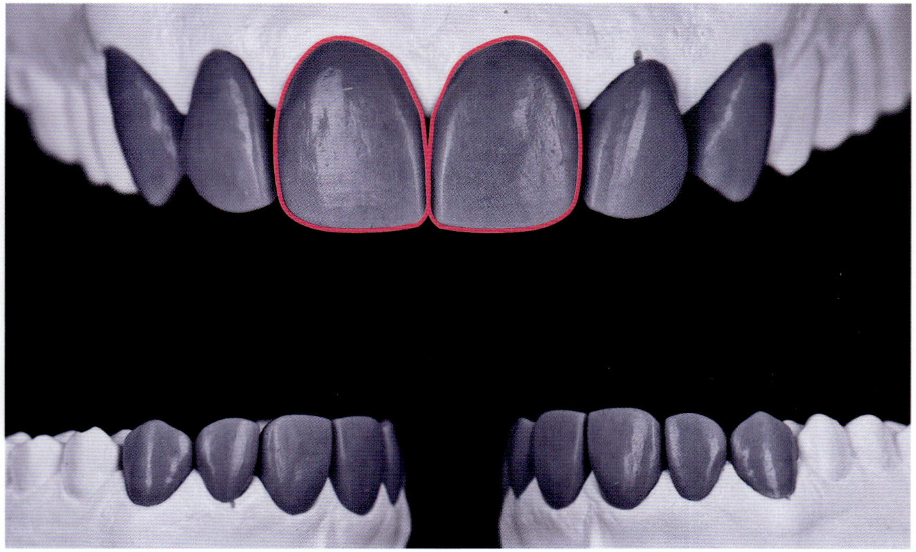

Fig 4-42
Schematic representation of central incisors' dominance and symmetry.

Symmetry and dominance of central incisors (Fig 4-42)

One factor determining the success of the esthetic treatment is the symmetry and domain of the central incisors, which should normally have the same shape and size and must be a mirror image of each other. Symmetry is the harmonious arrangement of several elements with respect to each other, which can be observed on both sides of a central axis. When the object presents a mirror image on both sides of the center, it can be said to have "static" symmetry; if it has two opposed halves very similar but not identical, it is said to have a "dynamic" symmetry. When we consider the whole smile, these minor irregularities and deviations will give it a more natural appearance.[6,41]

> **TIP**
>
> Dynamic symmetry is acceptable for the rest of the teeth but not for central incisors.

Regarding dominance, Lombardi stated that, "Just as unit is the prime requisite of a good composition, dominance is the prime requisite to provide unity." The central incisor must be larger enough than the lateral incisor to dominate the composition and bring order and coherence.[27]

Proportion (Fig 4-43)

In order to search for the best esthetic result, several authors have proposed the use of mathematic proportions to help establish the tooth forms and sizes.

In 1973, Lombardi proposed that the esthetic was optimized when the central to lateral width and lateral to canine width were proportionally repeated when the patient is viewed from the front. He introduced the use of the "golden proportion" in dentistry. He concluded that the lateral incisor was 62% of the central incisor, and the visible part of the canine in a frontal view was 62% of the lateral incisor.[27] In 1978, Levin revised and developed the golden proportion concept and recommended the golden proportion for optimal esthetic achievement. He developed a special caliper that always extend to the golden proportion, which was suggested to be useful in designing a proportional dental rehabilitation. He also developed a grid to evaluate what is esthetically wrong in the anterior proportional relationship and guide the clinicians in the dental rehabilitation of the anterior dental sector from central incisors to first pre-molar.[41]

Preston in 1993 reported that the golden proportion between maxillary central and lateral incisors was found in only 17% of the casts he studied when viewed from the front.[42]

Ward in 2001 proposed the use of the Recurring Esthetic Dental (RED) proportion, in which he states that the idea of a continuous proportion or repeated ratio as defined by Lombardi opens up the idea of using a continuous proportion not limited by the 62% proportion. The RED proportion states that the proportion of the successive widths of the teeth as viewed from the frontal should remain constant as one moves distally. The author states that although he prefers a RED proportion of approximately 70%, the RED proportion should be modified to fit the face, skeletal structure, and general body type of the patient.[43]

Snow considered a bilateral analysis of apparent individual tooth width as a percentage of the total apparent width of the six anterior teeth. He proposed the golden percentage where the proportional width of each tooth should be: 10% for each canine, 15% for each lateral incisor, and 25% for each central incisor, of the total distance across the anterior segment to achieve an esthetically pleasing smile.[40]

Fayyad et al compared the results of the three methods (golden proportion, RED proportion, and golden percentage) and concluded that only the golden percentage presented consistent results relative to the width of teeth, although with some deviations in the percentage values for each tooth (23% central incisor, 15% lateral incisor and 12% canine), which may be due to ethnic differences.[44,45]

Vestibular axial inclination of anterior teeth (Fig 4-44)

This refers to the direction of anterior teeth when they are related to the vertical midline. The long axis of anterior teeth in an esthetic smile follows a progression as the teeth move away from the midline, and when compared with it, they have a mesioinclination toward incisal and a distoinclination toward apical. This situation is gradually accentuated from the central incisors to the canines.[24]

> **TIP**
>
> This axial inclination should be symmetrical with the contralateral teeth, especially central incisors.

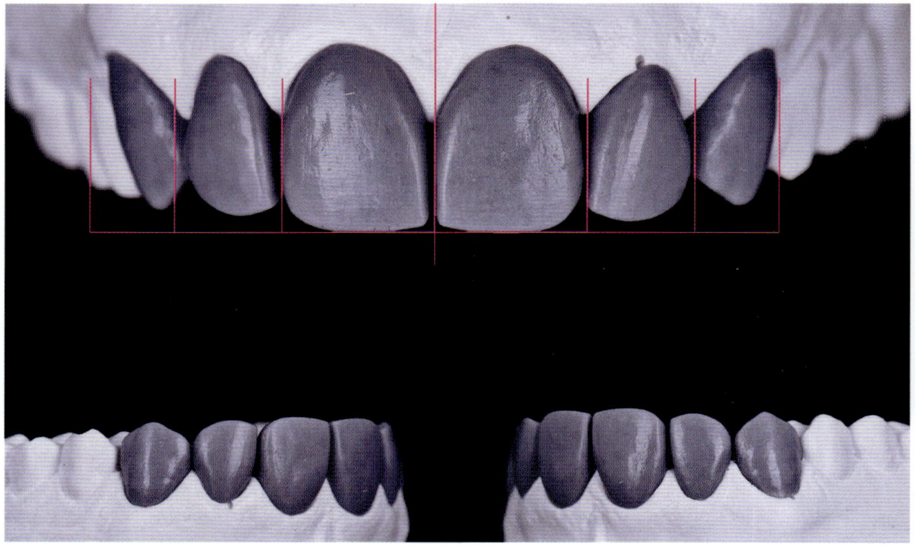

Fig 4-43
Schematic representation of dental proportion from canine to canine.

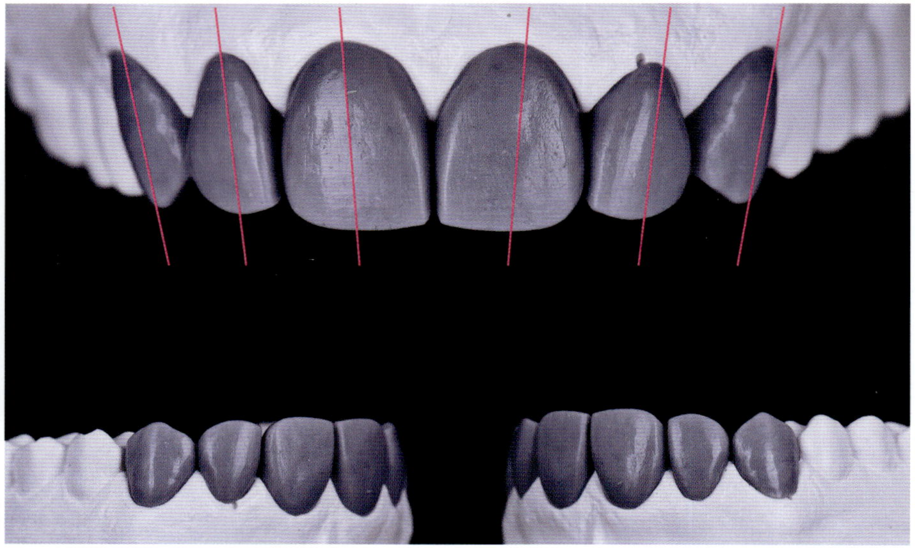

Fig 4-44
Schematic representation of axial inclination of anterior teeth.

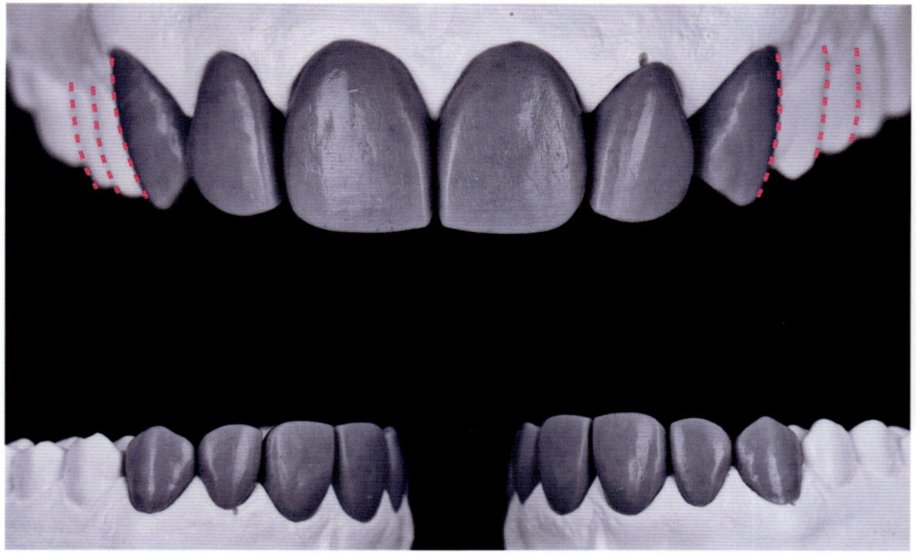

Fig 4-45
Schematic representation of axial inclination of posterior teeth. Here we can see how the inclination of the canine gives the inclination to all the posterior teeth.

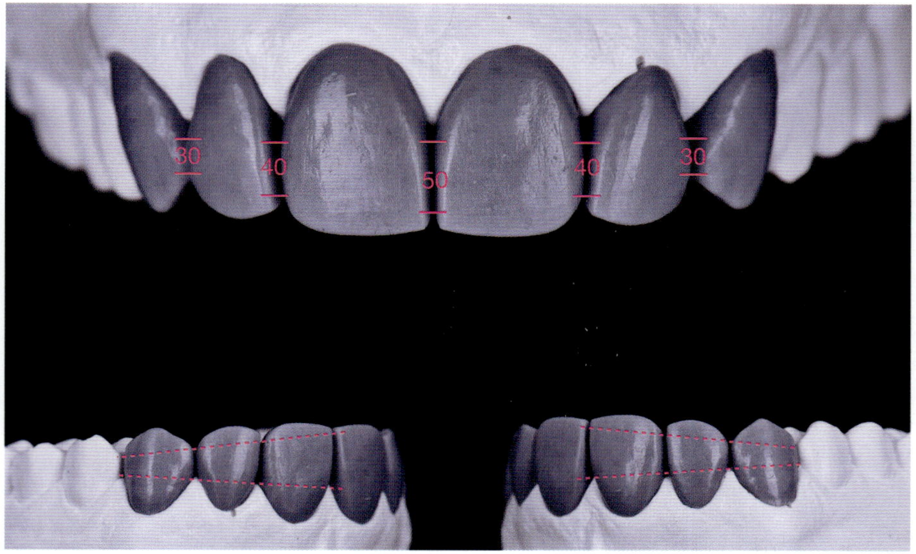

Fig 4-46
Schematic representation of the position of the contact areas.

Vestibular axial inclination of posterior teeth (Fig 4-45)

The exhibition of posterior teeth is regressive, which means that it is gradually minor in a distal direction or in an anteroposterior way due to the curvature of the dental arch. The canine is the tooth that gives the axial inclination of all the posterior teeth. They must follow it to fill the buccal corridor in an esthetic and pleasant way.[6,45]

This parameter compromises the medial-lateral width of a smile, and it can play an important role in a maxillary fixed prosthetic rehabilitation. An inadequate lateral and posterior tooth extension can produce a "black space" leading to an esthetic compromise. By measuring the width of a smile, we can predict the number of restorations and the amount of lateral exposition that we will need for each tooth in order to fulfill the buccal corridor, and not compromise esthetics.[34,46,47]

It has been studied that most patients (89%) had a smile that extended to both pre-molars.[47,48]

TIP

The canine is the tooth that dictates the axial inclination of the posterior teeth. The amount of each tooth that is exposed is dictated by the width of the patient smile.

Contact areas (Fig 4-46)

These are the greatest heights of contour or location of the greatest bulges on the proximal surfaces of the tooth, where one tooth touches the adjacent tooth. They have the function of stabilizing the position of teeth within the arch, preventing food importation, and protecting the interdental papilla. We must consider them as areas, not points; they are gradually more apical from central incisor to canine, forming an ascending line toward distal, and they are determined by both papillary and incisal embrasures.

An esthetic relationship exists between the anterior teeth, known as the 50-40-30 rule. This rule defines that the ideal contact area between the central incisors should be 50% of their length, between the maxillary lateral incisor and the central incisor should be 40% of the length of the central incisor, and between a canine and a lateral incisor should be 30% of the length of the central incisor[28]:

- Central incisors: normally located in the incisal third
- Central incisor and lateral incisor: between the medium and incisal third of each
- crown
- Lateral incisor and canine: in the medium third of the lateral and the union of
- The medium and incisal third of the canine[8,49,50]

TIP

In cases where the teeth are too long, it may be good to increase the contact area and keep the embrasures as narrow as possible, both cervical and incisal. This will enhance the perception of a relatively wider and, therefore, shorter tooth.

Interproximal spaces/cervical embrasures (Fig 4-47)

This is a triangular embrasure space between adjacent teeth located cervically to their contact area. They are formed by the contact of the proximal surfaces of teeth and are normally occupied by papilla. The anatomy of teeth determines their size and shape. The more rounded the tooth, the bigger the cervical embrasures.[50]

REMEMBER

To close these embrasures in cases of missing papilla, we can increase the length of the contact point apically. That way, we will fill the black space produced by the missing papilla and give an esthetic rehabilitation to our patient. It is important to remember that by increasing the length of the contact point, we will alter the tooth shape, making it appear to have a squared shape.

Incisal embrasures (Fig 4-48)

These are formed by the edges and separations between the teeth and the dark background of the mouth and follow a pattern that develops between central incisors and then progresses laterally. Their size and volume between teeth increase as the dentition progresses away from the midline. This means that the incisal embrasure space between the lateral incisor and the central incisor should be larger than the incisal embrasure between the central incisors, and that the incisal embrasure between the canine and the lateral incisor should be larger than the incisal embrasure between the lateral and central incisors.[28]

They individualize the anterior dentition and give efficiency to mastication (allows an escape route reducing the forces applied by mastication and avoids food impaction), and their width is determined by the position of the contact area. The bigger the contact area, the smaller the incisal embrasures. The design of the contact areas and incisal and cervical embrasures is also dependent on the shape and alignment of the teeth.[49]

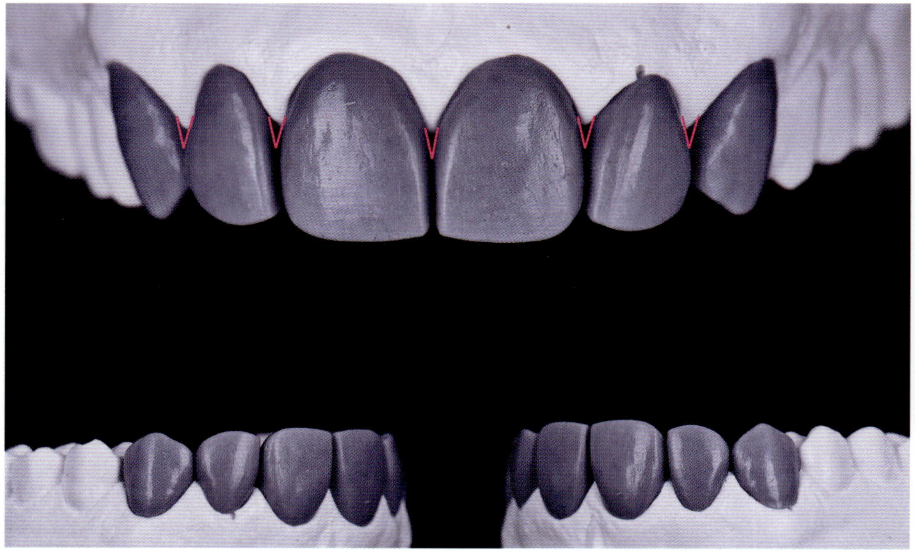

Fig 4-47
Schematic representation of the position of the interproximal spaces/cervical embrasures.

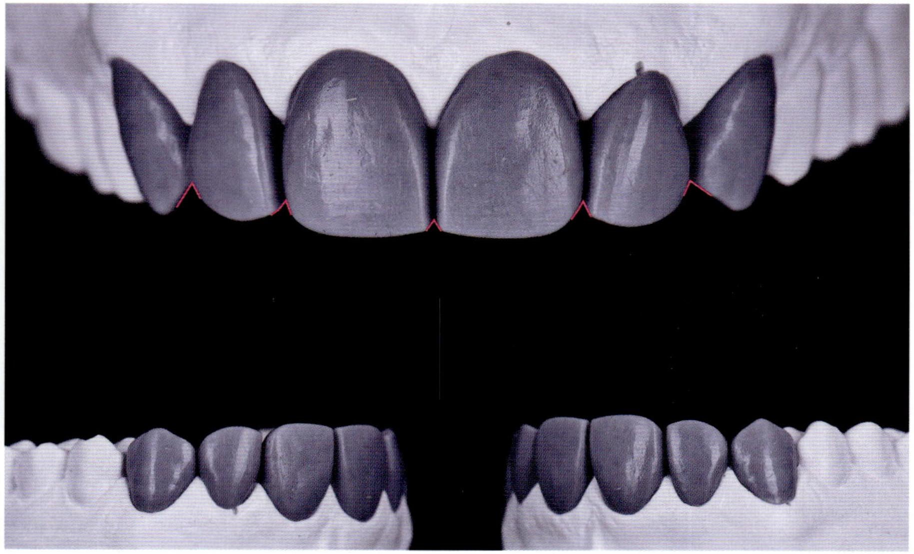

Fig 4-48
Schematic representation of the position of the incisal embrasures.

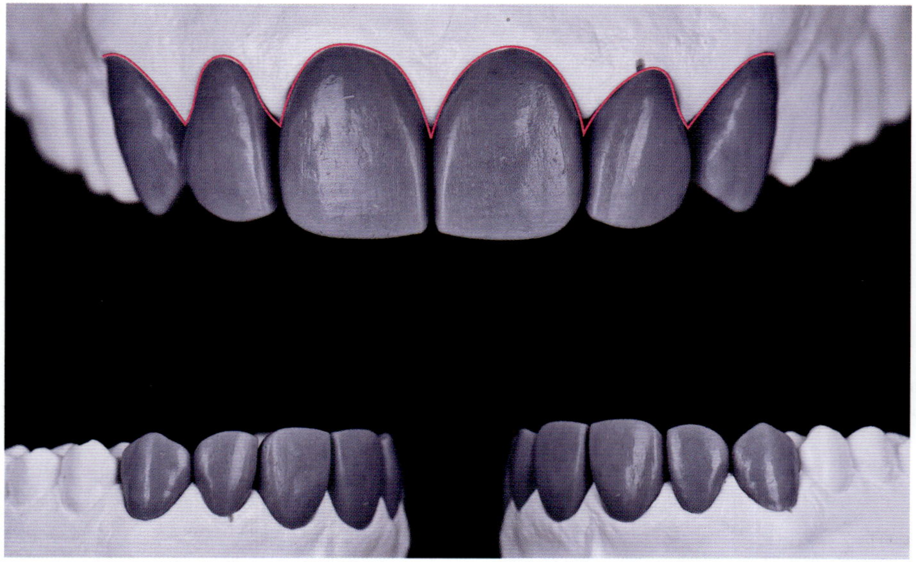

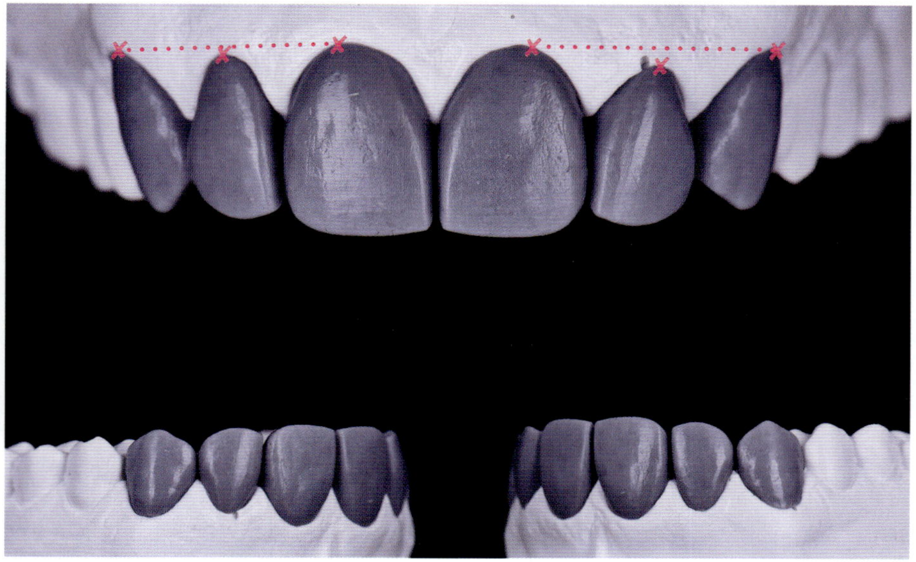

Figs 4-49 and 4-50
Schematic representation of the zenith position (left) and interproximal papilla position (right).

TIP

The position of the incisal embrasures move apically as they proceed toward the posterior area.

Gingival margin and zenith position (Figs 4-49 and 4-50)
Gingival esthetics has always been an important component of a healthy and beautiful prosthetic rehabilitation. The gingival margin and papilla must be healthy, and its morphology plays an important role in creating an esthetically pleasing smile. The gingival profile must have a knife-edge gingival margin tightly adapted to the teeth, interdental grooves, and pyramid-shaped interdental papilla.[51–53]

The gingiva is normally pale in color and can vary in degree of vascularization, epithelial keratinization, pigmentation, and in the thickness of the epithelium. It extends to the cementoenamel junction, forming a static frame for the teeth. The level of healthy gingiva is always dictated by the position of the alveolar bone beneath it, and it lies approximately 3 mm away from the intact bone. If the health of this tissue is compromised, every prosthodontic treatment should be postponed until it is sufficiently reinstated.[6]

Kokich and Spear refer that for gingival assessment the dentist should evaluate four criteria[52]:

1. Gingival level of both central incisors
2. Gingival margin of the lateral incisors (should be 0.5 mm coronal to the central incisor) and canines (same as the central incisors)
3. Gingival contour of the labial gingival margin of each tooth (which should follow the contour of the cementoenamel junction)
4. Interproximal papilla

The interdental appearance of the papilla in an apicocoronal location is crucial for an esthetic result.

Nordland and Tarnow classified a normal interdental papilla as one that fills the embrasure space to the apical extent of the interdental contact area.[54]

It is not easy to fill the interproximal cervical area with a papilla when we are performing fixed restorations on teeth; it requires a very good planification and provisionalization of the overall treatment. Tarnow et al, in 1992, concluded that when the measurement from the contact point to the crest of bone was 5 mm or less, the papilla was present in almost 100% of the cases. When the distance was 6 mm, the papilla was present in 56% of the cases, and when the distance was 7 mm or more the papilla was present in 27% or less of the cases.[55]

Cho et al confirmed the data obtained by Tarnow and also suggested that the increase of the interproximal distance between the tooth roots has a significant decreasing influence on the papilla presence.[56]

Chu measured 240 papillae heights, both mesial and distal interdental papilla, in the anterior maxillary teeth (including the central incisors, lateral incisors, and canines). The measurements were made from the level of the gingival zenith of the corresponding tooth to the tip of the papilla. The proportion of those measurements with the length of the correspondent clinical crowns was calculated. He has concluded that the average mesial papilla proportion and distal papilla proportion of the three groups of teeth studied were on average 40%.[57]

The zenith point is the most apical point of the gingival architecture of each tooth. Their positions are determined by the anatomy of the root, the cemento-enamel junction (CEJ), and the osseous crest.

Chu, in 2009, concluded that the mean location of the zenith point from the vertical bisected midline (VBM) of the clinical crown of central incisors, lateral incisors and canines was 1 mm distally, 0.4 mm distally, and 0 mm, respectively. And in an apical-coronal direction, the zenith of lateral incisors relative to the gingival tangential zenith joining adjacent central incisor and canine was approximately 1 mm.

Both central incisors' zeniths must be located 1 mm distally to their midline.

REFERENCES

1. De Azevedo A, da Rosa WL, da Silva AF, Correa MB, Torriani MA, Lund RG. Comparative effectiveness of dental anatomy carving pedagogy: a systematic review. J Dent Educ 2015;79:914–921.
2. De Azevedo A, Correa MB, Torriani MA, Lund RG. Optimizing quality of dental carving by preclinical dental students through anatomy theory reinforcement. Anat Sci Educ 2018; 11:377–384.
3. Abu Eid R, Ewan K, Foley J, Oweis Y, Jayasinghe J. Self-directed study and carving tooth models for learning tooth morphology: Perceptions of students at the University of Aberdeen, Scotland. J Dent Educ 2013;77:1147–1153.
4. Lone M, McKenna JP, Cryan JF, Downer EJ, Toulouse A. A survey of tooth morphology teaching methods employed in the United Kingdom and Ireland. Eur J Dent Educ 2018;22:e438–e443.
5. Kina S, Bruguera A. Restauraciones Estéticas Cerámicas. Maringá, Brazil: Dental Press Editora, Chapter 1, 2008.
6. Gürel G. The Science and Art of Porcelain Veneers. London: Quintessence Publishing, Chapter 2, 2003.
7. Ferraris M, Muñoz A. Histologia y Embriología bucodental, ed 2. Editorial Medica Panamericana, page Capitulo 8, 9 y 10.
8. Ash M, Nelson S. Wheeler's Anatomy Physiology and Occlusion, ed 8. Amsterdam: Elsevier, Chapter 13, 2006.
9. Schweiger J, Edelhoff D, Stimmelmayr M, et al. Automated production of multilayer anterior restorations with digitally produced dentin cores. QDT 2015;207–220.
10. Bazos P, Magne P. Bio-emulation: biomimetically simulating nature utilizing a histo-anatomic approach; structural analysis. Eur J Esthet Dent 2011,6:8–19.
11. Goldberg M. The dentino-enamel junction revisited. Connect Tissue Res 2002;43: 482–489.
12. Kraus BS. Morphologic relationships between enamel and dentin surfaces of lower first molar teeth. J Dent Res 1952;31:248–256.
13. Skinner M, Wood BA, Boesch C, et al Dental trait expression at the enamel-dentine junction of lower molars in extant and fossil hominoids. J Hum Evol 2008;54:173–186.
14. Scheid R, Weiss G. Woelfel's Dental Anatomy, ed 8. Wolters Kluwer, Part 1, 2001.
15. Brisban AS. Esthetics: a comparison of dentists' and patients' concepts. J Am Dent Assoc 1980;100:345–352.
16. Williams JL. A new classification of human tooth forms with special reference to a new system of artificial teeth. Dent Cosmos (n.d.) 6:627–628.
17. Frush JP, Fisher RD. How dentinogenics integrate the sex factor. J Prosthet Dent 1956;6:160–172.
18. Frush JP, Fisher RD. How dentinogenics integrate the personality factor. J Prosthet Dent 1956;6:441–449.
19. Frush JP, Fisher RD. The age factor in dentinogenics. J Prosthet Dent 1957;7:5.
20. Paolucci B, et al. Visagism: the art of dental composition. QDT 2012:187–200.
21. Fradeani M. Esthetic Rehabilitation in Fxed Prosthodontics. Volume 1: Esthetic analysis. Chicago, IL: Quintessence, Chapters 3 and 5, 2004.
22. Magne P, Belser U. Restauraciones de Porcelana Adherida En Los Dientes Anteriores: Método Biomimetico. Barcelona: Quintessence, Chapter 2, 2004.
23. Chiche G, Pinault A. Esthetics of Anterior Fxed Prosthodontics. Chicago, IL: Quintessence, 1993.
24. Rufenacht CR. Fundamentals of Esthetics. Chicago, IL: Quintessence, 1990.
25. Goldstein RE. Esthetics in Dentistry, ed 2. Hamilton, ON: BC Decker, 1998.
26. Miller EC, Bodden WR, Jamison HC. A study of the relationship of the dental midline to the facial median fine. J Prosthet Dent 1979;41:657–660.
27. Lombardi RE. The principles of visual perception and their clinical application to denture esthetics. J Prosthet Dent 1973;29:358–382.
28. Morley J, Eubank J. Macroesthetic elements of smile design. J Am Dent Assoc 2001;132: 39–45.
29. Johnston CD, Burden DJ, Stevenson MR. The influence of dental midline discrepancies on dental attractiveness ratings. Eur J Orthod 1999;21:517–522.
30. Kokich V, Kiyak HA, Shapiro PA. Comparing the perception of dentists and lay people to altered dental esthetics. J Esthet Dent 1999;11:311–324.
31. Pereira B, Jiménez-Castellanos E, Martinez-de-Fuentes R, Fernandez AA, Chu S. Perception of maxillary dental midline shift in asymmetric faces. Int J Esthet Dent 2015;10:588–596.
32. Pereira B, Jiménez-Castellanos E, Martinez-de-Fuentes R, Greenberg JR, Chu S. Laypersons' perception of facial and dental asymmetries. Int J Periodontics Restorative Dent 2013;33:e162–e171.
33. Ahmad I. Anterior dental aesthetics: dentofacial perspective. Br Dent J 2005;199:81–88.
34. Nold S, Horvath SD, Stampf S, Blatz MB. Analysis of select facial and dental esthetic parameters. Int J Periodontics Restorative Dent 2014;34:623–629.
35. Rosenstiel SF, Ward DH, Rashid RG. Dentists' preferences of anterior tooth proportion – a web-based study. J Prosthodont 2000;9:123–136.
36. Magne P, Gallucci GO, Belser UC. Anatomic crown width/length ratios of unworn and worn maxillary teeth in white subjects. J Prosthet Dent 2003;89:453–461.
37. Wolfart S, Thormann H, Freitag S, Kern M. Assessment of dental appearance following changes in incisor proportions. Eur J Oral Sci 2005;113:159–165.
38. Parnia F, Hafezeqoran A, Mahboub F, et al. Proportions of maxillary anterior teeth relative to each other and to golden standard in Tabriz Dental Faculty students. J Dent Res Dent Clin Dent Prospects 2010;4:83–86.
39. Wolfart S, Quaas AC, Freitag S, Kropp P, Gerber WD, Kern M. Subjective and objective perception of upper incisors. J Oral Rehabil 2006;33:489–495.
40. Snow SR. Esthetic smile analysis of anterior tooth width: the golden percentage. J Esthet Dent 1999;11:177–184.
41. Levin EI. Dental esthetics and the golden proportion. J Prosthet Dent 1978;40:244–252.
42. Preston JD. The golden proportion revisited. J Esthet Dent 1993;5:247–251.
43. Ward DH. Proportional smile design using the recurring esthetic dental (RED) proportion. Dent Clin North Am 2001;45:143–154.
44. Ali Fayyad M, Jamani KD, Agrabawi J. Geometric and mathematical proportions and their relations to maxillary anterior teeth. J Contemp Dent Pract 2006;7:62–70.

REFERENCES

45. Davis N. Smile design. Dent Clin Nort Am 2007,51:299–318.
46. Bidra A. Three-Dimensional esthetic analysis in treatment planning for implant-supported fixed prosthesis in the edentulous maxilla: review of the esthetics literature. J Esthet Restor Dent 2011;23:219–236.
47. Tjan AH, Miller GD, The JG. Some esthetic factors in a smile. J Prosthet Dent 1984;51: 24–28.
48. Dong JK, Jin TH, Cho HW, et al. The esthetics of a smile: a review of some recent studies. Int J Prosthodont 1999;12:9–19.
49. Stappert C, Tarnow DP, Tan JH, Chu SJ. Proximal contact areas of the maxillary anterior dentition. Int J Periodontics Restorative Dent 2010;30:471–477.
50. Chow YC, Eber RM, Tsao YP, Shotwell JL, Wang HL. Factors associated with the appearance of gingival papillae. J Clin Periodontol 2010;37:719–727.
51. Prichard J. Gingivoplasty, gingivectomy and osseous surgery. J Periodontol 1961;32: 275–282.
52. Kokich VG, Spear F. Guidelines for managing the orthodontic restorative patient. Semin Orthod 1997;3:3-20.
53. Garber DA, Salama MA. The aesthetic smile: diagnosis and treatment. Periodontol 2000; 1996;11:18–28.
54. Nordland WP, Tarnow DO. A classification system for loss of papillary height. J Periodontol 1998;69:1124–1126.
55. Tarnow DP, Magner AW, Fletcher P. The effect of the distance from the contact point to the crest of bone on the presence or absence of the interproximal dental papilla. J Periodontol 1992;63:995–996.
56. Chu HS, Jang HS, Kim DK, et al. The effects of interproximal distance between roots on the existence of interdental papillae according to the distance from the contact point to the alveolar crest. J Periodontol 2006;77:1651–1657.
57. Chu S, Tan J, Steppart C, Tarnow D. Gingival zenith positions and levels of the maxillary anterior dentition. J Esthet Restor Dent 2009;21:113–121.

CHAPTER 5

PHOTOGRAPHY COMMUNICATION

LOUIS HARDAN

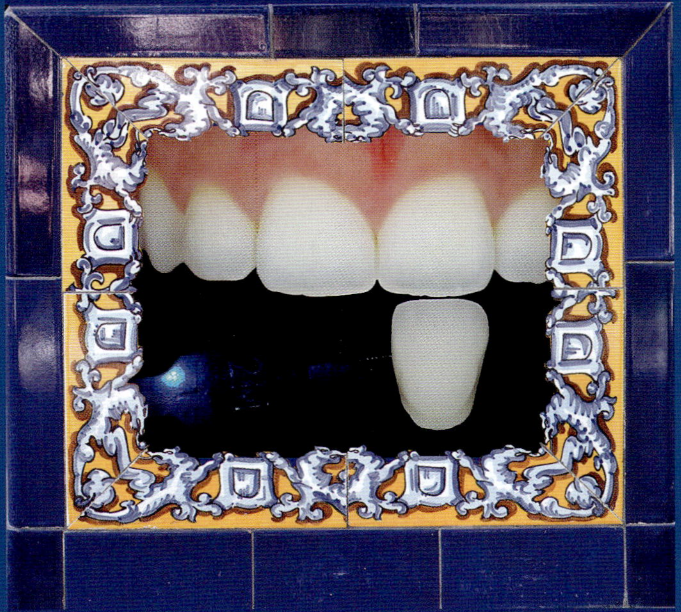

Communication with
the patient is always a winning
and well-appreciated strategy.
A happy patient will promote
the dentist's work in a very
efficient way ...

Photography Communication

With the constant evolution of digital technology, new and innovative instruments continue to emerge, allowing improved communication efficiently and easily. In dental practice, one of the most important prerequisites to a case's success is good communication with the lab technician, the patient, and even with colleagues of different specialties.

PHOTOGRAPHY: DIAGNOSTIC AND TRAINING IMPORTANCE

When a patient comes to the dental clinic, the dentist should study the case, diagnose, and start the treatment accordingly. Sometimes, the diagnosis is not evident from the start, and a specialist's opinion is required. In the past, the patient was referred from one doctor to another, which took a significant amount of time. Today, with the technological evolution, a simple photograph can be sent to a designated specialist who can request the appropriate tests and sometimes, the diagnosis is directly determined.[1]

The photographs in Fig 5-1 show an odd-looking lesion of the tongue. The diagnosis can be critical and should be approached delicately. On the one hand, the diffused light used for the first photograph eliminates hard light reflection and shows the anatomic appearance of the structure. On the other hand, the polarized light used for the second photograph eliminates the glare, which allows more detail to be shown since the expansion of the lesion becomes clearer.[2]

Sharing photographs between colleagues can prove their importance when transferring a patient from one practitioner to the other, especially when either the dentist or the patient is traveling or moving to another area.

Photographs are tremendously appreciated in the academic field because they represent an otherwise theoretical concept. They can be used to enrich scientific articles and to clarify clinical cases in lectures or workshops.[3] A photograph can show a case on a much bigger scale where even the slightest details can be discussed and analyzed; it allows us to explain the drawbacks of any work and how to fix them (Figs 5-2 and 5-3).

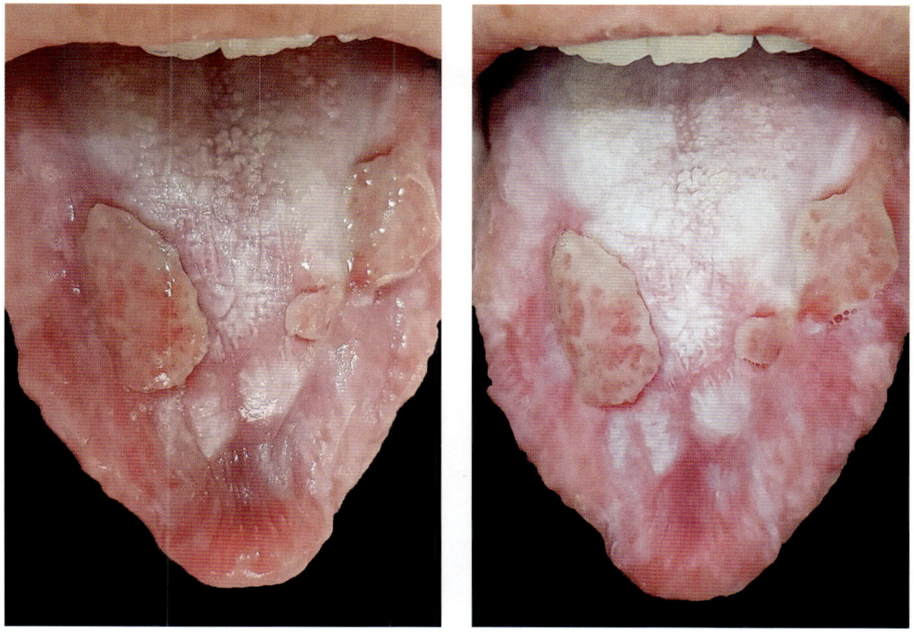

Fig 5-1
Photographs of a peculiar tongue lesion. On the left, the picture is taken under diffused light, while on the right, the picture is taken under polarized light.

PHOTOGRAPHY: DENTIST'S COMMUNICATION WITH THE DENTAL TECHNICIAN

Another important communication in the dental field is the dentist's communication with the dental technician. It is a crucial step in the treatment plan, especially in the domain of esthetic dentistry. High-quality photographs and videos can be analyzed to determine the esthetic association between the face, teeth, and lips. Full information can be transferred via videos since they capture the dynamics of lip movement and facial muscles contractions and their effect on teeth perception.[4]

No matter how much the dentist explains and describes the case and the outcome they seek, it will not be as efficient as a photograph. The SmileLite MDP (Mobile Dental Photography) device forms an easy and practical approach to photography, enabling dentists to take high-quality photographs and videos using their mobile phones (Fig 5-4). Information can then be directly sent to the lab technician using a social media application. With today's technologies and the introduction of the digital smile design concept, these tools are now, more than ever, essential instruments in the dental practice. They allow the dentist and their lab technician to design the smile and visualize treatment outcomes before initiation. Several digital smile design software suites already exist, like Digital Smile Design (DSD) and Rebel Dental.[5] A standardized set of photographs is required for each case, and after analyzing these photographs, a new smile is digitally designed. Then, a mock-up can help the patient see what they would expect at the end of the treatment (Fig 5-5).[6]

Photographs can help the technician visualize the dental environment in which their work will integrate. A large amount of information is transferred through photographs, such as color, shape, alignment, personalization, translucency, opalescence and the halo effect of adjacent teeth.[7]

The SmileLite MDP device emits a light similar to daylight, ensuring ideal conditions for taking a picture. It is also an interesting tool for enabling reliable, simple, and efficient shade matching (Fig 5-6).

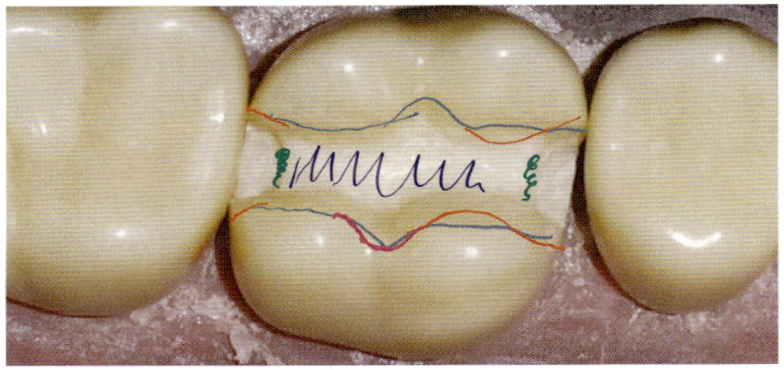

Fig 5-2
A student's preparation with sketching shows how to improve the tooth.

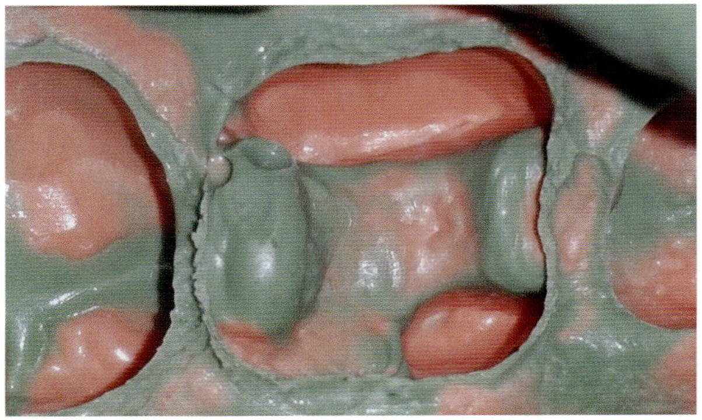

Fig 5-3
A photograph showing the defects of a student's impression.

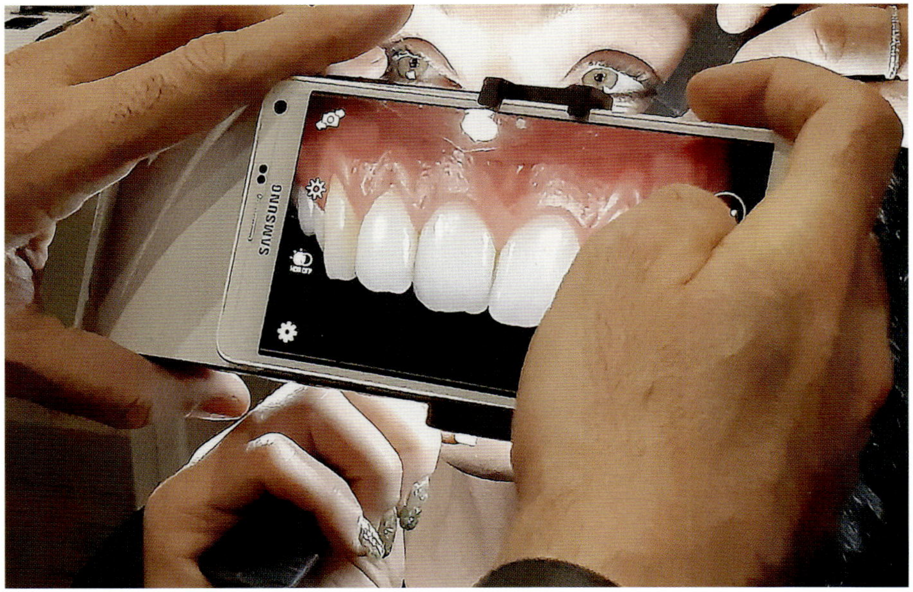

Fig 5-4
The SmileLite MDP (Mobile Dental Photography) device forms an easy and practical approach to photography, enabling dentists to take high-quality photographs and videos using their mobile phones.

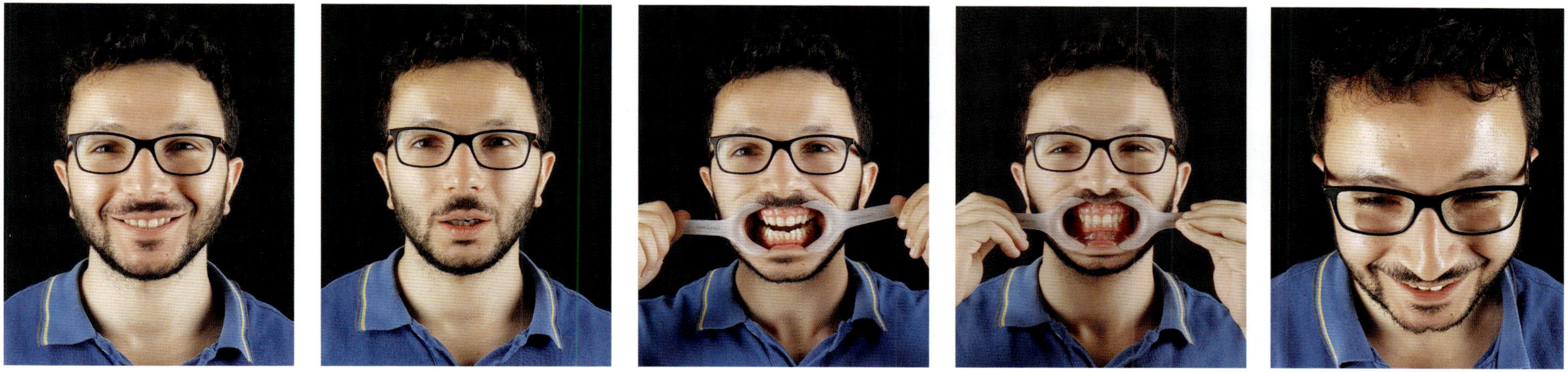

Fig 5-5
Five photographs are required to make a smile design project (REBEL); these photographs can be easily done using a smartphone and uploaded to the software with other data. These photographs are: smiling, lips at rest, retracted open, retracted closed, and 12 o'clock position.

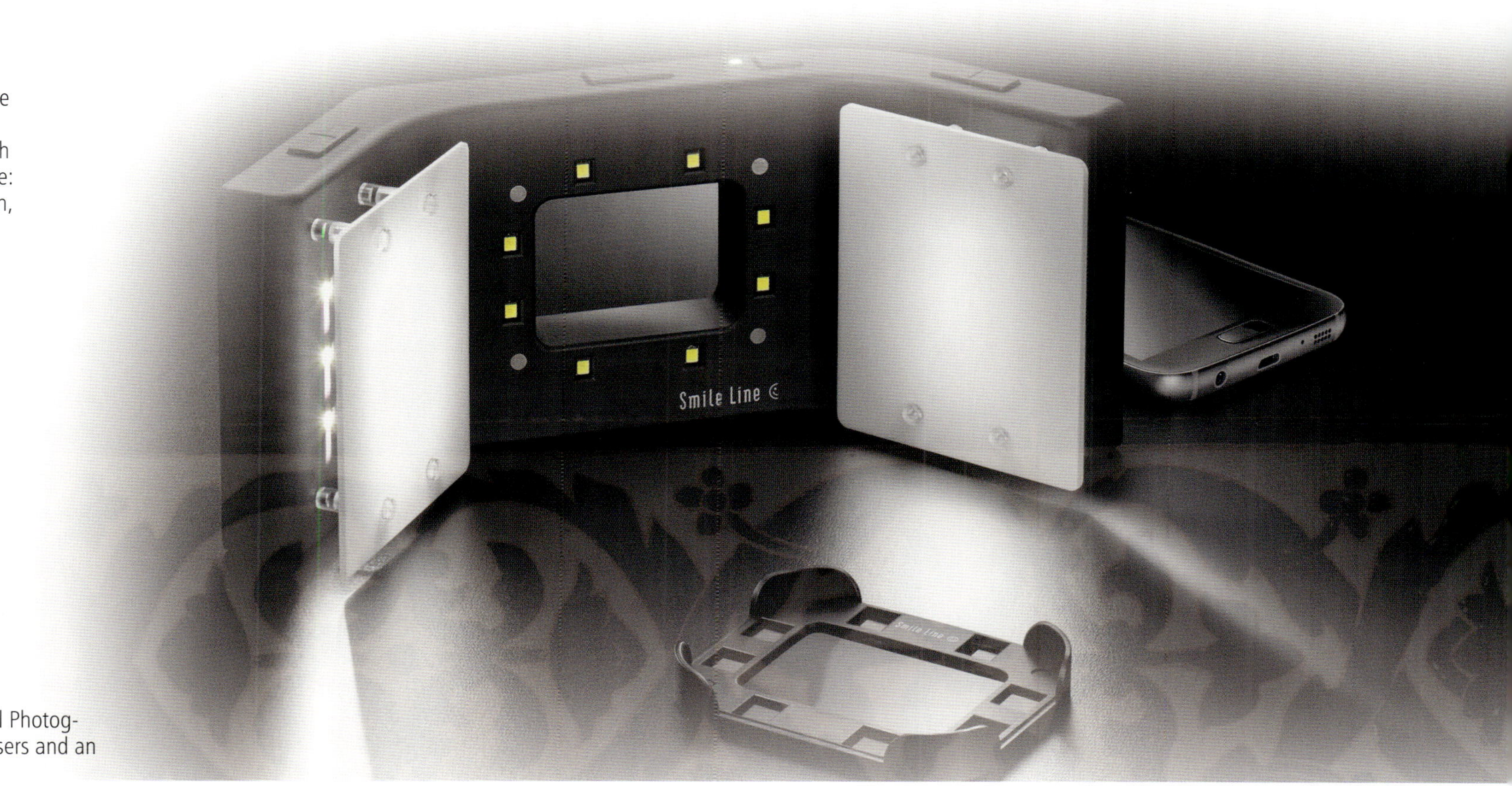

Fig 5-6
The SmileLite MDP (Mobile Dental Photography) device with mounted diffusers and an unmounted polarizing filter.

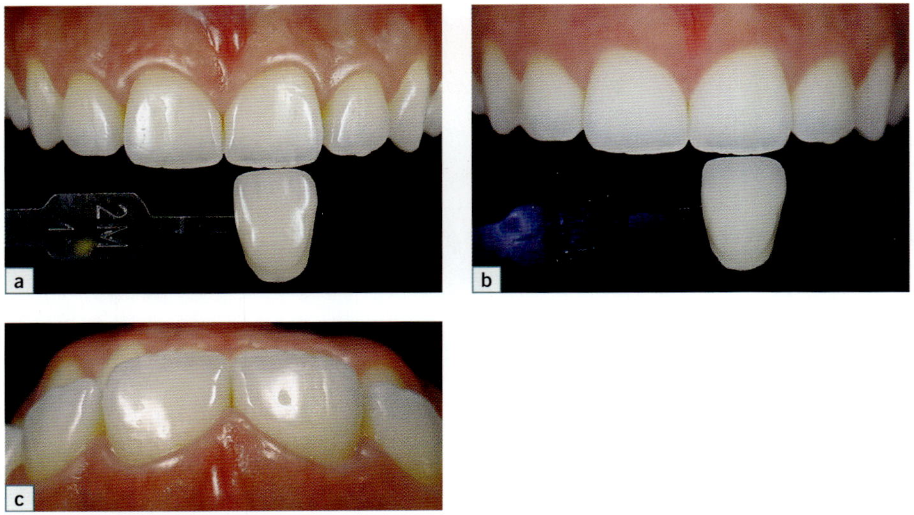

Fig 5-7
Using the different accessories of the SmileLite MDP device, three photographs can be enough to communicate with the lab technician. (a) With diffused light, one photograph should depict an edge-to-edge shade guide with a normal tooth to show the difference between the shade guide and the natural teeth. (b) With polarized light, the same photograph should be repeated (edge to edge) to show the extension of the translucency and its location in the incisal edge, some details like white spots and the difference in color with the artificial shade guide. (c) With the light coming from an opposite side of the camera, a photograph should be taken to show the secondary and tertiary anatomy, because esthetic is not only hue chroma and value but also anatomy.

CORRECT TOOTH SHADE SELECTION

To grasp shade matching, one must first comprehend the concept of color. Color is a subjective notion created in the brain by psychosensory and neurophysiological phenomena following the action of light on retinal receptors. Therefore, color perception is the complex result of physiological, psychological, and emotional phenomena. It is a very personal experience, depending on the training of the observer's eye and can be affected by an existing physiopathology. Thus, shade matching can be a subjective procedure and can vary depending on the individual.[8]

Thus, color perception varies according to the practitioner. Still, it can also vary individually for the same practitioner depending on psychological disposition, age, eye fatigue, saturation of retinal photoreceptors, or chromatic adaptation.
In addition to the parameters related to the practitioner, other factors can influence the perception of colors like lighting conditions, colors in the surroundings, patient position, and angle of vision.

To get reliable shade matching results, shade should be treated as an objective science.[9] By using photography, it can be estimated following objective criteria. An MDP device produces a standardized set of conditions suitable for the dental practice; it ensures a light analogous to daylight, the best light for color perception. Photographs can be analyzed to determine the shape and structure of a tooth, and according to black and white exposure, color values can be detected.

Using the different accessories of the SmileLite MDP device, three photographs can be enough to communicate with the lab technician and give them all the necessary information for the conception of an esthetic and well-integrated restoration (Fig 5-7).

Shade matching can also be achieved for resin composite restorations using the button technique. It consists of placing buttons of resin composites of different shades on a tooth and then taking a polarized photograph. When studying the photograph, the shade of the button that does not appear on the incisal edge is the enamel shade, and the shade of the button that does not appear in the cervical region is the dentin shade (Fig 5-8).

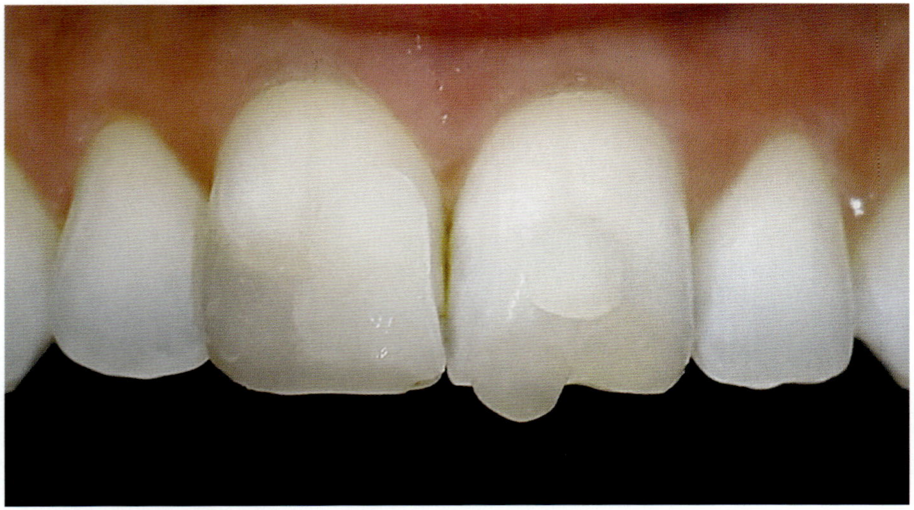

Fig 5-8
A photograph under polarized light for shade matching, using the button technique.

PHOTOGRAPHY: COMMUNICATION WITH THE PATIENT

It is important to note that communication with the patient is also essential, but it requires a unique approach since the patient is likely unfamiliar with medical terms. When talking to a patient, the dentist must find a common communication ground. A photograph is the simplest way to ensure easy and clear communication.[10] Images leave an impression on the patient and motivate them to start the treatment.

Patients are getting more involved in decision-making regarding their treatment plan. Dentists can display the current state of the mouth using photographs to explain what needs to be done. When a patient sees, for example, a fractured tooth or caries or any other problem, they understand the issue and appreciate the needed treatment (Fig 5-9).[11]

The treatment procedure remains a mystery for patients. Now that they know what is wrong and what needs to be done, they remain curious about the potential result and how to attain it. In this field, photographs of previous cases can give tremendous help. Patients can see "before and after" photographs and, as a result, they can visualize the outcome and even the steps of the procedure (Fig 5-10).[12] For example, if a patient is anxious about the preparation of a veneer or an inlay, they can see how much tooth structure is removed and how the tooth is restored. Even photographs of simple procedures, like a composite resin restoration, can help calm and reassure patients that do not know what to expect.

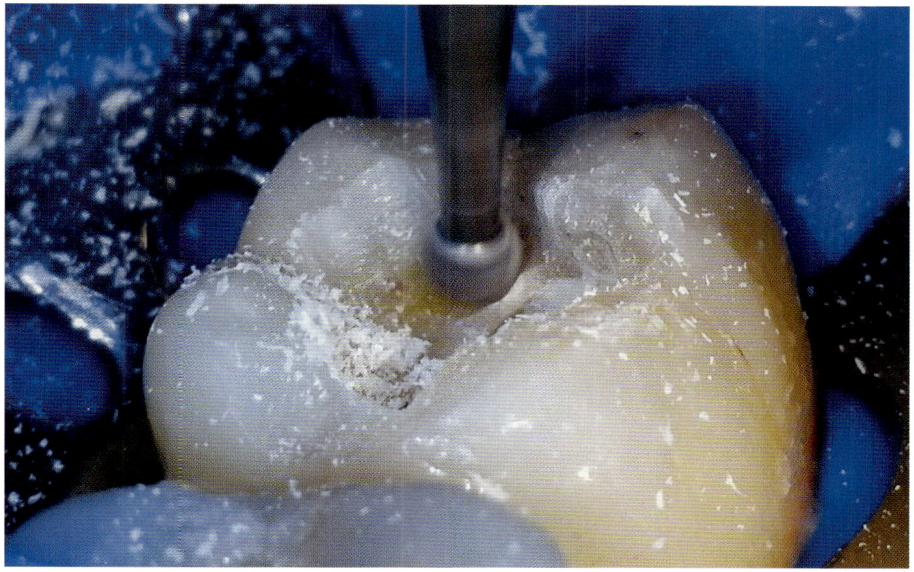

Fig 5-9
Showing the patient a picture of caries removal will make them more confident about the proposed treatment and better understand the procedure that the dentist is performing.

REMEMBER

When talking to a patient, the dentist must find a common communication ground. A photograph is the simplest way to ensure easy and clear communication. Images leave an impression on the patient and give them the motivation to start the treatment

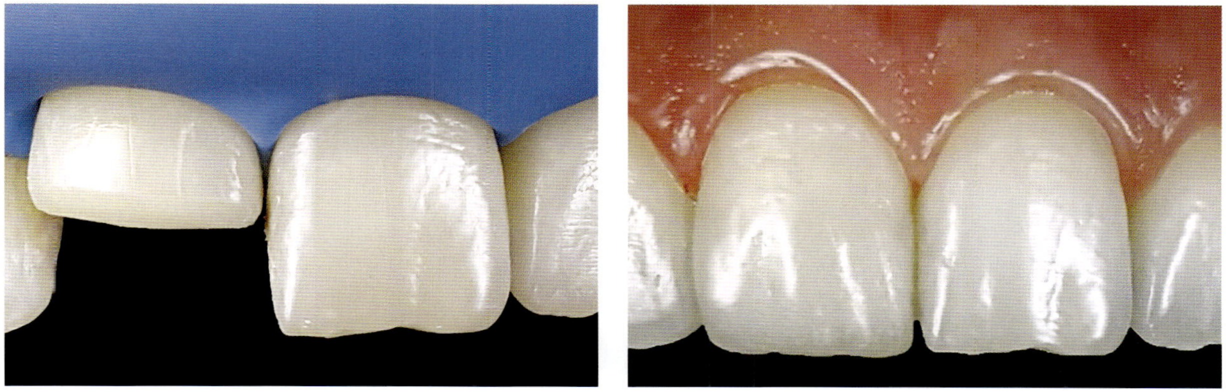

Fig 5-10
"Before and after" photographs of a direct restoration.

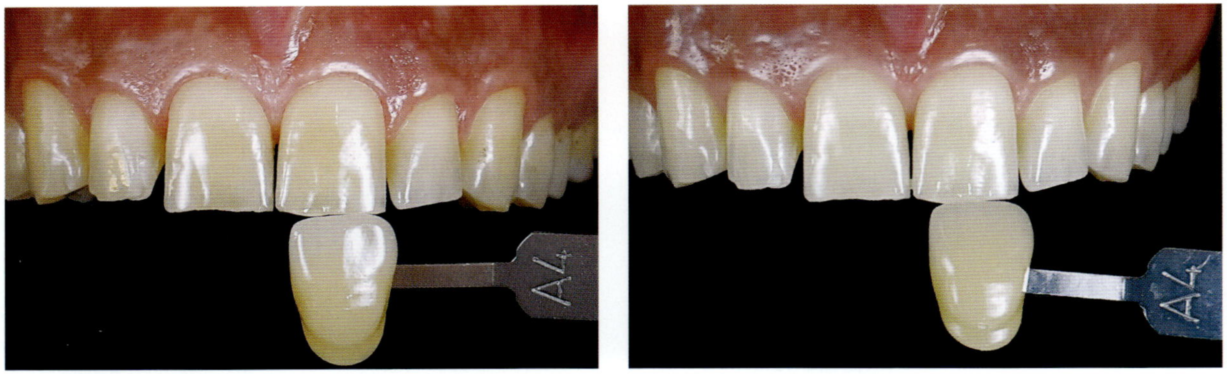

Fig 5-11
"Before and after" photographs after a whitening treatment.

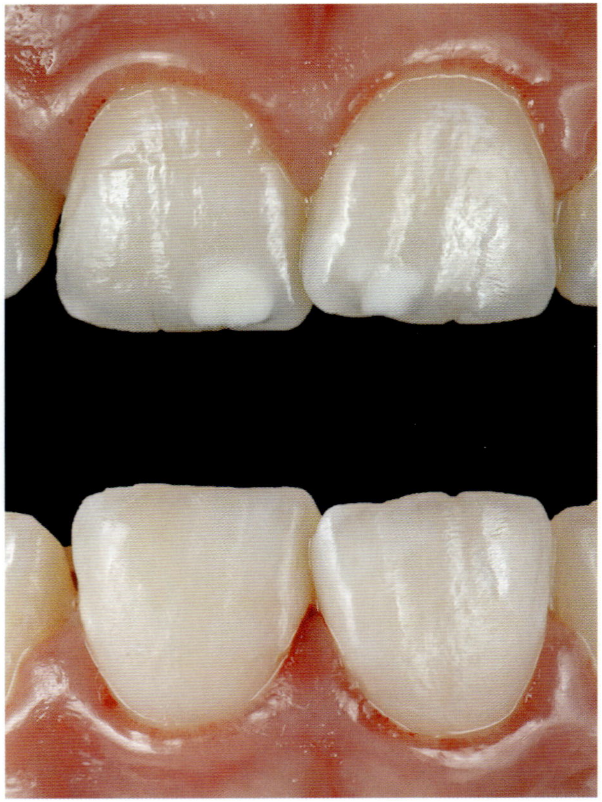

Concerning drastic changes in a patient's smile, most people like to consult with others before making important decisions. They seek the advice of people who are close to them to be sure of their next step. This has become more accessible now that the potential result can be seen before starting the treatment. Of course, they can see "before and after" photographs of other patients, but it is much more intriguing to visualize the result on the patient; this is now possible with the new technology of digital smile design. With a few photographs, we can simulate the potential results, and patients can perceive the changes in their smiles and faces before undergoing the treatment. Usually, they are fascinated by what they see; the whole digital experience, followed by a mock-up in the dental clinic, has a "wow effect" on the patients and the people with them. We can also talk about photography as proof of a treatment's evolution. For instance, sometimes at the end of a "whitening" session, the patient is slightly disappointed with the result, simply because they do not remember how their teeth were before the treatment. Patients seek and expect a white color, even if their dentist has already explained that the color will simply be lighter.

A comparison between before and after treatment photographs will convince the patient of the difference that has been made (Fig 5-11).

Another example where it is possible for the patient to not appreciate the evolution of his case is white lesion treatment; even when the appearance of a white spot has tremendously lessened, patients sometimes need to see the proof of this improvement (Fig 5-12). Any dentist can confront the same issue in different circumstances, and it is with the help of photography that the patient is convinced and satisfied.

When the treatment is done, and when the patients are satisfied, they share their new smile on social media for all to see. Patients now have an active contribution to the dentist's work and can greatly help promote and spread this work among their friends and family (Fig 5-13).[13]

Fig 5-12
"Before and after" photographs for a white lesion treatment.

Fig 5-13
Communication with the patient is always a winning strategy and is so appreciated. In the end, a happy patient will promote our work very efficiently.

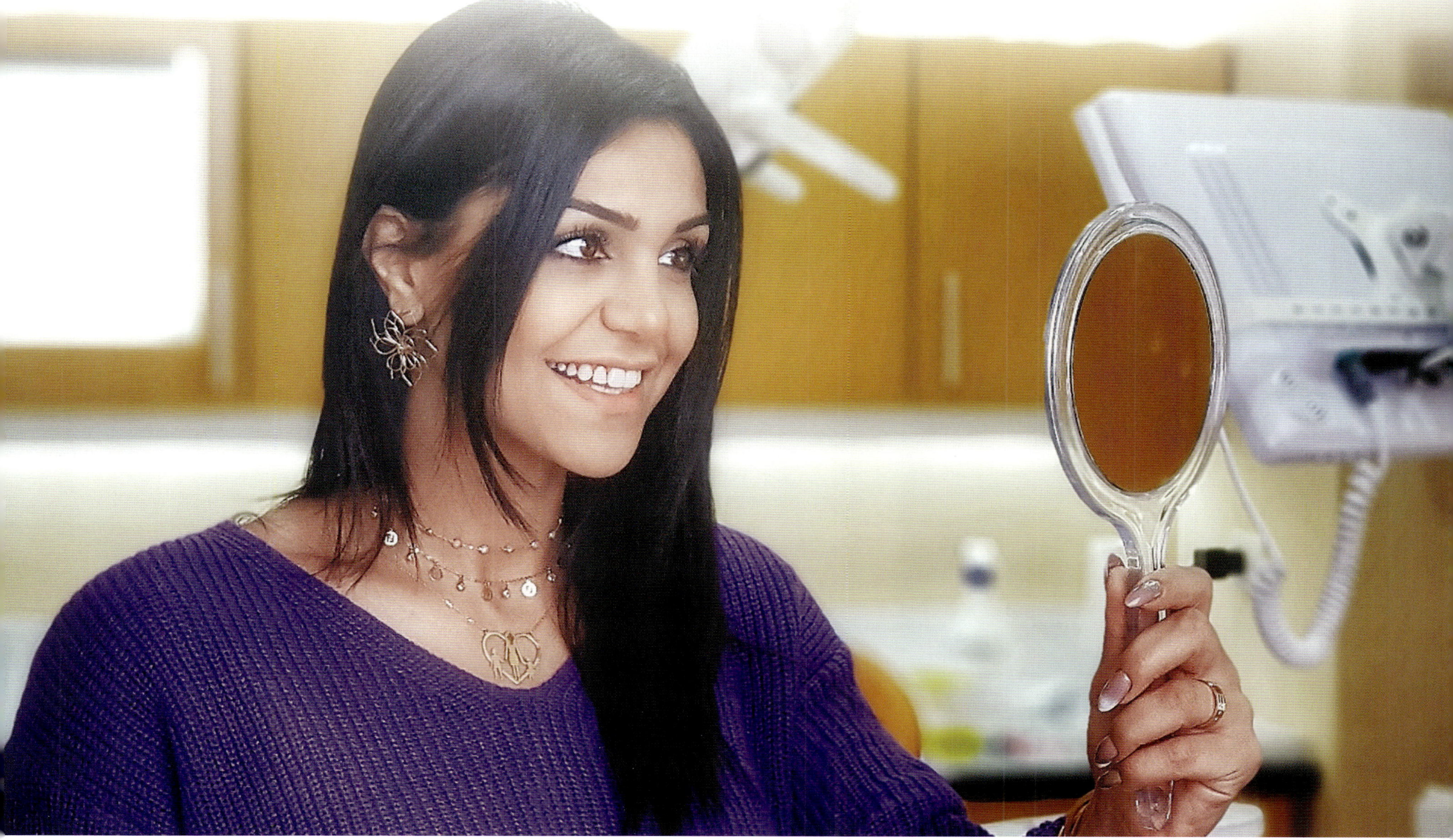

REFERENCES

1. Desai V, Bumb D. Digital dental photography: a contemporary revolution. Int J Clin Pediatr Dent 2013;6:193–196.
2. Lazar R, Culic B, Gasparik C, Lazar C, Dudea D. The accuracy of dental shade matching using cross-polarization photography. Int J Comput Dent 2019;22:343–351.
3. Binder J, Krautz C, Engel K, et al. Leveraging medical imaging for medical education – a cinematic rendering-featured lecture. Ann Anat 2019;222:159–165.
4. Sousa Dias N, Tsingene F. SAEF – Smile's Aesthetic Evaluation form: a useful tool to improve communications between clinicians and patients during multidisciplinary treatment. Eur J Esthet Dent 2011;6:160–176.
5. Levi YL de AS, Cota LV de S, Maia LP. Digital smile design for gummy smile correction. Indian J Dent Res 2019;30:803–806.
6. Da Cunha LF, Fernandes ABF, Baechtold MS, Correr GM, Gonzaga CC. Cara smile: use of planning software to facilitate esthetic dental treatment in a case. Indian J Dent Res Publ Indian Soc Dent Res 2019;30:964–969.
7. Pollini A, Morton D, Arunyanak SP, Harris BT, Lin W-S. Evaluation of esthetic parameters related to a single implant restoration by laypeople and dentists. J Prosthet Dent 2019;11:18.
8. Jain M, Jain V, Yadav NR, et al. Dental students' tooth shade selection ability in relation to years of dental education. J Fam Med Prim Care 2019;8:4010–4014.
9. Liberato WF, Barreto IC, Costa PP, de Almeida CC, Pimentel W, Tiossi R. A comparison between visual, intraoral scanner, and spectrophotometer shade matching: a clinical study. J Prosthet Dent 2019;121:271–275.
10. Gude T, Tyssen R, Anvik T, et al. Have medical students' attitudes towards clinical communication skills changed over a 12-year period? A comparative long-term study. BMC Med Educ 2020;20:11.
11. Kale S, Kakodkar P, Shetiya SH. Assessment of mother's ability in caries diagnosis, utilizing the smartphone photographic method. J Indian Soc Pedod Prev Dent 2019;37:360–364.
12. Carlsson GE, Wagner IV, Odman P, et al. An international comparative multicenter study of assessment of dental appearance using computer-aided image manipulation. Int J Prosthodont 1998;11:246–254.
13. Alalawi A, Aljuaid H, Natto ZS. The effect of social media on the choice of dental patients: a cross-sectional study in the city of Jeddah, Saudi Arabia. Patient Prefer Adherence 2019;13:1685–1692.

CHAPTER 6

PREPARATION – IMPRESSION – PROVISIONAL VENEERS

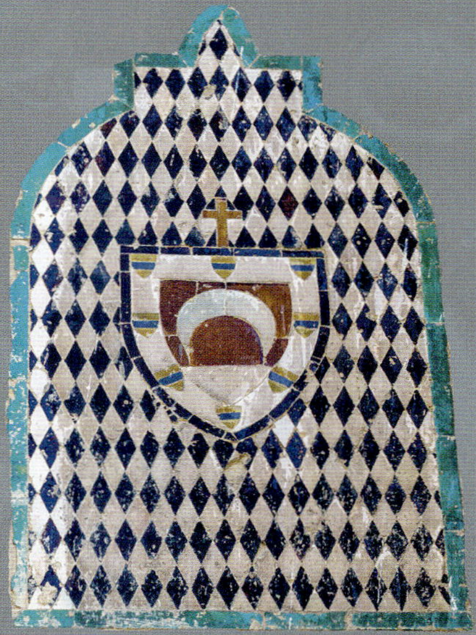

MACIEJ ŻAROW

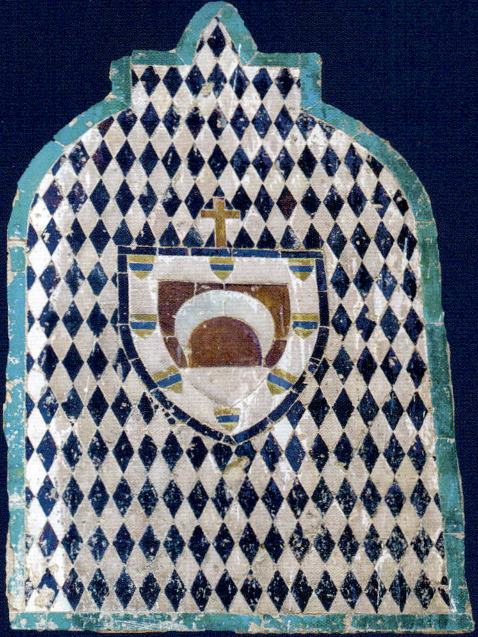

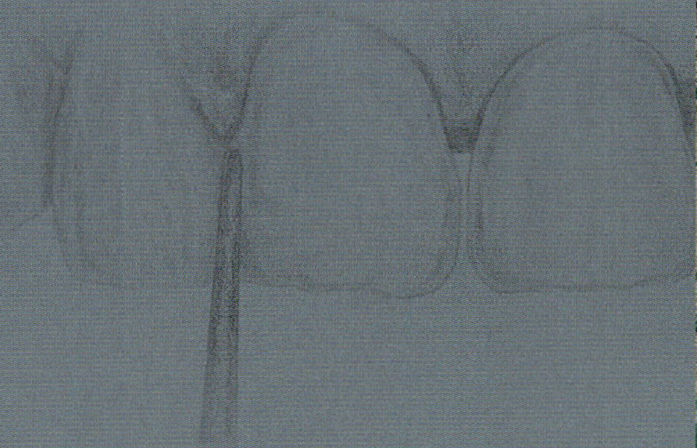

Preparation should be closely related to the esthetic treatment planning ... Conservative preparation means preserving the enamel, better adhesion, and durability of the veneers. Provisional veneers? They can be relatively simple for a dentist and remain in place until the next appointment if they are made according to the presented procedures ...

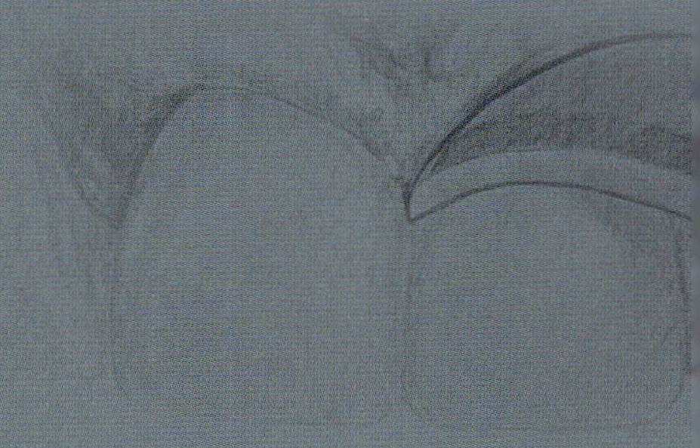

Preparation – Impression – Provisional Veneers

Porcelain veneers went through tremendous evolution due to reduced tooth preparation. This is possible due to the proper planning and tooth preparation through the mock-up, utilizing magnification and new developments in ceramic materials. This chapter describes the steps to a successful preparation, accurate impression, and provisional veneers.

STARTING THE PREPARATION

If the patient accepts the drive-test of the smile (mock-up) and decides to follow the dentist's treatment plan (including the cost estimate), you can start the tooth preparation for the veneers (Fig 6-1). Before the patient's visit, the dental assistant arranges the study casts, the casts with diagnostic wax-up, the silicone index, which is made from the laboratory silicone (for control of the preparation), and the index made from a traditional silicone (for provisional veneers fabrication).

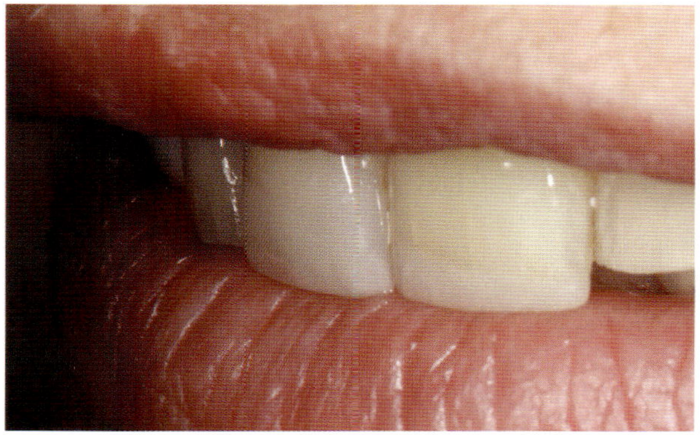

Fig 6-1a
A 41-year-old female patient presented to the dental clinic seeking a better esthetic outcome for the maxillary central incisors.

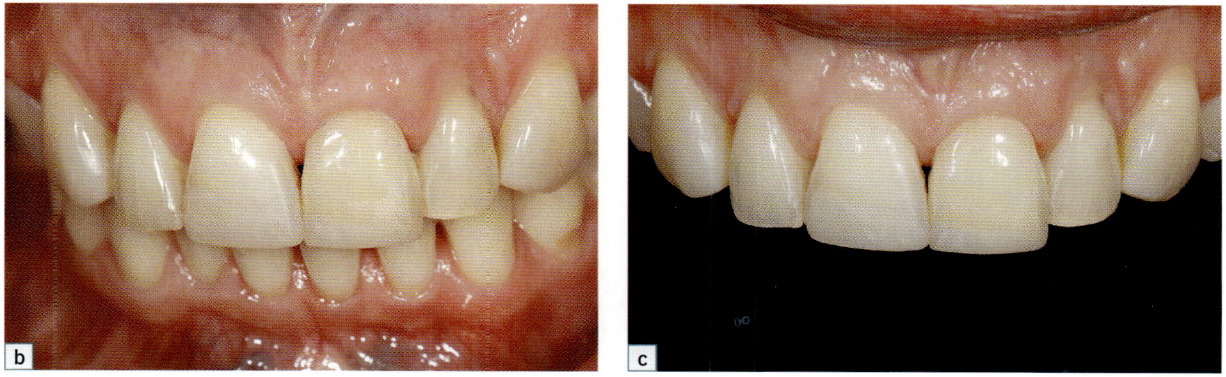

Figs 6-1b and 6-1c
Tooth 11 with extensive composite restoration, tooth 21 after root canal treatment (in the past internally bleached), with slight discoloration. The patient expected a change in teeth esthetics, preferably by making porcelain veneers.

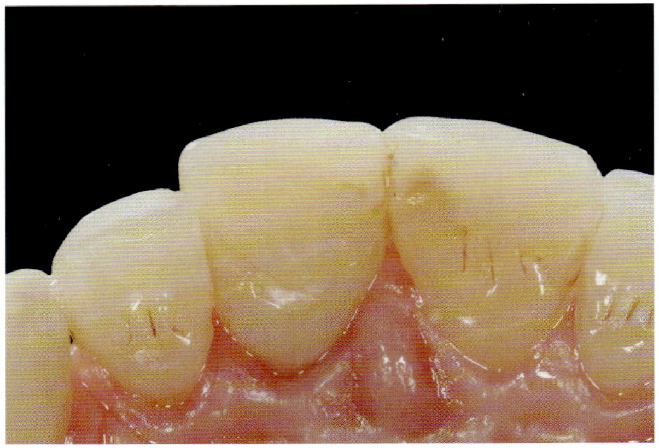

Fig 6-1d
Palatal view showing the outline of the restorations.

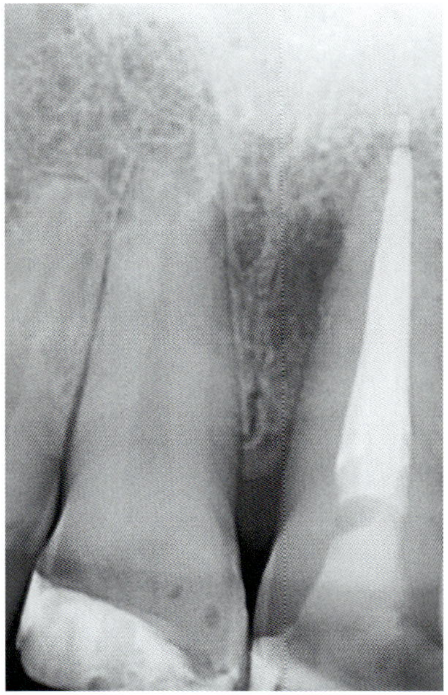

Fig 6-1e
Radiograph of teeth 11 and 21.

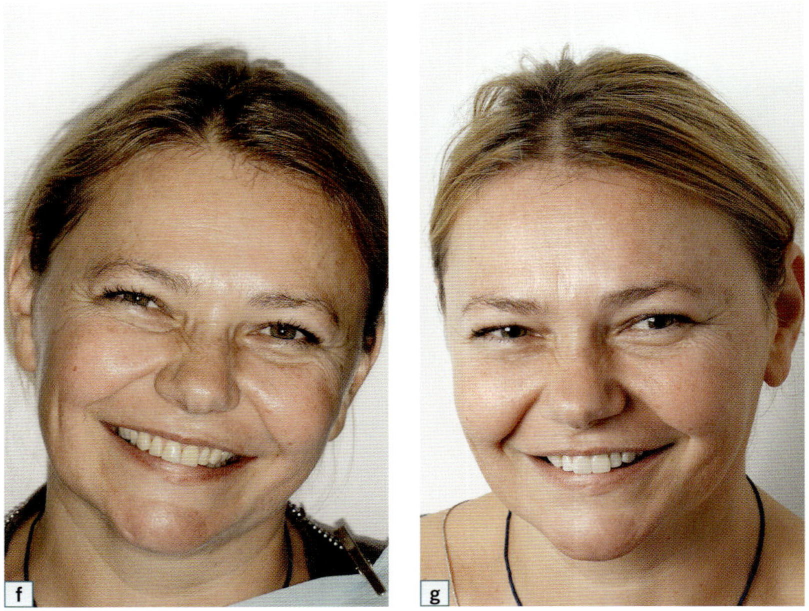

Figs 6-1f and 6-1g
Clinical situation (f) before and (g) after the mock-up.

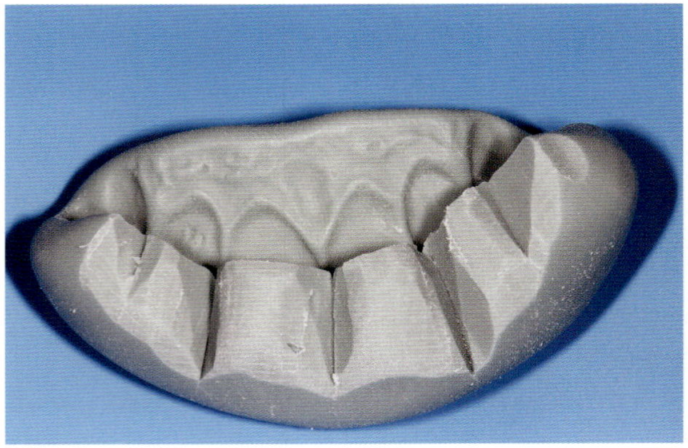

Fig 6-1h
The silicone index is taken from the diagnostic wax-up and cut along the gingival margin.

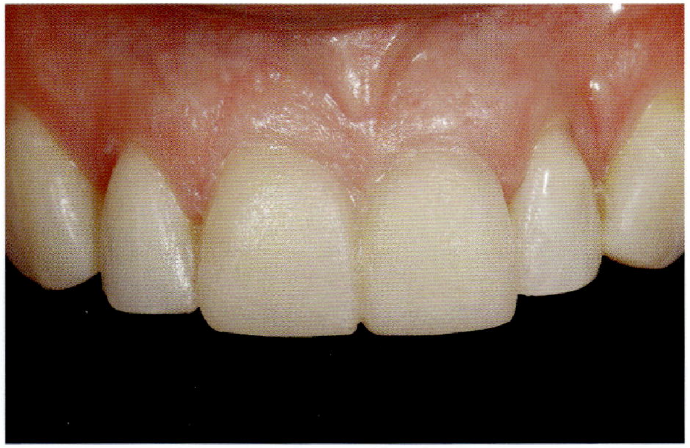

Fig 6-1i
The mock-up obtained from the silicone index based on the diagnostic wax-up.

THE VENEERS DRIVE-TEST (MOCK-UP) BEFORE PREPARATION

Veneer preparation needs to be performed through the mock-up (test-drive veneers). Why should we prepare on the test-drive veneers? Suppose we start the preparation on the natural teeth. In that case, there is a very high risk of dentin exposure. The thickness of the enamel is often different from what we find in an anatomy book and different from the dentist's expectations.[1–7]

The patient may have enamel wear due to the use of hard-bristle toothbrushes or abrasive toothpaste, or may have erosions or enamel defects. The mock-up preparation considers the definitive contour desired for the veneers. In most cases, exposure of the dentin can be avoided.

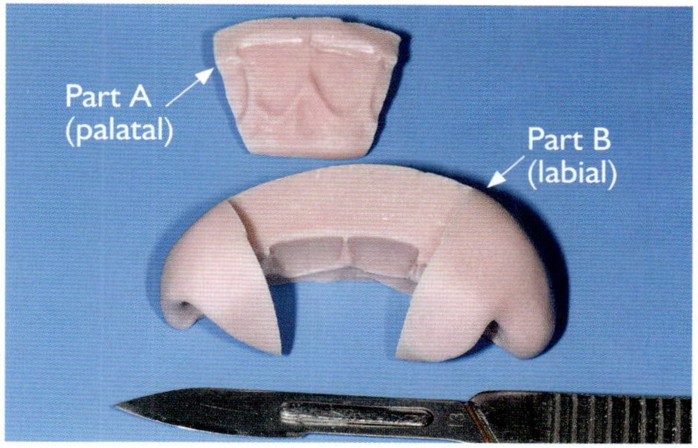

Fig 6-2a
The silicone index should be cut into two parts for veneer preparation control using a scalpel no. 13.

Silicone index as a template for preparation control

The silicone index is based on the diagnostic wax-up from the hard silicone and should be cut into two parts (Fig 6-2a). The palatal one will be used to control the space necessary for the incisal edge of the veneer (Fig 6-2b), and the labial one to control the volume for the veneer from the labial side (Fig 6-2c).

When cutting the silicone index, a scalpel no. 13 should be utilized, and the procedure should be obtained in a glass pad. Cutting the index without the solid base may result in injury to the dentist's fingers. The outline of the cutting line should be performed along the incisal edge – a bit more toward the buccal side (Fig 6-2a), so that way the incisal edge remains in the palatal part of the index. The cutting outline should include at least the teeth intended for preparation. Then, from the incisal cut, make a transverse cut toward the palatal part, dividing the index into two separate parts: palatal (part A) and labial (part B).

Then the incisal part of part B should be shortened, not to interfere with the visibility during the preparation control. Now part A can be used to control the reduction of the incisal edge and part B to control the reduction of the labial tooth structure.

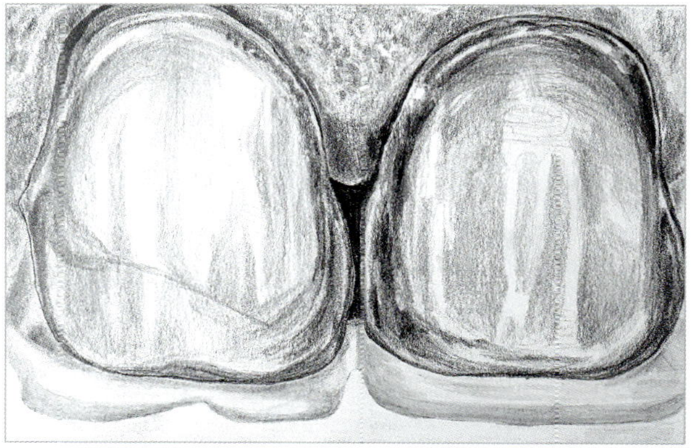

Fig 6-2b
The palatal part of the silicone index is used to control the reduction on the incisal edge.

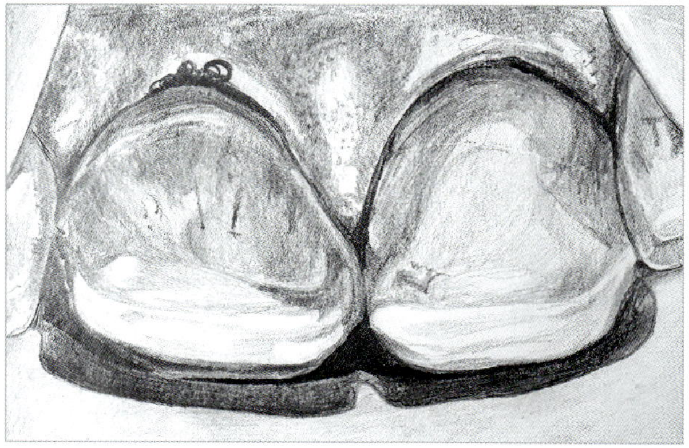

Fig 6-2c
Labial part of the silicone index is used to control space for the veneer from the labial side.

TEN STEPS FOR A SUCCESSFUL PREPARATION

Step 1: The horizontal grooves (preparation through the mock-up)

The horizontal grooves are created on the labial surfaces and the incisal edge of the tooth (Fig 6-3a).[8] On the labial surface, the grooves must have a depth of approximately 0.4 mm (bur no. 868B018), while on the incisal edge, we use a bur placed perpendicularly to the tooth axis to obtain 1.5 mm grooves (bur no. 68016). To better estimate the real tissue reduction, we mark the bottom of the grooves with a pencil (Fig 6-3b). Then we remove the test-drive veneers (mock-up; Fig 6-3c).

Step 2: The outline of the preparation

With the preparation outline with a round ball diamond bur (bur no. 801012), the preparation outline all around the labial surface is obtained (Fig 6-3d). Preparation is carried out very gently, not too deep toward the tooth tissues and not too close to the gingiva (remember that this is the initial outline only!) If we prepare too deeply, we can achieve "a gutter" – like chamfer. Remember to make only a slight outline margin! Accordingly, the preparation will be shallow, and it could be deepened in any step of the further preparation if necessary. The tapered bur no. 6844014 can be utilized as well to create the outline of the preparation.

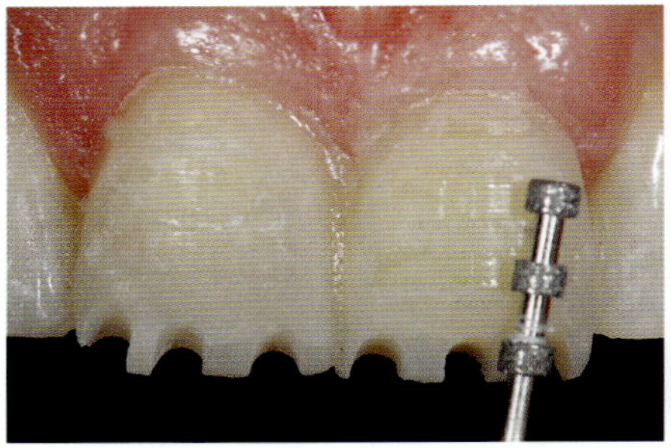

Fig 6-3a
The horizontal depth grooves on the labial surface and the incisal grooves (always through the mock-up).

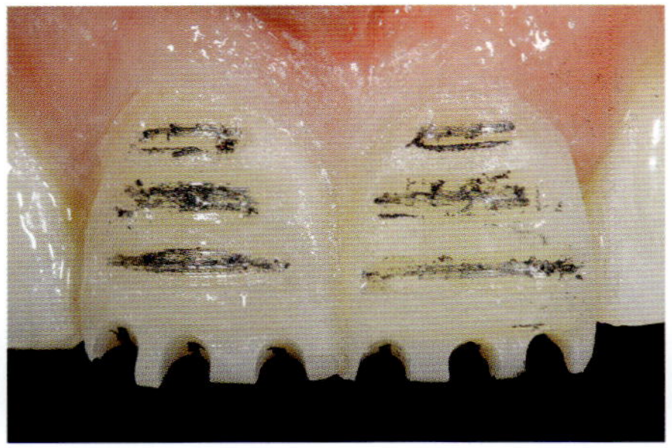

Fig 6-3b
Marking the horizontal grooves with a pencil helps identify where sufficient tooth structure has been removed.

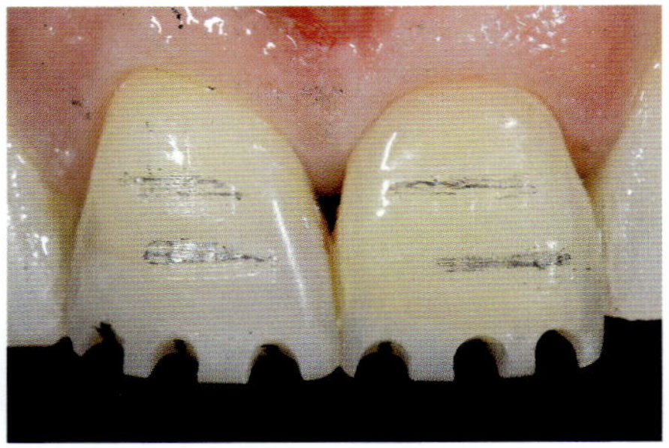

Fig 6-3c
After removing the test-drive veneers, we can see how minimal the amount of the actual tooth structure has been removed.

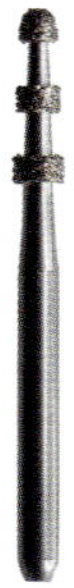

Bur no. 868B018 (0.4 mm)

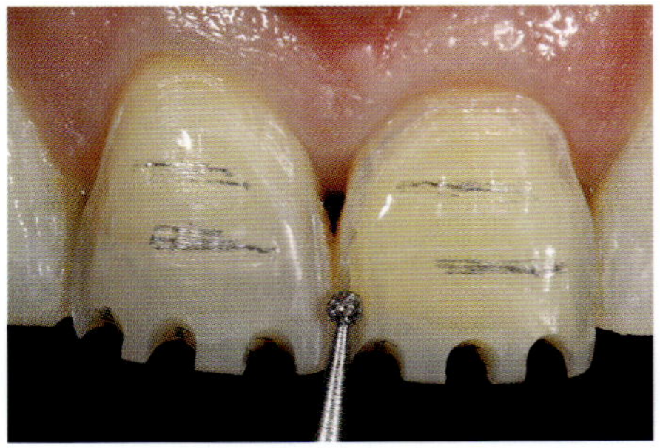

Fig 6-3d
The preparation outline on the labial surface was created with a round ball diamond bur.

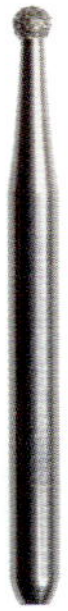

Bur no. 801012

Video: Preparation through the mock-up
https://books.dentist.com.pl/veneers/5

TIP

The initial outline margin of the preparation should be very gentle and not too deep. Also, it should not be too close to the soft tissues. Any additional deepening or shifting of the preparation toward the gingiva should be performed within the next stages of preparation.

Step 3: The incisal reduction

The incisal edge is reduced by 1.5 to 2 mm in relation to the planned final length of the veneer.[9–11] The bur should be placed perpendicularly toward the axis of the tooth while cutting the incisal edge. Do not prepare a chamfer finishing line on the palatal surface. The preparation on the incisal edge should be finished with a butt joint – this type of preparation remains preferable by the authors (to see more, check page 128).

Step 4: The definitive reduction of the labial surface

In the next step, the labial surface reduction is obtained by the preparation of the structure situated between the horizontal grooves (Fig 6-3e). The leveling of the surface must be performed in three different inclinations, depending on which part of the tooth is prepared: the cervical, the middle, or the incisal (Fig 6-3f).[12–14]

When preparing the labial surface, the bur must always be positioned to obtain three separate surfaces with different angles: the cervical, the middle, and the incisal.

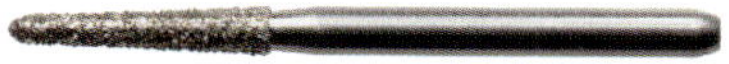

Bur no. 868016

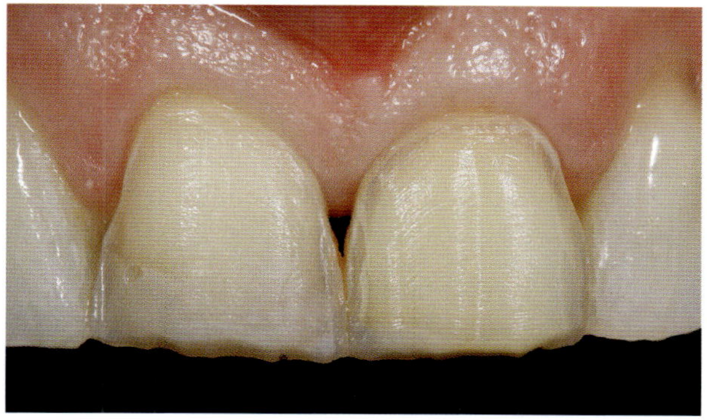

Fig 6-3e
The clinical situation after reducing the incisal edge and preparation after removing the horizontal grooves.

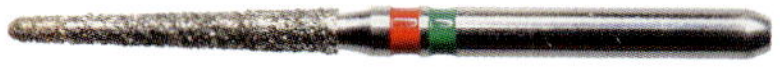

Bur no. 6844014

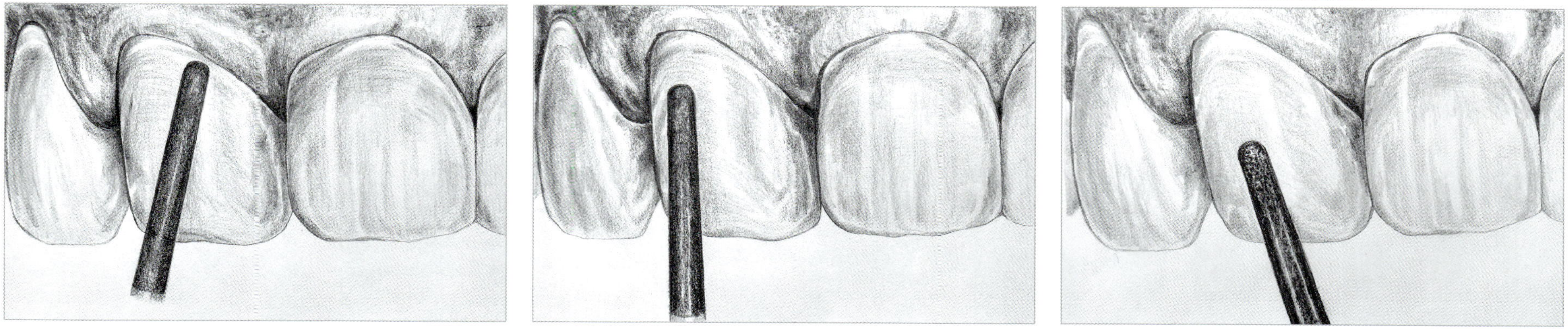

Fig 6-3f
During the veneer preparation, the inclination of the bur should differ, depending on which part of the surface we are working on: the cervical, the middle, or the incisal (bur no. 6844014).

Step 5: The 45-degrees preparation ("elbow" preparation)

When the proximal surface consists of a healthy tooth structure, usually there is no need to pass with the bur toward the palatal surface; however, it is important to prepare the embrasure space situated under the contact area to hide the veneer margin. To achieve this, the bur needs to be placed at an angle of 45 degrees, and a gentle outline needs to be prepared under the proximal contact (Fig 6-3g). The operator should always control the tooth preparation by viewing the prepared teeth from different angles: from the front, left, and right profiles (Fig 6-3h).

Step 6: Stripping of the proximal surfaces

If the proximal contact is loose, 45-degree preparation is usually sufficient. In the case of strong contact points, slightly loosening the proximal surfaces with an abrasive metal strip should be performed (Fig 6-3i). The purpose of loosening the proximal surfaces is to create a space for the impression material to freely enter the proximal contact and show the margin of the preparation. The loosening of the proximal surfaces should not be confused with the releasing of the proximal surfaces, which is a separate technique described in the next step.[15–17]

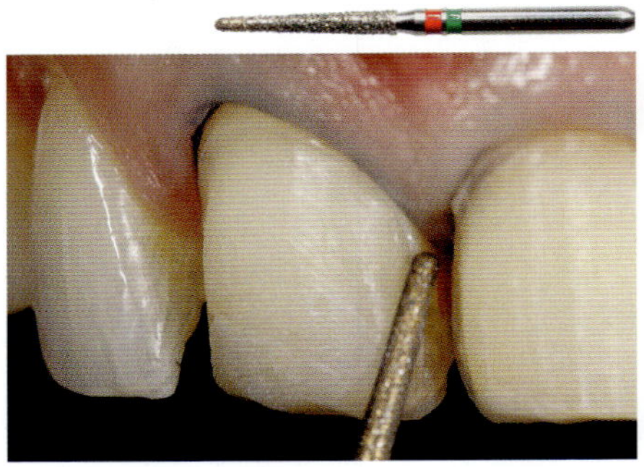

Bur no. 6844014

Fig 6-3g
Preparation of the tooth structure under the proximal contact with a bur at an angle of 45 degrees.

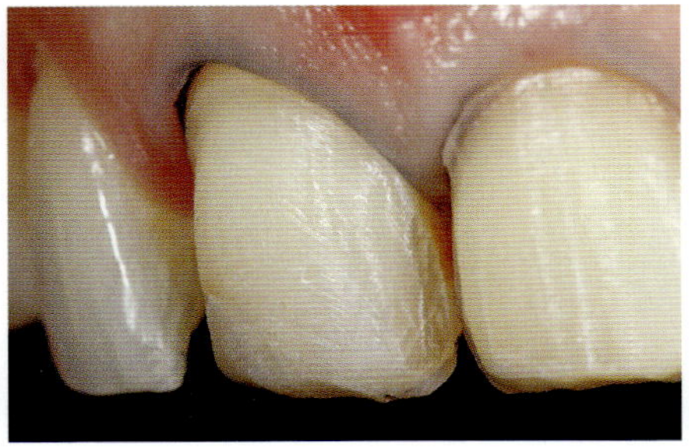

Fig 6-3h
To confirm the 45 degrees preparation, you should view the prepared tooth from the patient's semi-profile. In this position, the preparation margin usually becomes visible, which may create an esthetic problem after veneer cementation.

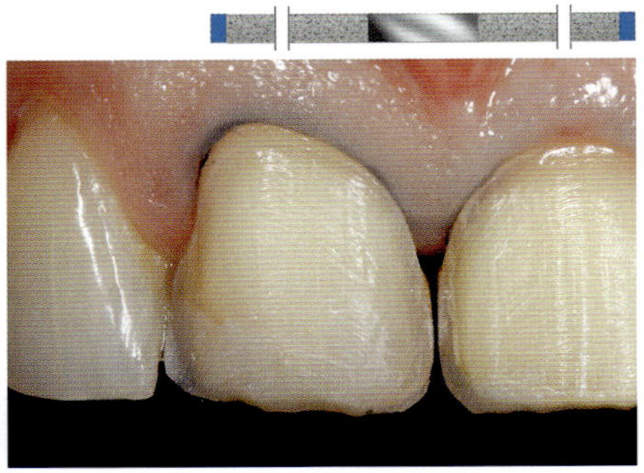

Metal abrasive diamond strip no. DS25

Fig 6-3i
Gentle stripping between the central incisors allows the dental technician to better visualize the preparation margin.

Video: The 45 degrees preparation
https://books.dentist.com.pl/veneers/6

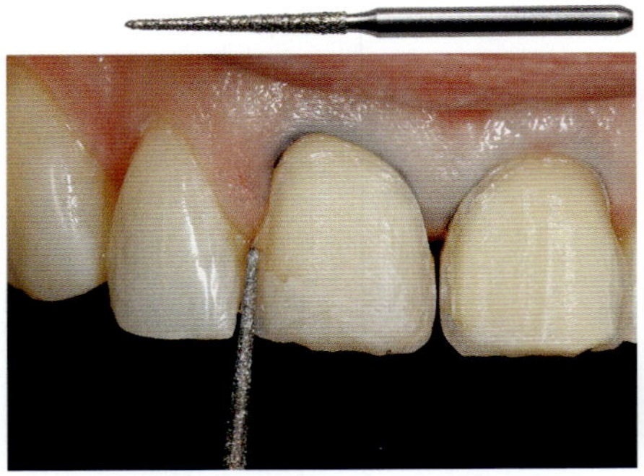

Bur no. 859010

Fig 6-3j
Preparation of the proximal surface due to the extensive restoration of tooth 11.

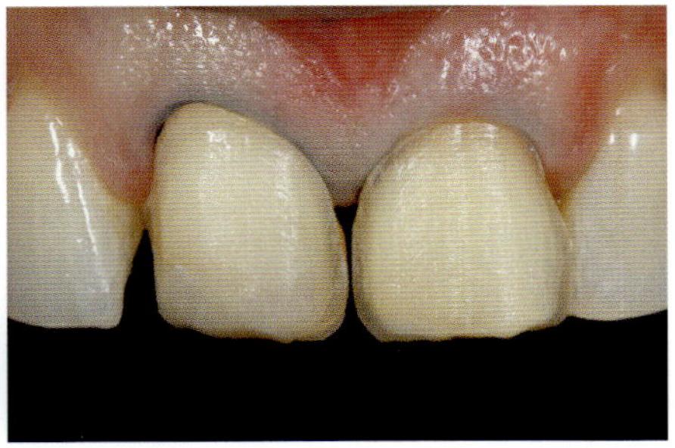

Fig 6-3k
Clinical situation after preparing the proximal surface of tooth 11.

Step 6 modified: Preparation of the proximal surfaces with an extension on the palatal surfaces

In some clinical situations, it is necessary to cover the entire proximal contact with a veneer.[18–22]

We will implement such a procedure when:

- There is an existing restoration on the proximal surfaces (Fig 6-3j)
- We plan to shift the line between the two adjacent teeth
- We plan to close the diastema
- It is necessary to correct the width of the individual teeth
- For this purpose, the proximal surfaces should be prepared so that the contact tooth veneer is relocated to the palatal surface (Fig 6-3k).

Step 7: Placing the first retraction cord

Suppose no retraction cord has been placed yet (for example, cord #000, Ultradent, not soaked in hemostatic agent). In that case, it is the right time to place it into the gingival sulcus for a minimal gingival retraction (Fig 6-3l).

Step 8: Shifting the preparation margin toward the gingival outline

The preparation margin should be brought closer to the gingiva, and the outline should be clearly marked for the dental technician (bur no. 6844014).

Step 9: Control of preparation with the silicone index and correction with a fine diamond bur

The silicone index should be positioned, and the preparation should be checked at the different levels of the labial surface (Fig 6-3m) and from the incisal edge (Fig 6-3n).[23,24] Places that need more preparation should be corrected with a bur no. 8868016 (Fig 6-3o) and checked again with the silicone index.

Step 10: Definitive smoothing of the surfaces

Finally, the surface is smoothed with a silicone polisher no. 9608 (Brownie Point, used in the past for amalgam polishing, 5000 rpm). Smoothing is carried out until the entire surface clearly reflects the light (Fig 6-3p). After polishing, all imperfections (such as sharp edges and unrounded angles) are clearly visible. If necessary, a correction can be made with a super fine diamond bur and polished with a polisher.

Fig 6-3l
The retraction cord #000 is placed in the gingival sulcus before the definitive modification of the preparation margin or at an earlier stage for the veneer.

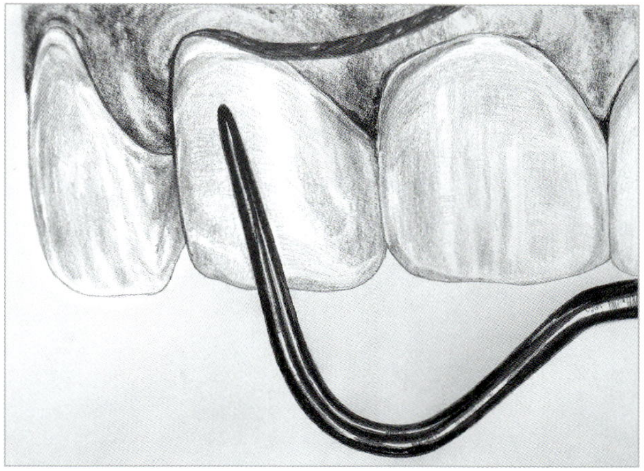

Video: Index check
https://books.dentist.com.pl/veneers/7

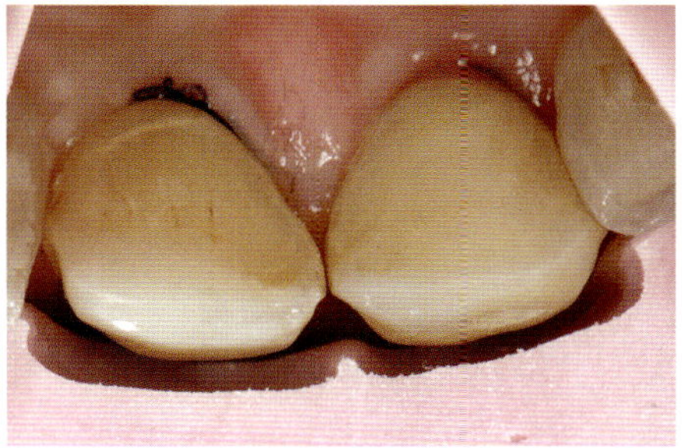

Fig 6-3m
Control of the labial surface preparation with a silicone index.

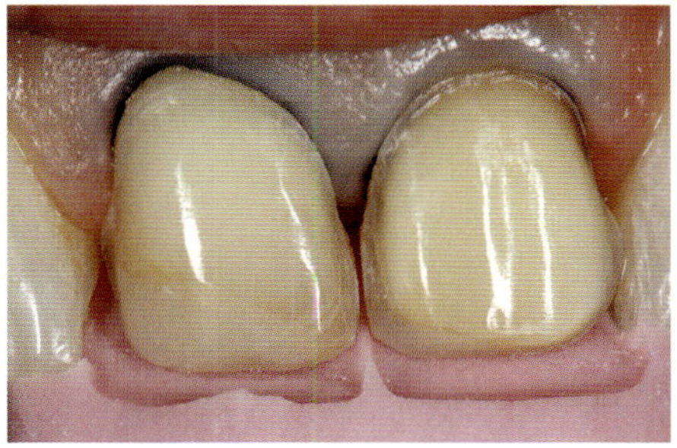

Fig 6-3n
Control of the incisal edge reduction.

Bur no. 8868016

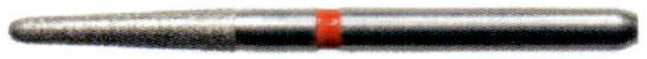

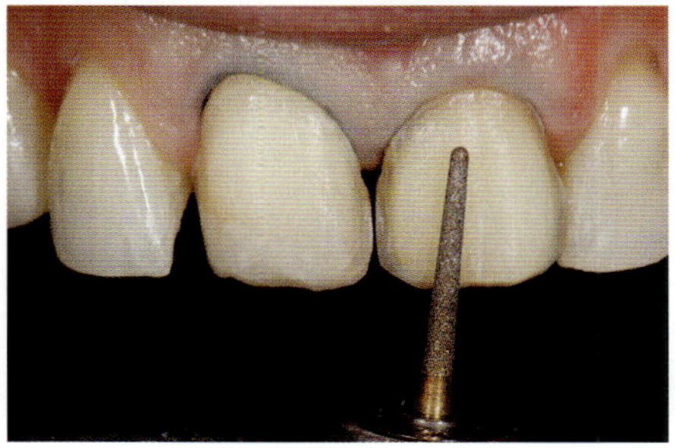

Fig 6-3o
Correction of the preparation with a bur.

Brownie Point no. 9608

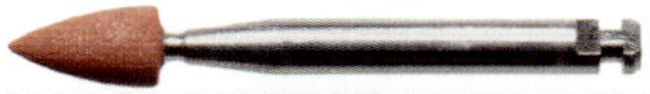

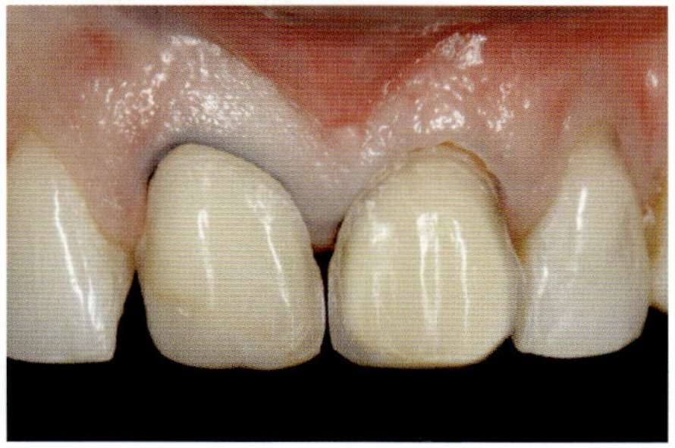

Fig 6-3p
The clinical situation after polishing the preparation surface. The gingival margin of tooth 21 was slightly corrected with electrosurgery. Tooth 11 was not prepared too close to the gingival margin to maintain the symmetry between the planned veneers.

SUMMARY OF PREPARATION

Fig 6-4a
The horizontal orientation depth grooves are prepared on the labial surfaces and the incisal edge (bur no. 868B018).

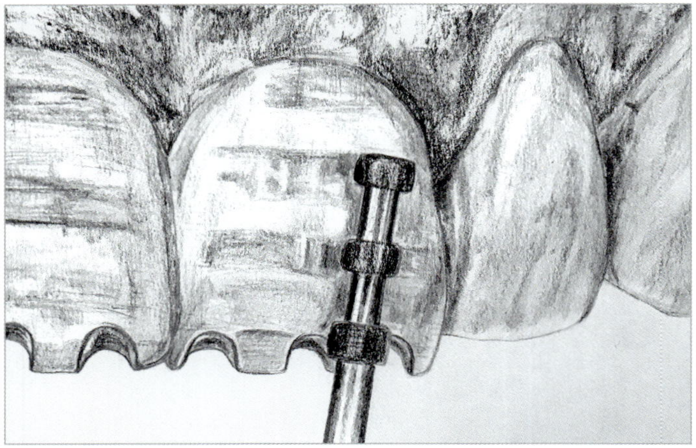

Fig 6-4b
Creating a gentle outline of the labial preparation with a round ball diamond bur (no. 801012).

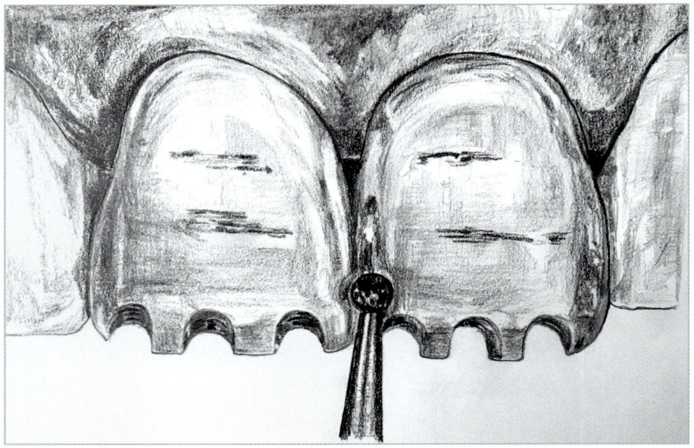

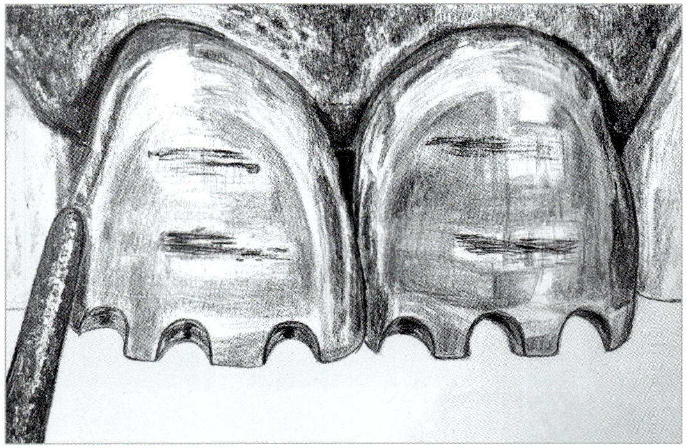

Fig 6-4c
If the round ball diamond bur appears too aggressive, we can use a chamfered diamond bur to outline the preparation.

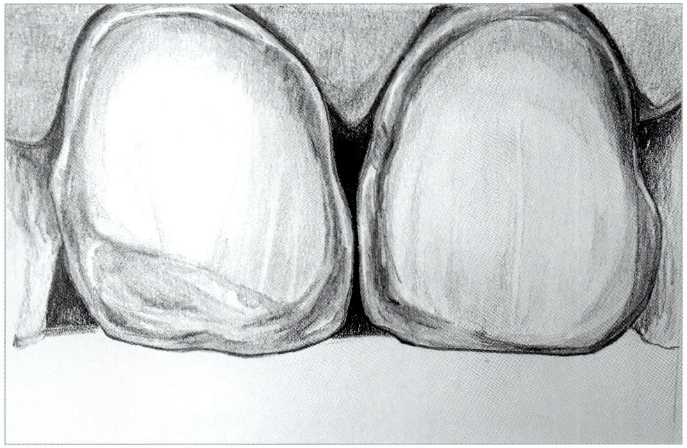

Fig 6-4d
A decision has to be taken whether the veneer will cover the proximal surface or if the proximal contact point will be maintained within the tooth structures.

Fig 6-4e
When the contact point remains in a healthy tooth structure, preparat on at the angle of 45 degrees must be carried out ...

Fig 6-4f
... in such a way that the preparation covers all the visible surfaces from the outside, including when looking from the semi-profile view.

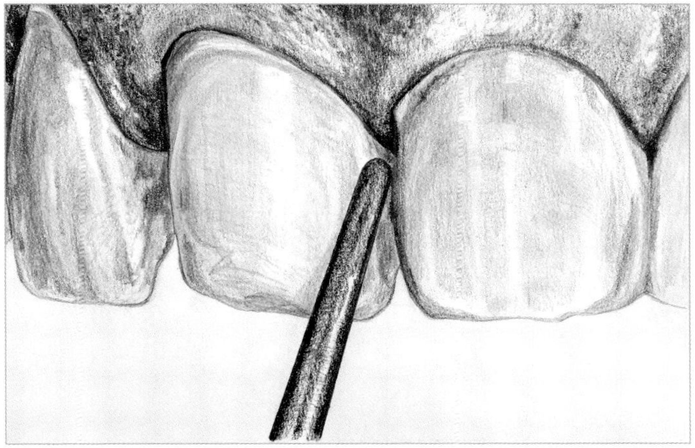

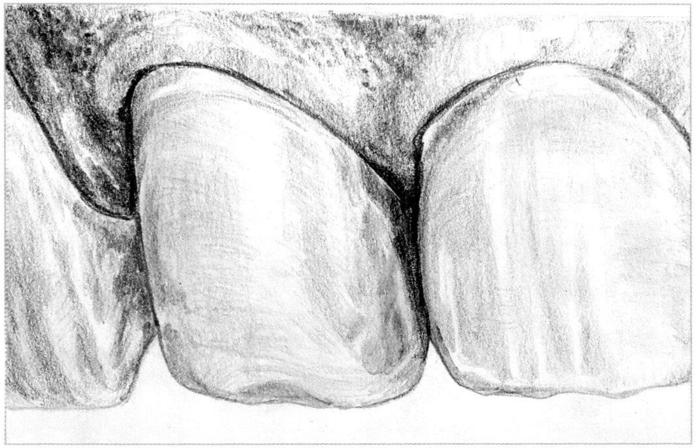

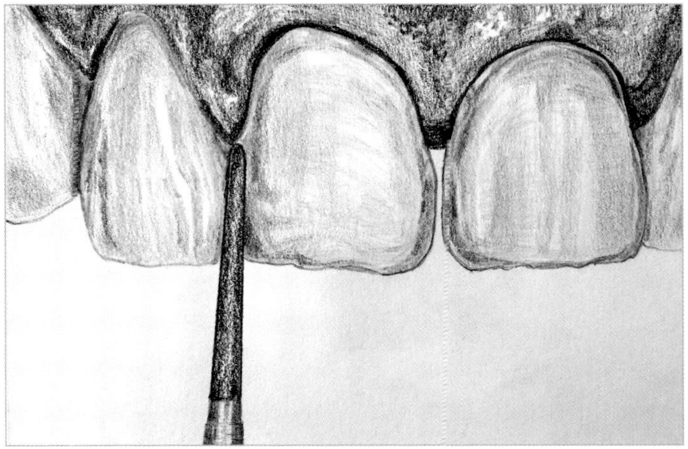

Fig 6-4g
In the event of an extended restoration on the proximal surface, the proximal reduction needs to be obtained with a narrow needle diamond, avoiding damage to the adjacent teeth.

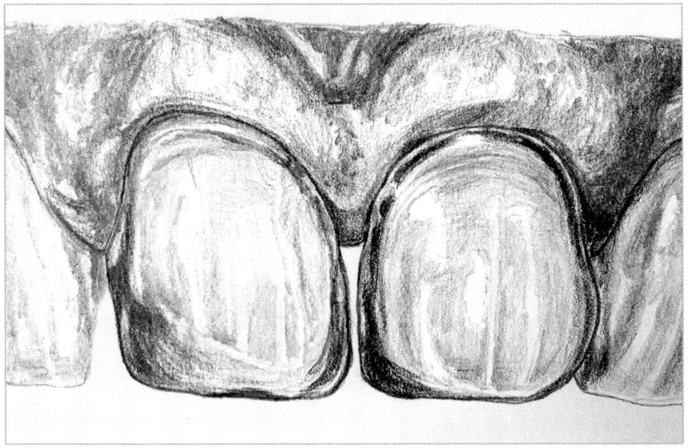

Fig 6-4h
Ensure that the preparation margin is clearly visible (especially on the proximal surfaces) and that the preparation surface is properly polished.

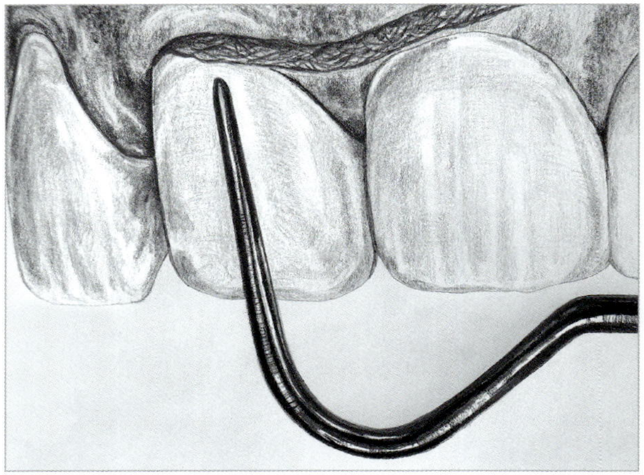

Fig 6-5a
The second gingival retraction cord should be a thicker one, so it will retract the soft tissues and allow the impression material to flow into the gingival sulcus (for example, cord #0).

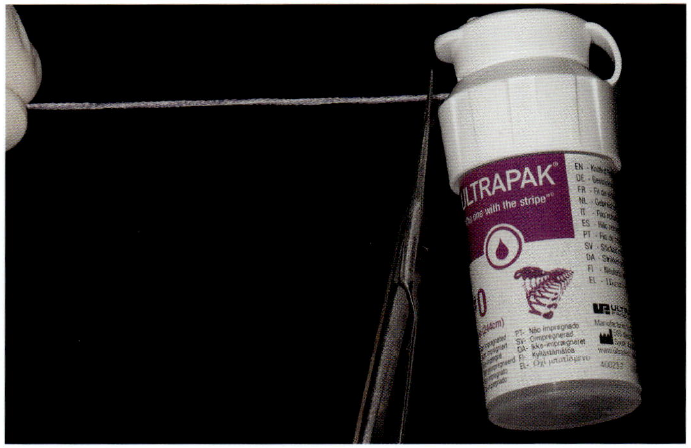

Fig 6-5b
The second retraction cord is usually cut in an unconventional way so that it is long enough to run along the gingival groove of all the prepared adjacent teeth for veneers.

Second gingival retraction cord

The first retraction cord, placed during step 7 of the preparation (Fig 6-3l), remains in the gingival sulcus. Its purpose is to seal the gingival sulcus and reduce the secretion of gingival fluid while taking the impression.

Next, the second retraction cord is placed (Fig 6-5a), soaked with a hemostatic agent (usually cord #0, Ultradent). The cord is cut to the appropriate length (Fig 6-5b) so that it can be placed in one piece on the entire labial side of the teeth prepared for veneers. The cord should be gently placed in the gingival groove. It should not be placed too deep, as its goal is to retract the gingiva outwards rather than inwards.

Positioning the cord in the gingival groove is usually achieved with a probe, and it should be left there for 5 to 10 minutes. While placing the retraction cord in the gingival sulcus (Fig 6-5c), moderate and gentle pressure should be applied on the cord with the instrument.

Holding the cord for a while in the gingival sulcus with an instrument allows the soft tissues to accept the cord inside the groove.

> **TIP**
>
> Never use excessive force, to avoid damaging the soft tissues and prevent bleeding.

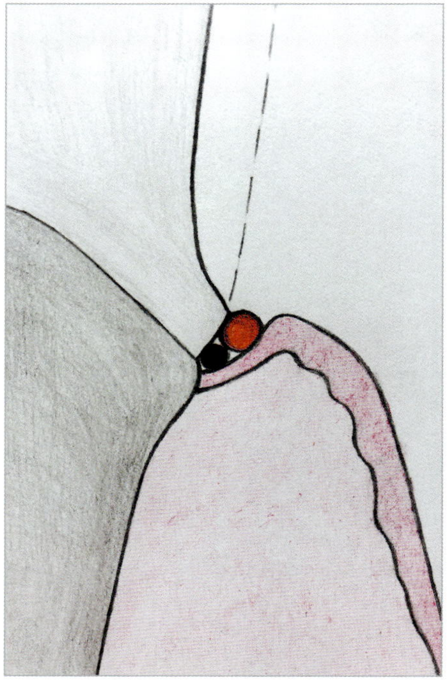

Fig 6-5c
The second retraction cord should not be placed deeply in the gingival groove. The purpose of placing this cord is to move the gingival tissue outwards, thus creating space for the impression material to flow into the gingival groove immediately after removing the cord.

FINAL IMPRESSION

Choice of impression material

To take an appropriate impression for the veneers, it is necessary to use a very precise impression material, such as polyether or polyvinyl siloxane.
A one-step/one-paste technique impression is taken with the polyether material, and usually a one-step/double-mix technique is required with polyvinyl siloxane material.

Taking a one-step/two-phase impression: double-mix technique

In this technique, the light body impression material (less viscous) is injected on the tooth directly after removing the retraction/deflection cord, while the heavy body impression material (with higher viscosity) is placed on the tray. How to choose an impression tray? It should not be too big or too small. The amount of the impression material around the prepared teeth must be sufficient to prevent the impression material from breaking in the area of the undercuts (Fig 6-5d).

Usually, two assistants are required to make a perfect impression. The second retraction cord should be placed in the gingival sulcus for 5 to 10 minutes to obtain a good retraction, giving us time to choose an impression tray and coat it with adequate adhesive for the polyether siloxane material (Fig 6-5e). The adhesive should be applied to the tray 5 minutes before taking the impression because it must dry for a sufficient adhesive effect.

FIVE STEPS FOR TAKING A ONE-STEP/TWO-PHASE IMPRESSION

Step 1: Rinse the teeth with a water-air spray, then dry them (the first dental assistant aspirates the excess water spray and saliva).

Step 2: Let the second dental assistant know that they can start applying the impression material on the tray. When the heavy body silicone paste (Fig 6-5f) begins to flow out of the Pentamix (or Dynamix) (for example, Variotime Heavy Tray), the assistant gives the dentist the signal: "Now." At this moment, we start to count the setting time of the impression material.

Video: Impression for the veneers
https://books.dentist.com.pl/veneers/8

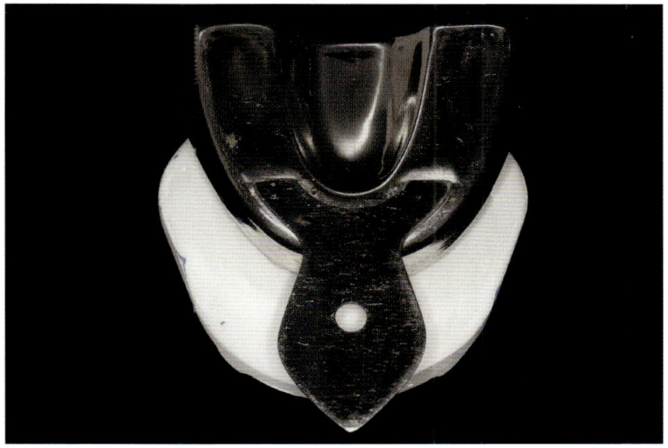

Fig 6-5d
The impression trays should be chosen in advance, for example, when the patient has been anesthetized before preparation. The impression trays should be neither too narrow nor too wide regarding the dental arch. The impression material should be of appropriate thickness to prevent it from tearing in the undercuts.

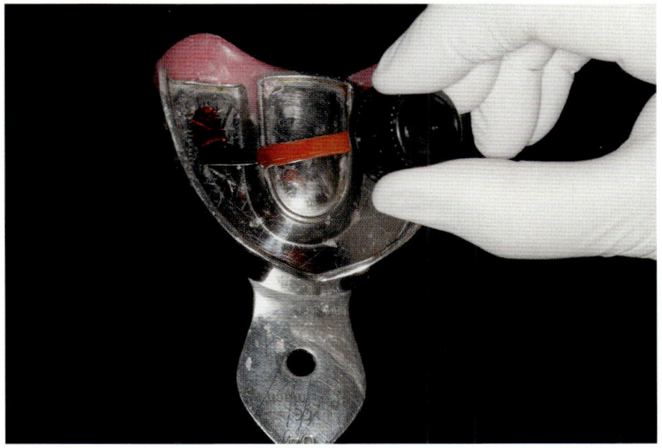

Fig 6-5e
The impression tray should be coated with an adhesive in advance (at least 5 minutes before taking the impression).

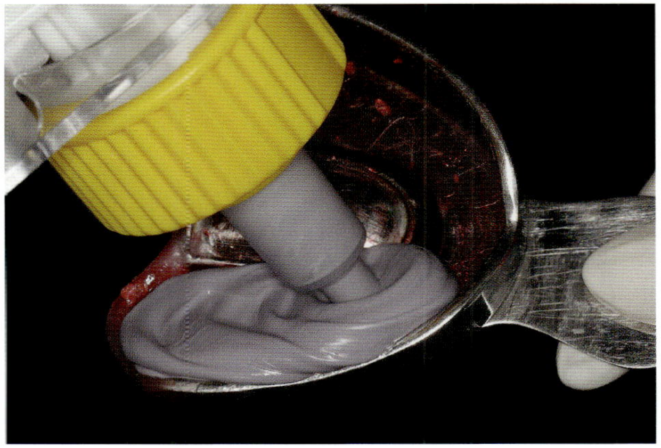

Fig 6-5f
Just before pulling out the cord from the gingival sulcus, we give a sign to the dental assistant to apply the heavy body mass in the impression tray.

Step 3: Now, the first assistant removes the thicker retraction cord from the gingival sulcus (Fig 6-5g), and the medium body silicone material (such as Variotime Medium Flow) is syringed directly from an automix system by the dentist (Fig 6-5h) along the gingival margin and on all the surfaces of the prepared teeth. It is important to apply the material continuously to avoid air bubbles.

Step 4: The impression tray is seated on the dental arch (Fig 6-5i) and stabilized without applying too much pressure. It is important to immobilize the impression tray in a stable position, especially during the first 90 seconds.

Step 5: Five minutes after Step 2, the impression material should be gently removed. The impression should be carefully inspected to understand whether there is a clearly defined finish line of the preparation, preferably using a magnification glass or under an operative microscope. It is important that the impression material exceeds the preparation margin, making it completely visible for the dental technician. In addition, the excess of impression material over the margin makes it easier to obtain a good emergence profile, compatible with the profile of the root beneath the preparation.

REMEMBER

Choosing the right size of impression tray is crucial for the final outcome of the impression. The impression tray should not touch the dental arch or the alveolar ridge, but at the same time, the space between the teeth and the impression tray should not be too big. The dentist should ensure that the front part of the tray covers a significant part of the gingival tissue above the preparation. If the shape of the tray does not make this possible, the impression tray should be customized, for example, by adding wax.

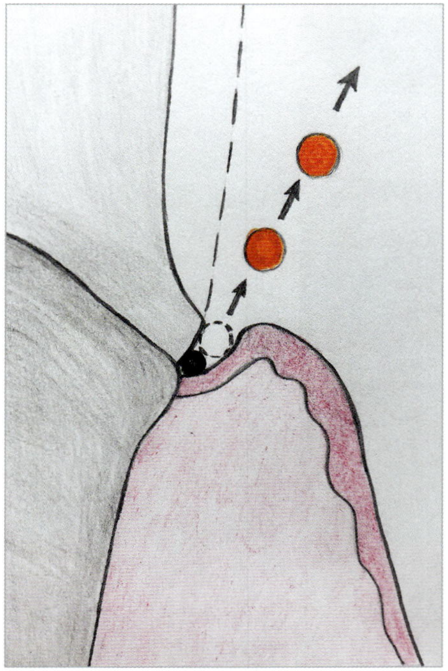

Fig 6-5g
The first assistant removes the thicker retraction cord from the gingival sulcus ...

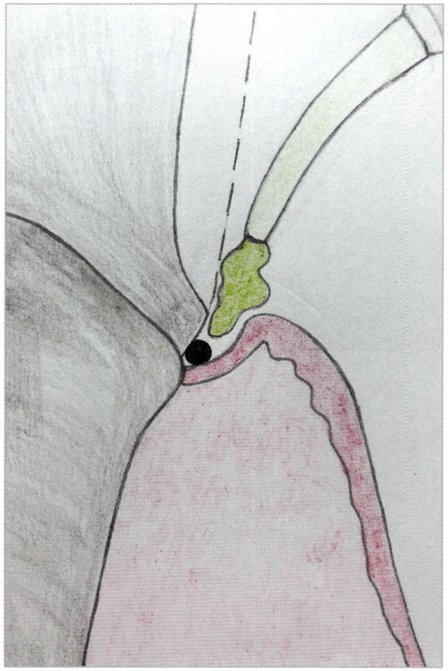

Fig 6-5h
... and the medium body impression material is syringed by the dentist in the gingival sulcus, millimeter by millimeter.

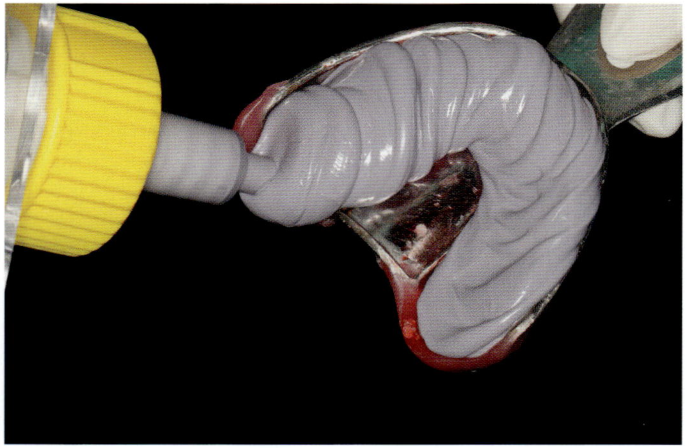

Fig 6-5i
The tray filled with the impression material – ready to be placed in the dental arch.

PROVISIONAL VENEERS

The fabrication of provisional veneers is a major problem for most practitioners. On the one hand, they should be as esthetic as possible and retain the prepared teeth until the next visit. On the other hand, they should be easily removable by the dentist. Veneers are prepared without any mechanical retention, which is typical for prosthetic crowns.

So how are provisional veneers supposed to last until the next appointment? The key to success is the dentist's skill and cleverness, and ensuring that the provisional material becomes wedged in the interdental spaces.

REMEMBER

Provisional veneers remain seated on the teeth thanks to material retention in the interproximal spaces; part of the material should be left in this area for adequate maintenance until the next visit. On the other hand, excess material around the gingival papilla can cause a gum recession. That is why major excess should be removed!

SIX STEPS FOR PERFORMING PROVISIONAL VENEERS

Step 1: Prepare the silicone index, from which the approved mock-up was made; it should be adjusted along the gingival margin so any possible excess of the temporary material can be removed from the interdental spaces (Fig 6-6a).

Step 2: If the provisional veneers are supposed to remain in the patient's mouth for an extended period, spot etching is recommended in the middle part of the labial surface (Fig 6-6b). A droplet of the bonding system is applied at the same limited surface area and polymerized.

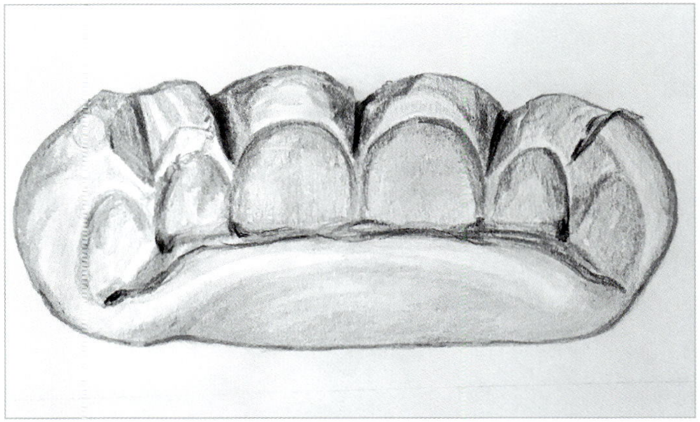

Fig 6-6a
The silicone index for provisional veneers should be properly trimmed in the interdental spaces to avoid the loss of the temporary composite.

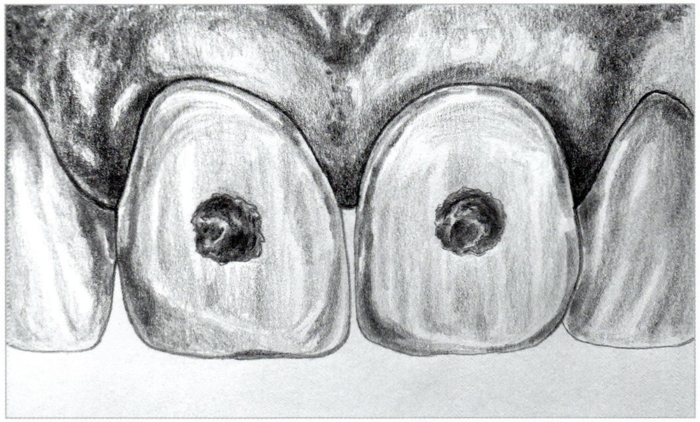

Fig 6-6b
If the provisional veneers are supposed to remain in the patient's mouth for more than a few days, it is recommended to perform spot etching on the labial surface, then spot a droplet of the bonding system and polymerize.

Step 3: A composite-based temporization material (such as Protemp) is directly syringed from an automix system and applied with the mixing tip placed at the deepest point of the silicone index (incisal edge; Fig 6-6c) by gradually extruding the material. In that way, the risk of air bubbles forming is reduced. Before the silicone index is inserted into the patient's mouth, it should be shaken to remove air bubbles.

Step 4: The silicone index is placed in the mouth (Fig 6-6d) (remember to mark the midline). Wait until the setting starts (approximately 60–90 seconds) before removing the composite excess. Now remove the excess from the interdental spaces with a flat spatula by moving it along the gingival margin.

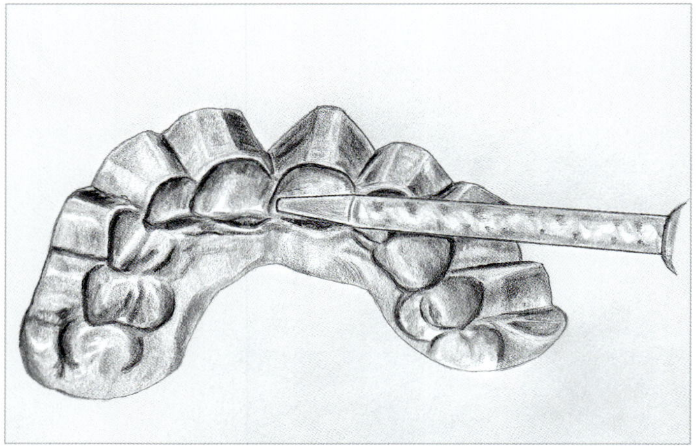

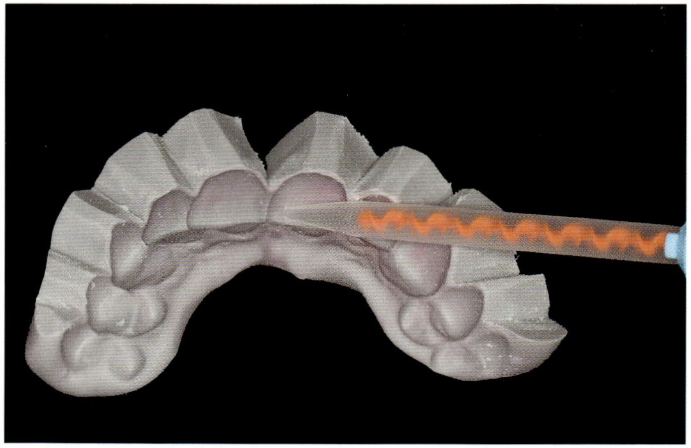

Fig 6-6c
Application of the temporary composite, applied from the mixing syringe directly into the silicone index. The mixing tip should be positioned at the deepest point of the silicone index so that no air bubbles can form.

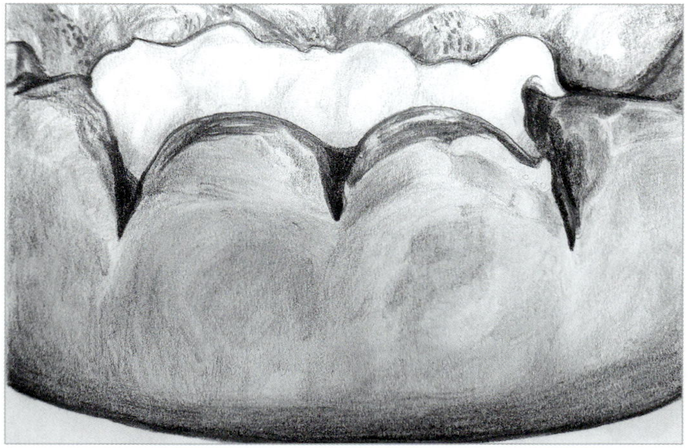

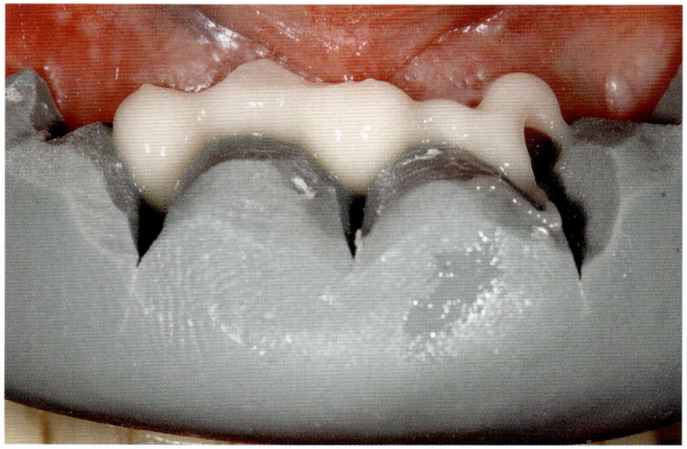

Fig 6-6d
The silicone index is placed on the prepared teeth (remember about the marked midline to facilitate the appropriate placement of the index on the teeth). After about 60 seconds, we start to remove the excess material.

Step 5: Remove the index and start removing the excess material from the palatal surface and the gingival margin (Fig 6-6e; scalpel no. 12, Excesso Style Italiano); the remaining excess should be gently removed with a bur no. 889540009 (Fig 6-6f), in such a way as to avoid bleeding from the gingiva. Leaving the excess temporary composite that compresses the gum is associated with a risk of recession, especially if the provisional veneers are placed for a longer period.

Step 6: Articulating paper is used to detect premature contacts and to remove them with a rugby ball-shaped bur. Any unevenness on the palatal surfaces is removed with a Sof-Lex disk. Eliminations of overloading will increase the chance of maintaining the provisional veneers.

Video: Provisional veneers
https://books.dentist.com.pl/veneers/9

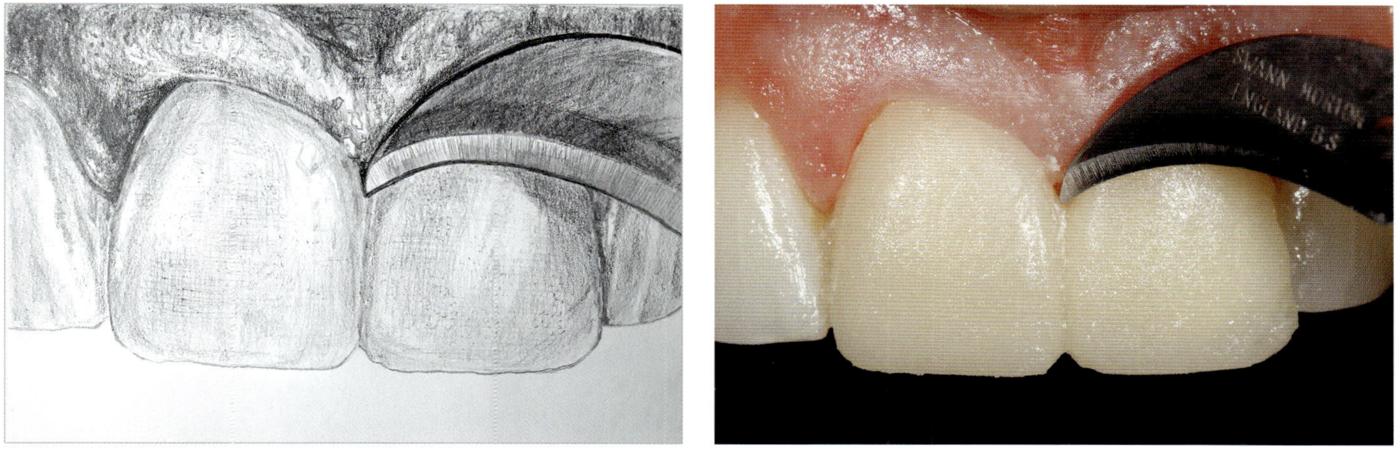

Fig 6-6e
After a few minutes, the silicone index is removed from the mouth and the polymerized resin excess can be gently removed with a scalpel no. 12. To avoid soft tissue damage, always hold the blade in the opposite direction to the gingiva.

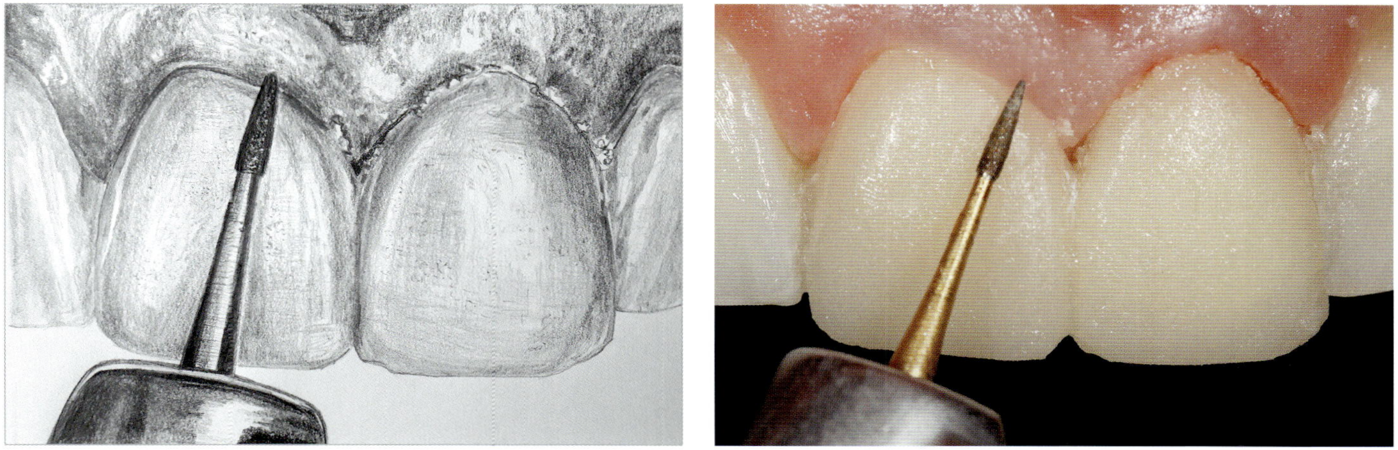

Fig 6-6f
If any additional excess material needs to be removed, use a bur no. 889540009.

INCISAL EDGE PREPARATION DILEMMAS

The subsection on preparation for porcelain veneers (step 3) describes the preparation of the incisal edge. The butt joint preparation (Fig 6-7c) is chosen as preferable by the authors where the incisal edge is covered with the veneer by 1.5 to 2 mm. This does not mean that you should always prepare 1.5 to 2 mm of the incisal edge because, in most cases, the aim of veneers is to extend the incisal edge. So, the preparation is performed from the mock-up, often without touching the actual tooth structures. 1.5 to 2 mm incisal coverage with a butt joint veneer is preferred for the following reasons:

- We can extend the incisal edges of the anterior teeth symmetrically, according to the new planned smile line
- Thanks to the new treatment plan, we gain the space for modeling the incisal edges, which from an esthetic point of view represents the most important detail exposed from the upper lip while smiling and in the rest position
- We gain a favorable path for veneer insertion from the labial side during the placement, which allows less invasive preparation (slight undercuts in the proximal and cervical area are not an issue anymore)
- The appropriate thickness of the ceramics strengthens the incisal edge
- Preparation without palatal extension decreases the risks of:
  - Constriction of the envelope of function (in case of thick porcelain)
  - Unpredictable preparation of the palatal surface, which is difficult for the dentist to repeat and can turn out to be too shallow
  - Chipping off the palatal part of the veneer
  - More invasive preparation due to the insertion path being in line with the long axis of the tooth
- This type of preparation has been confirmed in studies as the most predictable for the long-term success of the veneers
- The dentist can easily perform it, and it is repeatable

What should be done if the palatal surface is worn or damaged by erosion? Should a palatal extension be performed for the veneer preparation?

The answer is: No! It is better to restore the damaged palatal surfaces with the composite resin and finish the preparation with a butt joint in this clinical situation. In Fig 6-7, four different types of preparation are shown.

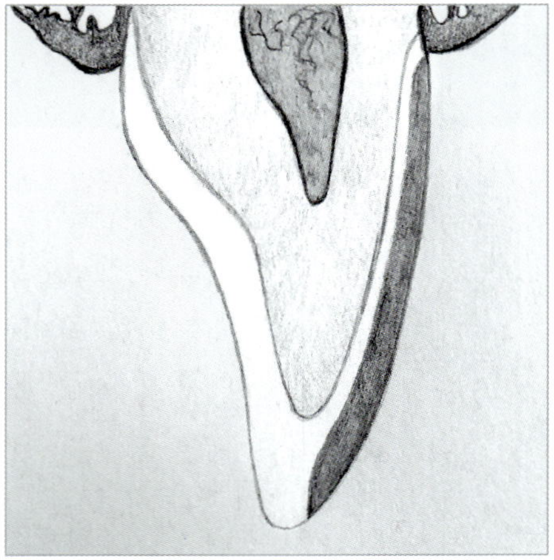

Fig 6-7a
The window preparation; the incisal edge remains intact.

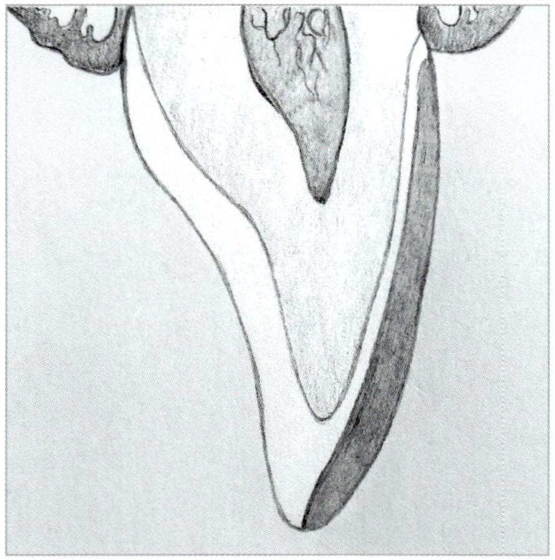

Fig 6-7b
The feather-edge preparation: the incisal edge is prepared labially but its length remains unchanged.

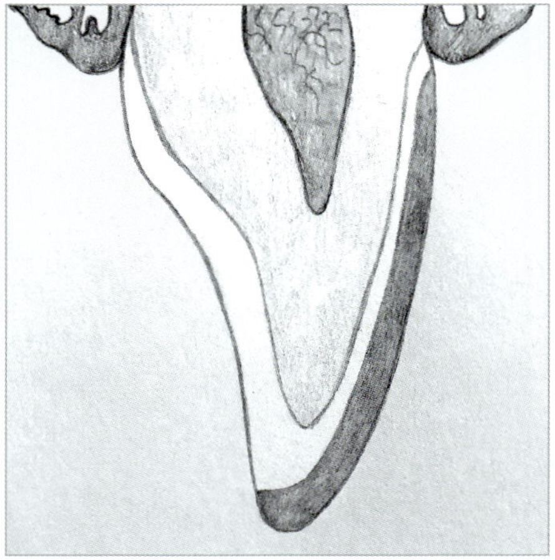

Fig 6-7c
The bevel or butt joint incisal preparation.

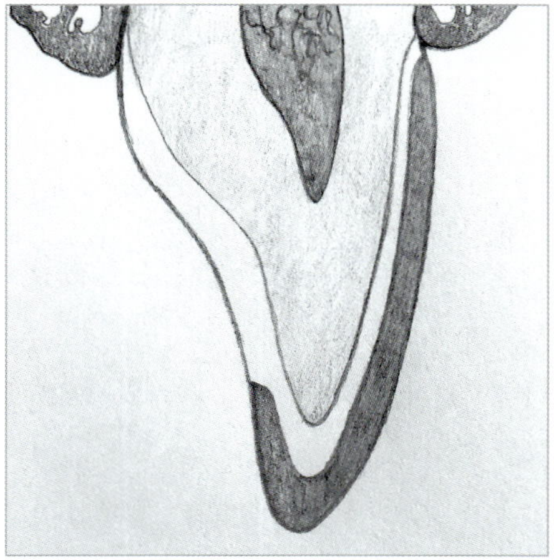

Fig 6-7d
The preparation with palatal extension.

PROXIMAL SURFACE PREPARATION DILEMMAS

The subsection on the preparation for porcelain veneers (step 5 and step 6 modified) concerns the preparation of the proximal surface. Several types of preparation can be distinguished here:

1. **Short-wrap design:** this is a preparation with a small interference range within the proximal surface. In this type of preparation, the proximal surface remains in its original position and is created by original tooth structures (the margin between the porcelain veneer and the hard tissues are visible; Fig 6-8a).

2. **Medium-wrap design**: this is a preparation with a medium range of interference within the proximal surface where its margin is moved more toward the interdental space (the margin between the porcelain veneer and the hard tissues are not visible) while maintaining the proximal surface within the original tooth structure (Fig 6-8b).

3. **Long-wrap design:** this is a preparation with a greater range of interference where the proximal surface is released and the original tooth structures are covered with the porcelain veneer that creates a completely new contact point (Fig 6-8c).

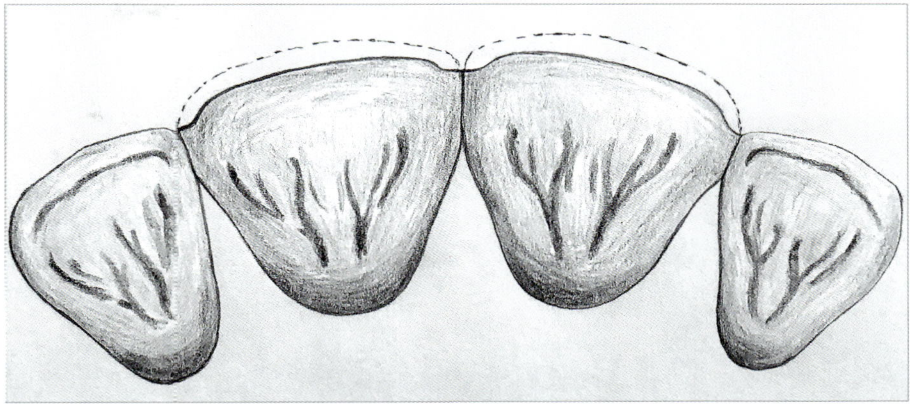

Fig 6-8a
Short-wrap design: a preparation with a small range of interference within the proximal surface.

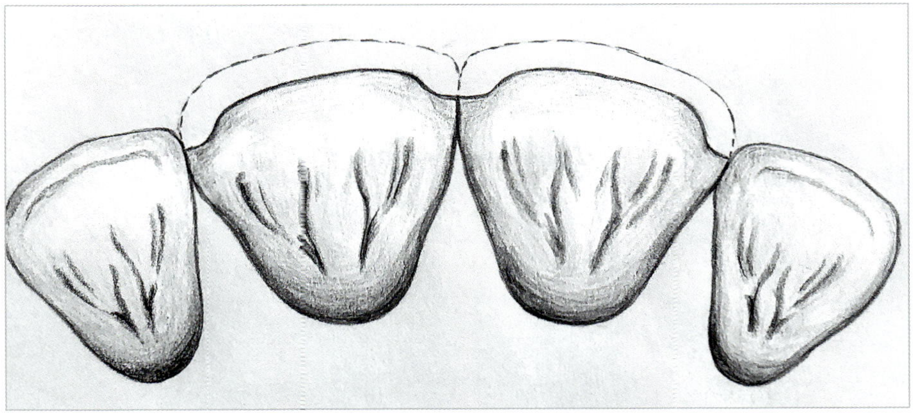

Fig 6-8b
Medium-wrap design: a preparation with a medium range of interference within the proximal surface (depending on the clinical situation, the proximal contact is made up entirely or partially by the hard tissues)

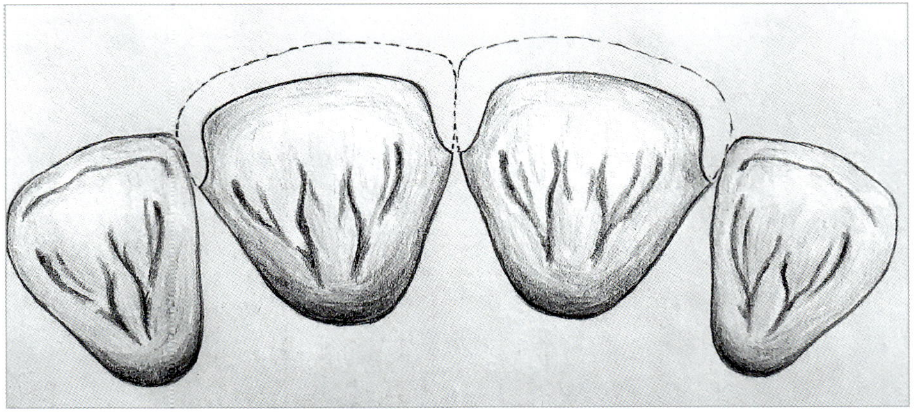

Fig 6-8c
Long-wrap design: a preparation with a greater range of interference where the proximal surface is completely released.

Analyzing the preparation of the proximal surfaces in the sagittal section, we can notice that the short-wrap and medium-wrap preparation does not release the original proximal contact point, but with "elbow" preparation they can interfere in the interdental space to cover the surface located directly below the contact point and visible from the profile (Fig 6-9).

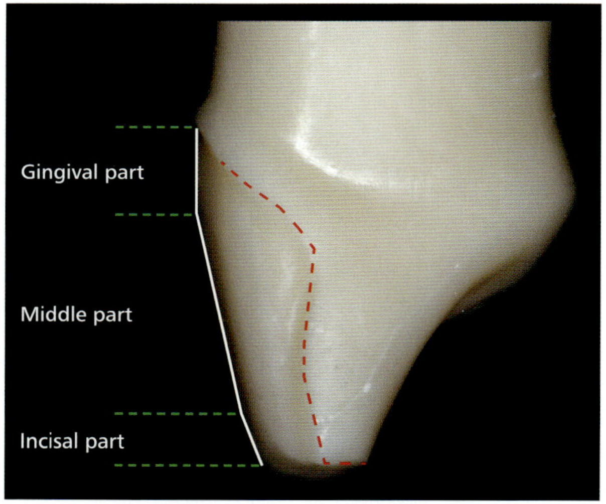

Fig 6-9a
Preparation for the porcelain veneers without eliminating the proximal surface, with "elbow" preparation entering the interdental space.

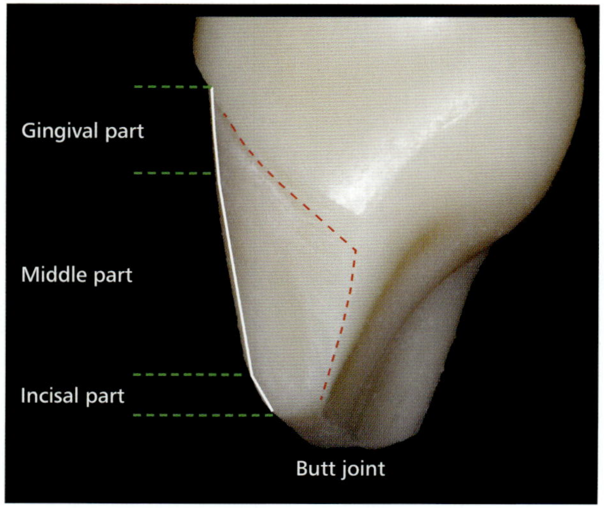

Fig 6-9b
Preparation for the porcelain veneers with the release of the original proximal surface (recommended, for example, when extensive composite restoration Class 3 or 4 is located on the proximal surface and should be covered with the veneer).

CANINE PREPARATION DILEMMAS

Preparation for the canines is exactly the same as for the incisors – the butt joint preparation of the incisal edge. Another case illustrates the preparation of the canines as part of comprehensive prosthetic therapy (Fig 6-10).

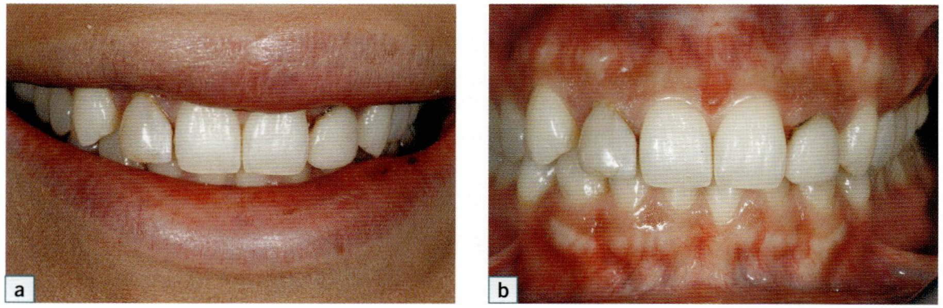

Figs 6-10a and 6-10b
The patient presented to the dental clinic seeking a better esthetic outcome for the maxillary dental arch.

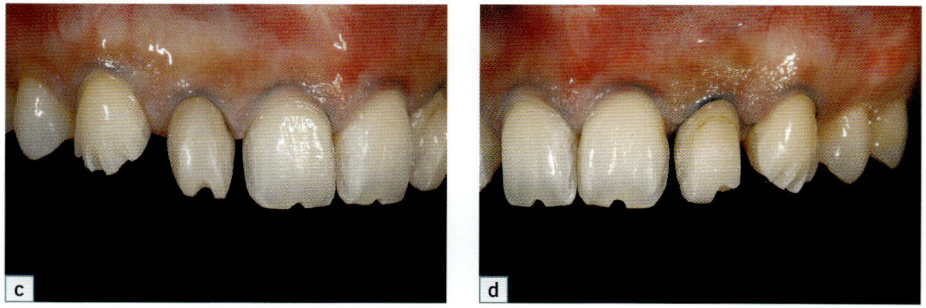

Figs 6-10c and 6-10d
After aligning the symmetry in the gingival margin, teeth 13–23 were prepared by obtaining the orientation grooves on the incisal edges (pay attention to the preparation of the incisal edges of the maxillary canines).

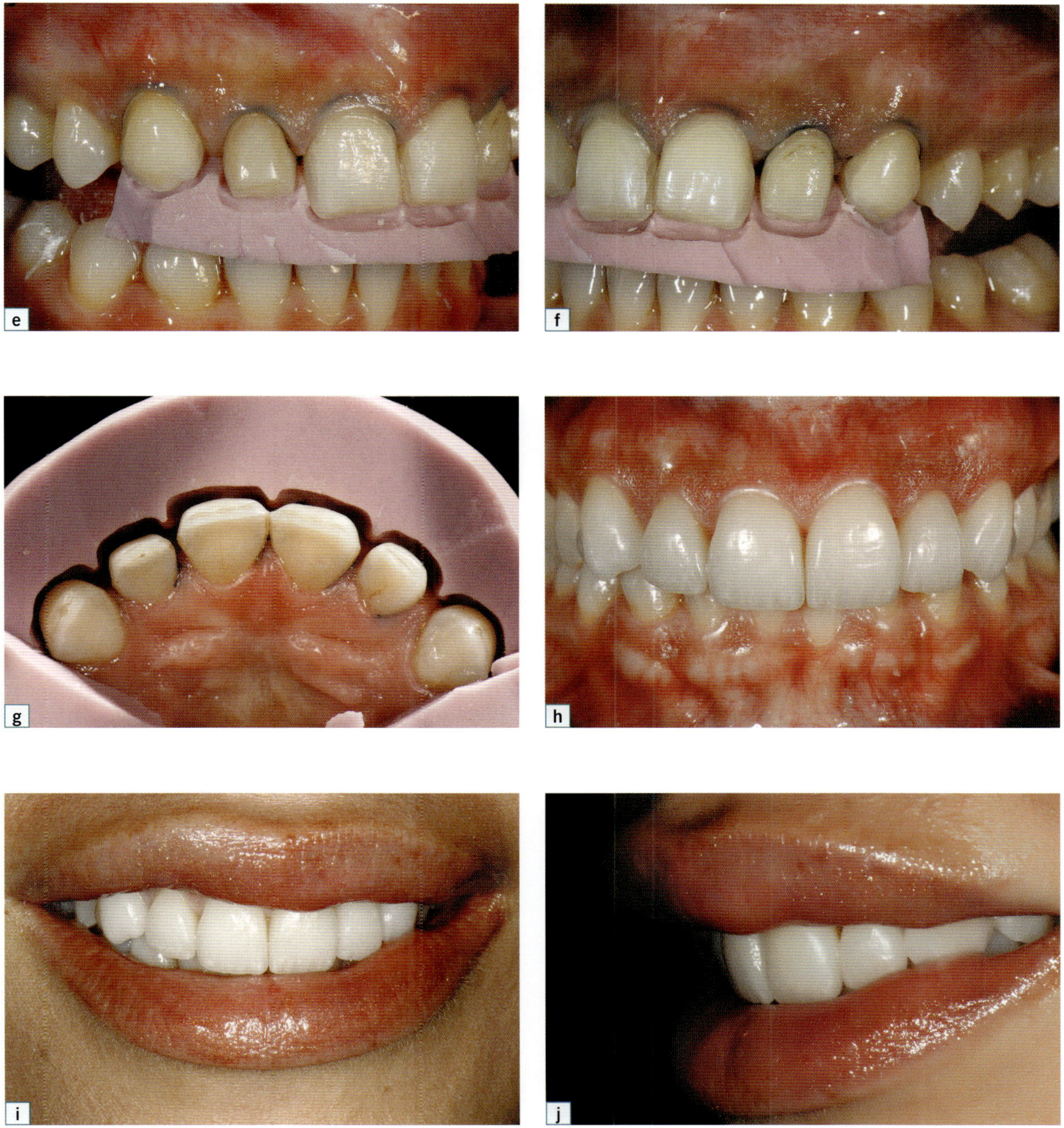

Figs 6-10e and 6-10f
Next, the reduction on the incisal edges was performed in accordance with the previously marked orientation grooves. The definitive preparation of the incisal edge was controlled with the adjusted silicone index.

Fig 6-10g
Control of the preparation depth on the labial surface.

Fig 6-10h
Clinical situation after veneer placement on teeth 13–23.

Figs 6-10i and 6-10j
The patient's smile after treatment.

PREMOLAR PREPARATION DILEMMAS

When preparing premolars, the preparation procedure includes the labial surface and partially the bucco-occlusal edge, preferably without interference with occlusion, in order not to increase the functional risk (Fig 6-11).

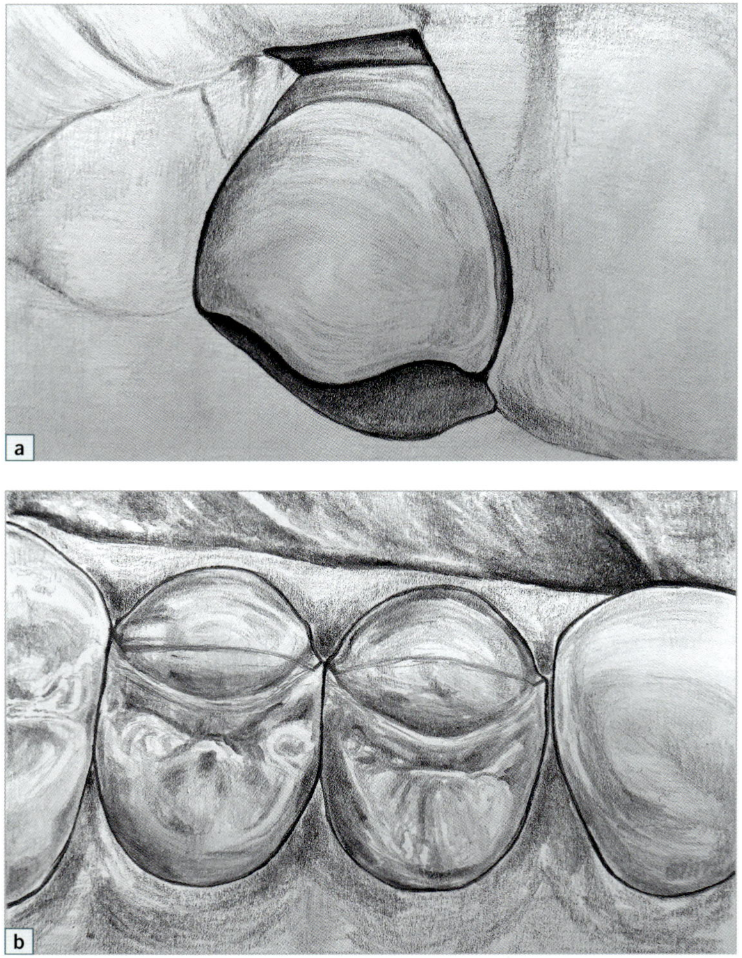

Fig 6-11
Preparation of the maxillary premolars: (a) labial view with a rubber dam; (b) occlusal view.

MANDIBULAR INCISOR PREPARATION DILEMMAS

The author of this chapter is not in favor of preparing mandibular teeth for porcelain veneers due to the small size of the mandibular incisors (and the associated risk of dentin exposure), and also because their labial surface is in contact with the palatal surface of the maxillary teeth during functional movements. Thickening the labial surfaces of the mandibular veneers often results in constriction of the functional envelope, which increases the functional risk significantly. The issue is broadly discussed in Chapter 8. However, sometimes there are favorable conditions to fabricate porcelain veneers in the mandibular dental arch (for example, when we reconstruct worn dentition occlusion or replace old veneers with new ones). The preparation steps are exactly the same: preparation through the mock-up, creating the orientation depth grooves, and butt joint preparation on the incisal edge with a 1.5 mm space reserved for the ceramic material. The case illustrated in Fig 6-12 shows mandibular arch porcelain veneer treatment accompanied by simultaneous increasing the occlusal vertical dimension (OVD).[25–33]

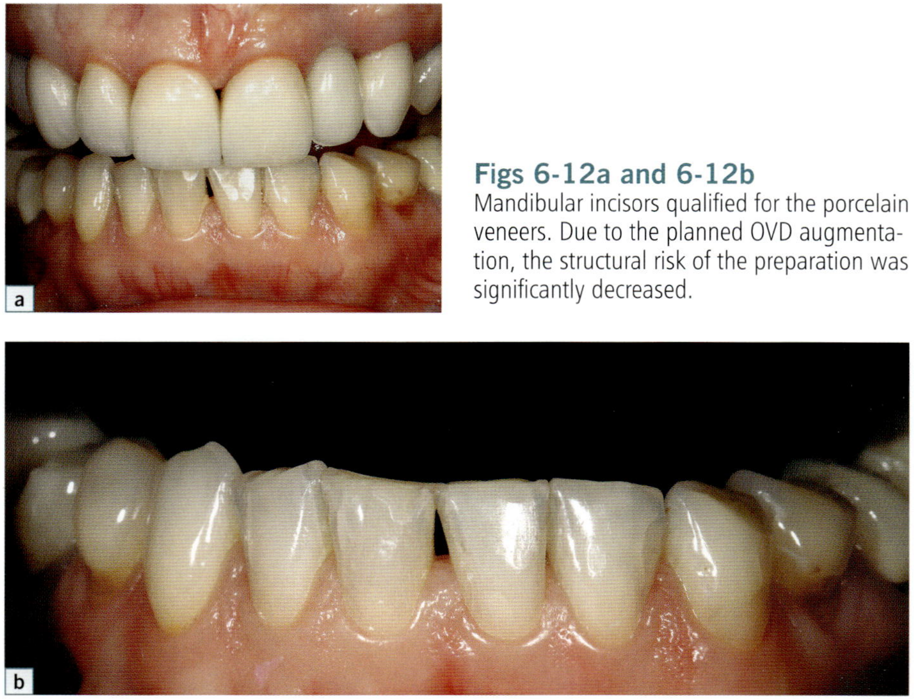

Figs 6-12a and 6-12b
Mandibular incisors qualified for the porcelain veneers. Due to the planned OVD augmentation, the structural risk of the preparation was significantly decreased.

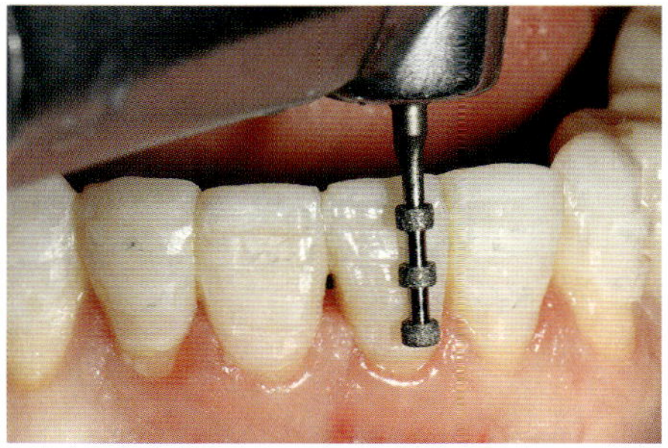

Fig 6-12c
The preparation was started through the mock-up (after increasing the OVD – in the first stage with the provisional restorations); orientation depth grooves on the labial surface were performed.

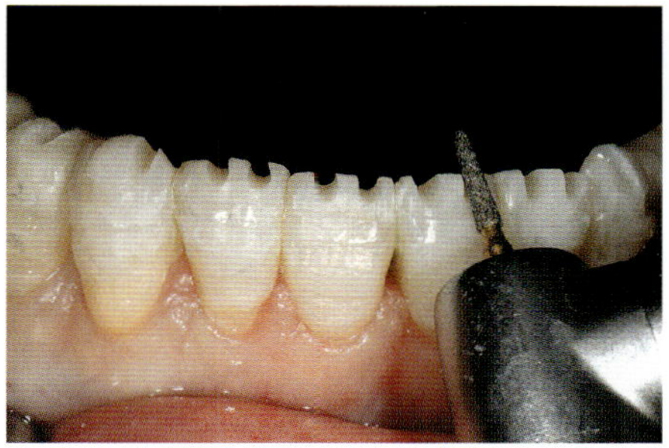

Fig 6-12d
The orientation depth grooves on the incisal edges.

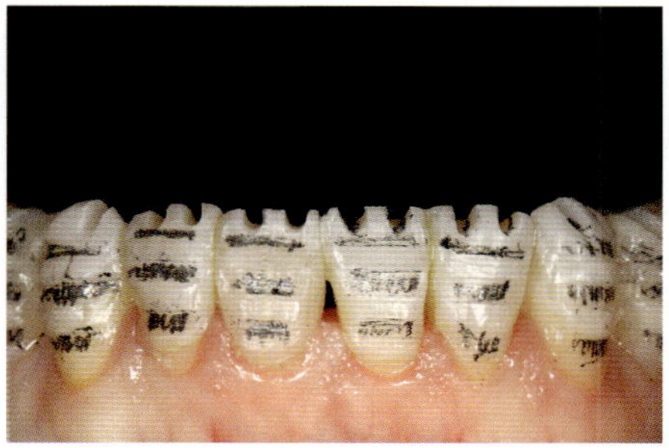

Fig 6-12e
The clinical situation after marking the orientation depth grooves with a pencil.

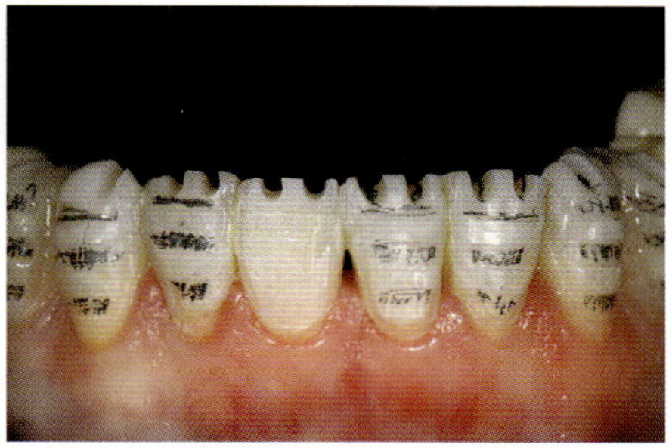

Fig 6-12f
The labial surface of tooth 41 was prepared accordingly to the orientation grooves.

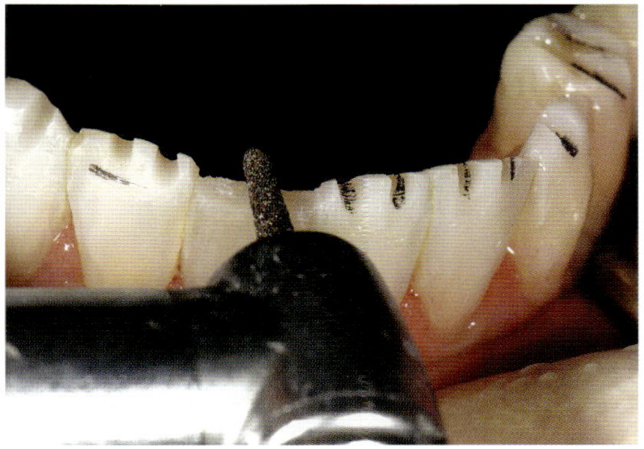

Fig 6-12g
A bur was positioned perpendicular to the tooth axis to reduce the incisal edge.

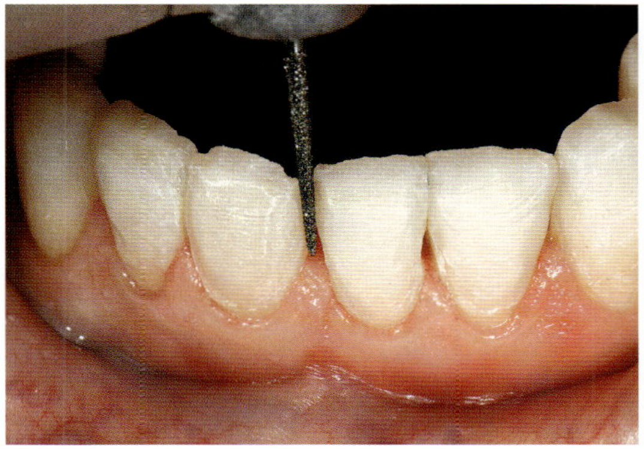

Fig 6-12h
The long axis of the tooth, which was deviated, required the preparation of the proximal surfaces. The dental technician could create a midline connecting the central mandibular incisors perpendicularly to the horizontal plane.

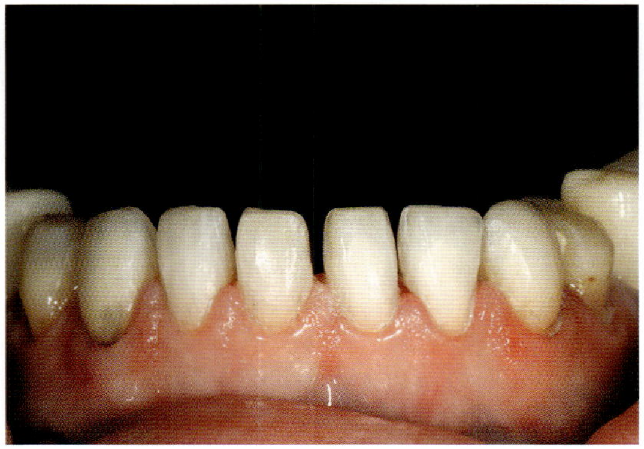

Fig 6-12i
Clinical situation after preparation of teeth 44–34.

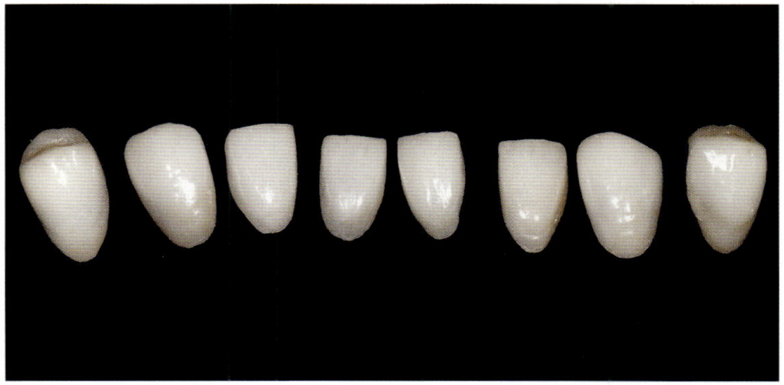

Fig 6-12j
Porcelain veneers on teeth 44–34, ready for cementation.

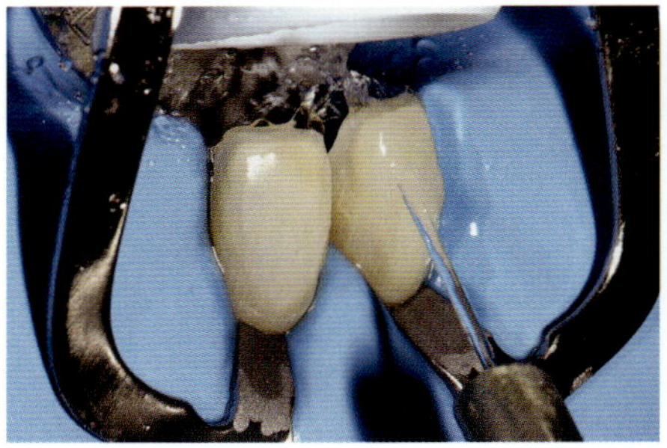

Fig 6-12k
Isolation of teeth 41 and 31 during adhesive preparation for the veneer cementation.

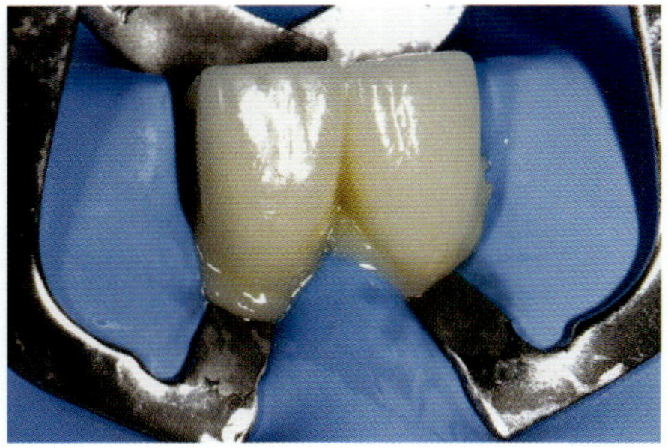

Fig 6-12l
Cementation of the veneers on teeth 41 and 31.

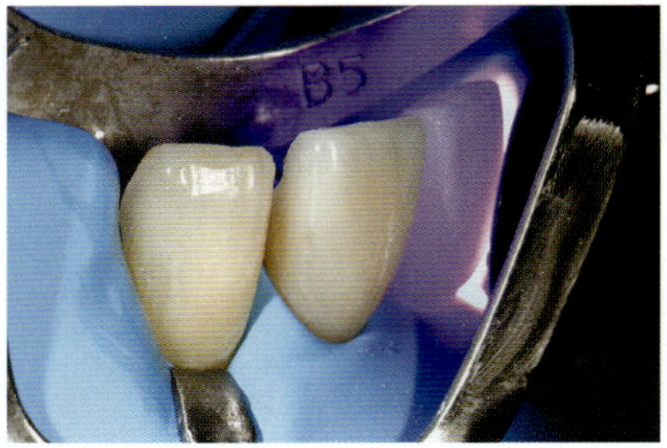

Fig 6-12m
Isolation of tooth 42 during adhesive veneer cementation.

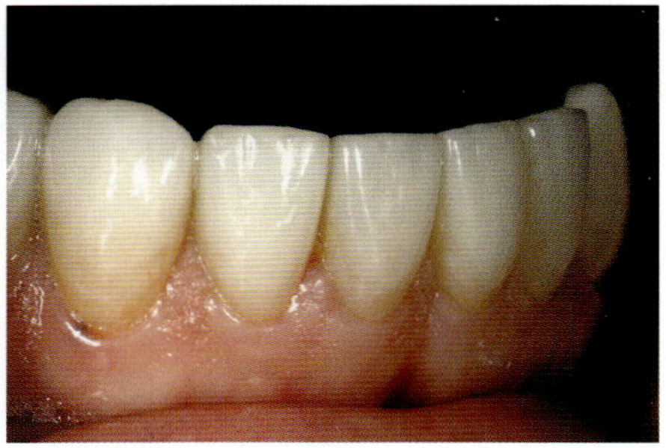

Fig 6-12n
Veneers after cementation.

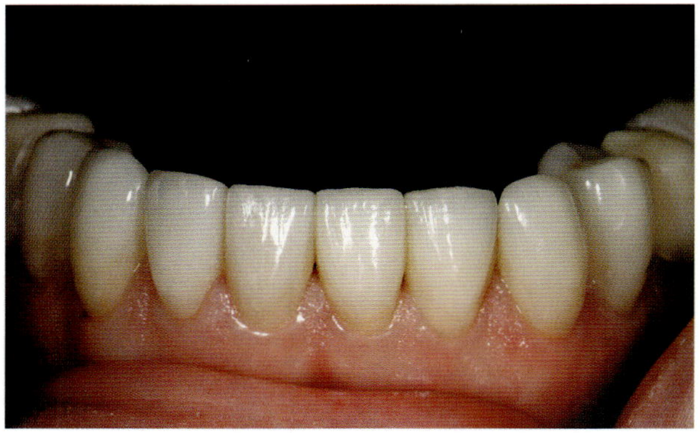

Fig 6-12o
Clinical control of the porcelain veneers in the mandibular arch 6 months after cementation.

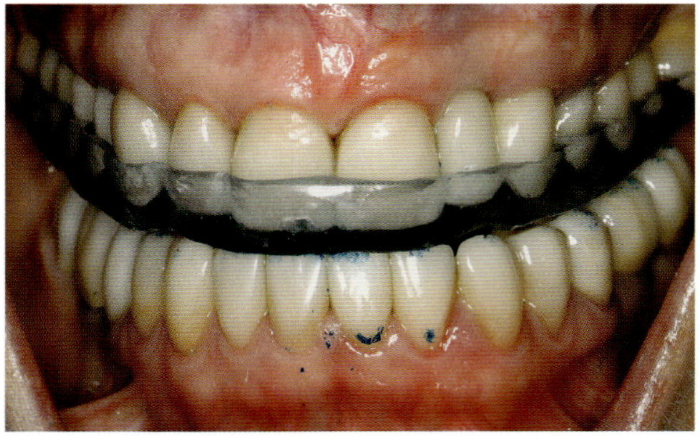

Fig 6-12p
Michigan splint made for the maxillary arch to protect the veneers.

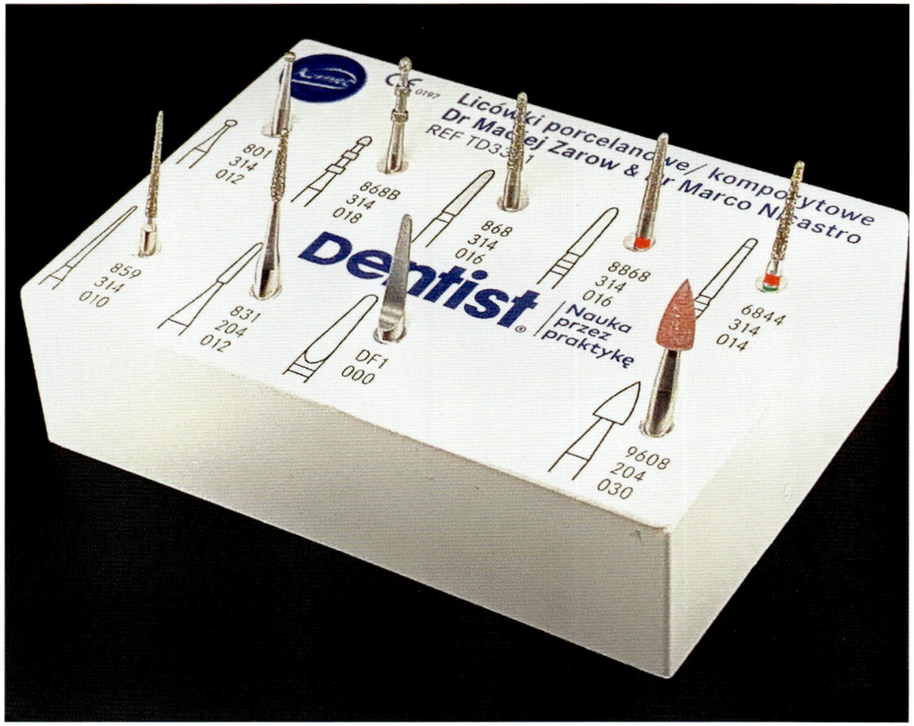

Fig 6-13
A set of burs for porcelain/composite veneer preparation and for the characterization of composite veneers (according to Dr. Żarow/Dr. Nicastro).

REFERENCES

1. Gürel G, Morimoto S, Calamita MA, Coachman C, Sesma N. Clinical performance of porcelain laminate veneers: outcomes of the aesthetic pre-evaluative temporary (APT) technique. Int J Periodontics Restorative Dent 2012;32:625–635.
2. Gürel G. Discovering the artist inside: a three-step approach to predictable aesthetic smile designs, Part 1. Dent Today 2013;32:74, 76–78.
3. Gürel G. Discovering the artist inside: a three-step approach to predictable aesthetic smile designs, Part 2. Dent Today 2013;32:126, 128–131.
4. Gürel G, Sesma N, Calamita MA, Coachman C, Morimoto S. Influence of enamel preservation on failure rates of porcelain laminate veneers. Int J Periodontics Restorative Dent 2013;33:31–39.
5. Oztürk E, Bolay S. Survival of porcelain laminate veneers with different degrees of dentin exposure: 2-year clinical results. J Adhes Dent 2014;16:481–489.
6. Gürel G. Porcelain laminate veneers: minimal tooth preparation by design. Dent Clin North Am 2007;51:419–431
7. Reshad M, Cascione D, Magne P. Diagnostic mock-ups as an objective tool for predictable outcomes with porcelain laminate veneers in esthetically demanding patients: a clinical report. J Prosthet Dent 2008;99:333–339.
8. Magne P, Belser UC. Novel porcelain laminate preparation approach driven by a diagnostic mock-up. J Esthet Restor Dent 2004;16:7–16.
9. Chai SY, Bennani V, Aarts JM, Lyons K. Incisal preparation design for ceramic veneers: a critical review. J Am Dent Assoc 2018;149:25–37.
10. Castelnuovo J, Tjan AH, Phillips K, Nicholls JI, Kois JC. Fracture load and mode of failure of ceramic veneers with different preparations. J Prosthet Dent 2000;83:171–180.
11. Akoğlu B, Gemalmaz D. Fracture resistance of ceramic veneers with different preparation designs. J Prosthodont 2011;20:380–384.
12. Magne P, Magne M, Belser UC. Adhesive restorations, centric relation, and the Dahl principle: minimally invasive approaches to localized anterior tooth erosion. Eur J Esthet Dent 2007;2:260–273.
13. Hong N, Yang H, Li J, Wu S, Li Y. Effect of preparation designs on the prognosis of porcelain laminate veneers: a systematic review and meta-analysis. Oper Dent 2017;42:197–213.
14. Albanesi RB, Pigozzo MN, Sesma N, Laganá DC, Morimoto S. Incisal coverage or not in ceramic laminate veneers: a systematic review and meta-analysis. J Dent 2016;52:1–7.
15. Magne P, Douglas WH. Design optimization and evolution of bonded ceramics for the anterior dentition: a finite-element analysis. Quintessence Int 1999;30:661–672.
16. Stappert CF, Ozden U, Gerds T, Strub JR. Longevity and failure load of ceramic veneers with different preparation designs after exposure to masticatory simulation. J Prosthet Dent 2005;94:132–139.
17. Peumans M, Van Meerbeek B, Lambrechts P, Vanherle G. Porcelain veneers: a review of the literature. J Dent 2000;28:163–177.
18. Rouse JS. Full veneer versus traditional veneer preparation: a discussion of interproximal extension. J Prosthet Dent 1997;78:545–549.
19. Harnois P. A new perspective on minimally invasive veneer techniques. Dent Today 2013;32:120, 124–125.
20. Nazarian A. Closing the gap with minimal preparation veneers. Dent Today 2006;25:70–71.
21. Priest G. Proximal margin modifications for all-ceramic veneers. Pract Proced Aesthet Dent 2004;16:265–272.
22. Edelhoff D, Frandtner O, Saeidi Pour R, Liebermann A, Stimmelmayr M, Güth JF. Anterior restorations: the performance of ceramic veneers. Quintessence Int 2018;49:89–101.
23. Magne P, Magne M. Use of additive waxup and direct intraoral mock-up for enamel preservation with porcelain laminate veneers. Eur J Esthet Dent 2006;1:10–19.
24. Magne P, Douglas WH. Additive contour of porcelain veneers: a key element in enamel preservation adhesion, and esthetics for aging dentition. J Adhes Dent 1999;1:81–92.
25. Acar Ö, Erkut S, Özçelik TB, Ozdemır E, Akçil M. A clinical comparison of cordless and conventional displacement systems regarding clinical performance and impression quality. J Prosthet Dent 2014;111:388–394.
26. Perakis N, Belser UC, Magne P. Final impressions: a review of material properties and description of a current technique. Int J Periodontics Restorative Dent 2004;24:109–117.
27. Hirsh LS, Marion LR. Esthetic provisionalization for a combined porcelain veneer and anterior single crown case. Compend Contin Educ Dent 2011;32:38–42.
28. Nixon RL. Provisionalization for ceramic laminate veneer restorations: a clinical update. Pract Periodontics Aesthet Dent 1997;9:17–28.
29. Calamia JR. Materials and technique for etched porcelain facial veneers. Alpha Omegan 1988;81:48–51.
30. Seebach C. Special considerations for mandibular anterior veneers. Oral Health. 2006. Available at https://www.oralhealthgroup.com/features/special-considerations-for-mandibularanterior-veneers/ [Accessed August 30, 2017].
31. da Costa DC, Coutinho M, de Sousa AS, Ennes JP. A meta-analysis of the most indicated preparation design for porcelain laminate veneers. J Adhes Dent 2013;15:215–220.
32. Guess PC, Selz CF, Voulgarakis A, Stampf S, Stappert CF. Prospective clinical study of press-ceramic overlap and full veneer restorations: 7-year results. Int J Prosthodont 2014;27:355–358.
33. Pini NP, Aguiar FH, Lima DA, Lovado JR, Terada RS, Pascotta RC. Advances in dental veneers: materials, applications, and techniques. Clin Cosmet Investig Dent 2012;4:9–16.

CHAPTER 7

VENEERS CEMENTATION

MACIEJ ŻAROW

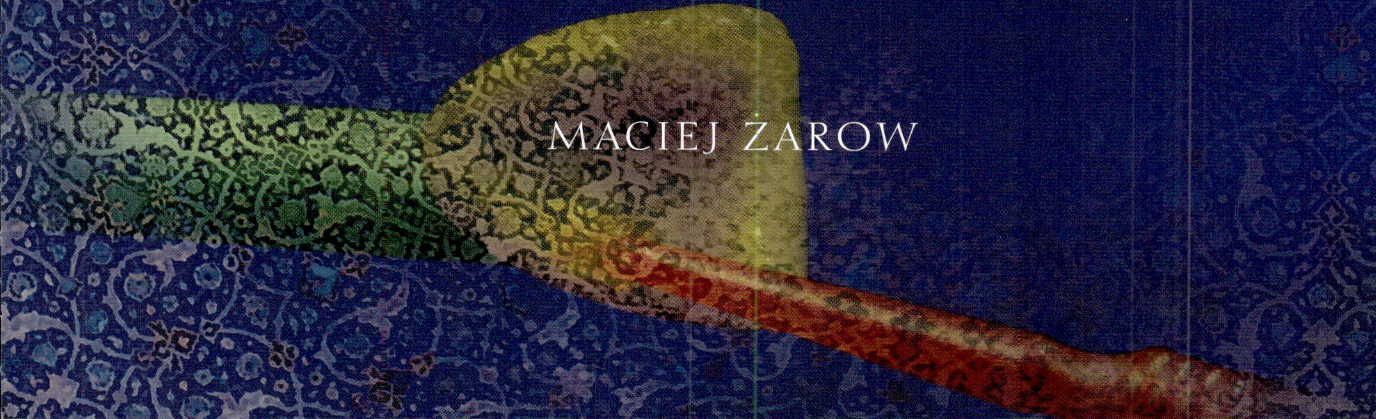

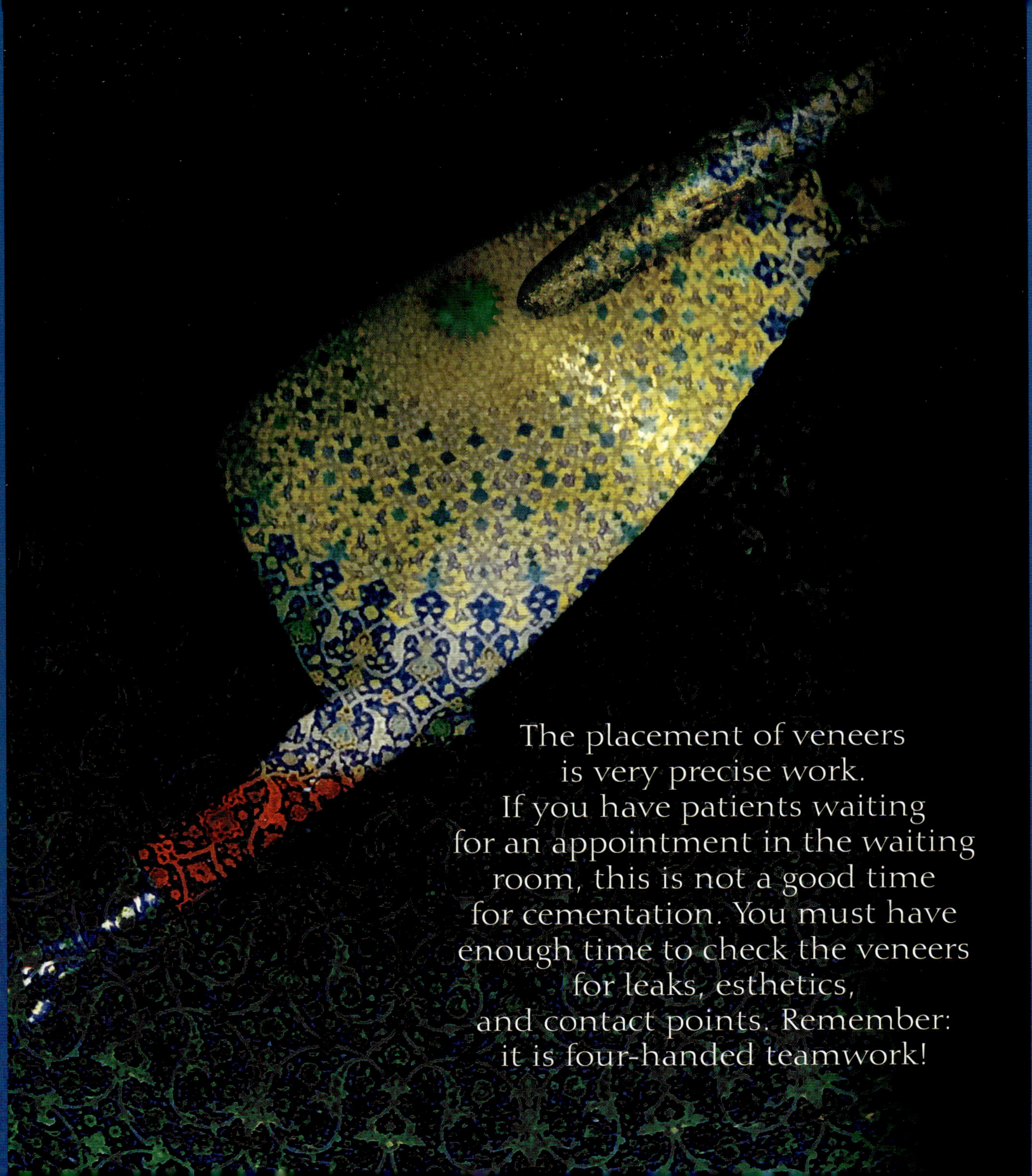

The placement of veneers
is very precise work.
If you have patients waiting
for an appointment in the waiting
room, this is not a good time
for cementation. You must have
enough time to check the veneers
for leaks, esthetics,
and contact points. Remember:
it is four-handed teamwork!

Veneers cementation

The cementing procedure will determine the durability of the veneers. When placing veneers, we must be sure about their marginal fit, color, shape, length, the composition in which they create a smile, their position in relation to the upper and lower lip, and of course, the patient's satisfaction. Perfect adhesive preparation will result in clinical success.

WHEN TO USE ANESTHESIA?

After receiving the porcelain veneers from the dental laboratory (Fig 7-1a), first check their marginal fit on the die stone. Then, you can start working with the patient.

It is important not to anesthetize the patient before the veneers are tried in, as they will not feel their lip, and the dentist will not be able to evaluate the actual smile. If the patient has a high level of hypersensitivity of the teeth, anesthesia should be performed from the palatal side (for example, with The Wand device) to prevent the upper lip from becoming immobilized (Fig 7-1b).[1,2] The Wand device is an interesting alternative for veneers due to the need to control the upper lip.

TIP

Veneers should be carried carefully from one place to another by a dental assistant to avoid accidents. A fall onto a ceramic floor will certainly crack the restoration.

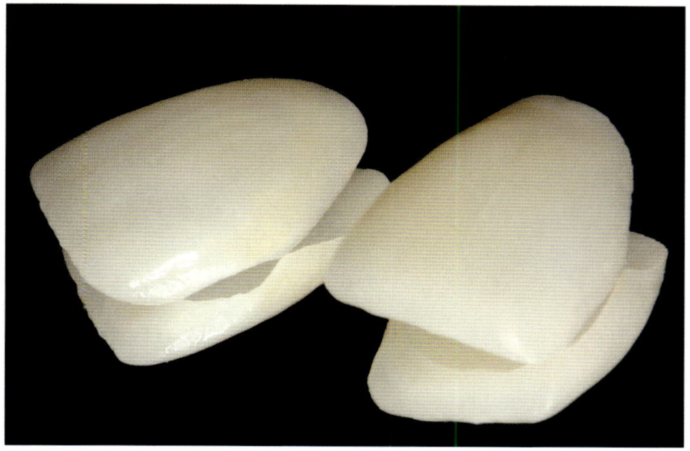

Fig 7-1a Veneers were fabricated in the dental laboratory. It is important to check their marginal integrity on the die stone before starting the work with the patient.

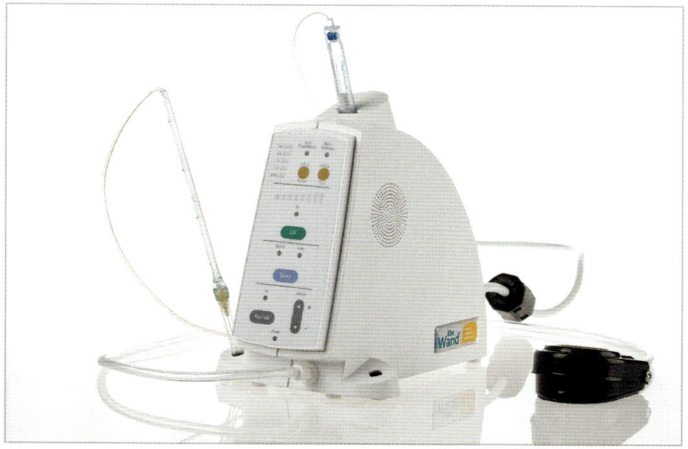

Fig 7-1b Anesthesia from the palatal side with The Wand device is an interesting alternative for veneers due to the need for upper lip control and the ability to control the smile and phonetics during the try-in.

CHECKLIST

Removing provisional veneers (Fig 7-2)

To remove provisional veneers, you can use curettes, which will no longer be used for scaling. You should pay special attention to the proximal surfaces, as the temporary composite may have invisible excesses (eg, ProTemp).

If the excess temporary material is not completely removed, the veneer cannot be seated in the correct position, and there can be a false impression that the veneer does not fit.

Trying in "dry" veneers

First, the veneers should be tried in "dry." The adaptation of the veneers has to be checked to see whether they are reaching the preparation margin. If not, there is likely a problem with the proximal surface, which is too convex and needs to be adjusted slightly.

Checking the adaptation of proximal surfaces (Fig 7-3)

You should always check that the proximal surfaces are properly contoured and connecting properly.[3]

When trying in veneers, the dental assistant places the articulation foil (8–12 μm) in the needle holder. Then, they place it between the proximal surfaces of the teeth (Fig 7-3a) before the dentist seats the veneers in the correct position. Now, the dentist presses the veneers slightly against the teeth, and the dental assistant gently pulls the foil toward the incisal edge.

If the articulation foil tears (Fig 7-3b) or becomes blocked, leaving a clear mark on the proximal surface of the veneer, it means that the contact point is too tight.

In such a case, the heaviest red marks on the interproximal surface are gently removed with a gray porcelain rubber placed on a straight handpiece (Figs 7-3c and 7-3d).

After gentle adjustment with a gray porcelain rubber, repeat the activity of pulling the articulation foil toward the incisal edge (and further adjustment with a porcelain rubber if necessary). This procedure can be repeated as often as required until the perfect proximal contact point/surface is achieved. This perfect fitting should be checked with dental floss. For example, the dentist holds the veneers with their fingertips while the dental assistant slides the dental floss between the contact points of the veneers. If the dental floss causes a significant displacement of the veneer, felt under the dentist's fingertips, it indicates too tight contact point.

Good adaptation of proximal contact point/surface is very important.[4] If necessary, it should be performed not once or twice, but even 15, 20, or more times. If the contact point is too tight, the veneer may crack or be cemented in the wrong position, resulting in a lack of marginal seal.

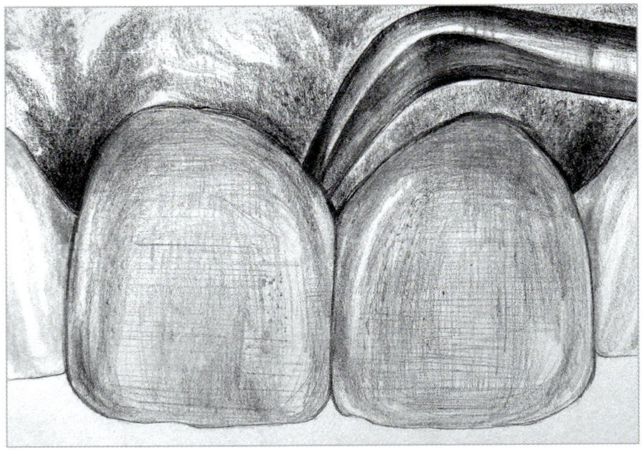

Fig 7-2
For the removal of provisional veneers, it is worth using a solid curette: pry up the veneers, which should easily detach from the hard tissues.

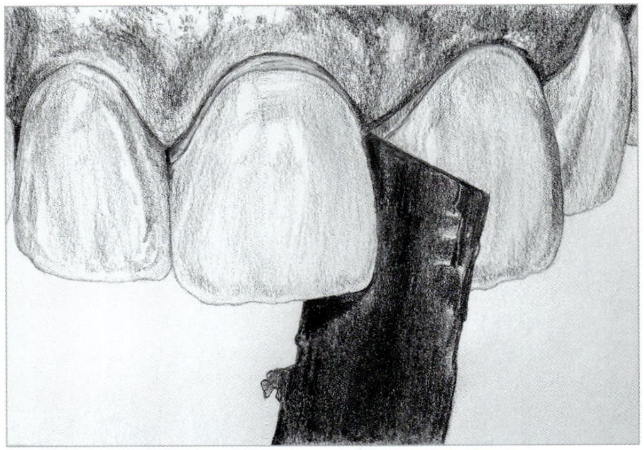

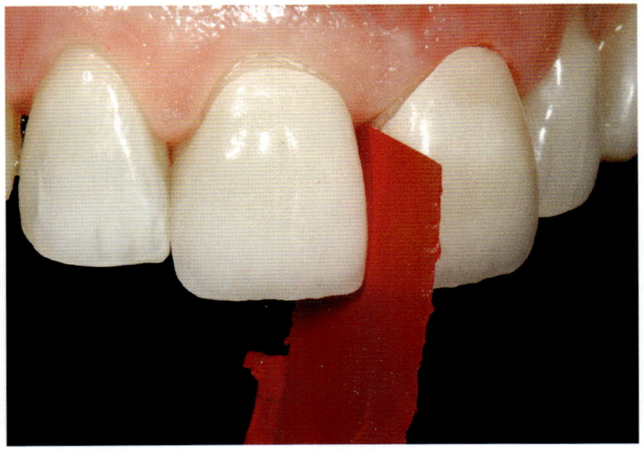

Fig 7-3a
An 8 μm articulation foil placed in the needle holder is a way to clearly mark places of interference on the proximal surface.

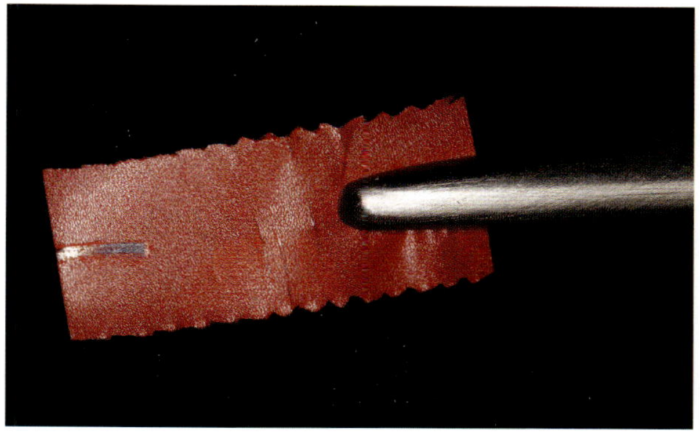

Fig 7-3b
A torn or heavily thinned articulation foil proves that the contact surface is too convex and must be modified.

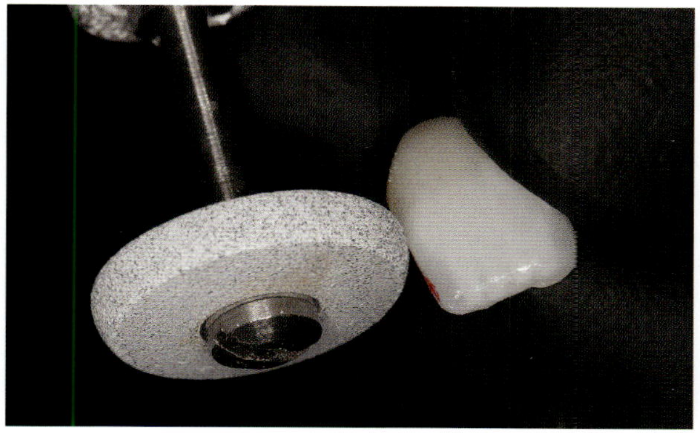

Fig 7-3c
A gray porcelain rubber (Diatech Polisher 230134AA) on the straight handpiece is used to correct the proximal surfaces.

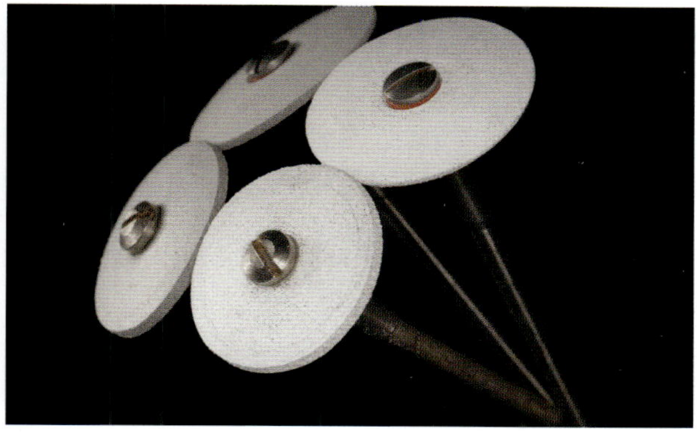

Fig 7-3d
Note: when correcting the proximal contact point with a gray porcelain rubber, blunt the new rubber so that its tip does not immerse into the porcelain (the porcelain rubber in the upper part of the photograph is new, and in the lower part it is blunt).

Evaluation of black triangles closure (Fig 7-4)

Check that there is no gum recession after provisional veneers. If something alarms you, for example, black triangles,[5] a periodontal examination should be performed: the closure of the proximal contact point should be located 4 mm from the alveolar bone.

If the proximal contact point is further away and black triangles are visible, extend the proximal surface by adding porcelain to the veneers. This can be inconvenient because the veneers have to be returned to the laboratory. Therefore, it is better to ask your dental technician to fabricate relatively longer contact surfaces.

In the case of proximal surfaces that are too long, modification with a porcelain rubber is simple enough to be carried out by a dentist. On the other hand, adding porcelain to the proximal contact point on the veneer is beyond the skills of a dentist – so a laboratory becomes necessary.[6,7]

Control of marginal seal and adaptation

If the palatal part of the incisal edge protrudes from the preparation margin, it is most likely that the veneer is not seated in its correct position. In such a case, check that any material from the provisional veneer is left in the interproximal space, and that the proximal contact point is not too convex, preventing passive placement of the veneer. Veneers should be seated passively! When the proximal contact point no longer interferes with the insertion of the veneer into place, the marginal seal and adaptation should be re-checked, especially on the proximal and palatal surfaces.

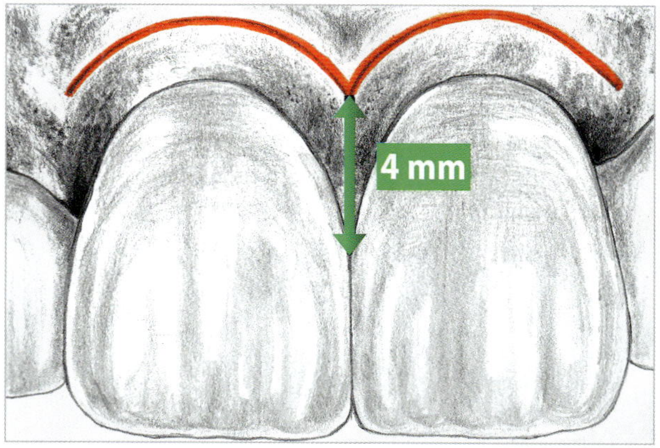

Fig 7-4
The closure of the proximal contact point should be located 4 mm from the alveolar bone. In order to be sure of the distance from the bone, anesthetize the patient and place the dental explorer subgingivally until the bone is reached. Perhaps the black triangle will not be closed at the cementing stage due to the effect related to the impression and provisional restorations. Still, during the healing stage, if measured correctly, the triangle will be closed with soft tissues.

Trying in "wet" veneers

How to check the color of porcelain veneers? Do they change color after cementation? In what light should you verify a color? These are all questions of concern to dentists. The most important aspects of color assessment are presented below.

THE MOST IMPORTANT STAGES OF COLOR VERIFICATION

1. The veneer should always be tried in daylight.

2. The color cannot be checked while trying in "dry" veneers. There is a layer of air between the veneer and tooth structure, which blocks light transmission deep into the tooth. In the presence of this layer, the veneers always appear brighter than they really are. Therefore, a layer of glycerin gel (for example, a glycerin gel for intimate hygiene that will easily rinse out with water) should be applied to the inner surface of the veneer before trying in. Due to the presence of the gel, one optical unit is generated, and the light is also absorbed by hard tissues and then diffused. This allows you to predict the definitive appearance of the veneers after cementing.[8,9]

3. Veneers are first evaluated by the dentist (Fig 7-5), and if possible, by the dentist with the technician. Only after the team's (dentist–technician) acceptance of the color and the shape can restorations be shown to the patient.

4. The patient must have time in an appropriate space to accept the veneers. Walls of a neutral color are important to avoid changes to light color, and patients need a room in which they can assess the veneers calmly.

Corrections

At this stage, it may turn out that the veneers need to undergo corrections, which can be divided into:

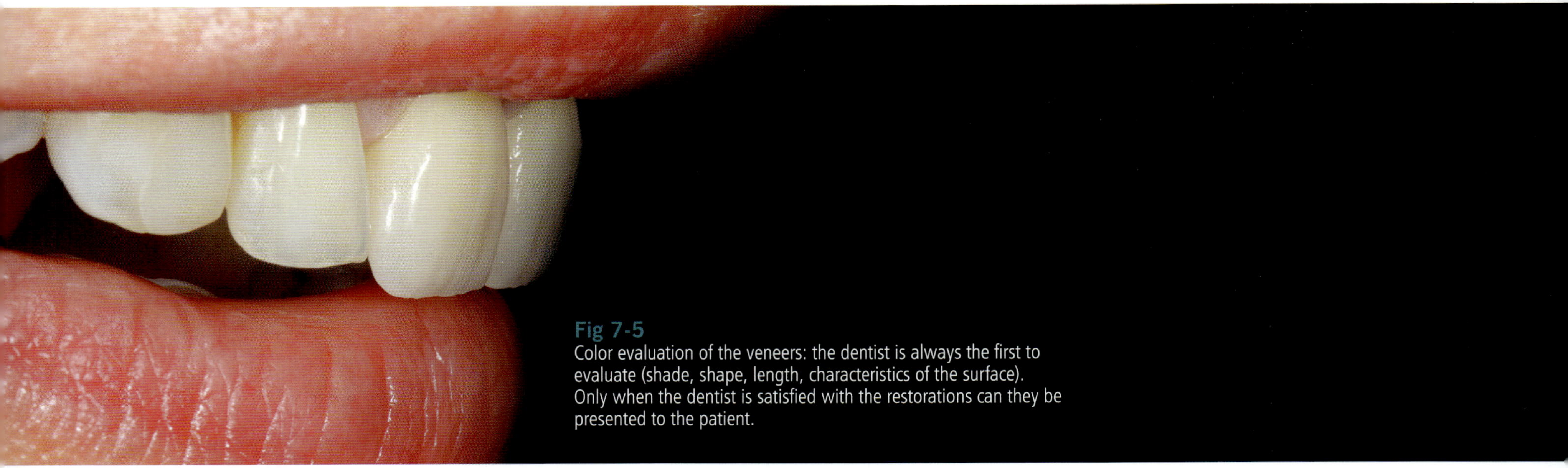

Fig 7-5
Color evaluation of the veneers: the dentist is always the first to evaluate (shade, shape, length, characteristics of the surface). Only when the dentist is satisfied with the restorations can they be presented to the patient.

- **Simple corrections without the need to return the veneers to the dental laboratory**

  The most common corrections concern reducing the length, width, changing the incisal angles, emergence profile or a slight correction of the tooth axis inclination. This is done with a gray, slightly abrasive rubber, applied to the straight handpiece.

- **Corrections requiring the use of a porcelain furnace**
  - **Color correction:** In some clinical cases, there is a need for color correction. That makes the participation of the dental technician and the use of a porcelain furnace necessary. The dental technician can modify the veneers by slightly staining them from the outside (Fig 7-6a) or by blocking penetrating tooth discoloration from the inside of the veneer (Fig 7-6b). This must be done in such a way as to avoid interferences during the clinical seating of the restoration.
  - **Shape modification:** In some cases, the veneers may need to be lengthened or widened, or black triangle closure may be required by adding porcelain to the veneer (Fig 7-6c).

REMEMBER

Laboratory corrections of the veneers are possible, but they require the presence of a dental technician and the use of laboratory equipment. Therefore, it is important to plan the restorations properly and to provide the laboratory with information that is as detailed as possible, such as:

- The length and shape of the teeth and the curvature of the mesial/distoincisal angle (wax-up)
- Precise information about where the proximal contact surface should meet (closing the black triangles 4 mm from the alveolar bone)
- Color map of final veneers
- Color of the tooth core after preparation
- The level of surface characterization
- The level of dominance of the central incisors in relation to the lateral incisors

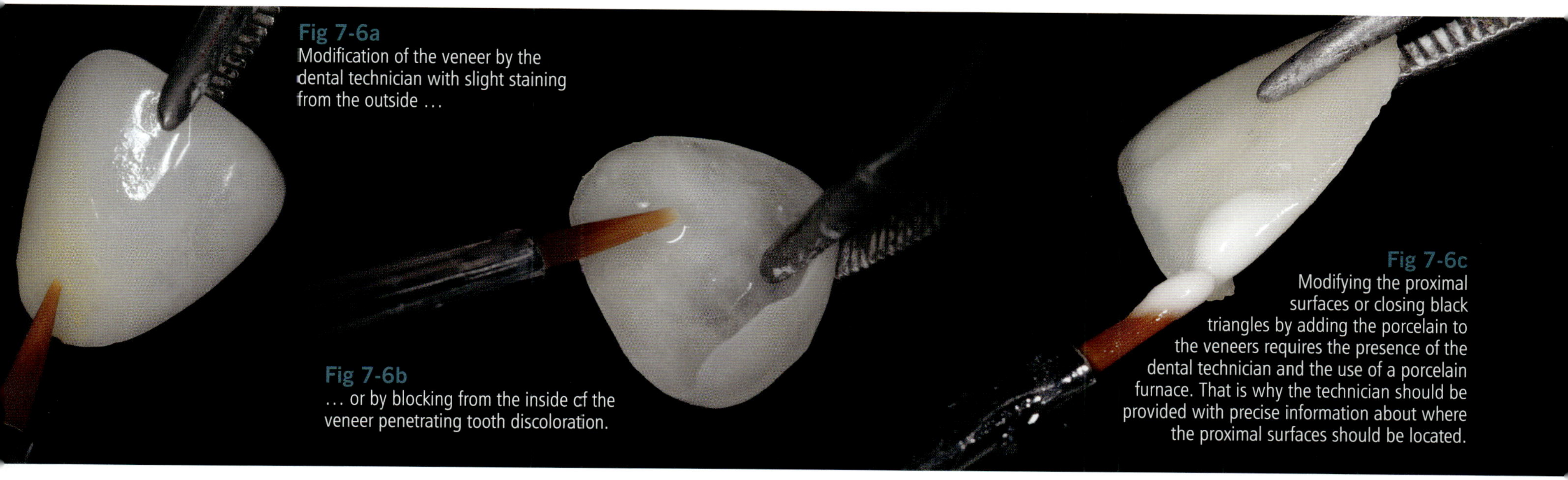

Fig 7-6a
Modification of the veneer by the dental technician with slight staining from the outside …

Fig 7-6b
… or by blocking from the inside of the veneer penetrating tooth discoloration.

Fig 7-6c
Modifying the proximal surfaces or closing black triangles by adding the porcelain to the veneers requires the presence of the dental technician and the use of a porcelain furnace. That is why the technician should be provided with precise information about where the proximal surfaces should be located.

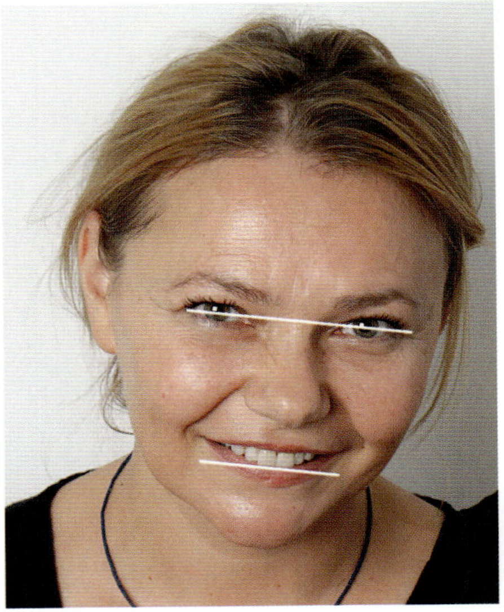

Fig 7-7a
During the esthetic evaluation of the veneers, check whether the incisal edges are parallel to the interpupillary line, and ...

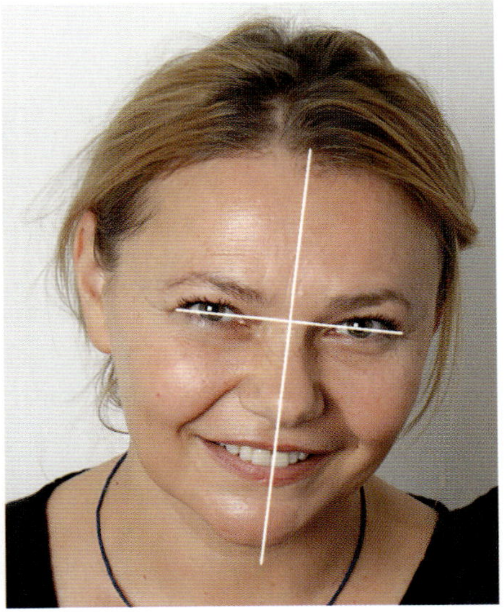

Fig 7-7b
... assess whether the line connecting the mesial proximal surfaces of the central incisors coincides with the facial midline.

VENEER ESTHETIC EVALUATION BEFORE CEMENTATION: CHECKLIST (FIG 7-7)[10–15]

A. The horizontal line	Evaluate whether the incisal edges are parallel to the interpupillary line (Fig 7-7a)
B. The midline	Evaluate whether the line connecting the mesial proximal surfaces of the central incisors coincides with the facial midline (Fig 7-7b)
C. Tooth axis	Evaluate whether the axes of the teeth with veneers tilt distally (in other words: whether consecutive teeth further away from the midline tilt more and more distally) (Fig 7-7c)

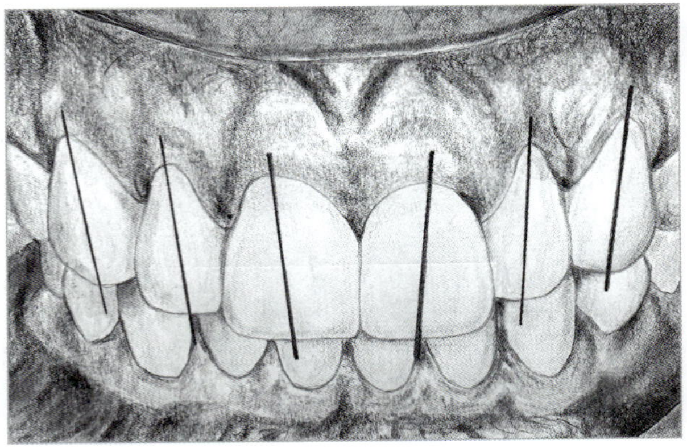

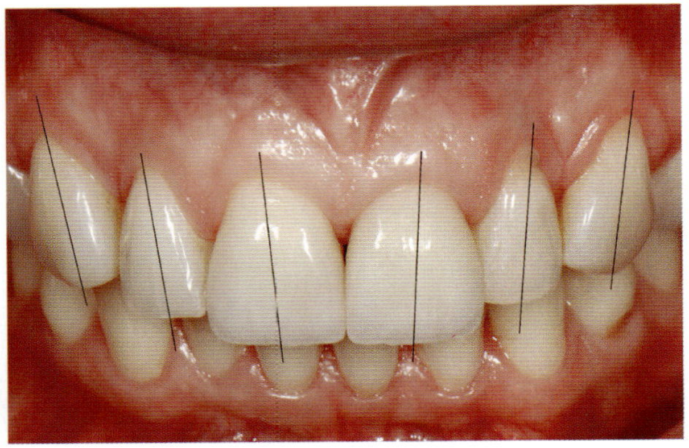

Fig 7-7c
Evaluate whether the axes of the teeth with veneers tilt distally and ...

D. Width of the central incisors	Evaluate whether the width of both central incisors is identical (Fig 7-7d)
E. Mesial and distoincisal angle	The mesial incisal angle should be more acute than the distal one. The mesial incisal angles of the maxillary central incisors should be identical (Fig 7-7e)
F. Exposure of the incisal edges from under the upper lip	According to the esthetic treatment plan, tested on mock-up (veneers test drive), the maxillary incisors should protrude 1–3 mm from under the upper lip in repose position (Fig 7-7f)
G. Veneer profile and inclination of the incisal part toward the oral cavity	When looking at the profile, one-third of the incisal part of the veneer should tilt toward the oral cavity, and the incisal edge should touch the border of the wet and dry part of the lower lip (the "Vermilion line")

H. Shape of the tooth crown	Evaluate the shape of the veneers (square, oval, triangular), their compliance with the treatment plan, diagnostic wax-up and patient's expectations
I. Emergence profile	Evaluate whether the gingival emergence profile is too convex, which could adversely affect periodontal health when the veneer is cemented. The transition between the root/cervical and the veneer should be smooth
J. Proximal contact surfaces/points	The proximal contact surfaces/points should give some resistance to floss, but the floss should not displace seated veneer held by the fingers
K. Black triangles	The closure of black triangles should be located 4 mm from the alveolar bone

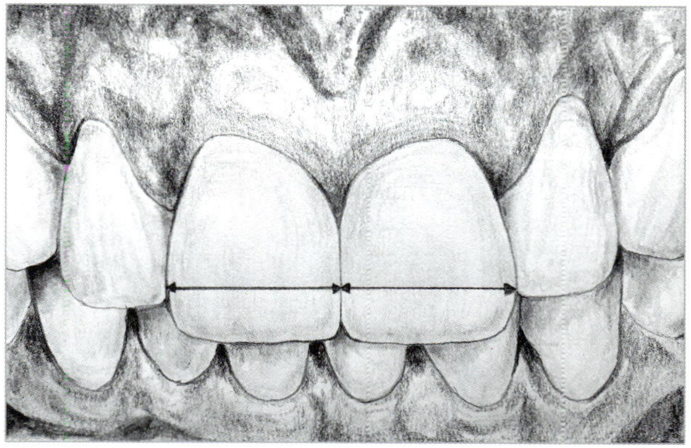

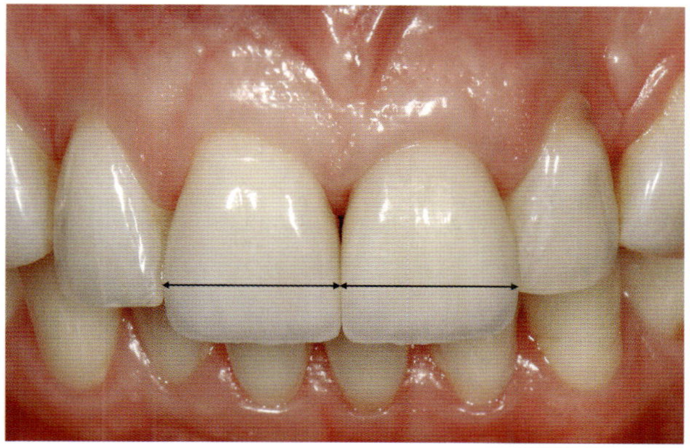

Fig 7-7d
… is the width of both central incisors similar (or preferably identical)?

Fig 7-7e
Evaluate whether the mesial incisal angle is more acute and the distal angle is more rounded (check whether it corresponds to what has been planned).

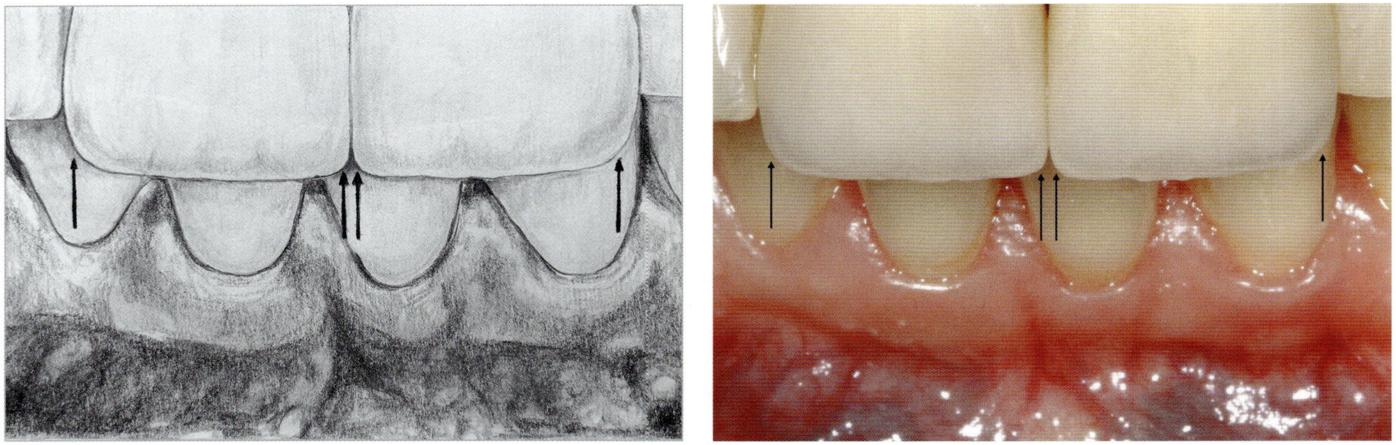

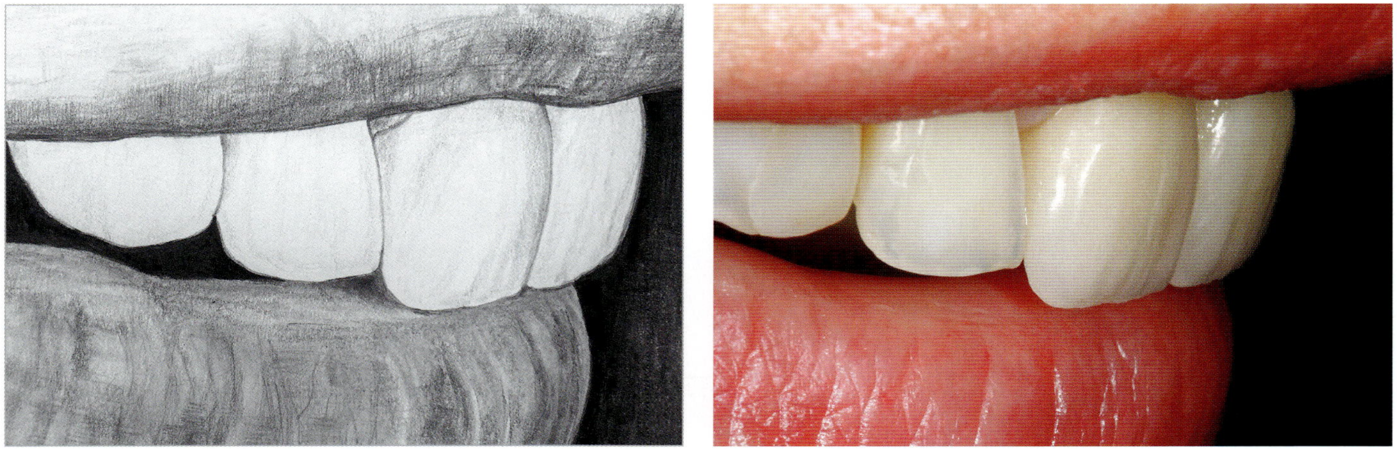

Fig 7-7f
During the esthetic evaluation of the veneers, it is necessary to check the exposure of the central incisors from under the upper lip in the repose position, and to verify the inclination angle of the incisal one-third of the veneer (the incisal edge of the veneer should meet the vermilion line of the lower lip).

ADHESIVE PREPARATION OF THE VENEERS

Step 1: Cleaning with 70% alcohol

After trying in and touching the veneer with your fingers, it is very important to clean it thoroughly with alcohol. In particular, the inner surface of the veneer should be clean and free from the articulation foil or any other contamination (Fig 7-8a).

Table 7-1 Recommended concentration of hydrofluoric (HF) acid and etch time

Feldspathic porcelain veneer	5–10% HF, 60–90 seconds
Lithium disilicate veneer (E.max)	5% HF, 20 seconds
Leucite-reinforced glass-ceramic veneers	5% HF, 20 seconds

Step 2: Etching with hydrofluoric acid

Etching the porcelain with hydrofluoric acid (HF) is one of the most important steps to ensure the correct adhesion of the veneer (Fig 7-8b). Hydrofluoric acid etching of the ceramics and increasing the surface gives a better chance of micro-mechanical bonding between the resin cement and the porcelain veneer surface (Table 7-1).

Traditionally, 10% HF is used for 60–90 seconds.[16–33]

However, keep in mind that hydrofluoric acid is a highly toxic substance (Fig 7-8c). The higher its concentration, the greater the health risk for the dental staff member carrying out the etching.[21,22]

Hydrofluoric acid can cause severe skin and nail burns, systemic toxicity, chemical eye burns, and breathing disorders leading to death. The symptoms caused by the activity of hydrofluoric acid are not related to the pH, but to its high toxicity. In 1982, a mistake occurred in a dental office in Japan when a dentist applied hydrofluoric acid to the teeth of a 3-year-old patient instead of sodium fluoride. This resulted in the death of the young patient.[23]

Since then, Japan has changed regulations and restricted the use of hydrofluoric acid in dental offices.[24]

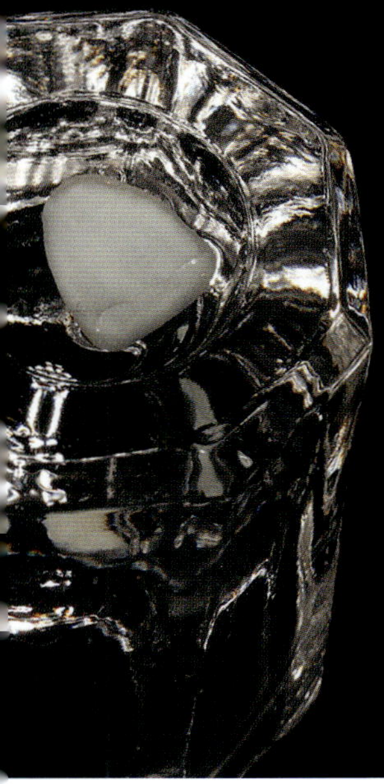

Fig 7-8a Bathing the veneer in alcohol. In the event of traces of articulation foil, make sure that the veneer has been properly cleaned.

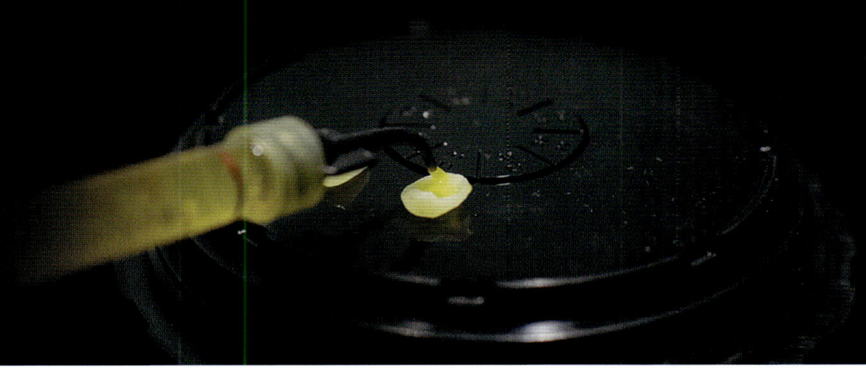

Fig 7-8b Hydrofluoric acid is applied to the inner surface of the veneer for a specific period, depending on the thickness of the veneer and the type of porcelain (20 to 90 seconds).

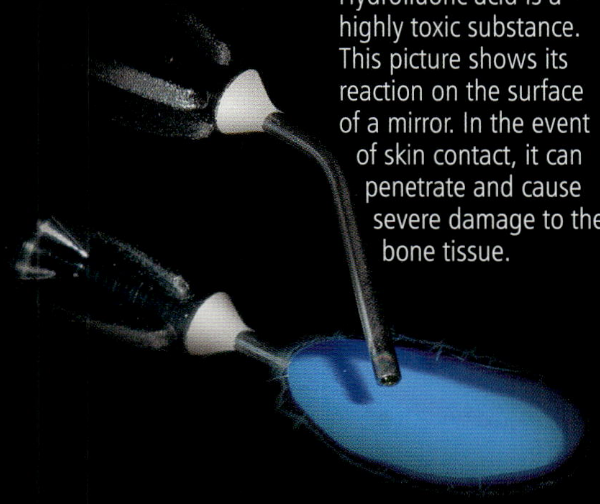

Fig 7-8c Hydrofluoric acid is a highly toxic substance. This picture shows its reaction on the surface of a mirror. In the event of skin contact, it can penetrate and cause severe damage to the bone tissue.

The person carrying out the etching procedure of the veneers should wear a protective visor and gloves, and avoid direct contact with HF at all costs, even when wearing gloves (Fig 7-8d). Besides the health risk to the dental team, there is a risk of over-etching the veneer, which may result in a reduction in its mechanical strength, especially in the case of very thin and less invasive restorations.

To reduce the risk of HF toxicity, over-etching, and weakening of the veneers caused by application beyond the recommended time, it is advised to use HF with a concentration of 5% while fabricating thinner veneers using new materials such as lithium disilicate[25–29]:

- 10% HF may have a weakening effect on leucite and lithium disilicate veneers, especially in the case of very thin restoration.[25]
- When cementing thin veneers, 10% concentration of HF will be too strong. It will lead to the dissolution of a large amount of the glassy phase causing large irregularities, which can damage the integrity of the material and probably lead to cracks.[30]

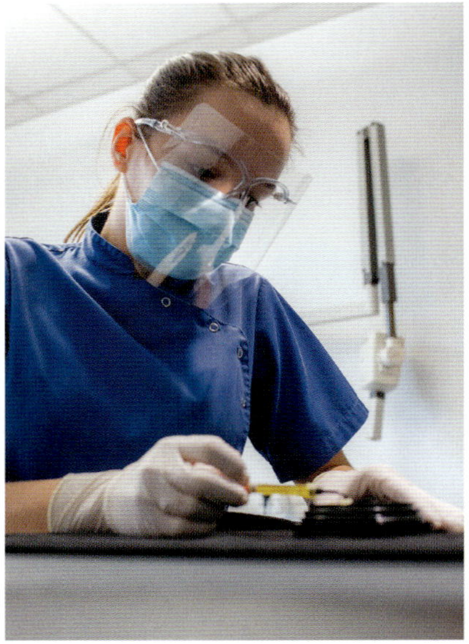

Fig 7-8d
Basic precautions should be followed when etching porcelain veneers with hydrofluoric acid. Mask, protective visors, and gloves are mandatory.

Video: Etching the veneers with hydrofluoric acid https://books.dentist.com.pl/veneers/10

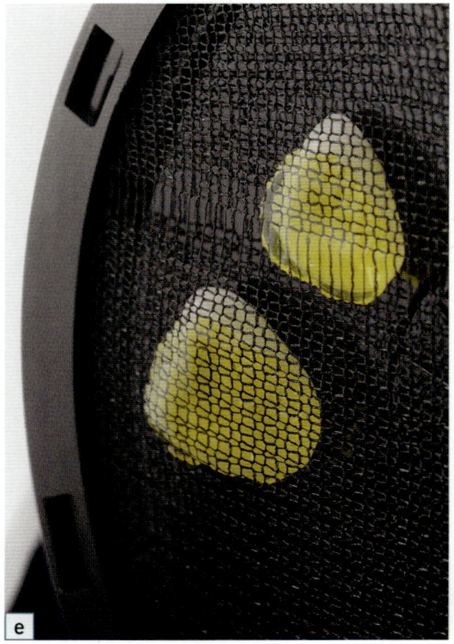

Figs 7-8e to 7-8g
The traditional concept of adhesive veneer preparation was to hold it in the fingers and to etch it. A special box is now available for safe etching and rinsing of the veneers (veneerME), developed by Style Italiano and Dr. Gürel, which is an important step toward facilitating adhesive preparation of the veneers. The etching is done when the veneers are placed on a sticky pad of the veneerME and then the membrane-frame is clipped on the base of the veneerME box to prevent the veneers from dropping onto the floor …

Video: Ultrasonic bath https://books.dentist.com.pl/veneers/13

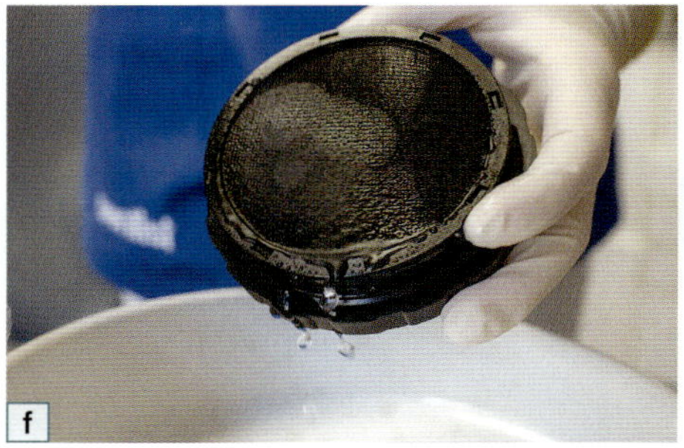

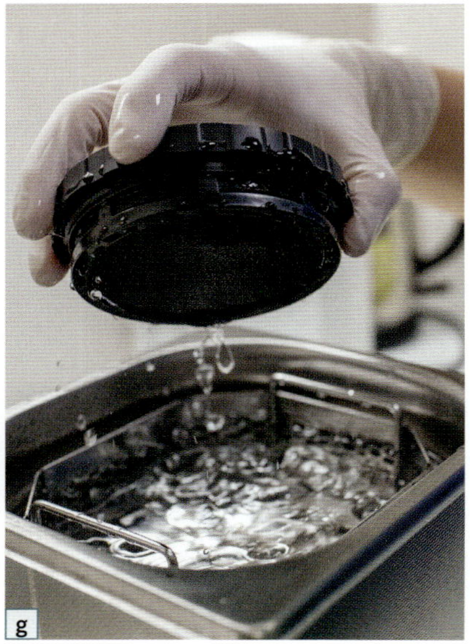

Video: Filling veneerME with alcohol https://books.dentist.com.pl/veneers/12

FROM THE LITERATURE REVIEW

Increased time of etching with HF reduces the flexural bond strength of the lithium disilicate porcelain.[34,35]

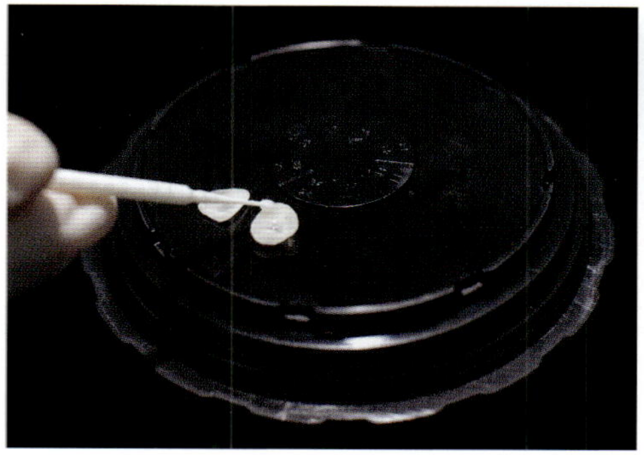

Fig 7-8h
After thorough drying, we apply the silane coupling agent, an important chemical compound that enables bonding of two completely different materials (ceramics, composite).

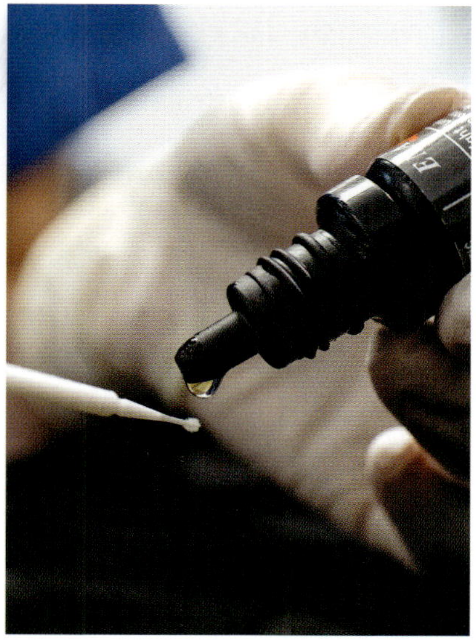

Fig 7-8i
Application of the adhesive system on the inner surface of the veneer.

Step 3: Rinsing the veneer

Thorough rinsing of hydrofluoric acid and etched ceramic is essential for the successful bonding of the veneer with the resin cement. First, rinse the hydrofluoric acid from the inner surface of the veneer with a water spray, holding the veneer between the fingers (while wearing gloves).

A better solution is to buy a special box with a sticky pad, to which the veneers are glued via their buccal surface, after which the inner surface is ready for acid application and then for safe rinsing (Figs 7-8e and 7-8f). The perfect solution for the final stage of cleaning is to place veneers in 95% ethyl alcohol or distilled water in an ultrasonic bath to eliminate residues of HF formed as crystalline deposits (Fig 7-8g) (some authors recommend cleaning the inner surface of the veneer with orthophosphoric acid before using the ultrasonic bath).[31–33]

Step 4: Drying the veneer

The veneer must be perfectly dry before applying the silane solution. This must be done with an air spray from the dental unit.

Step 5: Silane application

The silane is applied for 60 seconds (Fig 7-8h), preferably in several layers. A source of warm air at about 50°C will significantly enhance the outcome of the silane (use, for example, a hairdryer or a more professional A-dec warm dryer). There are bonding systems on the market that contain silane solution, but research shows that, when used separately, silane creates a much more stable bonding.

FROM THE LITERATURE REVIEW

Studies have shown that, after etching porcelain with HF acid, crystalline deposits are formed on the inner surface of the veneer, which can be removed with an ultrasonic bath.[31–33]

Step 6: Adhesive system application

Then, the adhesive system (Fig 7-8i) is applied as one layer spread on the inner surface of the veneer. We never light-cure the bonding system on the veneer. The veneer should also be protected from strong light sources to avoid accidental activation of polymerization of the applied adhesive system.

Video: Initial veneer rinsing
https://books.dentist.com.pl/veneers/11

Video: Final veneer rinsing
https://books.dentist.com.pl/veneers/14

Video: Final veneer drying
https://books.dentist.com.pl/veneers/15

ADHESIVE PREPARATION OF THE TOOTH SURFACE

Step 1: Isolating the teeth with a rubber dam

When cementing two or more veneers, this procedure should be started with two central incisors, which requires the isolation of two or four incisors (Fig 7-9a). For this purpose, we can use:

- Hygenic B5 or B6 (butterfly) clamps cut in half, so they can be applied simultaneously on two central incisors (Figs 7-9b and 7-9c). Their advantage is that they provide sufficient space for the fingers during seating. Their disadvantage is the frequent loss of retention, although this can be reactivated with Krampon forceps (Fig 7-9d).

  Other possible clamps for isolation while cementing veneers are Brinker clamps, which show good subgingival retention. Their disadvantage is the lack of space for fingers during the veneer placement procedure.

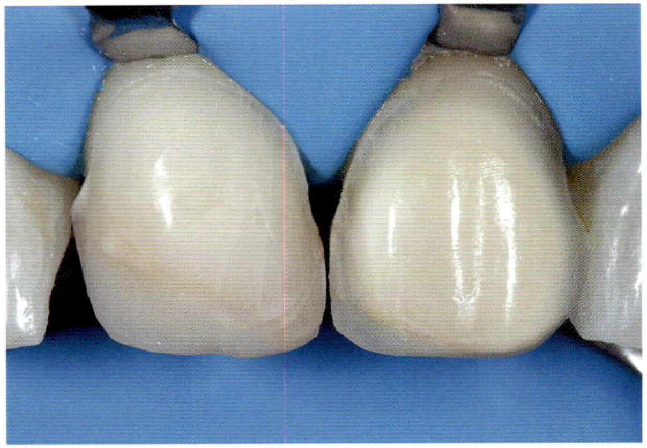

Fig 7-9a
The placement of the veneers should always be started with the two central incisors. For this purpose, it is best to isolate two adjacent teeth with a rubber dam.

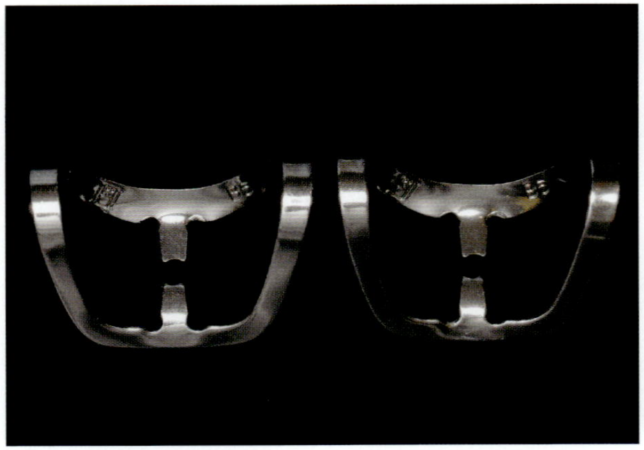

Fig 7-9b
Clamps no. B5 and B6 (Hygenic, Coltene) are suitable for the isolating teeth prepared for veneers. For their simultaneous placement on two central incisors, it is necessary to...

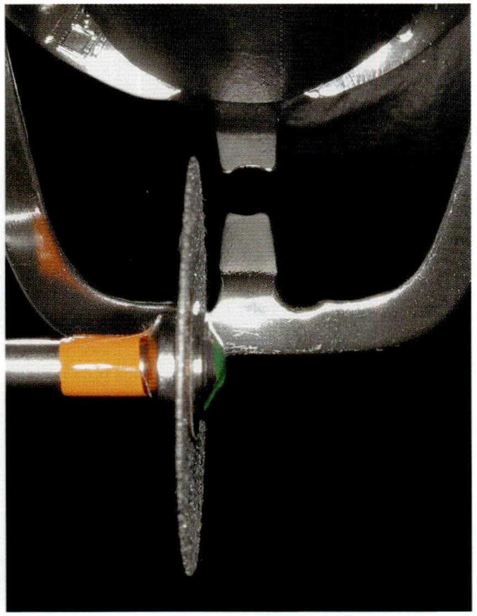

Fig 7-9c
... modify them by cutting one of the "wings of the butterflies" with a metal separating disk on the straight handpiece (but watch your fingers while cutting).

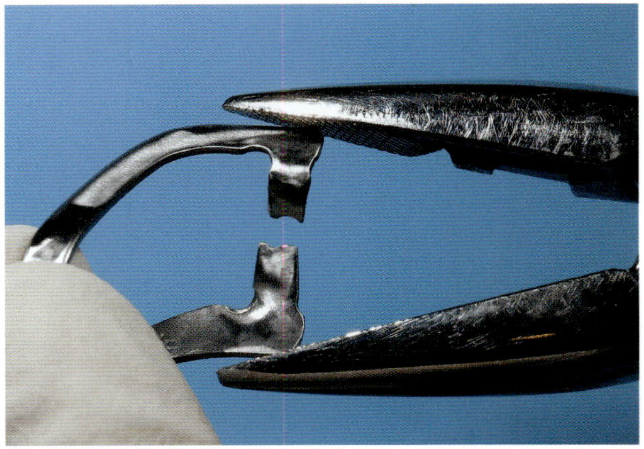

Fig 7-9d
The Krampon forceps can be used as an easy way to activate the clamps.

Step 2: Airborne-particle abrasion of the tooth hard tissues (micro-abrasion)

Airborne-particle abrasion with an abrasive unit (Fig 7-10a) is a perfect means of removing contaminations such as blood, dental plaque, materials used for provisional veneers, and so on, from the tooth surface (Fig 7-10b). It is recommended to use 27 μm aluminum oxide sand, and the pressure of the airborne-particle abrasion unit should be 40 PSI.[36,37]

It has been proven that air abrasion significantly improves the bonding strength of the adhesive system to the tooth's hard tissues. After airborne-particle abrasion, carefully blow out with air spray the isolated area to get rid of sand particles, then rinse with water spray and dry again.

Step 3: Trying in veneers with a rubber dam in place

It is important to try in veneers on the isolated teeth to ensure that the clamps or rubber of the rubber dam do not interfere with the correct placement of the veneers.

Step 4: Etching with orthophosphoric acid

Orthophosphoric acid with the consistency of a gel should be applied over the entire preparation surface and actively spread for 20 seconds (Fig 7-10c). Then, the gel should be meticulously rinsed for 10–20 seconds

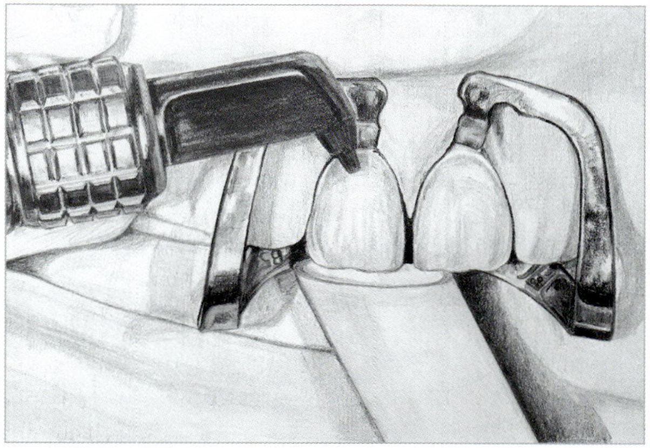

Fig 7-10a
Using an airborne-particle abrasion unit to clean the tooth surface before etching and applying the bond system. The abrasion nozzle should be kept 2–3 cm from the tooth surface.

Video: Veneers cementation – preparation of the tooth hard tissues
https://books.dentist.com.pl/veneers/16

TIP
The assistant should keep the end of the suction as close as possible, to be able to remove the excess sand.

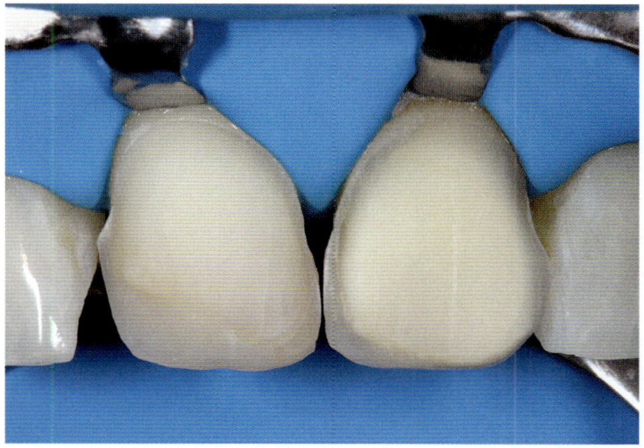

Fig 7-10b
Perfectly cleaned tooth surface after airborne-particle abrasion.

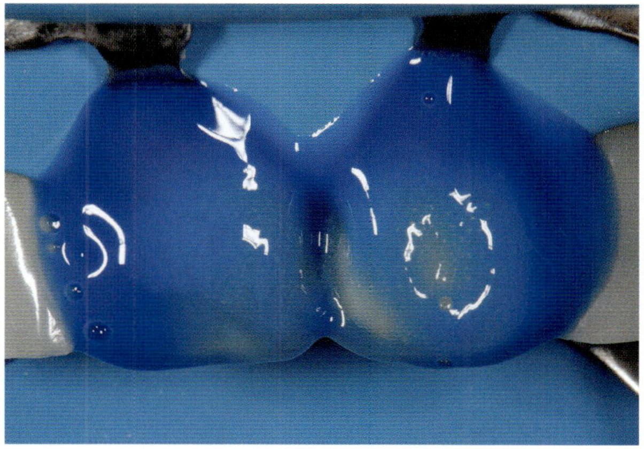

Fig 7-10c
Precise etching of the entire preparation surface with orthophosphoric acid (for 20 seconds) is important for adhesive preparation.

Step 5: Application of the adhesive system

The adhesive system must be applied precisely to the entire preparation surface (Fig 7-11), preferably by rubbing in two successive layers, then thoroughly blown to a thin layer before polymerization.[38] The adhesive system should be polymerized, paying attention to whether the tip of the optical fiber is located perpendicularly to the preparation surfaces and that it light-cures 100% of the surface to which the veneer will be cemented. Note: adhesive systems of thin consistency should be used because they will not interfere with the correct seating of the veneers after polymerization.

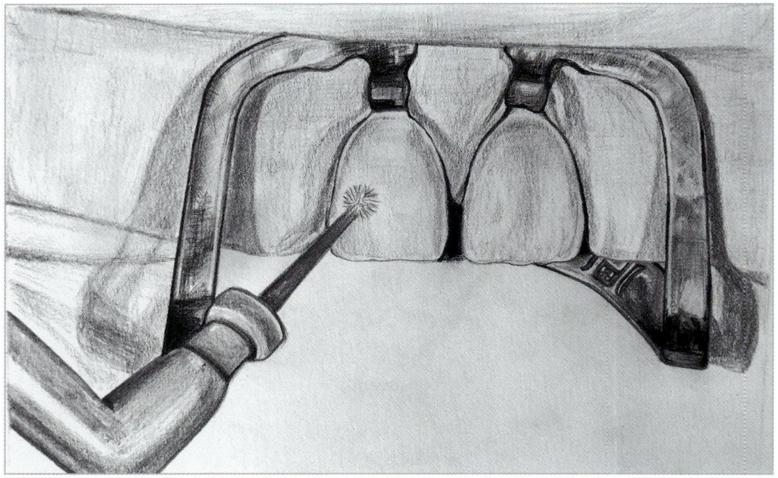

Fig 7-11a
Apply a coat of the adhesive system twice, then blow thoroughly with the air spray to obtain a thin layer …

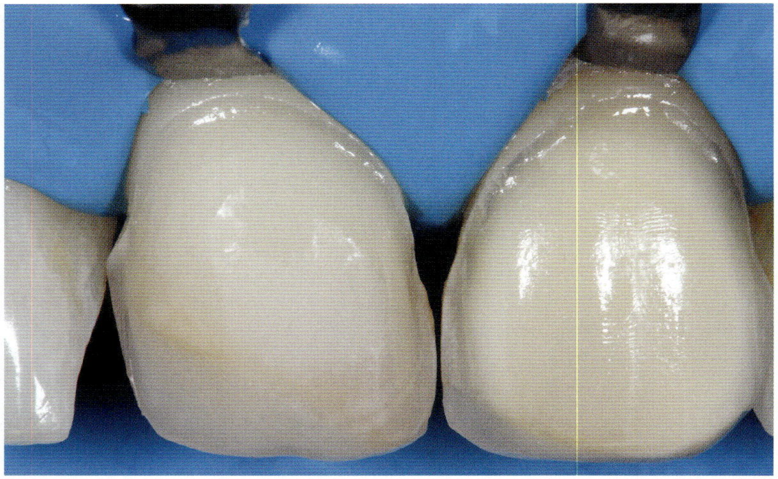

Fig 7-11b
… now, the bonding system can be light-cured for a minimum of 20 seconds by holding the light perpendicularly to the tooth surface. Take into account the size of the tooth surface in relation to the cross-section of the optical fiber curing light, so the entire tooth surface is well exposed.

PORCELAIN VENEERS CEMENTATION PROCEDURES

Porcelain veneers can be cemented with four different types of luting cement (Table 7-2). Below are presented the most common options for placing veneers. The author of this chapter divides the veneers depending on their thickness, which will be decisive in choosing a cementing method.

Veneers thicker than 0.5 mm

When we have veneers thicker than 0.5 mm, they are more resistant to damage during cementation, and they can be cemented on a heated conventional composite, for example, Enamel Plus.[38]

1. Heat the composite in a heater designed especially for the composite (Fig 7-12a). The heating of the composite should be started about 60 minutes before cementing, due to the time needed to warm up the material and achieve the consistency necessary for cementing.
2. Check the consistency of the composite (Fig 7-12b): Will it allow the veneer to be seated easily into place?
3. Apply a thin layer of the heated composite on the entire inner surface of the veneer (Fig 7-12c); if there is a problem with spreading the composite, a disposable applicator should be used, lightly moistened in unfilled resin to evenly spread the composite (Fig 7-12d).

Table 7-2 Types of luting cement for placing porcelain veneers

Luting cement	Example	Advantages	Disadvantages
Conventional light-cured composite	Enamel Plus (Micerium)	• Does not require haste when cementing • Easy to remove excess • Low abrasion (high content of fillers) • Fills the gaps perfectly in the case of micro-gap	• Requires long polymerization • Requires preheating • For an inexperienced dentist – risk of veneer fracture
Flowable light-cured composite	G-aenial Universal Flow (GC)	• Does not require haste when cementing • High abrasion resistance (high filler content) • No risk of veneer cracking • No need to preheat	• More difficult to remove excess due to the "flow" effect
Light-cured luting cement	Variolink Esthetic LC (Ivoclar)	• Does not require haste when cementing • Easy to remove thanks to pre-polymerization to the gel phase • No risk of veneer fracture, especially for thin restorations • Possibility to check the color effect of luting cement before final cementation (Try-In Paste)	• Necessity to purchase the whole kit
Dual cure luting cement	Rely X Unicem (3M)	• Simplified formula (self-etching cement)	• Limited amount of time for material removal • In the case of a micro-gap, the high liquidity of the material could be a reason for incomplete closure and concavity in the surface • Low filler content

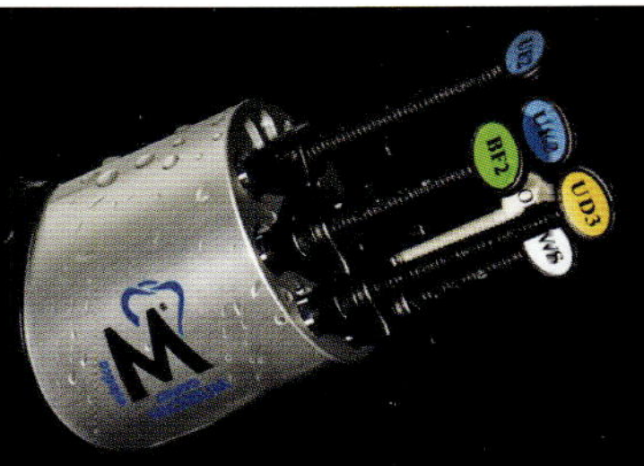

Fig 7-12a
Heating a conventional composite in a heater designed for this purpose. Heating should start early enough (as much as 60 minutes) before cementing the veneers (photograph: Dr. Dawid Pisuk).

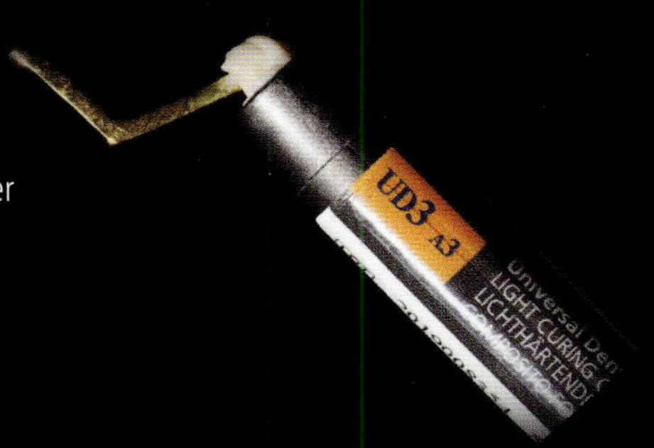

Fig 7-12b
The consistency of the composite should always be checked before applying to the inner surface of the veneer.

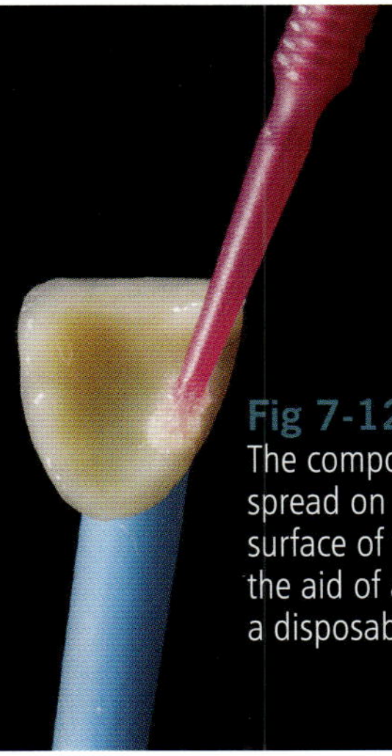

Fig 7-12c
The composite should be spread on the entire inner surface of the veneer with the aid of a flat plastic or a disposable applicator …

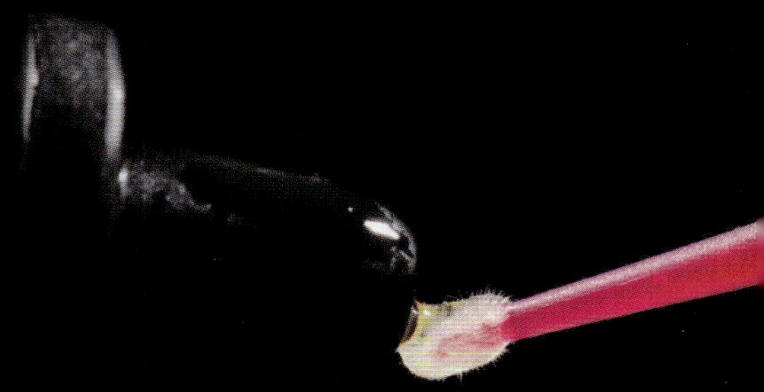

Fig 7-12d
… additionally, the disposable applicator can be moistened with unfilled resin to make it easier to spread the composite.

4. Place the veneers on the corresponding teeth and press them repeatedly with your fingers until the excess composite resin stops extruding around all margins of the veneer.

5. Remove the excess luting composite using a dental probe wetted with unfilled resin (Fig 7-12e). Removal of the excess should not be problematic, as the material sticks easily to the instrument. With one circular motion, you remove most of the excess from the labial surface and then from the palatal surface.

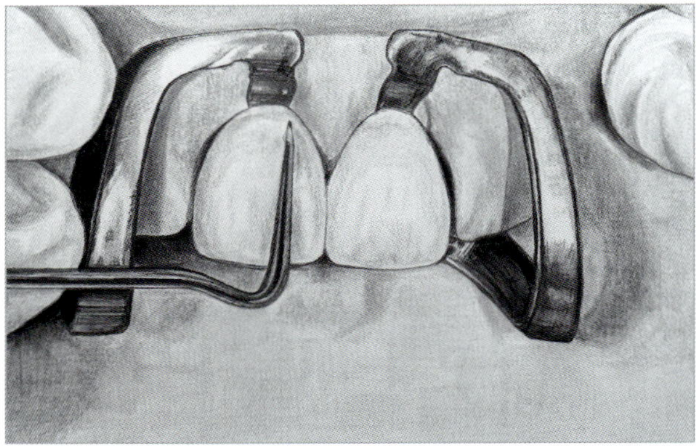

Fig 7-12e
The dental probe wetted with unfilled resin is an excellent instrument for removing excess luting cement.

6. The excess material on the proximal surface is removed with dental floss: the dentist stabilizes the veneer with their fingers, and the dental assistant gently pulls the floss along the curvature of the proximal surface from the incisal edge toward the gums, then takes it out from the palatal surface.

7. Once sure that the veneer is in the right position, polymerize for three seconds from the labial side and start again to remove excess material, especially from the proximal and palatal surfaces.

8. Cover all the margins with glycerin gel and proceed with the final polymerization for 60 seconds on each side (60 seconds from the labial side gingivally, 60 seconds at the incisal edge, and 60 seconds from the palatal side). During the final polymerization, pay attention to the orientation of the curing light (it is not uncommon for the dental assistant to place the light at an oblique angle, decreasing its curing efficiency) and to the risk of overheating the tooth (the new curing light models, due to their small size, tend to overheat).

9. After the final polymerization, remove the excess composite resin with scalpel no. 12, with motions from the gingival margin toward the coronal part of the tooth, cutting off all possible excess. The veneer is like glass, thanks to which the scalpel moves over the veneer and will not scratch it; it will only remove the polymerized composite (Fig 7-12f). As part of the polymerized composite is located under the clamp, it is then necessary to remove it, pull away the rubber dam with your fingers, and continue removing excess with a scalpel or curette (Fig 7-12g).

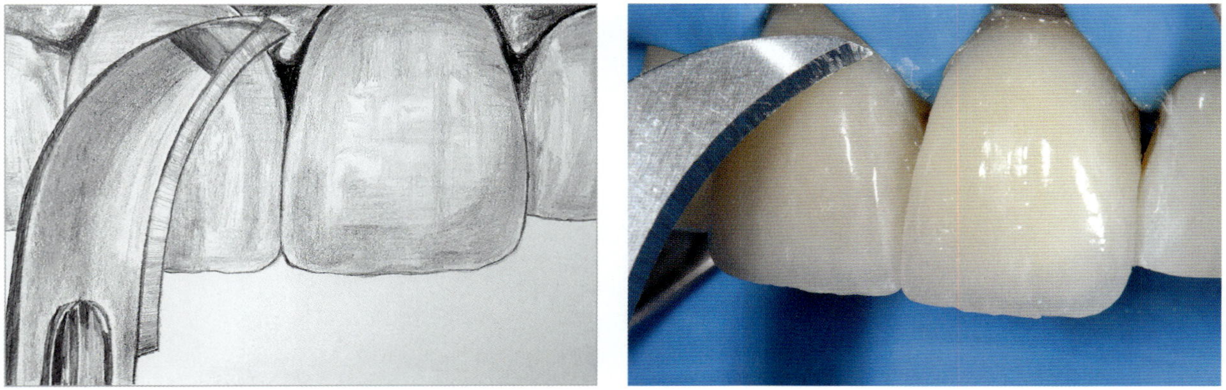

Video: Placing veneers – cementation procedure
https://books.dentist.com.pl/veneers/17

Fig 7-12f
Removal of excess polymerized composite using a scalpel no. 12.

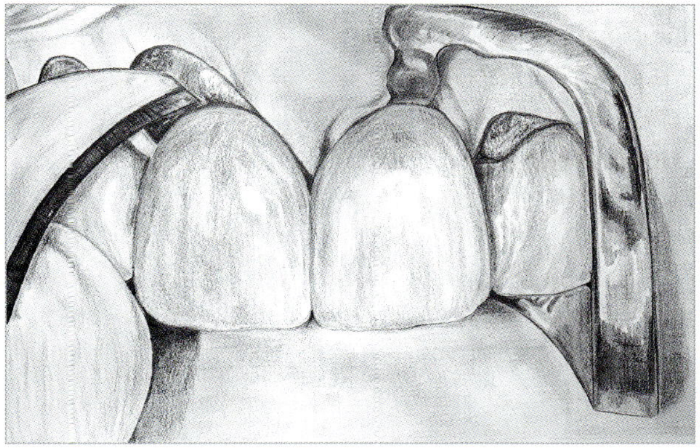

Fig 7-12g
Pull back the rubber dam with your fingers to expose the excess material and remove it with a scalpel.

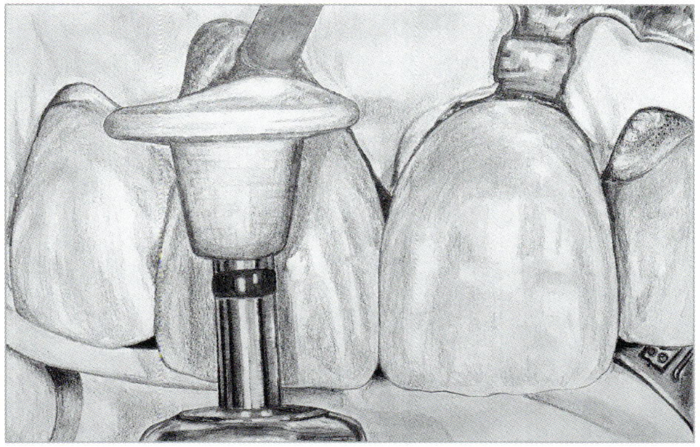

Fig 7-12h
Polishing veneers tooth transition.

10. Next, with a new rubber no. KE0309 (Kenda Nobilis), perform the polishing procedure at low speed (a completely new rubber has the flexibility to be perfectly adjusted to the preparation margin during polishing Fig 7-12h).

11. Before removing the rubber dam, make sure that excess material does not remain on the palatal surface, and use a red Sof-Lex disk to remove any excess present.

12. After removing the rubber dam, check again for excesses and, if necessary, use a scalpel, curette, rubber, or Sof-Lex disk from the palatal surfaces.

13. Seat the patient in an upright position and re-check the smile esthetics. Check the veneer/veneers in occlusion and during articulating movements.

14. The next step is to arrange a follow-up visit in 7 days, when the presence of any excess, occlusal overloads and final esthetics should be investigated (Figs 7-12i and 7-12j).

Veneers thinner than 0.5 mm

In this type of veneer, especially those made of feldspathic porcelain, there is a reduced mechanical strength before the veneers are cemented.[39,40] Therefore, without appropriate experience, you should not risk cementing on a heated composite. Instead, you should use a flowable composite or light-cured luting cement.

Figs 7-12i and 7-12j
(i) Evaluate the veneers and the patient's smile;
(j) during the control visit.

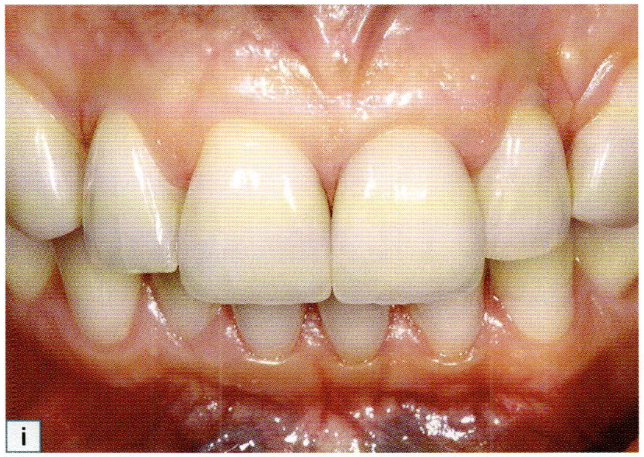

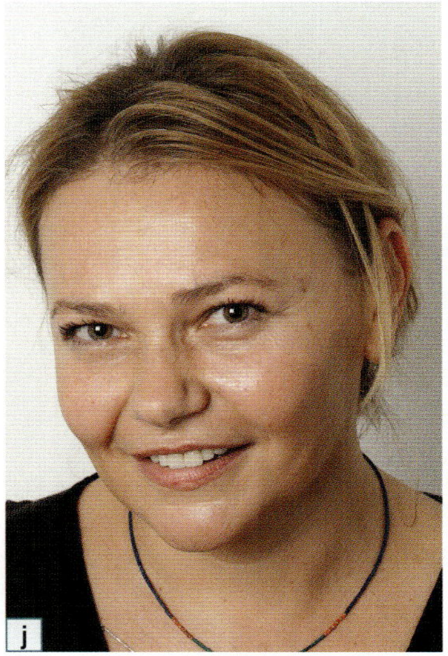

Flowable light-cured composite

When using flowable composite (for example, G-aenial Universal Flow, Fig 7-13a), we have the same procedures as for veneer cementation with the heated composite (described above), except the heating procedure, which we skip.[41,42]

Light-cured luting cement

When using an extensive kit for veneer cementation, the color of the luting cement should be chosen before the adhesive preparation of the veneer. In general, the color does not have a special meaning when placing thicker veneer, but may play a big role when cementing very thin veneer,[43–44] especially in the case of discolored tooth structure. When using a light-curing luting cement (for example, Variolink Esthetic LC, Fig 7-13b), test the selected color by using the try-in test paste (Fig 7-13c).

1. Evaluate the shade of the veneer seated on the try-in paste: if accepted, a composite cement corresponding with the try-in paste should be used.

2. After adhesive preparation of the tooth (in the rubber dam) and the inner surface of the veneer, a luting cement is applied on the entire inner surface and seated on the prepared tooth. After ensuring that the restoration is seated in the correct position and reaches the preparation margin, press it with your fingertips and light-cure, moving the light along the preparation margin for a few seconds (try to polymerize each surface for three seconds) (Fig 7-13d). Pre-polymerization allows the gel phase to be reached, which will help easy removal of the cement excess with a curette along the preparation margin (Fig 7-13e) and with dental floss from the interdental spaces.

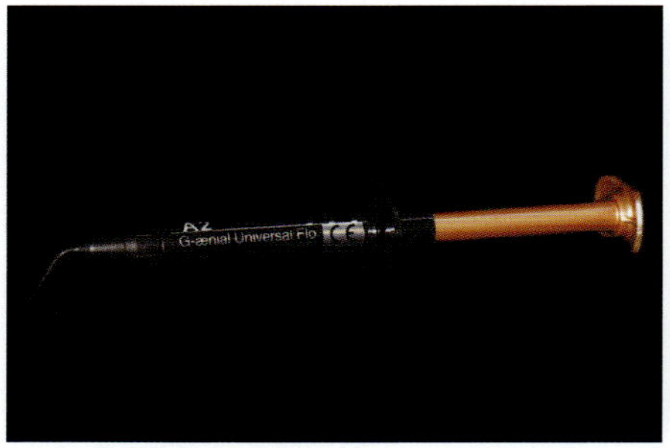

Fig 7-13a
An example of a flowable composite that will work well for thin veneers cementation.

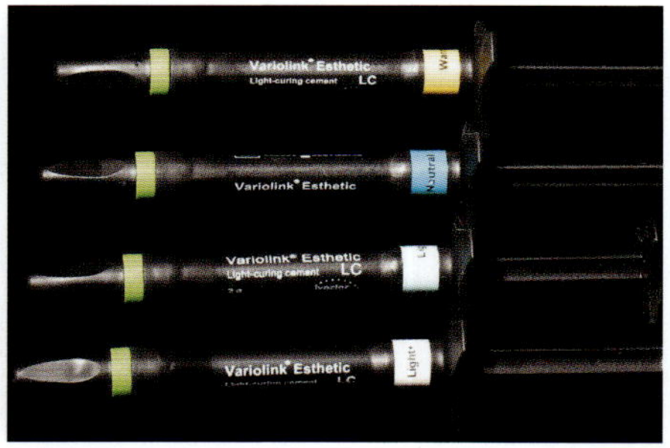

Fig 7-13b
A kit for porcelain veneers cementation, containing a ready-made try-in paste to evaluate the final color of the veneer after cementation.

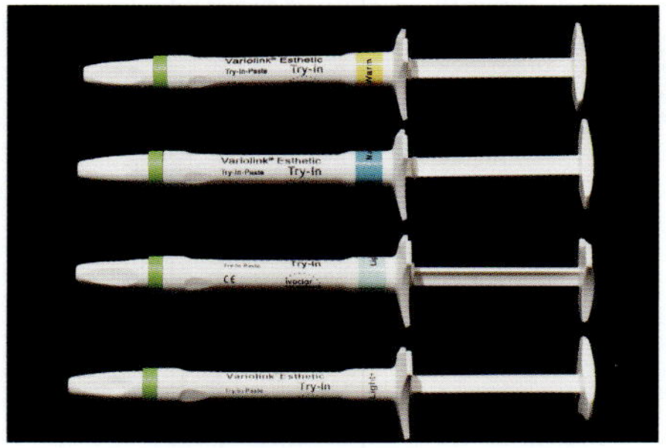

Fig 7-13c
Every try-in paste has a corresponding color for the luting cement.

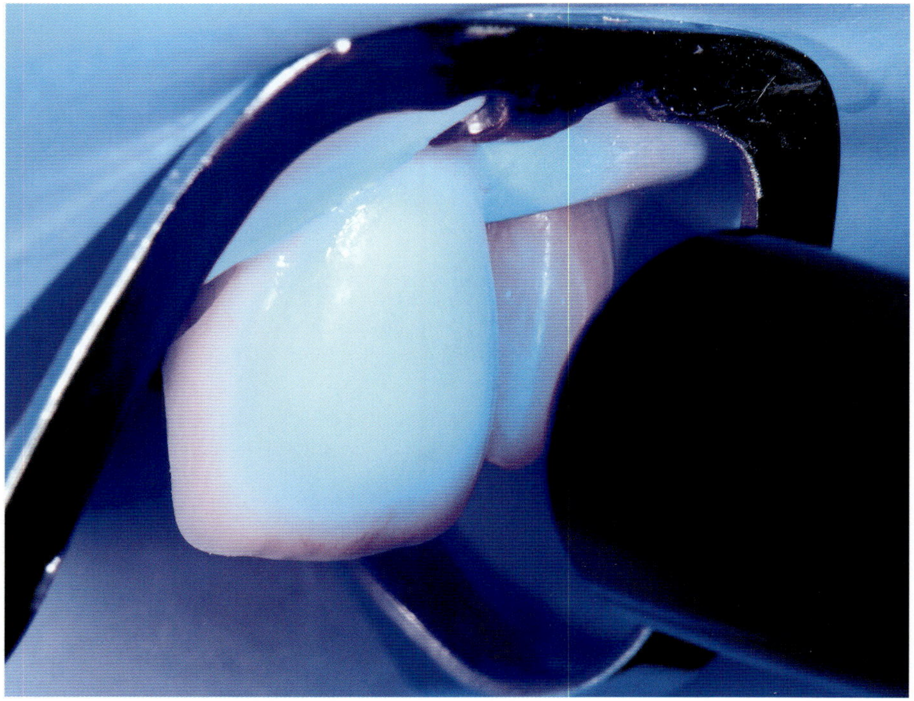

Fig 7-13d
When using conventional light-curing luting cement after a short (three-second) polymerization time …

3. Application of glycerin gel (Fig 7-13f) (protection against oxygen-inhibition layer) and final polymerization of the veneer for 60 seconds on each side (Fig 7-13g).

4. Remove the composite excess with a blade no. 12 (Fig 7-13h) and polish the preparation margin (Fig 7-13i).

TIP

When removing composite excess with a scalpel no. 12, use the blade toward the crown of the tooth to avoid damaging the gums. The dental assistant should be asked to protect the patient's lower lip in the event of accidental closure of the mouth. With the scalpel, we make gentle cutting movements. Do not worry about the porcelain – the blade will not scratch it!

Fig 7-13e
... initial removal of the cement excess with a curette.

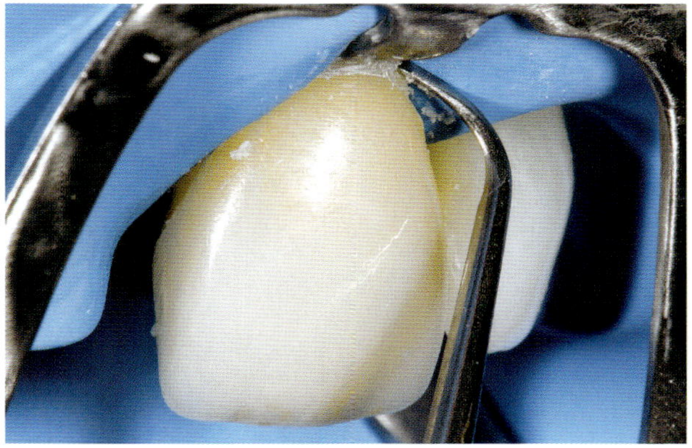

Fig 7-13f
Application of glycerin gel to protect against oxygen-inhibition layer ...

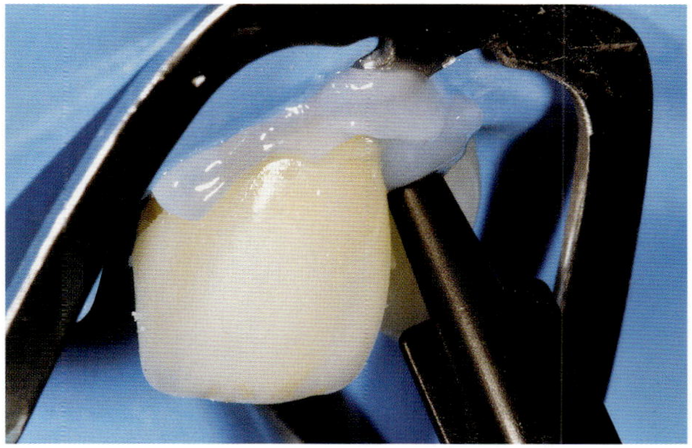

Fig 7-13g
... and polymerization for 60 seconds on each side.

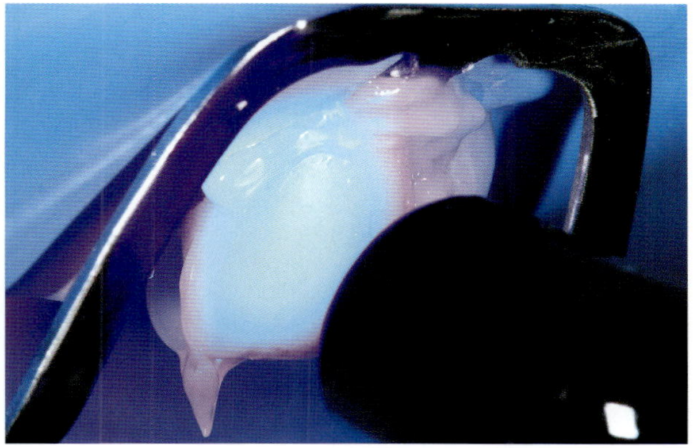

Fig 7-13h
After final polymerization, remove cement excess with a blade no. 12 ...

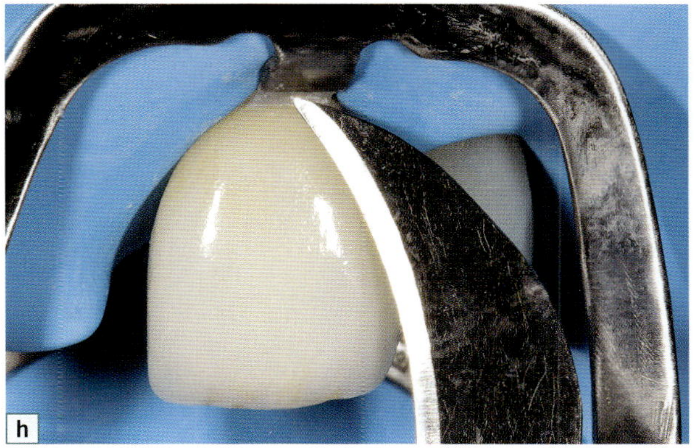

Fig 7-13i
... and gently polish the preparation margin.

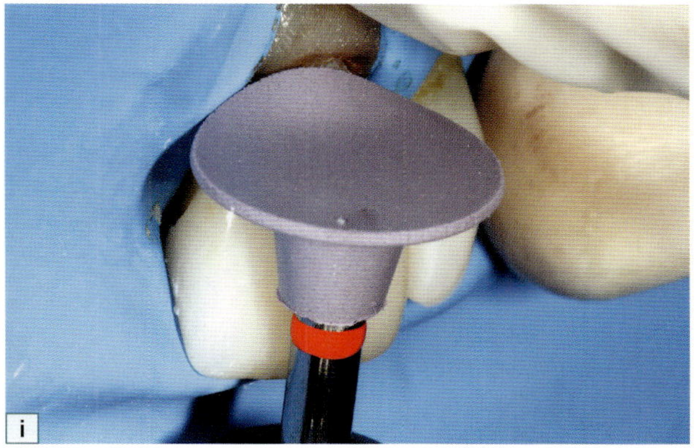

PROCEDURES AFTER VENEERS CEMENTATION

1. Control of cement excess

This is a very important step after cementing veneers. Check the presence for any excess before removing the rubber dam. With gingival retraction, any excess is very clearly visible. Immediately after removing the rubber dam, the gingiva very quickly returns to its place, making it impossible to notice any small excess. Therefore, the removal of excess should be carried out HERE AND NOW, immediately after cementing veneers.

2. Control of anterior overload

Seat the patient in position 45 degrees, put your fingertips on the teeth with veneers, then ask the patient to bite several times. If finger vibrations are detected, you must start correcting the premature contacts immediately. Vibration is an important indicator of anterior overload, which should be corrected immediately after veneers have been cemented.

3. Finding premature contacts

A 200 μm horseshoe articulating paper is used to detect premature contacts; it provides a "base" for the thin and more accurate 8–20 μm red articulation foil (Fig 7-14a). The contact points, marked on the front teeth with red and blue articulating paper, are removed (the thin red articulating paper marks very clearly on the blue background of 200 μm articulating paper).

4. Kois chewing test

Seat the patient upright in position 90 degrees, place a 200 μm horseshoe articulating paper between their teeth, and then ask them to chew as if they were chewing a beefsteak. This test is supposed to simulate real chewing while eating.[45] Any extensive blue surfaces (representing attrition between the maxillary and mandibular anterior teeth) that appear on the front teeth, especially those that are present on the palatal surfaces of the veneers, have to be eliminated.

You should strive to achieve delicately marked blue lines and eliminate the large, heavily marked areas.

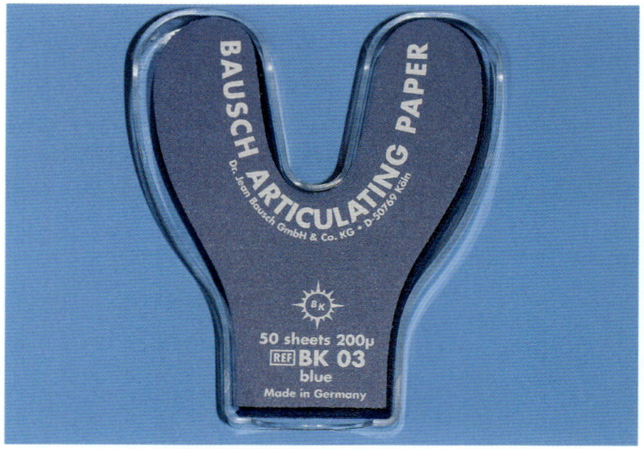

Fig 7-14a
The blue horseshoe-shaped articulating paper, 200 μm thick, is designed to dry the tooth surface and prepares for the use of thinner and more accurate articulating paper (red tracing paper, 20 μm thick, which is very precise in detecting premature contacts).

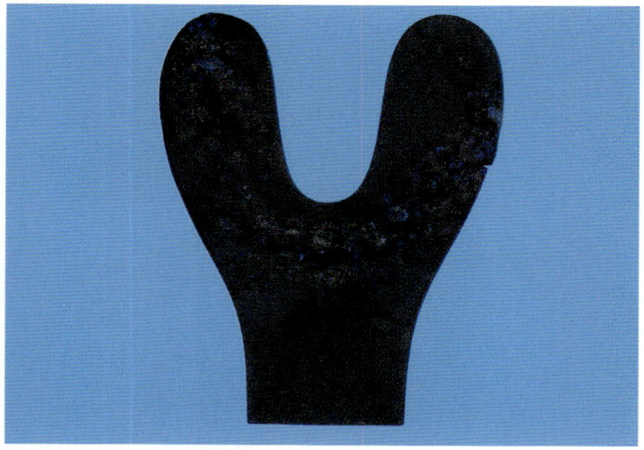

Fig 7-14b
The chewing test with 200 μm articulating paper developed by Dr. J. Kois can detect friction between opposing teeth, which is not good for temporomandibular joints, tooth structures, or restorative materials.

> **REMEMBER**
> The blue surfaces which occur on the palatal surface of porcelain veneers after the chewing test (Fig 7-14b) indicate the presence of attrition while chewing. Attrition is dangerous to porcelain restorations, and can lead to fracture or chipping of the veneers …

REFERENCES

1. Primosch RE, Brooks R. Influence of anesthetic flow rate delivered by the Wand Local Anesthetic System on pain response to palatal injections. Am J Dent 2002;15:15–20.
2. Ogle OE, Mahjoubi G. Advances in local anesthesia in dentistry. Dent Clin North Am 2011;55:481–499.
3. Calamia V, Pantzis A. Simple case treatment planning: diastema closure. Dent Clin North Am 2015;59:655–664.
4. Krämer N, Lohbauer U, Frankenberger R. Adhesive luting of indirect restorations. Am J Dent 2000;13(Spec No):60D–76D.
5. Bamashmous MS. Veneer or interproximal enamel reduction? J Contemp Dent Pract 2018;19:749–751.
6. Kois JC. The restorative-periodontal interface: biological parameters. Periodontol 2000. 1996;11:29–38.
7. Kois JC. The gingiva is red around my crowns – a differential diagnosis. Dent Econ 1993;83:101–102.
8. Turgut S, Bagis B. Effect of resin cement and ceramic thickness on final color of laminate veneers: an in vitro study. J Prosthet Dent 2013;109:179–186.
9. Turgut S, Bagis B. Colour stability of laminate veneers: an in vitro study. J Dent 2011;39 Suppl 3:e57–e64.
10. Fradeani M. Evaluation of dentolabial parameters as part of a comprehensive esthetic analysis. Eur J Esthet Dent 2006;1:62–69.
11. Small BW. Location of incisal edge position for esthetic restorative dentistry. Gen Dent 2000;48:396–397.
12. Frese C, Staehle HJ, Wolff D. The assessment of dentofacial esthetics in restorative dentistry: a review of the literature. J Am Dent Assoc 2012;143:461–466.
13. Magne P, Gallucci GO, Belser UC. Anatomic crown width/length ratios of unworn and worn maxillary teeth in white subjects. J Prosthet Dent 2003;89:453–461.
14. Duarte S Jr, Schnider P, Lorezon AP. The importance of width/length ratios of maxillary anterior permanent teeth in esthetic rehabilitation. Eur J Esthet Dent 2008;3:224–234.
15. Hasanreisoglu U, Berksun S, Aras K, Arslan I. An analysis of maxillary anterior teeth: facial and dental proportions. J Prosthet Dent 2005;94:530–538.
16. Roulet JF, Söderholm KJ, Longmate J. Effects of treatment and storage conditions on ceramic/composite bond strength. J Dent Res 1995;74:381–387.
17. Fabianelli A, Pollington S, Papacchini F, et al. The effect of different surface treatments on bond strength between leucite reinforced feldspathic ceramic and composite resin. J Dent 2010;38:39–43.
18. Soares CJ, Soares PV, Pereira JC, Fonseca RB. Surface treatment protocols in the cementation process of ceramic and laboratory-processed composite restorations: a literature review. J Esthet Restor Dent 2005;17:224–235.
19. Jardel V, Degrange M, Picard B, Derrien G. Surface energy of etched ceramic. Int J Prosthet 1999;12:415–418.
20. Jardel V, Degrange M, Picard B, Derrien G. Correlation of topography to bond strength of etched ceramic. Int J Prosthet 1999;12:59–64.
21. Burd A. Hydrofluoric acid-revisited. Burns 2004;30:720–722.
22. Ozcan M, Allahbeickaraghi A, Dündar M. Possible hazardous effects of hydrofluoric acid and recommendations for treatment approach: a review. Clin Oral Investig 2012;16:15–23.
23. Hagiwara Y. Die strafrechtliche Verantwortung des Zahnarztes. Chuo Gakuin Univ Rev Fac Law 2013:26:75–112. (In Japanese)
24. Kameyama A, Haruyama A, Tanaka A, et al. Repair bond strength of a resin composite to plasma-treated or UV-irradiated CAD/CAM ceramic surface. Coatings 2018;8:230.
25. Hooshmand T, Parvizi S, Keshvad A. Effect of surface acid etching on the biaxial flexural strength of two hot-pressed glass ceramics. J Prosthet 2008;17:415–419.
26. Naves LZ, Soares CJ, Moraes RR, Gonçalves LS, Sinhoreti MA, Correr-Sobrinho L. Surface/interface morphology and bond strength to glass ceramic etched for different periods. Oper Dent 2010;35:420–427.
27. Sundfeld Neto D, Naves LZ, Costa AR, et al. The effect of hydrofluoric acid concentration on the bond strength and morphology of the surface and interface of glass ceramics to a resin cement. Oper Dent 2015;40:470–479.
28. Murillo-Gómez F, Palma-Dibb RG, De Goes MF. Effect of acid etching on tridimensional microstructure of etchable CAD/CAM materials. Dent Mater 2018;34:944–955.
29. Bajraktarova-Valjakova E, Grozdanov A, Guguvcevski L, et al. Acid etching as surface treatment method for luting of glass-ceramic restorations. Part 1: Acids, application protocol and etching effectiveness. Open Access Maced J Med Sci 2018;6:568–573.
30. Ramakrishnaiah R, Alkheraif AA, Divakar DD, Matinlinna JP, Vallittu PK. The effect of hydrofluoric acid etching duration on the surface micromorphology, roughness, and wettability of dental ceramics. Int J Mol Sci 2016;17:822.
31. Canay S, Hersek N, Ertan A. Effect of different acid treatments on a porcelain surface. J Oral Rehabil 2001;28:95–101.
32. Chen JH, Matsumura H, Atsuta M. Effect of different etching periods on the bond strength of a composite resin to a machinable porcelain. J Dent 1998;26:53–58.
33. Magne P, Cascione D. Influence of post-etching cleaning and connecting porcelain on the microtensile bond strength of composite resin to feldspathic porcelain. J Prosthet Dent 2006;96:354–361.
34. Wong ACH, Tian T, Tsoi JKH, Burrow MF, Matinlinna JP. Aspects of adhesion tests on resin glass ceramic bonding. Dent Mater 2017;33:1045–1055.
35. Zarow M. Licówki porcelanowe na zębach po leczeniu endodontycznym – zmodyfikowana metoda izolacji koferdamem. Medycyna Praktyczna. Stomatologia 2012;1:93–99.
36. D'Amario M, Piccioni C, Di Carlo S, De Angelis F, Caruso S, Capogreco M. Effect of airborne particle abrasion on microtensile bond strength of total-etch adhesives to human dentin. Biomed Res Int 2017; Article ID 2432536.
37. Chaiyabutr Y, Kois JC. The effects of tooth preparation cleansing protocols on the bond strength of self-adhesive resin luting cement to contaminated dentin. Oper Dent 2008;33:556–563.
38. D'Arcangelo C, De Angelis F, Vadini M, D'Amario M. Clinical evaluation on porcelain laminate veneers bonded with light-cured composite: results up to 7 years. Clin Oral Investig 2012;16:1071–1079.

REFERENCES

39. Tuğcu E, Vanlıoğlu B, Özkan YK, Aslan YU. Marginal adaptation and fracture resistance of lithium disilicate laminate veneers on teeth with different preparation depths. Int J Periodontics Restorative Dent 2018;38(Suppl):87–95.
40. Perroni AP, Kaizer MR, Della Bona A, Moraes RR, Boscato N. Influence of light-cured luting agents and associated factors on the color of ceramic laminate veneers: a systematic review of in vitro studies. Dent Mater 2018;34:1610–1624.
41. D'Arcangelo C, De Angelis F, D'Amario M, Zazzeroni S, Ciampoli C, Caputi S. The influence of luting systems on the microtensile bond strength of dentin to indirect resin-based composite and ceramic restorations. Oper Dent 2009;34:328–336.
42. Sampaio CS, Barbosa JM, Cáceres E, et al. Volumetric shrinkage and film thickness of cementation materials for veneers: an in vitro 3D microcomputed tomography analysis. J Prosthet Dent 2017;117:784–791.
43. Archegas LR, Freire A, Vieira S, Caldas DB, Souza EM. Color stability and opacity of resin cements and flowable composites for ceramic veneer luting after accelerated ageing. J Dent 2011;39:804–810.
44. Edelhoff D, Prandtner O, Saeidi Pour R, Liebermann A, Stimmelmayr M, Güth JF. Anterior restorations: the performance of ceramic veneers. Quintessence Int 2018;49:89-101.
45. Kois JC, Hartrick N. Functional occlusion: science-driven management, J Cosmetic Dent 2007;23:53–57.

CHAPTER 8

ATLAS OF CLINICAL PROCEDURES

MACIEJ ŻAROW

Are porcelain veneers a challenge
for the dentist in terms
of comprehensive esthetic
treatment, ensuring the patient
beauty and harmony of life?
Probably yes, but in most cases,
it depends on following the rules
that will lead to success.

Atlas of clinical procedures

In hundreds of clinical situations that I have encountered in everyday practice, one can find an extensive set of experiences, regularities, and rules that allow the formulation of effective treatment procedures for porcelain veneers. This chapter will help you understand how to proceed in different clinical situations to accomplish the planned treatment.

VENEERS AND TEETH WITH MULTIPLE DIRECT RESTORATIONS

It can be assumed that the larger the tooth surface area covered by composite restorations, the worse the prognosis will be for porcelain veneers. On the other hand, it is difficult to find ideal cases for veneers in everyday practice as those often shown in books, at lectures by famous dentists, or in advertising brochures. In everyday practice, the dentist expects the dental technician's help by fabricating porcelain veneers in cases where it is difficult to perform perfect restorations due to their number, shape, or match the color to the adjacent teeth. It can be assumed that veneers can be performed when more than 50% of the tooth structure remains after preparation.[1]

Of course, the more structure of the tooth is present, the more predictable veneer will be. The more enamel remains on the preparation margin, the better the future veneer adhesion and its final prognosis.[2–4] All this should be properly explained to the patient. After that conversation, a final, well-thought-out decision should be made about whether to remake only the previous restorations, perform porcelain veneers, or maybe decide on more invasive treatment, like all-ceramic crowns.

The principle is simple: the quantity and quality of the tooth structure contribute to good adhesion and prognosis of the veneer. The lack of predictable adhesion prompts us to plan indirect restorations based on mechanical retention, such as prosthetic crowns.

RULES WHEN PERFORMING VENEERS ON TEETH WITH MULTIPLE COMPOSITE RESTORATIONS

1. Replacement of all leaking and "suspicious" restorations with new ones
2. Tooth whitening has to be carried out at least 1 month before the planned treatment so that the color of the veneer can be matched to the new, stable one and also allow the bonding system to have optimal adhesion to the tooth
3. In the case of an extensive composite restoration on the proximal surface, preparation should include the entire contact surface in order to cover the composite resin with the indirect veneer[5,6]
4. In the juxtagingival area, the preparation margin should not "meet" the composite resin restoration (what is acceptable in the case of posterior indirect partial restorations)

REMEMBER

Do not hesitate to replace all the restorations that do not meet the appropriate marginal adaptation standards. Leaving leaking composite resin under the veneer can cause discoloration, inflammation of the gums, or weakening of the final veneer adhesion …

Case 1: Veneers and teeth with multiple composite restorations

A 33-year-old female patient presented to the dental office seeking porcelain veneers for her anterior maxillary teeth. The patient did not like the color of her teeth and the occurrence of many composite restorations that became discolored over time.

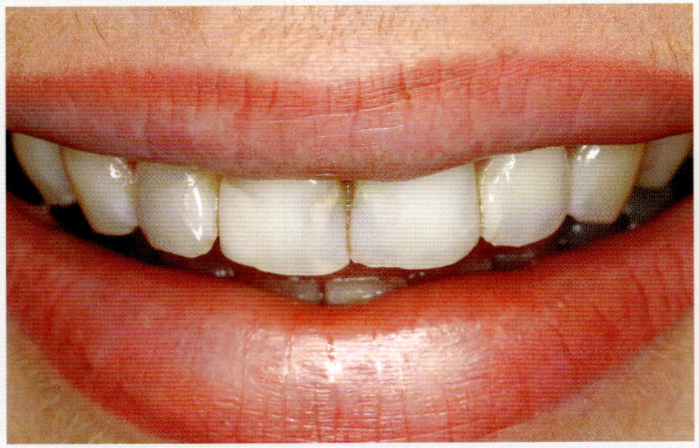

Fig 8-1a
Patient's smile before starting the treatment.

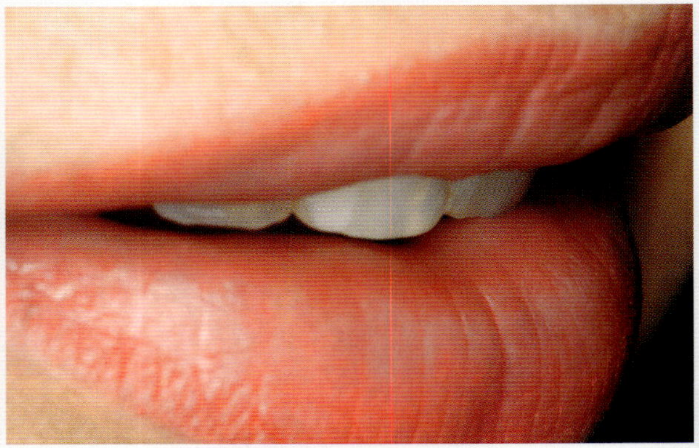

Fig 8-1b
Location of the incisal edges of the maxillary teeth in relation to the upper lip in repose.

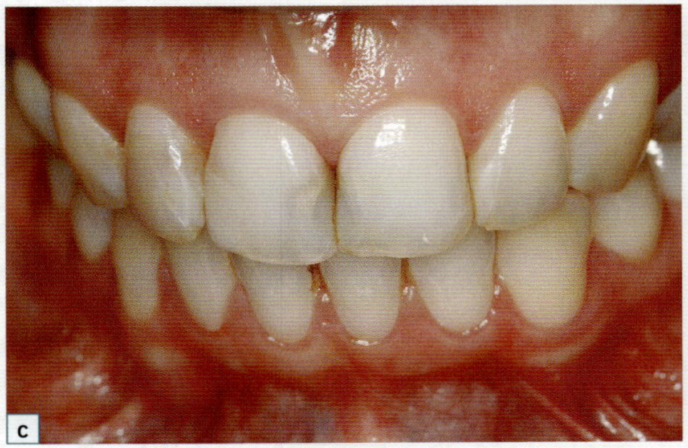

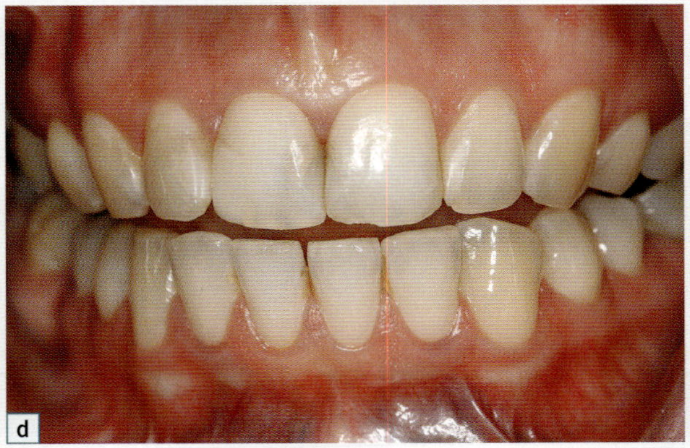

Figs 8-1c and 8-1d
Intraoral photographs of the anterior teeth – extensive composite restorations are clearly visible.

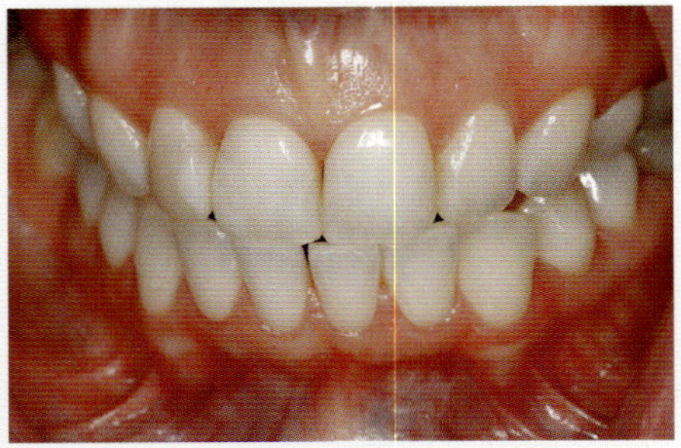

Fig 8-1e
Situation after teeth whitening and replacing the restorations.

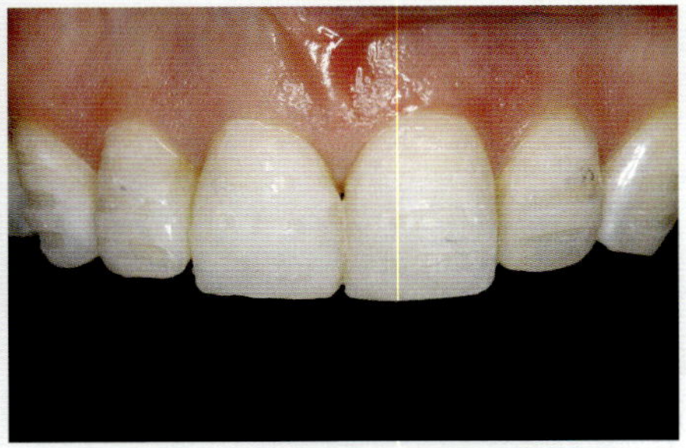

Fig 8-1f
Porcelain veneer preparation from a mock-up level, created on the basis of the diagnostic wax-up.

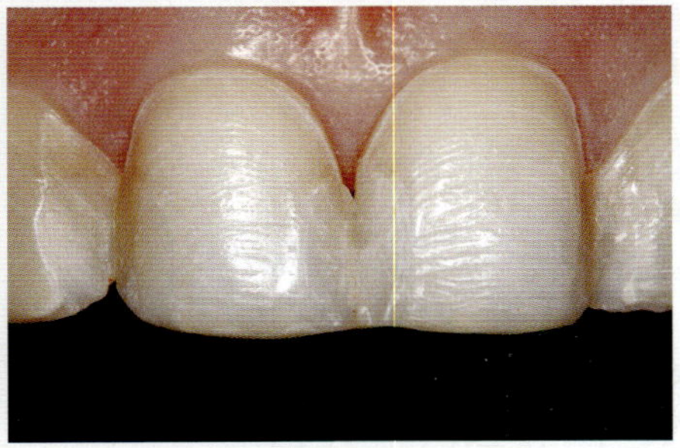

Fig 8-1g
Initial preparation on the labial surface shows the extension of Class 3 and 4 restorations in teeth 12, 11, 21, and 22.

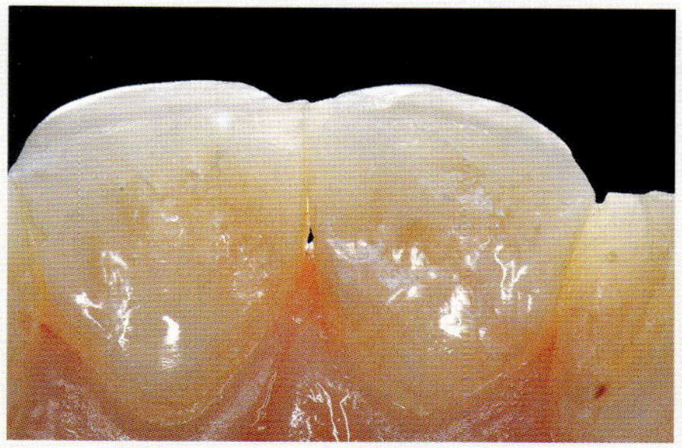

Fig 8-1h
Anterior teeth – palatal view.

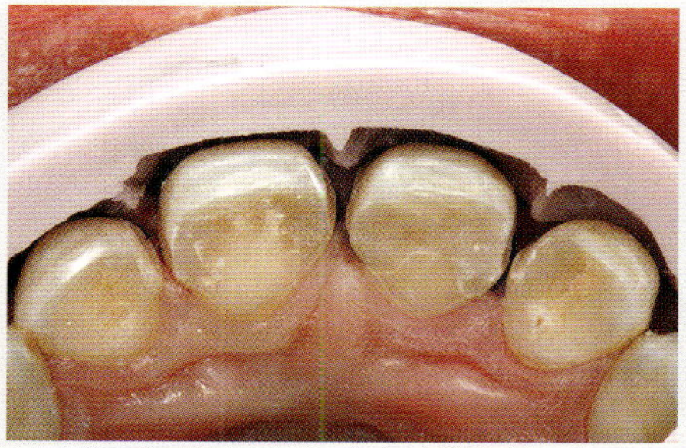

Fig 8-1i
Depth of the preparation was controlled with a silicone index made on the basis of the diagnostic wax-up model.

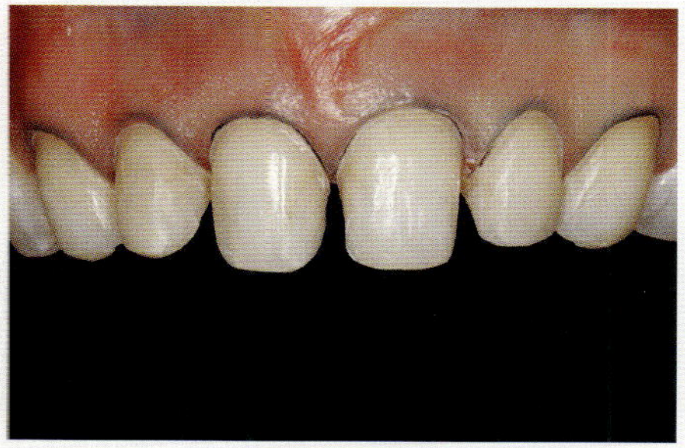

Fig 8-1j
Clinical situation after veneer preparation on teeth 13–23. Note: preparation on tooth 12 mesial, 11 mesial and distal, 21 mesial and distal, and 22 mesial was extended to the proximal surface.

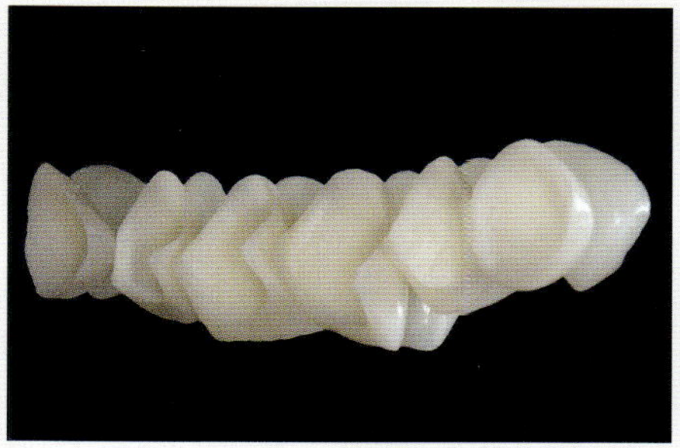

Fig 8-1k
Feldspathic porcelain veneers 13–23 were fabricated in the dental laboratory.

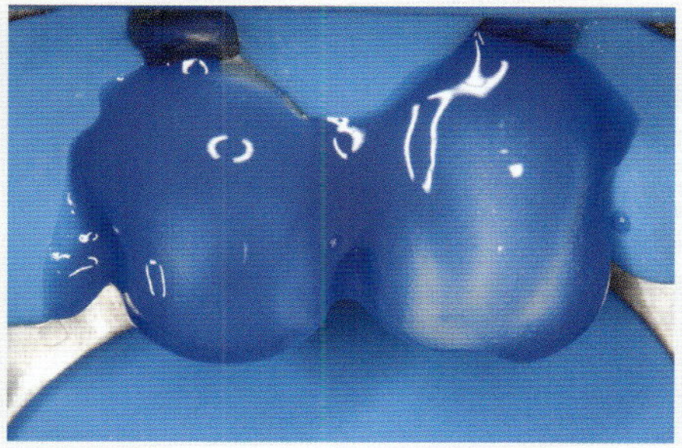

Fig 8-1l
Teeth 11 and 21 etched with phosphoric acid in rubber dam isolation.

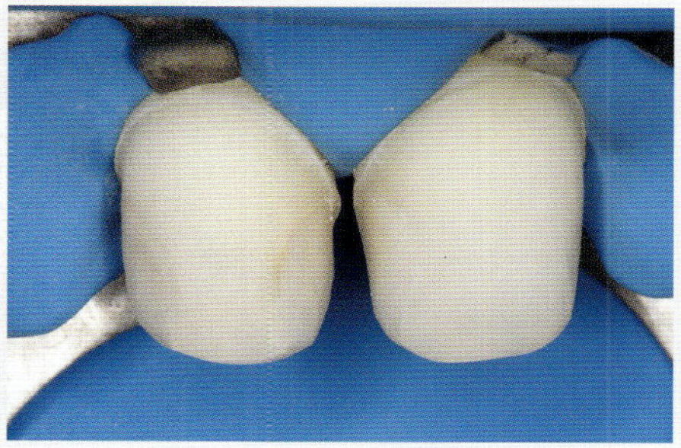

Fig 8-1m
Situation after etching the teeth surface …

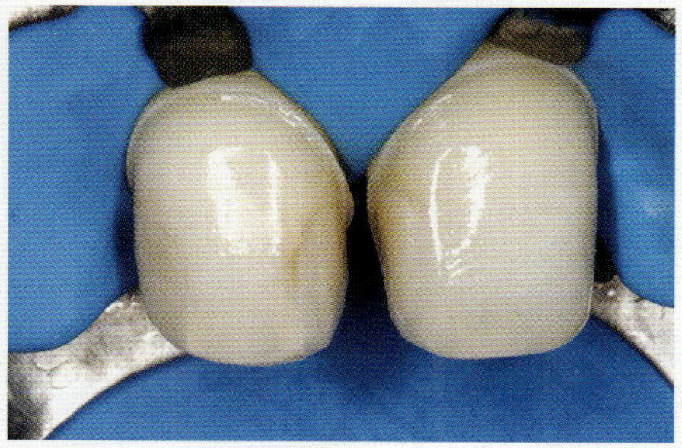

Fig 8-1n
… and after application of the bonding system and polymerization.

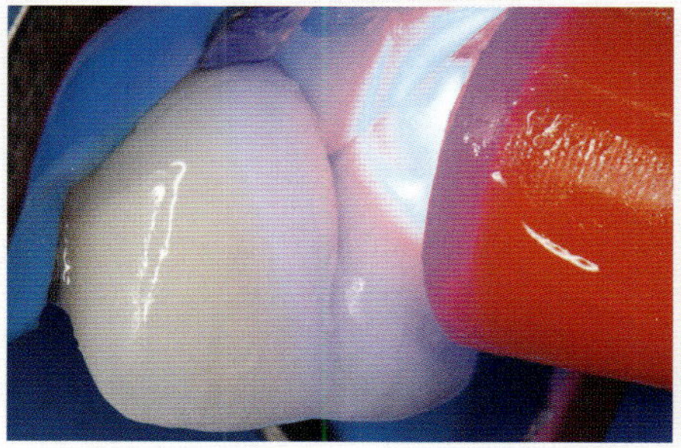

Fig 8-1o
Simultaneous cementation of two veneers on teeth 11 and 21.

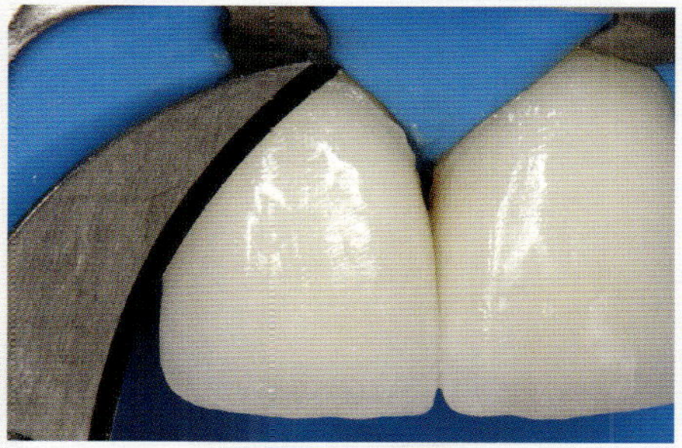

Fig 8-1p
Removing polymerized composite resin excess with a scalpel no. 12.

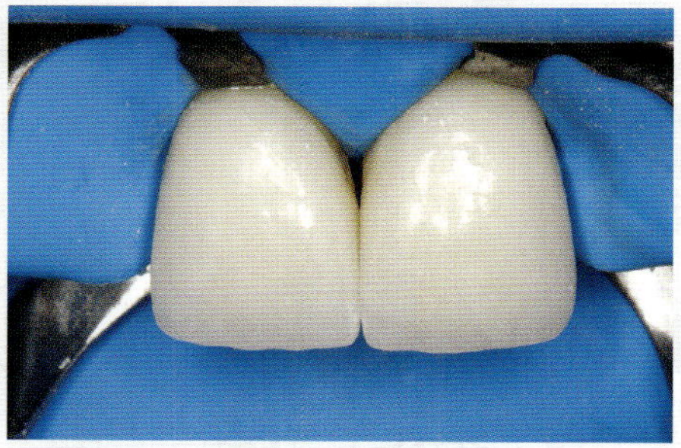

Fig 8-1q
Situation after cementation of two porcelain veneers in rubber dam isolation and removing the excess material.

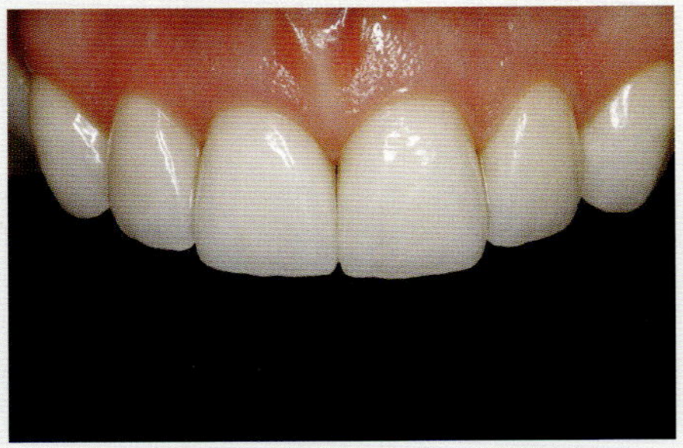

Fig 8-1r
Integration of the porcelain veneers with gingival tissues a few weeks after cementation.

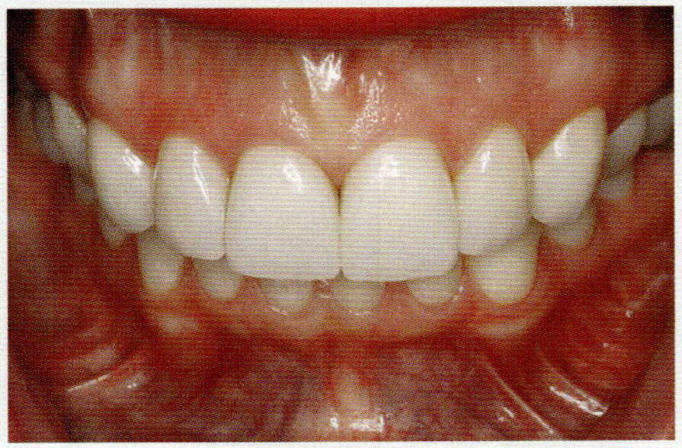

Fig 8-1s
Color compatibility with the remaining teeth of the maxillary and mandibular arches.

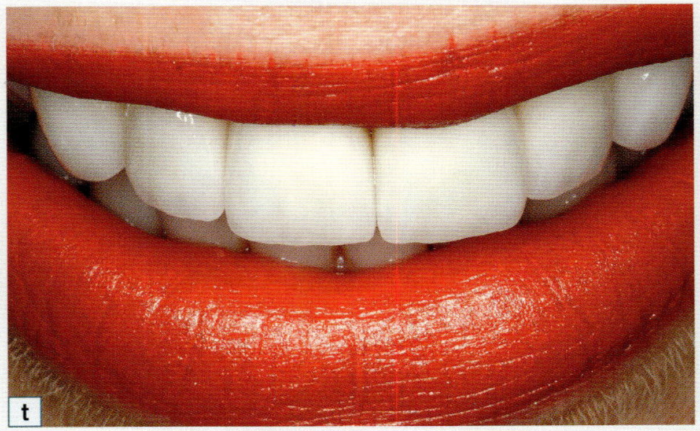

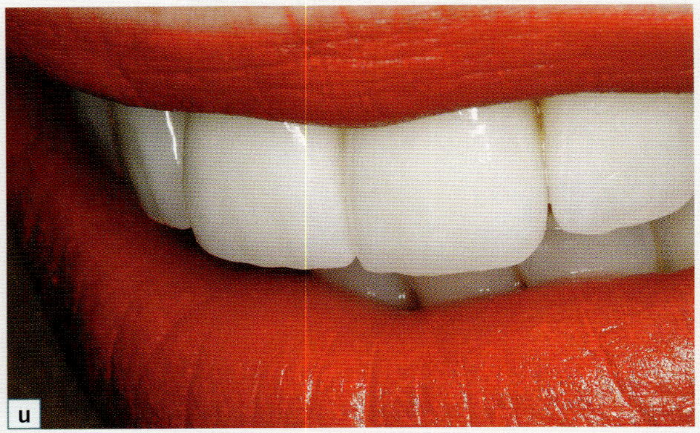

Figs 8-1t to 8-1v
Patient's smile: perfect integration with the upper and lower lip.

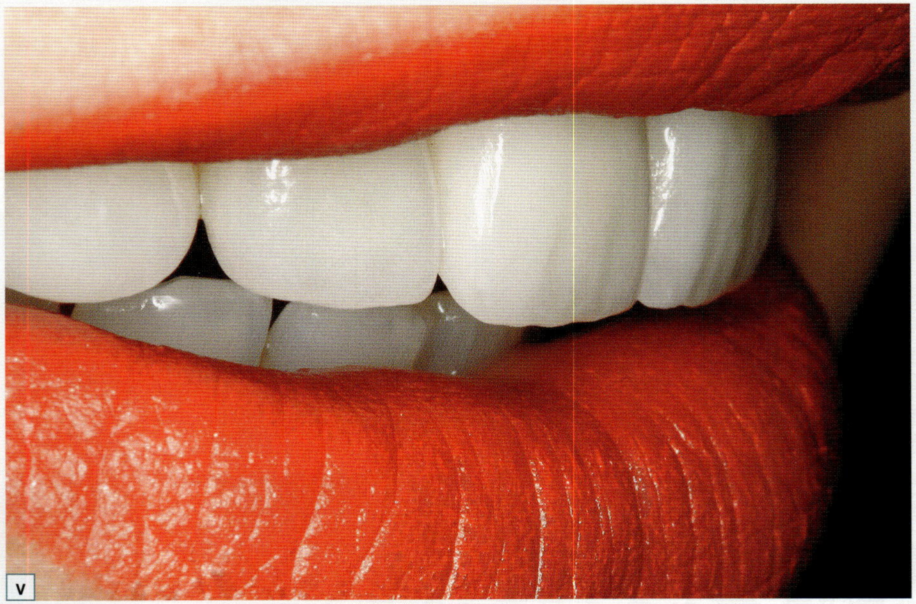

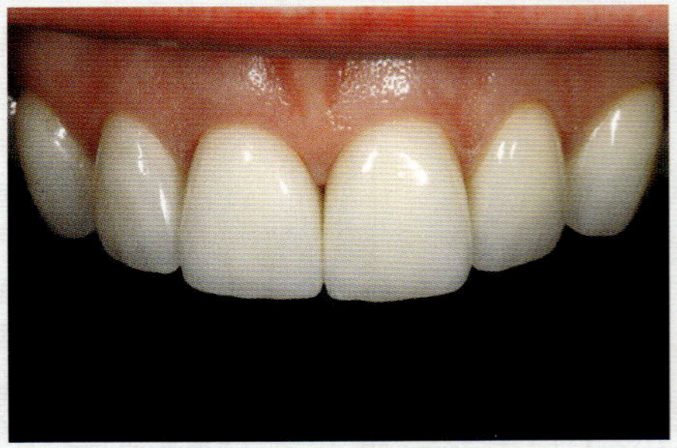

Fig 8-1w
Clinical follow-up 6 years after veneers cementation.

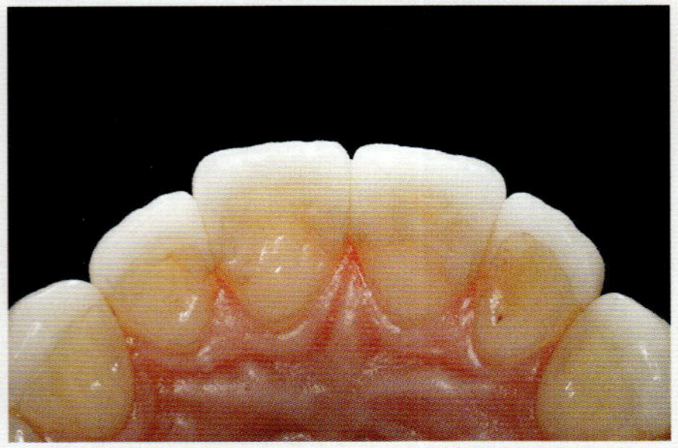

Fig 8-1x
Clinical situation 6 years after veneers cementation – palatal view.

Case 2: Veneers on the teeth with multiple composite restorations, 25-years follow-up

How long can veneers last? Dentists and patients often ask this question. A 25-year observation of porcelain veneers performed on teeth with multiple, extensive restorations is presented below. Follow-up over 25 years showed perfect integration of the veneers with tooth structure, soft tissues, and esthetic harmony with the patient's smile. This case shows that following strict adhesion procedures can lead not only to great esthetic results, but also to long-lasting restorations.

(With permission of Dr. Marco Nicastro)

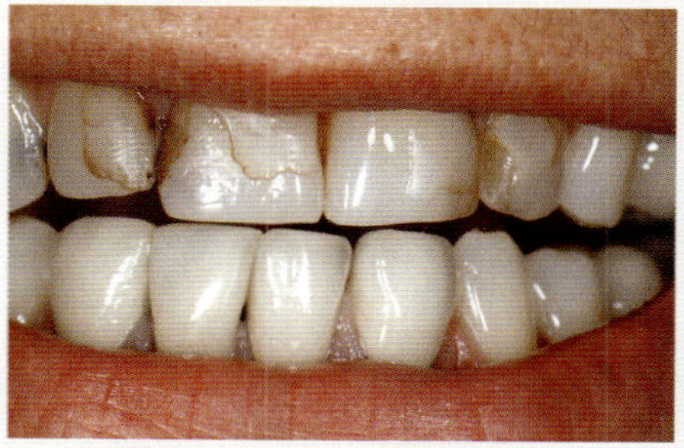

Fig 8-2a
A 27-year-old female patient with extremely unesthetic old restorations presented to the office seeking esthetic treatment.

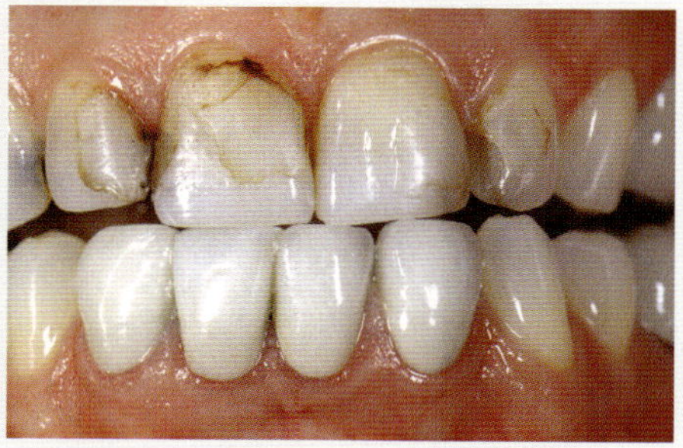

Fig 8-2b
Clinical situation before treatment.

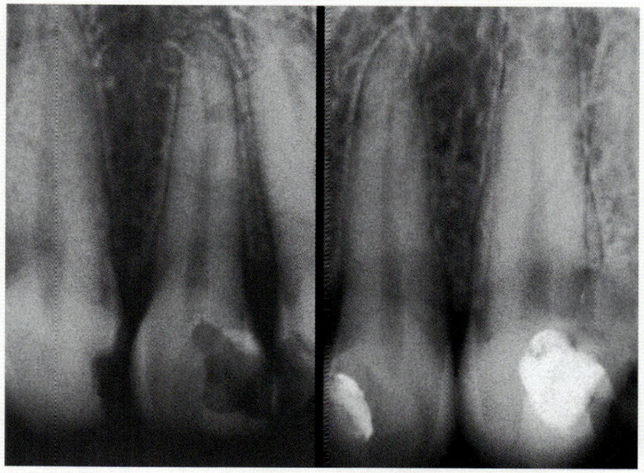

Fig 8-2e
Radiographs showing the extension of composite restorations.

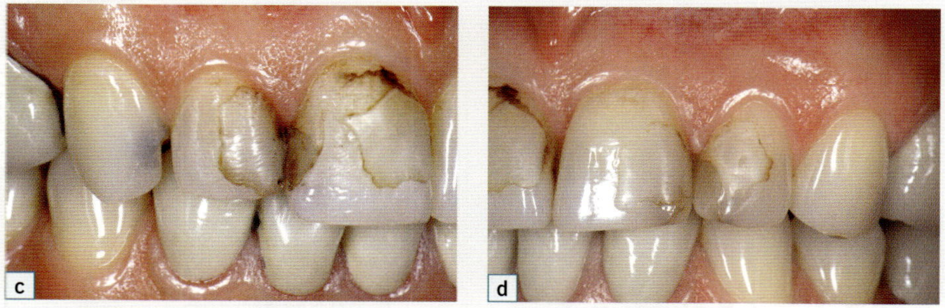

Figs 8-2c and 8-1d
Close-up of the discolored restorations in the maxillary arch.

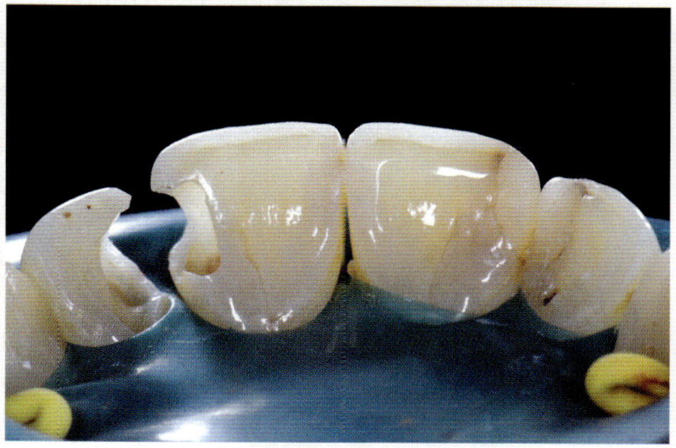

Fig 8-2f
After removing the old restorations in teeth 11 and 12 – palatal view.

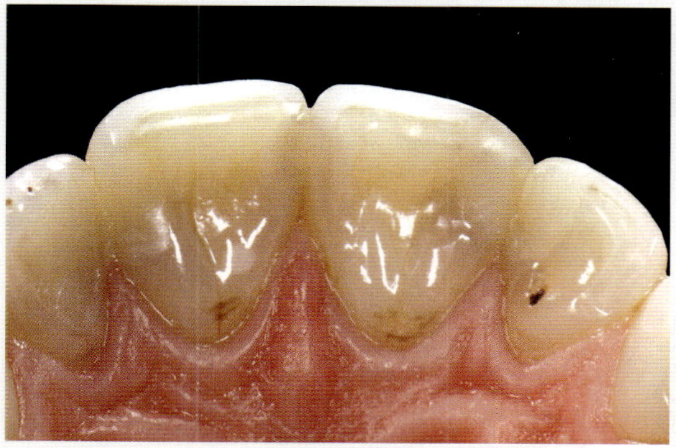

Fig 8-2g
After replacing the restorations with new ones – palatal view.

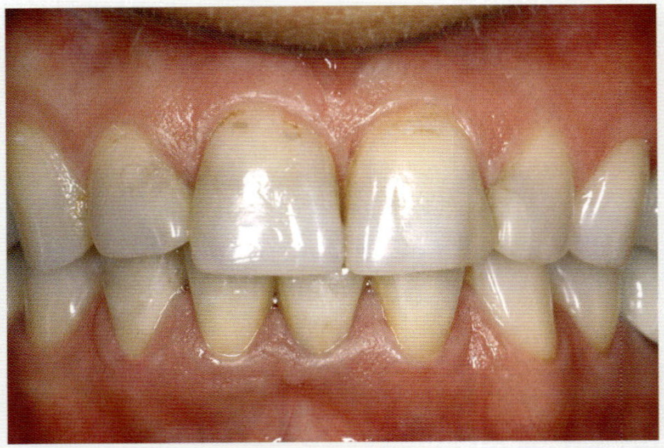

Fig 8-2h
Clinical situation after replacing the old composite restorations.

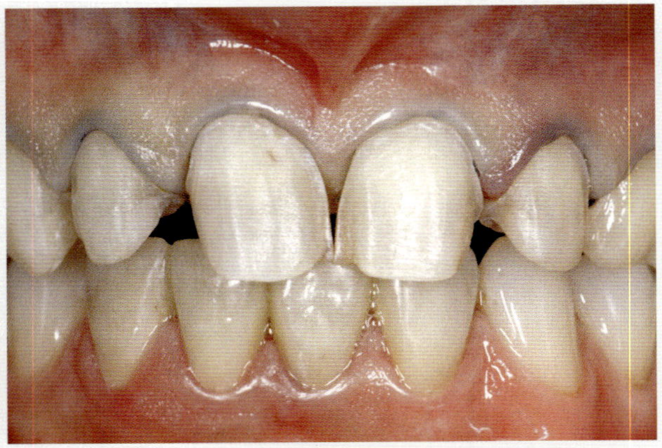

Fig 8-2i
Clinical situation after teeth preparation. Note: The proximal surfaces with extensive composite restorations are included in the preparation to allow them to be covered with porcelain.

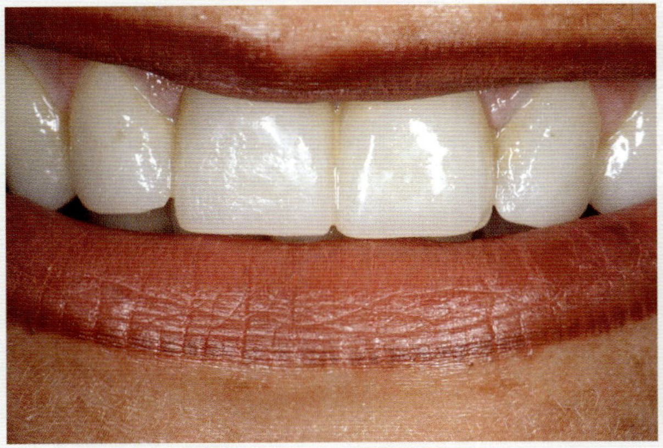

Fig 8-2j
After taking the impressions, provisional veneers were placed to protect the teeth.

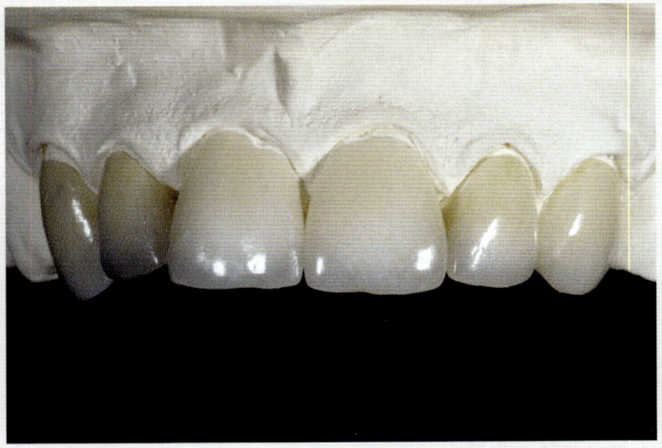

Fig 8-2k
Feldspathic porcelain veneers were fabricated in the dental laboratory.

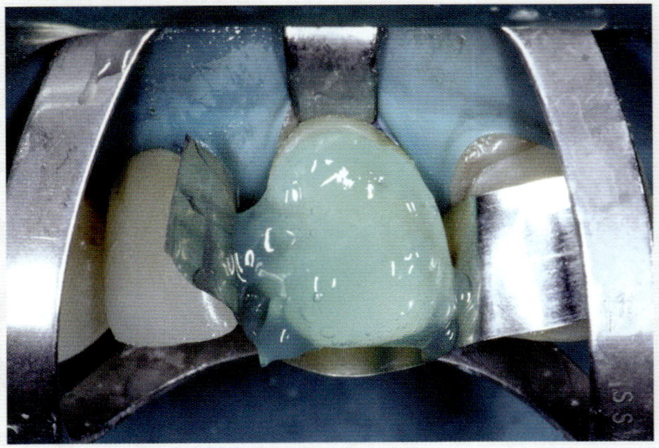

Fig 8-2l
After the try-in and acceptance of the veneers, adhesive cementation was obtained in the isolation of a rubber dam.

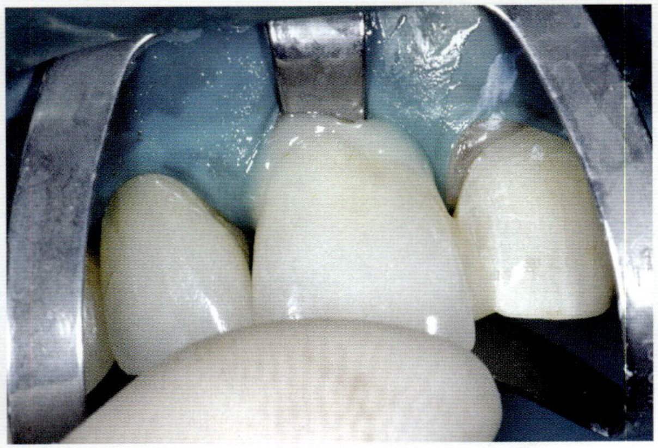

Fig 8-2m
Porcelain veneers were cemented individually with a dual-cure luting cement (restorations made 25 years ago).

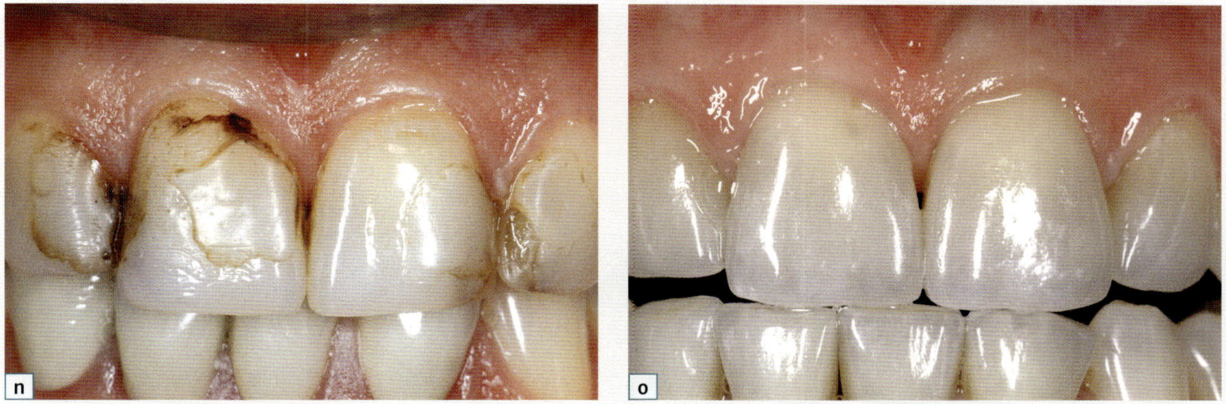

Figs 8-2n and 8-2o
Clinical situation (n) before and (o) after treatment with porcelain veneers.

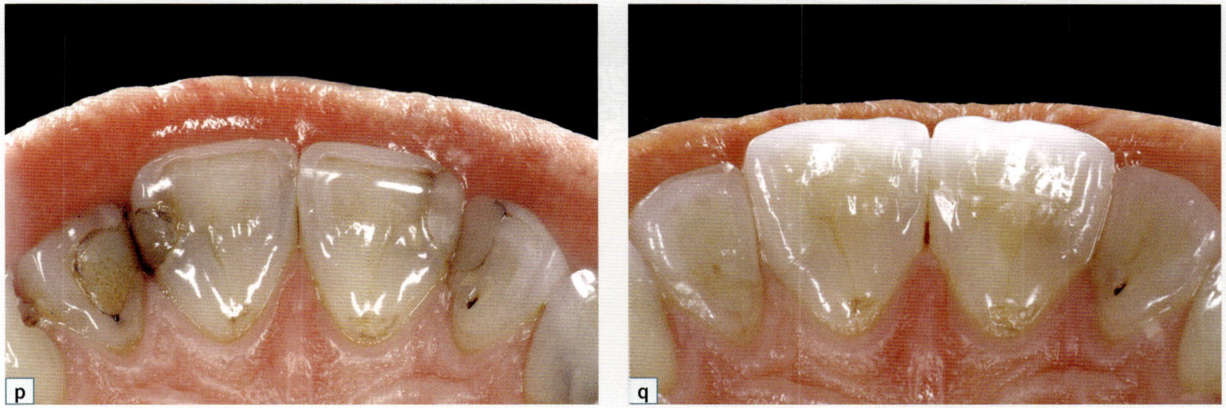

Figs 8-2p and 8-2q
Clinical situation (p) before and (q) after treatment – palatal view.

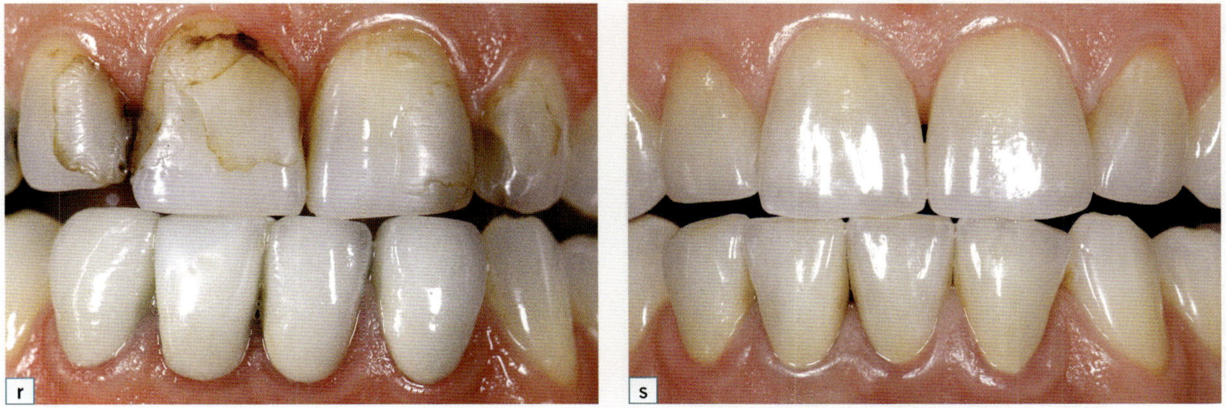

Figs 8-2r and 8-2s
Anterior teeth (r) before and (s) after treatment.

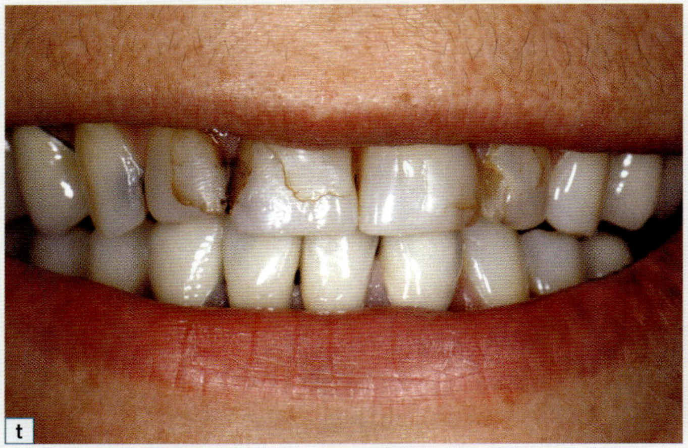
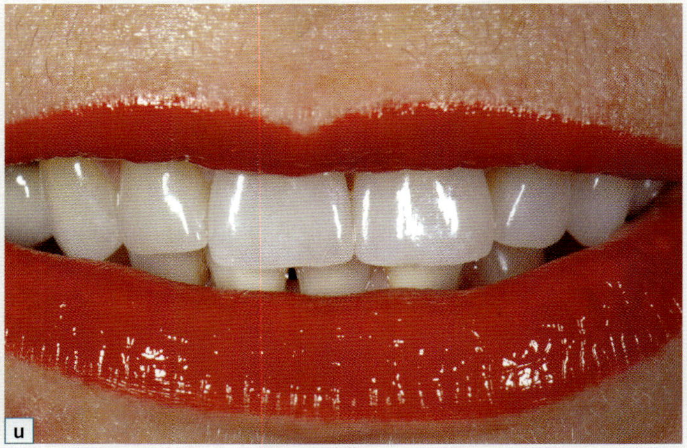

Figs 8-2t and 8-2u
Patient's smile (t) before and (u) after treatment.

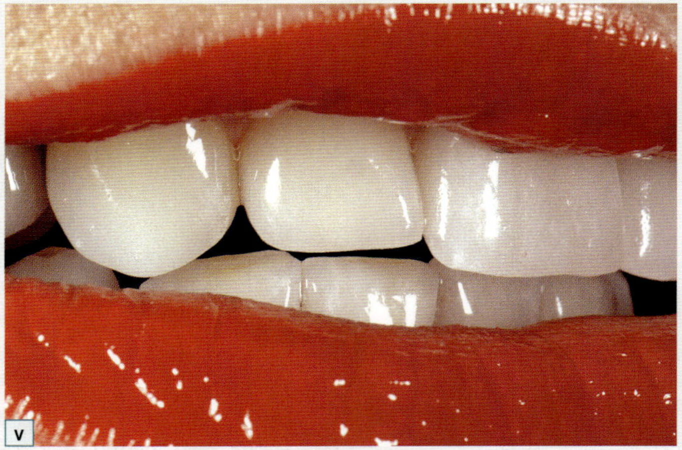
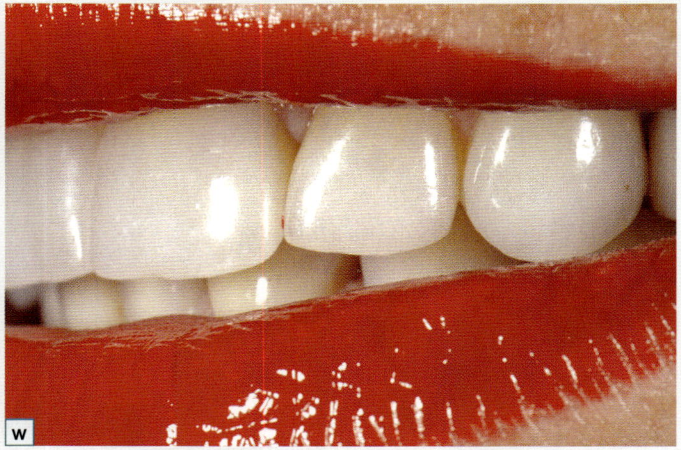

Figs 8-2v and 8-2w
Patient's smile from the (v) right and (w) left semi-profile.

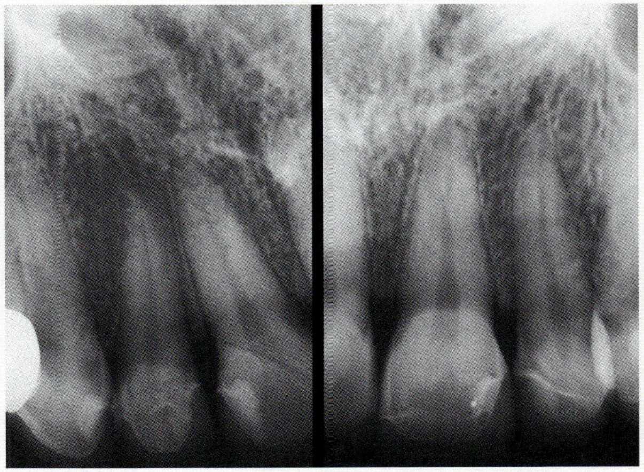

Fig 8-2x
Radiographs after porcelain veneers cementation.

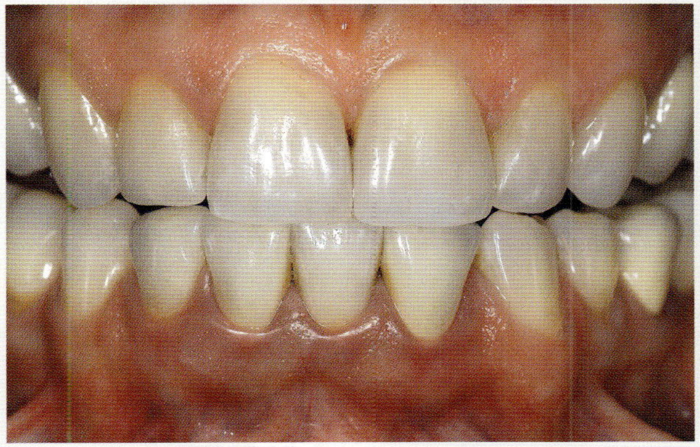

Fig 8-2y
Clinical situation 10 years after porcelain veneers cementation.

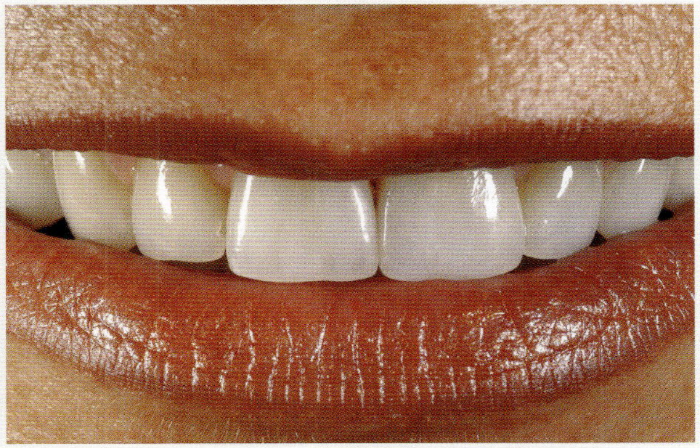

Fig 8-2z
Patient's smile 10 years after porcelain veneers cementation.

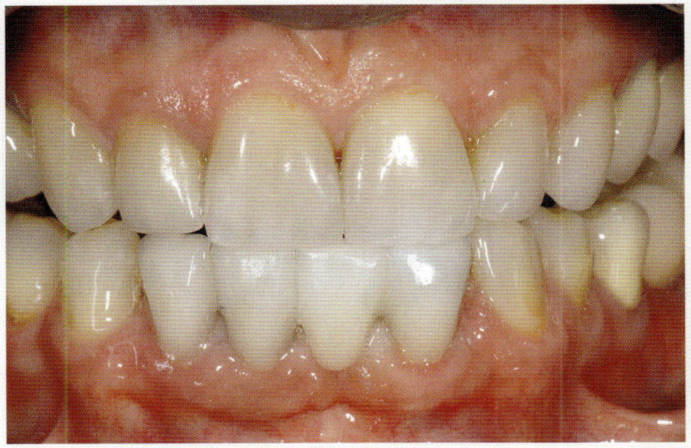

Fig 8-2aa
Clinical situation 25 years after porcelain veneers cementation (in the meantime, the patient lost a tooth in the mandibular arch, and the prosthetic restoration in the mandible was replaced).

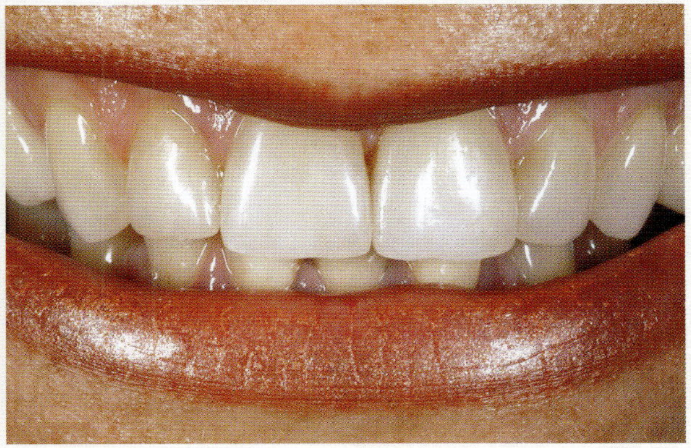

Fig 8-2bb
Patient's smile 25 years after porcelain veneers cementation.

VENEERS AND DISCOLORED TEETH AFTER ROOT CANAL TREATMENT

A discolored tooth after root canal treatment poses a serious challenge for the dentist. Of course, it would be best to whiten it internally using the walking bleach technique, and then choose the type of treatment,[7–9] but bleaching is not always possible due to:

- Subgingival microcracks (risk of external cervical resorption)
- Post and core in the root canal (risk of additional loss of hard substance when removing the post)
- Risk of tooth fracture or perforation related to the removal of old restorative material located in the pulp chamber
- Major tooth damage in the cervical area[9]

If there is even a slight chance to change the color of the tooth to a brighter one, take advantage of bleaching – a dental technician will have a much easier task when they do not have to use a masking opaque material for tooth discoloration. The greater the masking of the discoloration, the more "opaque" the veneer will look without letting light inside the tooth, which may lead to the impression of an "artificial" restoration.

Extensive discoloration is often associated with extended preparation of the tooth, because the dental technician will need more space to cover the discoloration. However, the deeper and more extended the preparation, the bigger the risk of exposing the dentin, which will negatively impact the future durability of the veneer adhesion and reveal an even darker layer of the tooth (dentin is darker than enamel).

In order to minimize the preparation, it is best to plan enlargement of the tooth labial volume with the mock-up.[10–11] If the additive mock-up is accepted, we gain 0.2–0.4 mm before the beginning of the preparation, which is crucial for the dental technician in order to cover the discoloration. This procedure significantly enhances the chance of enamel preservation during the preparation.

"Additive" veneers, ie, enlarging the labial volume of the tooth, have completely changed the approach to tooth preparation planning. In the past, in the case of discoloration, the veneer preparation performed by the dentist was supposed to be deep. By "entering" the dentin with the bur, the dentist unconsciously exposed the dark tooth structure, so the dental technician faced an even greater challenge to mask the discoloration with the restoration.

RULES WHEN PERFORMING VENEER ON DISCOLORED TOOTH AFTER ROOT CANAL TREATMENT

1. Consider internal bleaching to change the color of the tooth to a brighter one (always remember about the contraindications for whitening!)[9,12]
2. When a decision is made to perform a veneer on the discolored tooth, plan two symmetrical veneers (this will reduce the risk of esthetic failure, and less of the discolored tooth structure will be removed due to additive veneers fabrication)[13]
3. Avoid single veneer preparation[13]
4. Check with a mock-up whether it is possible to enlarge the labial volume and extend the incisal edge; if so, the preparation will be less invasive[10,11]
5. The preparation should always be performed from the mock-up level[10,11]
6. Avoid exposing the dentin, so the dark layer of the tooth is not revealed and the durability of the veneer adhesion with the tooth structure is not weakened.

REMEMBER

Paradoxically, when performing two veneers, we remove less hard tissues than in the case with one veneer – because by planning two symmetrical veneers, it is possible to symmetrically increase their external volume. It will also be much easier for a dental technician to achieve the desired esthetic result. We often pander to patient pressure by making one asymmetrical veneer – which significantly increases the risk of esthetic failure.

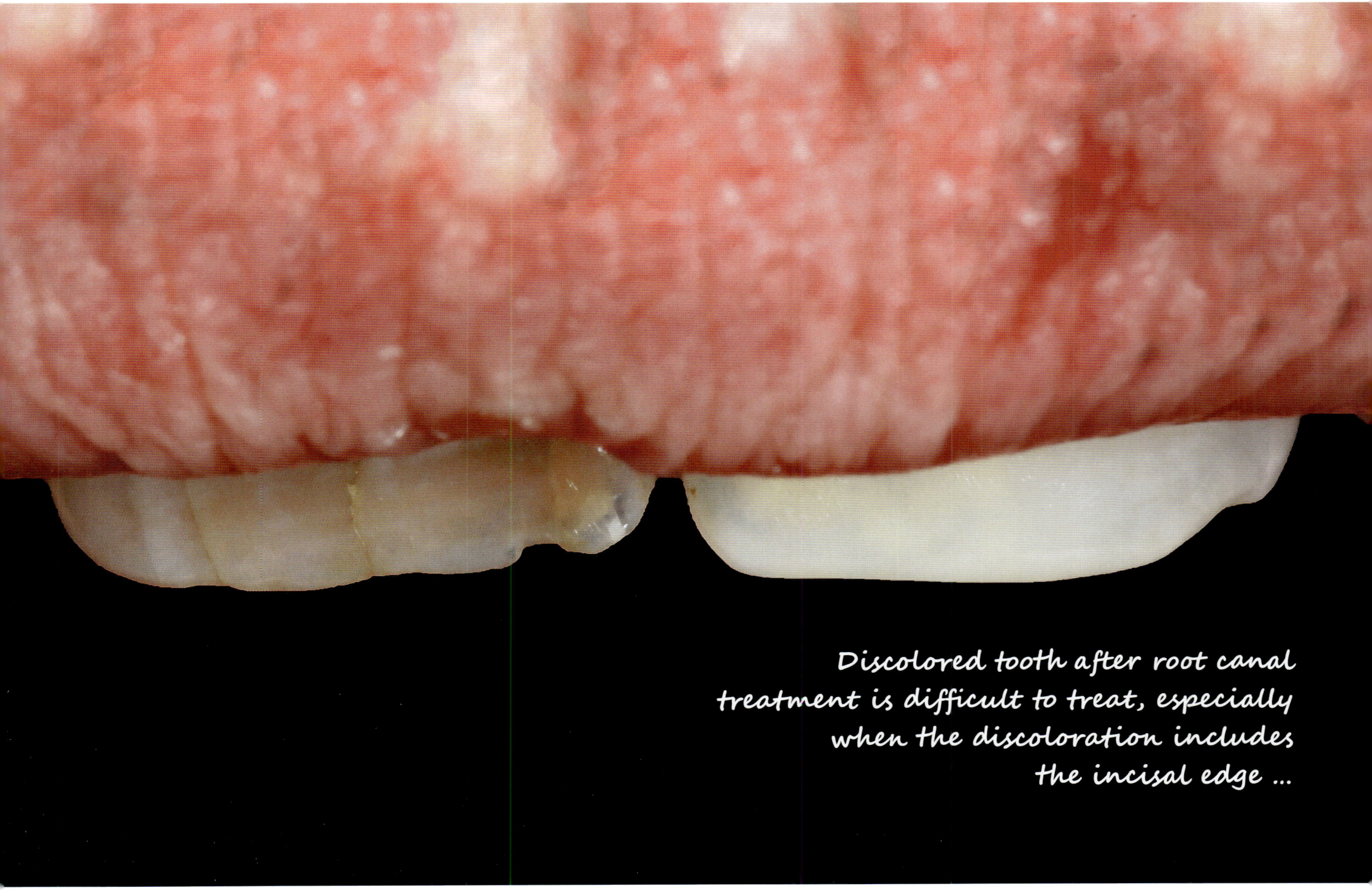

Discolored tooth after root canal treatment is difficult to treat, especially when the discoloration includes the incisal edge ...

Case 3: Discolored tooth after root canal treatment with contraindication for internal bleaching

A 31-year-old patient presented to the dental office to improve the esthetics of tooth 11 (Figs 8-3a to 8-3d). The tooth was significantly discolored due to trauma and pulp necrosis many years ago. In the past, tooth 11 had root canal treatment and a fiberglass post was cemented (Fig 8-3c), which disqualifies internal bleaching. It is unreasonable to take the structural risk by removing the fiber post and composite resin from the tooth chamber. This can result in additional tooth structure loss and the risk of creating cracks or fractures. The patient was offered treatment with two porcelain veneers on the central maxillary incisors (Fig 8-3e). For this purpose, a diagnostic wax-up was created and a mock-up based on it (Figs 8-3f to 8-3h), which was presented to the patient by means of photographs.

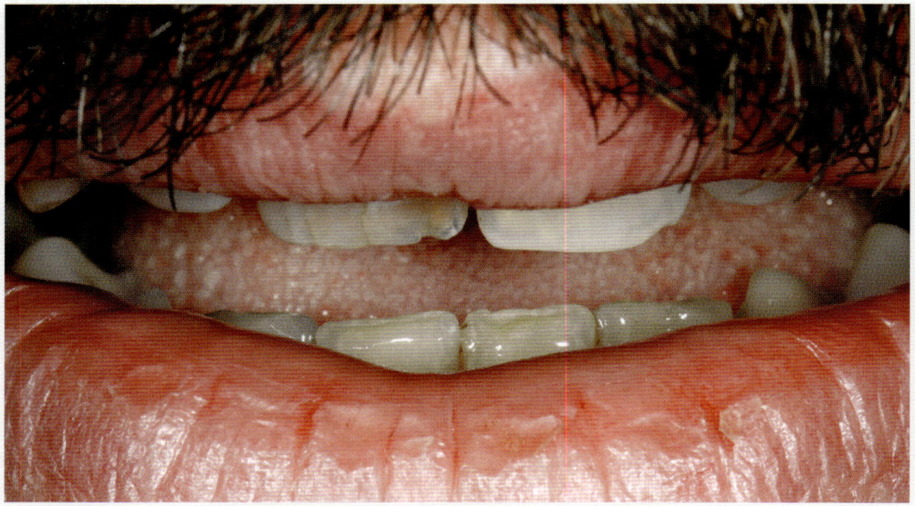

Fig 8-3a
Extraoral photograph with lips in repose – taken to assess the current position of the incisal edges of the maxillary teeth in relation to the upper lip.

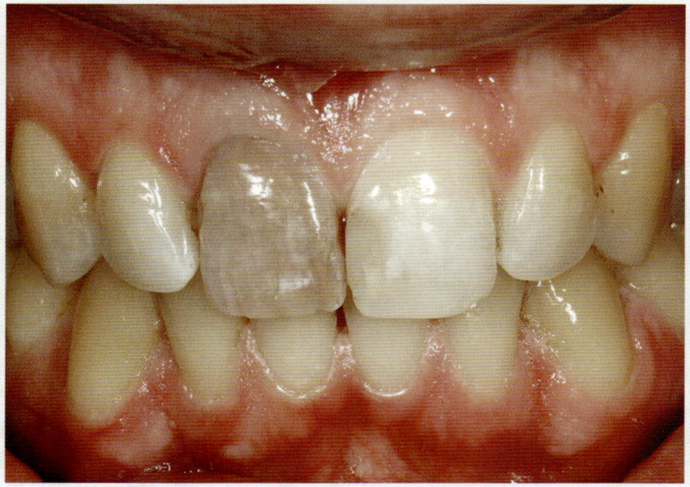

Fig 8-3b
Discolored tooth 11. Intraoral photograph in the position of maximum intercuspation.

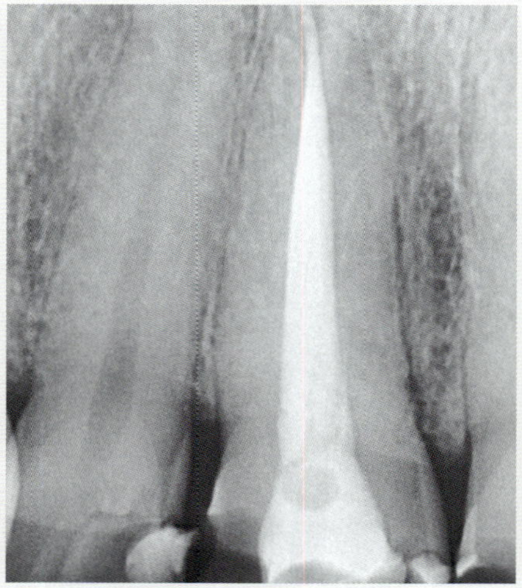

Fig 8-3c
Radiograph of tooth 11: visible root canal filling and fiberglass post slightly deviating from the root canal axis.

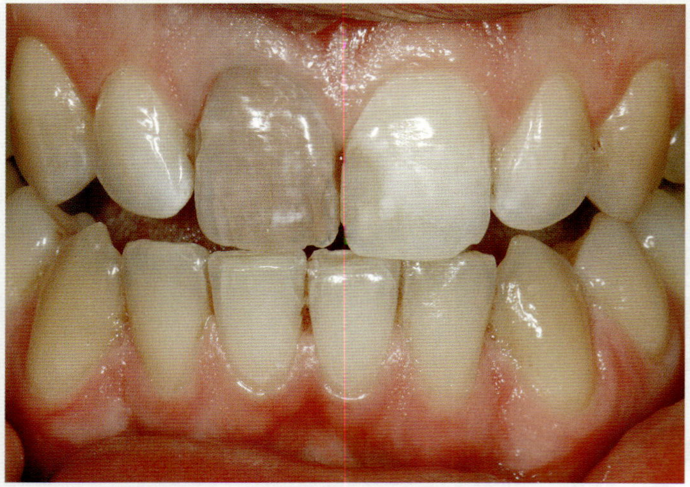

Fig 8-3d
Discolored tooth 11. Intraoral photograph taken in the anterior guidance.

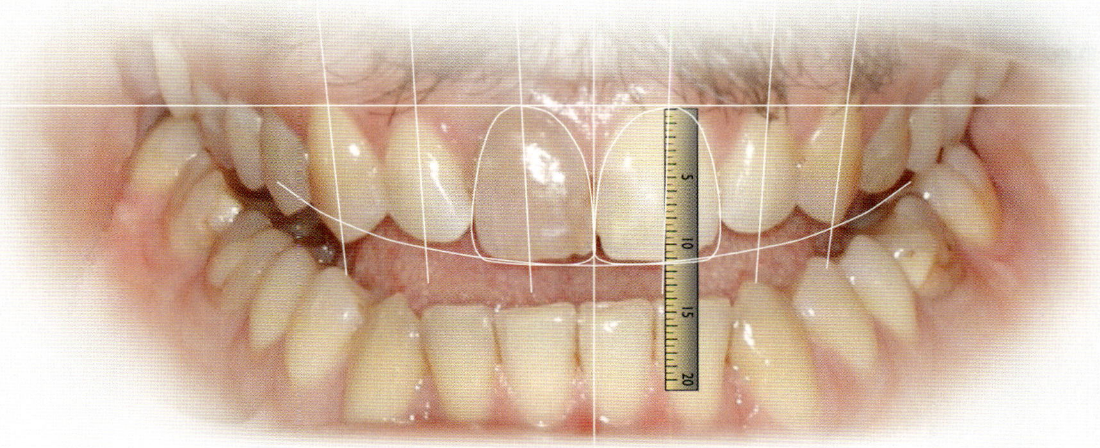

Fig 8-3e
Digital Smile Design (DSD) planning of the new shape of the teeth to transfer information to the dental laboratory and perform a mock-up.

Video: Performing mock-up
https://books. dentist.com.pl/veneers/18

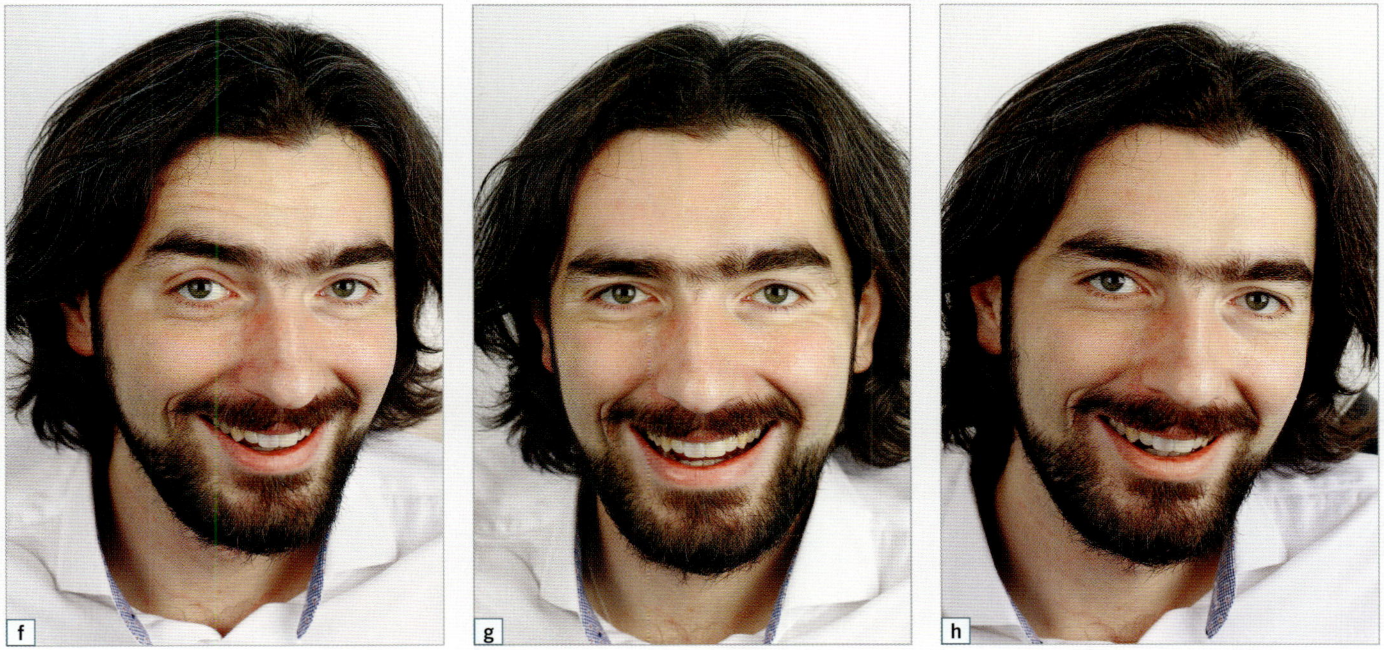

Figs 8-3f to 8-3h
Photographs of the patient's smile with a mock-up made according to DSD and diagnostic wax-up. Thanks to the photographs, the patient can see the visualization of the treatment plan integrated into his full face and smile.

Why was it indicated to cover two central incisors symmetrically with veneers in this case?

- Performing two symmetrical veneers increased the chance of esthetic success (it is more difficult to notice the difference when two veneers are covering the teeth symmetrically).
- Planning veneers that are slightly bigger than the current size of the teeth made it possible to minimize the depth of preparation.
- By fabricating two symmetrical restorations, it was possible to obtain a more predictable bond strength for the veneer (exposure of the dentin was significantly reduced).

At the next appointment, veneer preparation was performed on teeth 11 and 21 through the mock-up (Fig 8-3i), which minimized the final tooth preparation. The preparation was controlled with a silicone index cut in two planes: horizontal to control the depth of preparation at different zones of the buccal surface (Figs 8-3j and 8-3k) and vertical to control the incisal reduction (Fig 8-3l).

The final preparation was obtained after inserting the #000 retraction cord, followed by placing a second #00 cord impregnated with Astrident (Fig 8-3m). After taking the impressions for porcelain veneers and opposite dental arch, the facebow registration has taken. Next, the teeth were covered with provisional veneers (Fig 8-3n). Their retention was ensured thanks to their mutual connection on the proximal surfaces and temporary resin mechanical interlock in the interdental spaces. The final feldspathic porcelain veneers were made in the dental laboratory. The dental technician obtained an excellent esthetic effect by blocking the discoloration from the inside of the veneer and additional external staining. After try-in with glycerin gel (Fig 8-3o), the veneers were adhesively prepared and cemented in rubber dam isolation. The final esthetic outcome and integration with the soft tissues were assessed a few weeks after cementation (Figs 8-3p to 8-3t). A comparison of the clinical situation and the patient's smile before and after treatment is presented in Figs 8-3u to 8-3x. Clinical follow-up after 4 years showed a perfect esthetic and biological integration of the veneers (Fig 8-3y).

Video: Preparation through the mock-up
https://books.dentist.com.pl/veneers/19

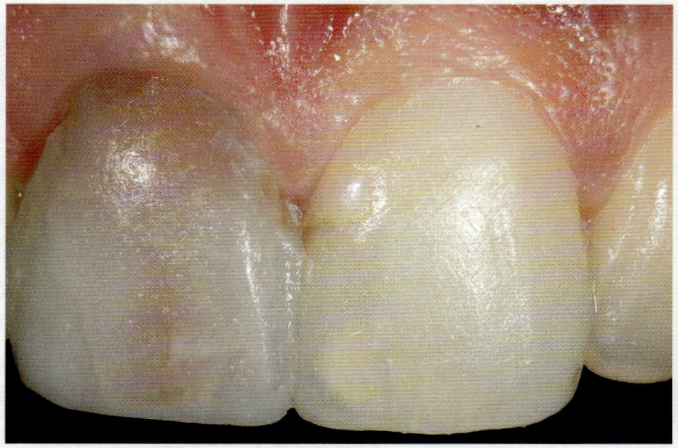

Fig 8-3i
Mock-up was applied with a silicone index directly before the preparation. (Mock-up is always supposed to be a starting point for minimally invasive veneer preparation.)

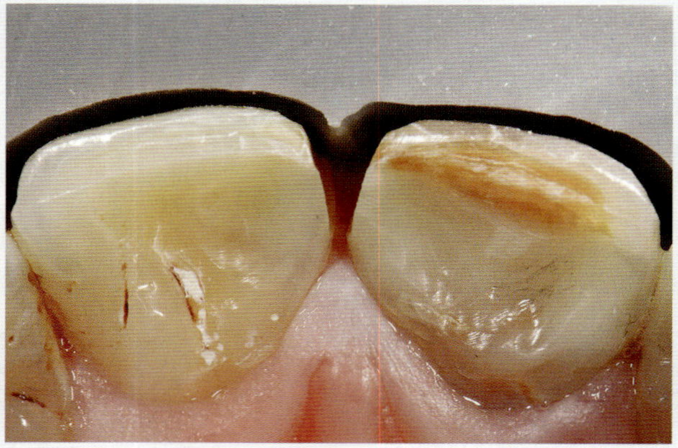

Fig 8-3j
Controlling the preparation depth with a silicone index.

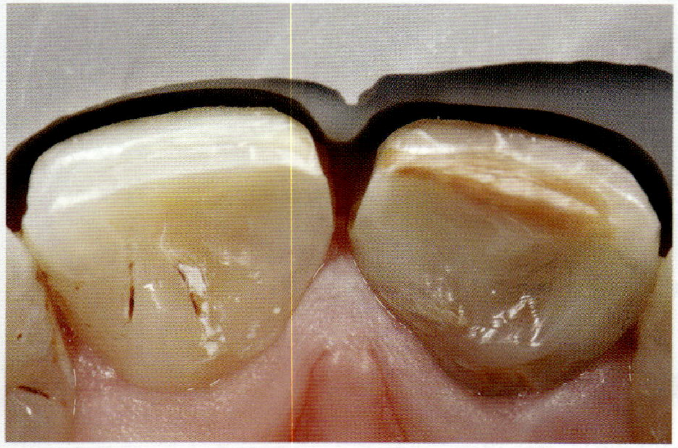

Fig 8-3k
Silicone index cut in "harmonica," making it possible to control the preparation depth on the labial surface at different levels.

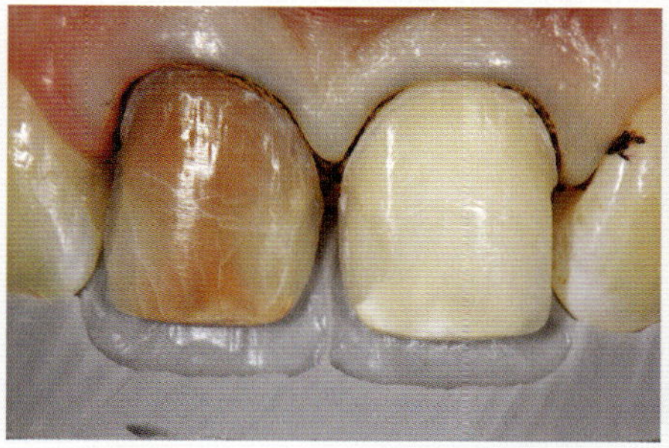

Fig 8-3l
Controlling the space for the porcelain at the incisal edge.

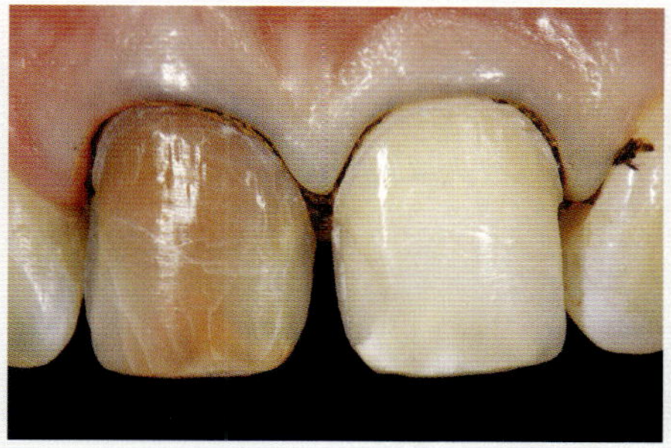

Fig 8-3m
Final veneer preparation on teeth 11 and 21 with retraction cords before an impression with a polyvinyl siloxane material.

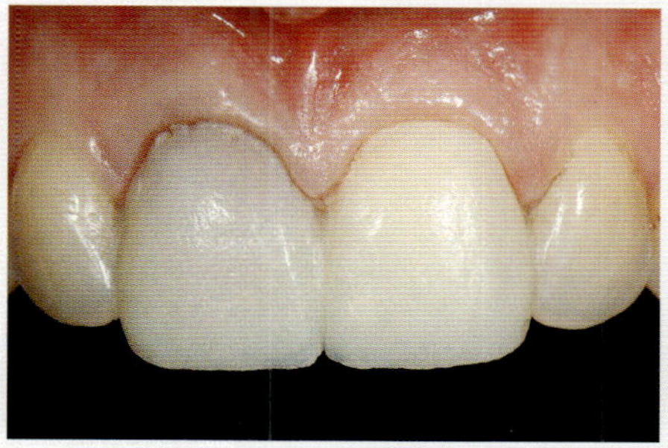

Fig 8-3n
Provisional veneers on teeth 11 and 21.

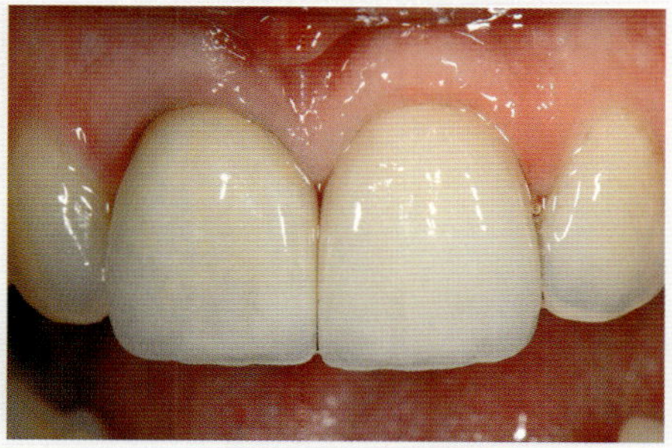

Fig 8-3o
Feldspathic veneers try-in with glycerin gel to simulate the final color that will be achieved after cementation.

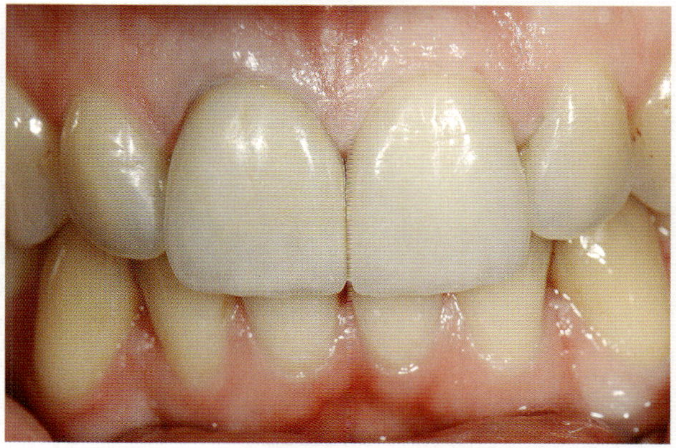

Fig 8-3p
Final esthetic outcome 3 weeks after veneers cementation.

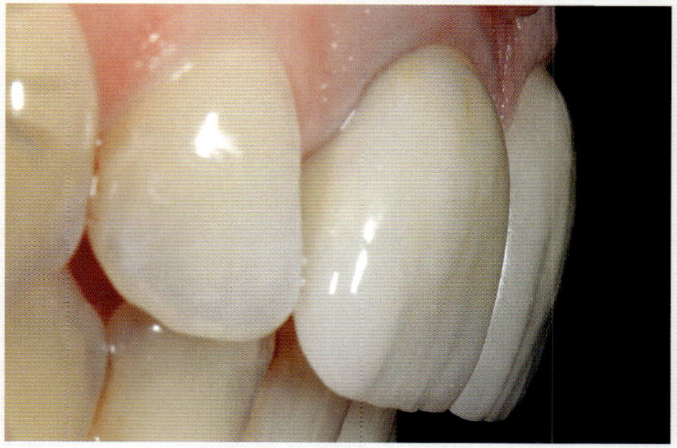

Fig 8-3q
Semi-profile intraoral photograph showing the perfect soft tissue integration and masking previous discoloration (laboratory work: DT Artur Nyga).

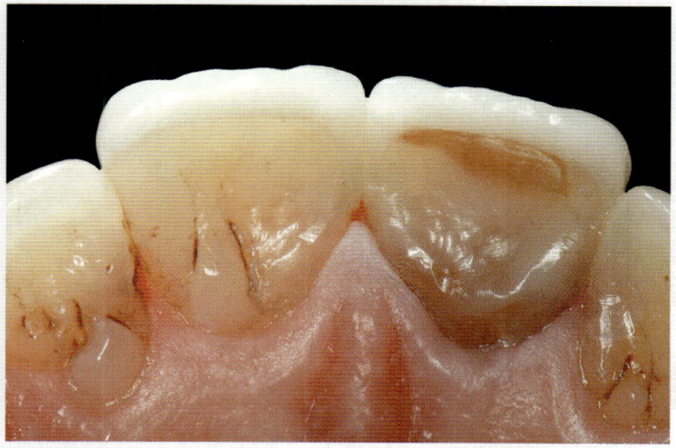

Fig 8-3r
Intraoral photograph from the palatal view – visible palatal margin of the veneer with a butt joint preparation, without interfering with the concave part of the palatal surface.

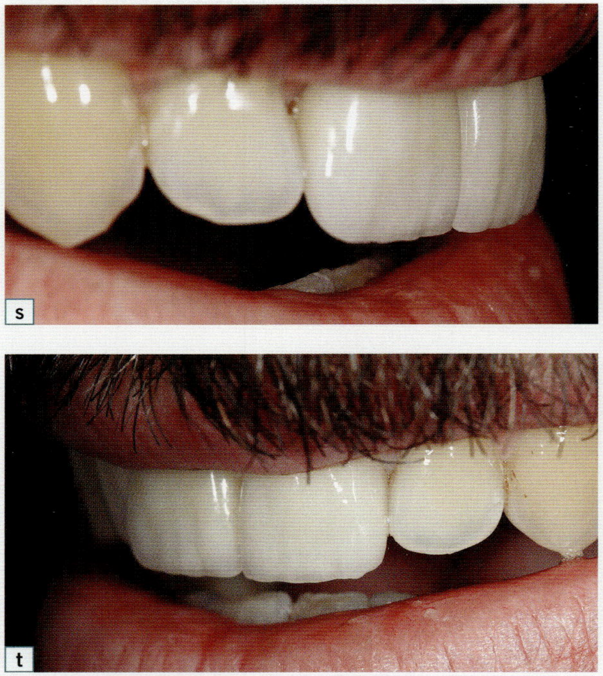

Figs 8-3s and 8-3t
Patient's smile 3 weeks after veneers' cementation.

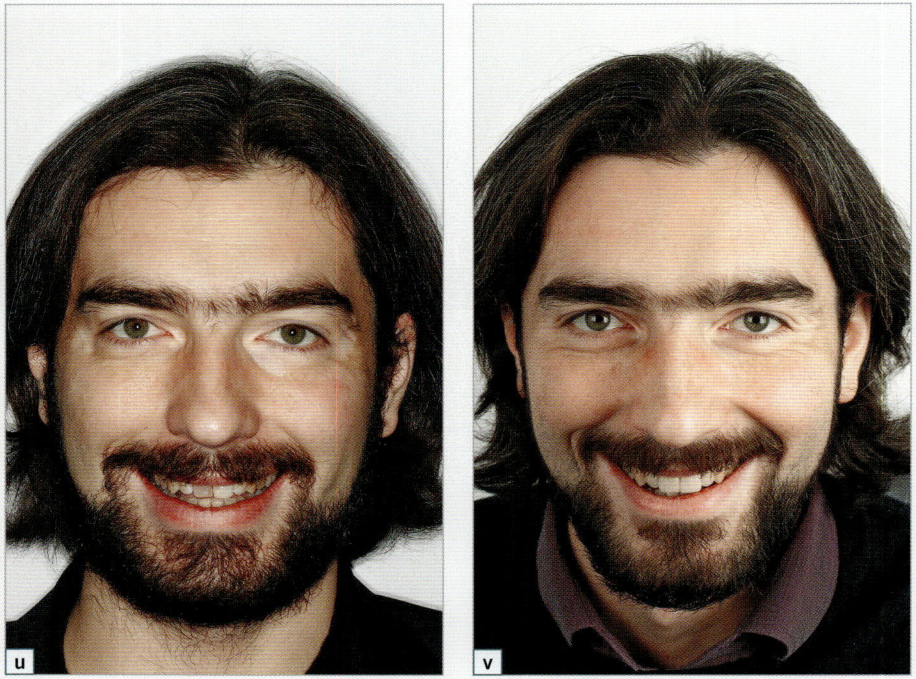

Figs 8-3u and 8-3v
Photographs of the patient (u) before and (v) after porcelain veneer treatment.

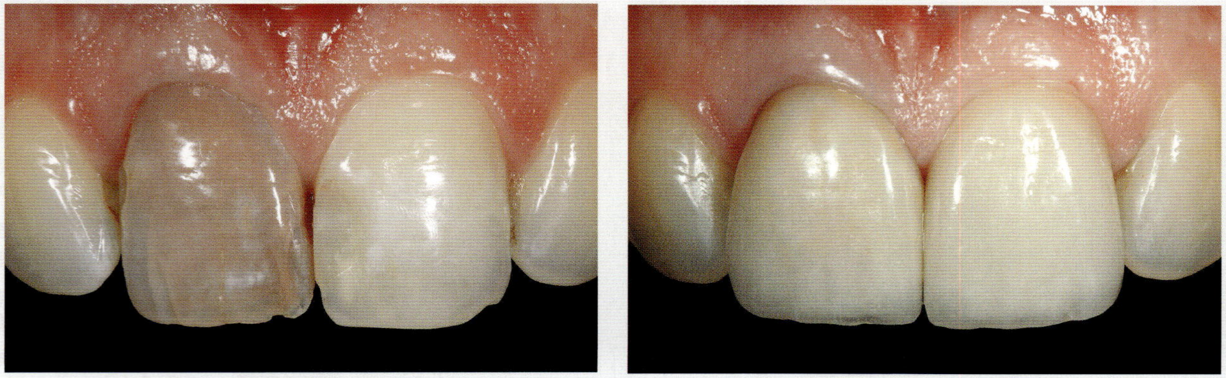

Figs 8-3w and 8-3x
Intraoral photographs of discolored tooth 11 (w) before treatment and (x) after veneer cementation.

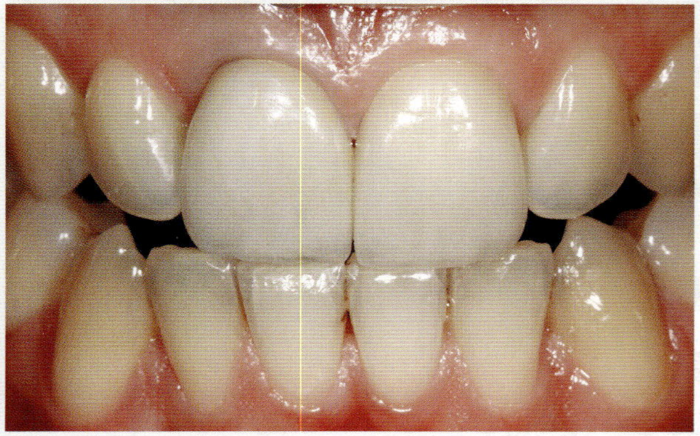

Fig 8-3y
Clinical follow-up 4 years after veneers cementation.

Case 4: Endodontically treated discolored tooth with contraindication for internal bleaching

A 37-year-old female patient presented to the dental office in order to improve the esthetics of her maxillary incisors due to tooth discoloration (tooth 11) and unpleasant restorations in the adjacent teeth (Figs 8-4a to 8-4f). Tooth 11 had a fiberglass post, placed many years ago, which is a contraindication for internal bleaching. As in Case 3 (see Fig 8-3), the structural risk of removing the old post was relatively high. The patient's tooth restorations had been replaced many times in the past. She wanted to achieve an equally esthetic and durable effect; therefore, teeth 12–22 were qualified for porcelain veneers.

Teeth were externally bleached in a conventional way (overnight whitening). Then composite restorations with marginal leakage and discoloration were replaced, and a Class 3 cavity in tooth 12 was prepared and filled (Figs 8-4g to 8-4j). Next, based on the diagnostic wax-up, a mock-up was made and, using photographs, the proposed changes were shown to the patient (Figs 8-4k and 8-4l). After the treatment plan acceptation, the mock-up through preparation was performed (Figs 8-4m and 8-4n) to reduce the tooth preparation to the necessary minimum.

Due to minor protrusive inclination of the maxillary incisors, control photographs of the prepared teeth were taken. Their relationship to the lower lip was analyzed so that the dental technician has enough space for the adequate profiling of the incisal part of the veneer (the incisal edge should reach the vermilion border of the lower lip during the phonetic tests; Fig 8-4o).

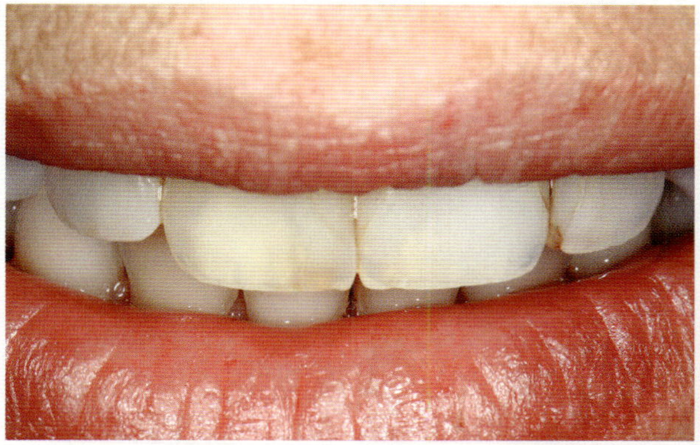

Fig 8-4a
Patient's lips in repose: significant exposure of the front teeth makes tooth discoloration uncomfortable for the patient.

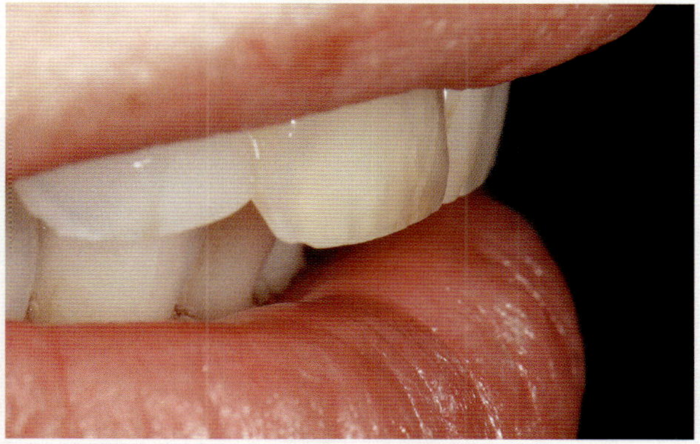

Fig 8-4b
Right semi-profile view of the teeth, upper and lower lip in repose.

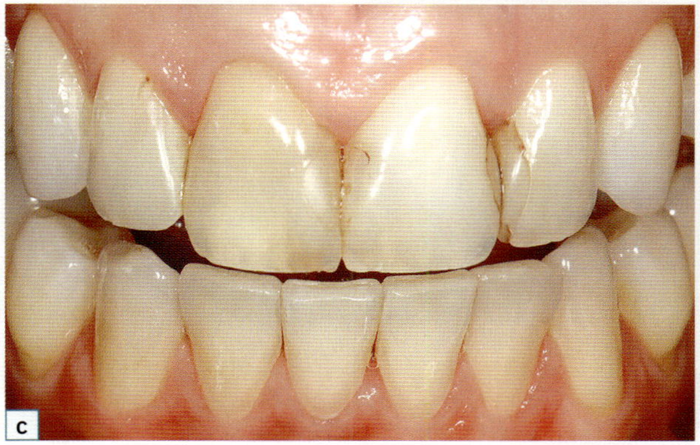

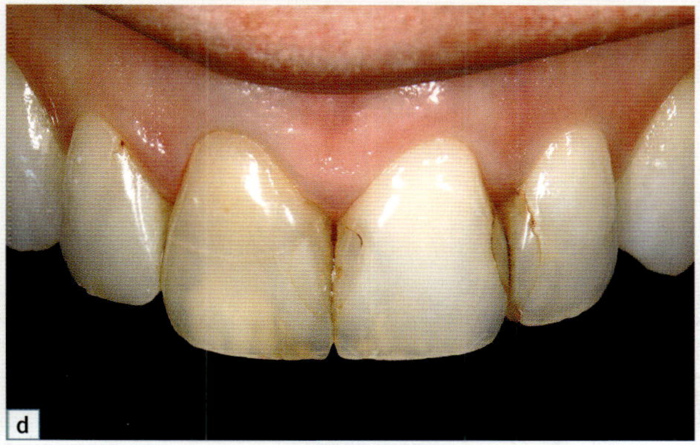

Figs 8-4c and 8-4d
Intraoral photographs of discolored maxillary anterior teeth: tooth 11 after root canal treatment; teeth 12, 21, and 22 with vital pulp, but their composite restorations need to be changed.

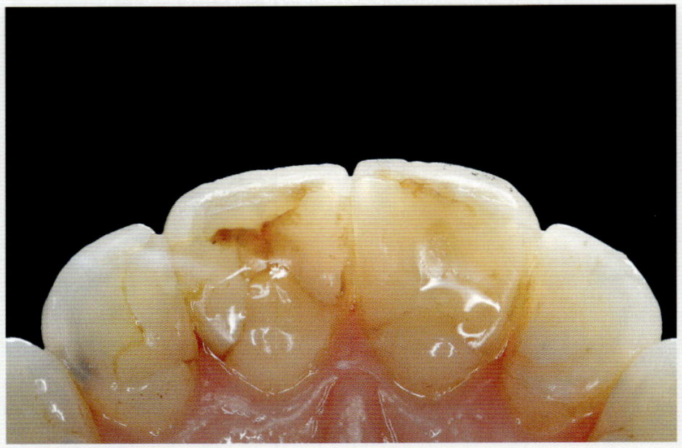

Fig 8-4e
Clinical situation prior to treatment – palatal view.

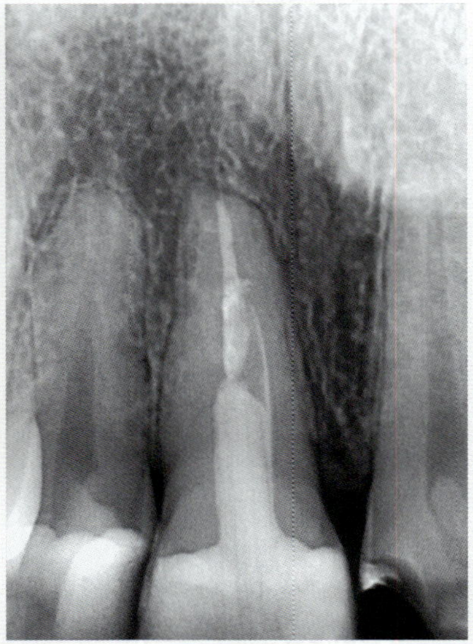

Fig 8-4f
Radiograph of tooth 11 after previous endodontic treatment: a visible fiberglass post is a contraindication for internal bleaching.

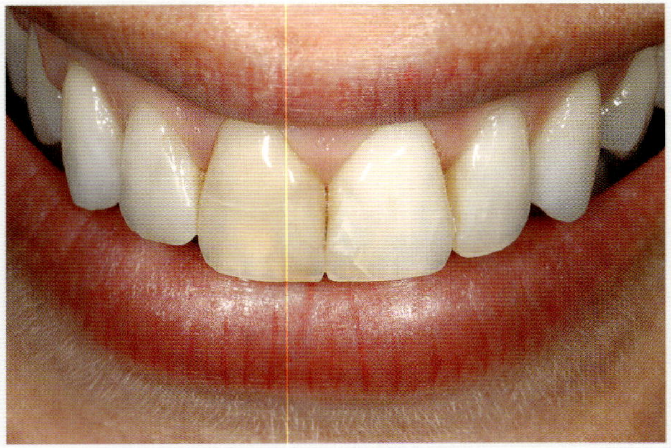

Fig 8-4g
Patient's smile after conventional, overnight tooth whitening and replacing the leaking restorations.

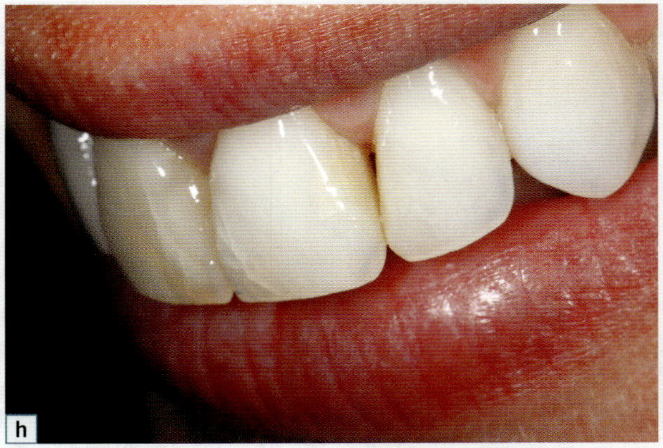

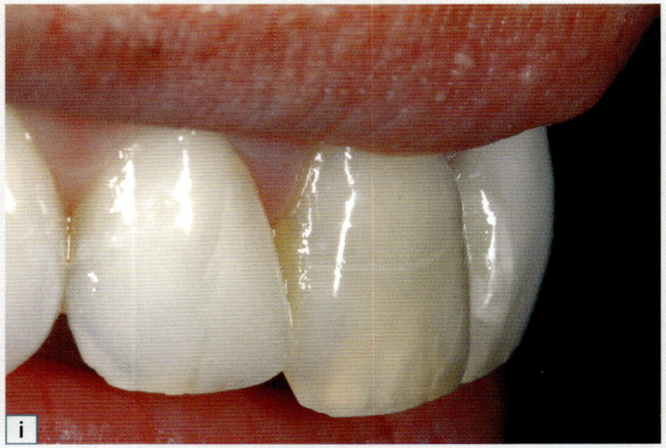

Figs 8-4h and 8-4i
Patient's smile from the (h) left and (i) right semi-profile after conventional overnight tooth whitening and replacing the leaking composite restorations.

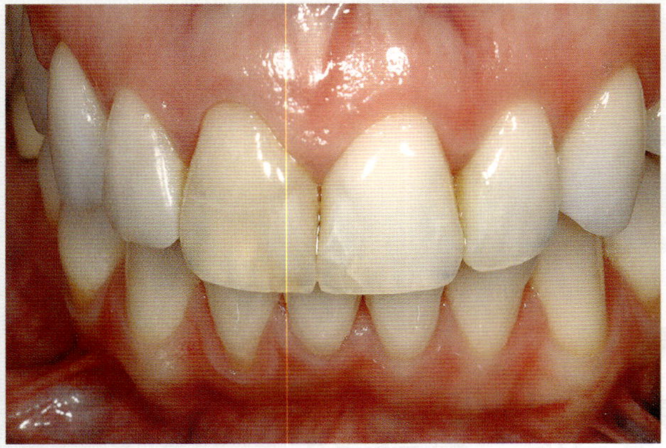

Fig 8-4j
Intraoral photograph after conventional overnight tooth whitening and replacing the leaking composite restoration.

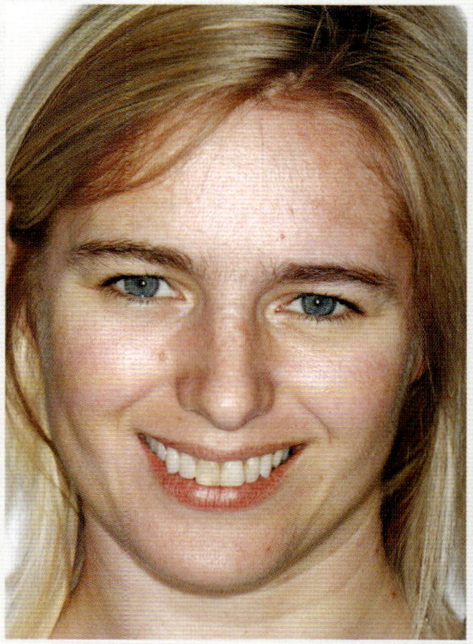

Fig 8-4k
Patient's face and smile before treatment.

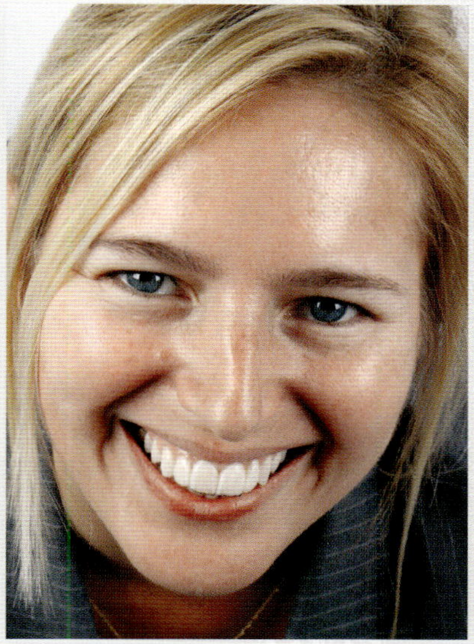

Fig 8-4l
Patient's face and smile after placing the mock-up on the anterior maxillary teeth (12–22).

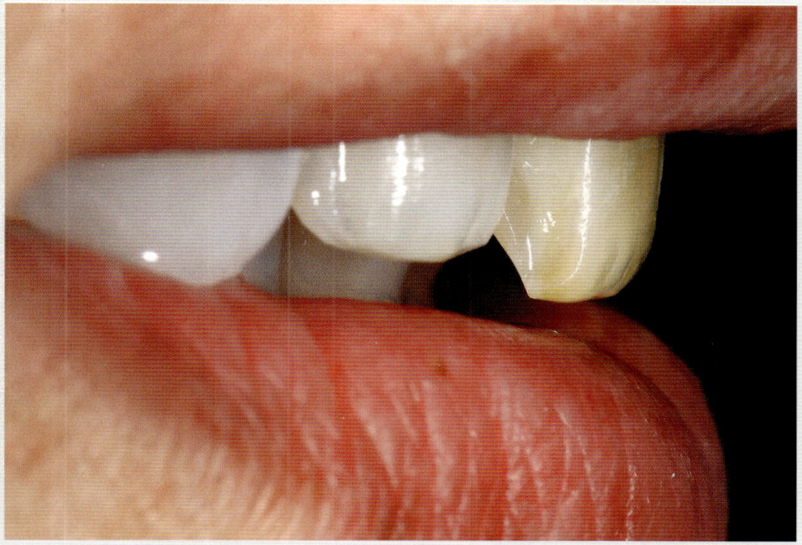

Fig 8-4o
Due to the relative protrusion of the maxillary incisors, their position was assessed in relation to the lower lip during the preparation, so the dental technician will have enough space for the incisal profile of the porcelain veneer (the incisal edge should reach the vermilion border of the lower lip).

REMEMBER

The incisal edge of the designed veneer should end on the border of the wet and dry red zone of the lower lip (ie, vermilion border) while pronouncing "F" or "V" sounds.

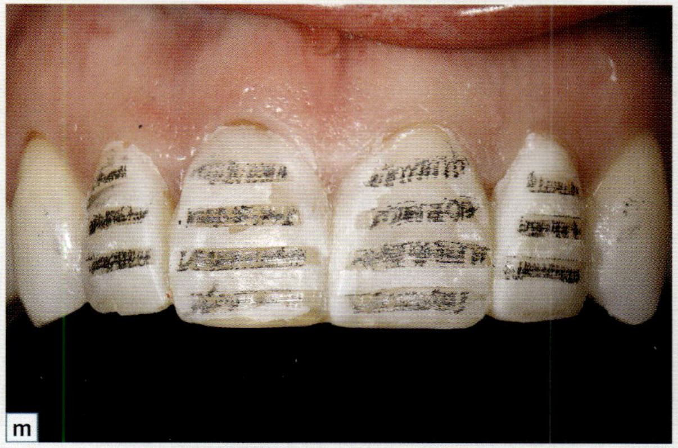

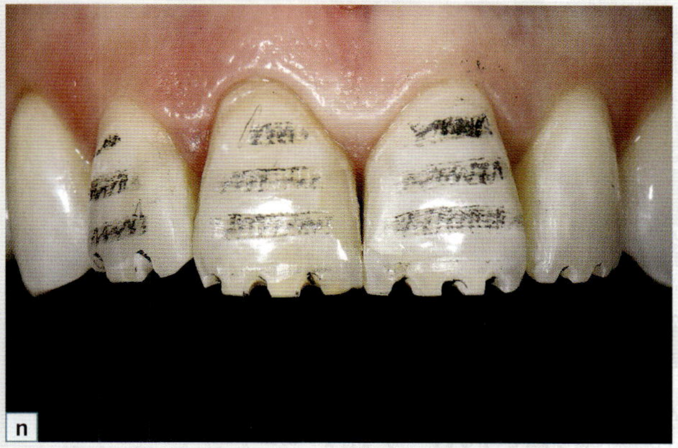

Figs 8-4m and 8-4n
Veneer preparation through the mock-up – in this way, the tooth preparation is reduced to the necessary minimum.

Depth of preparation was controlled with the silicone index (Fig 8-4p). The preparation included extensive restorations on the proximal surfaces, thanks to which the future border between the veneer and composite filling was shifted to the palatal surface (easier to control, as the composite restorations can be replaced in the future if needed, without damaging the veneer). After the preparation was completed, a second retraction cord (so-called deflection cord) – soaked in a hemostatic agent – was placed (Fig 8-4q), and impressions were taken after 5 to 10 minutes. Feldspathic porcelain veneers were fabricated in a dental laboratory (Fig 8-4r).

Their seating and marginal fit were checked on their original stone die and in the patient's mouth at the next appointment. Next, the proximal relationships and then color, shape, and esthetics in relation to the upper and lower lip were assessed. After approval by the dentist and the patient, rubber dam isolation was carried out, and the tooth surface was conditioned for adhesive cementation (Figs 8-4s and 8-4t). The veneers were cemented with a light-cured composite resin. After removing the composite resin excess, the preparation margin was covered with glycerin gel and finally polymerized (Fig 8-4u). After cementing two porcelain veneers on the maxillary central incisors, the rubber dam isolation was changed to adjacent teeth, and further veneers were cemented on the lateral incisors (Fig 8-4v). The final appearance immediately after cementing veneers and a few weeks later are shown in Figs 8-4w to 8-4bb.

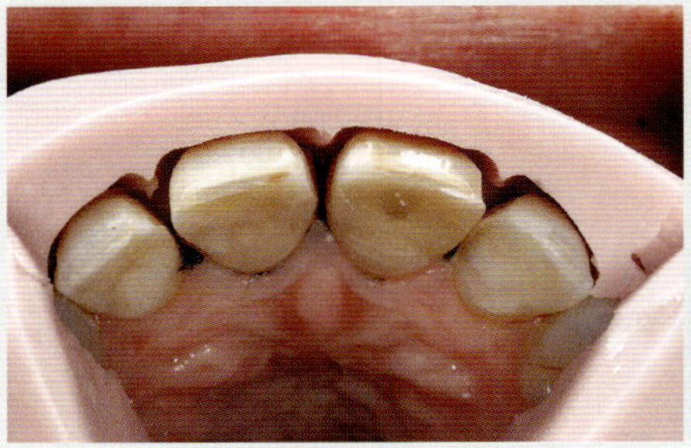

Fig 8-4p
Controlling preparation depth with a silicone index.

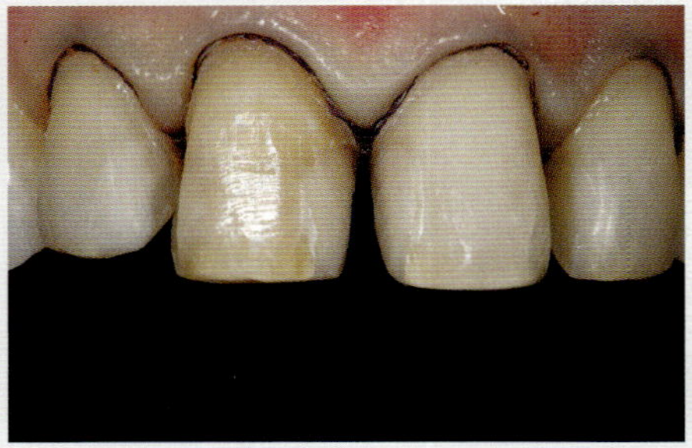

Fig 8-4q
After the preparation was completed, a second retraction cord soaked in a hemostatic agent was placed, and impressions were taken after 5 to 10 minutes.

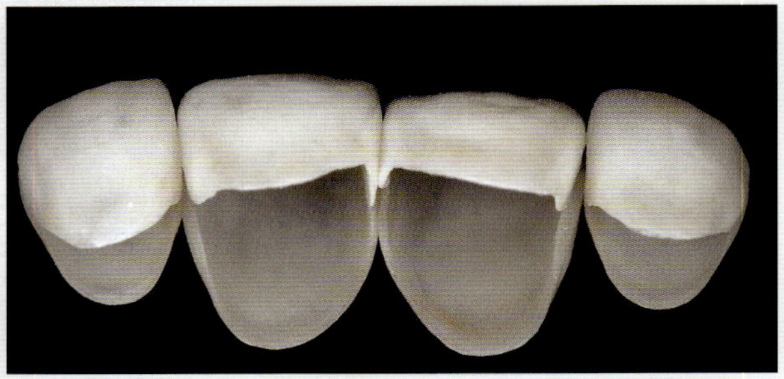

Fig 8-4r
Feldspathic porcelain veneers.

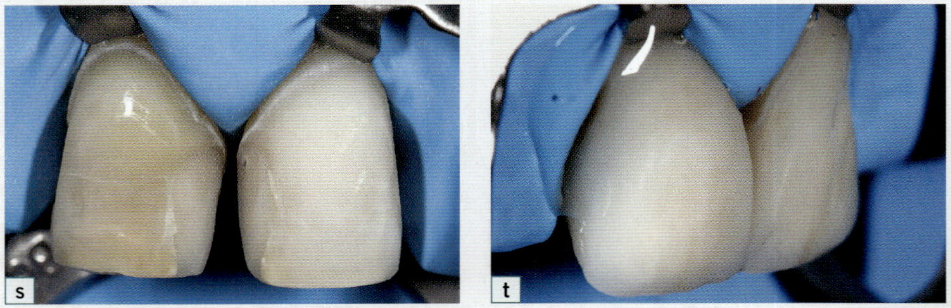

Figs 8-4s and 8-4t
After the dentist and patient accepted the color, shape, and esthetics of the veneers, the teeth were isolated with a rubber dam, and the tooth surface was conditioned for adhesive cementation.

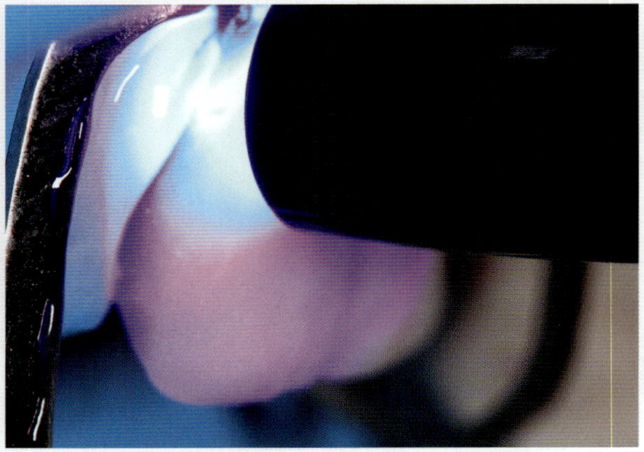

Fig 8-4u
Veneers were cemented, and after removing the composite resin excess, the margins were then covered with glycerin gel and finally cured.

Fig 8-4v
Veneers cemented in pairs in rubber dam isolation.

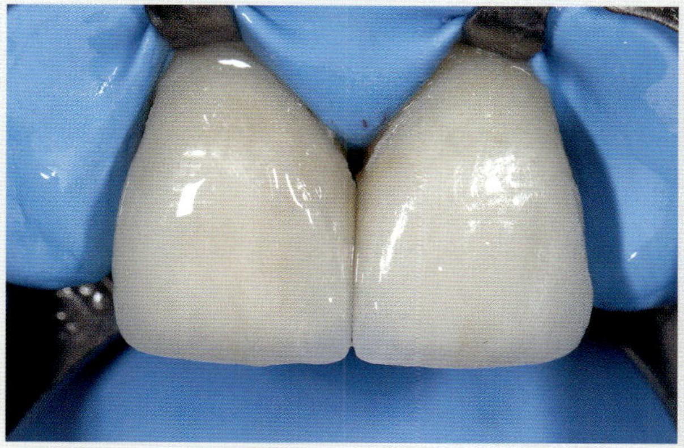

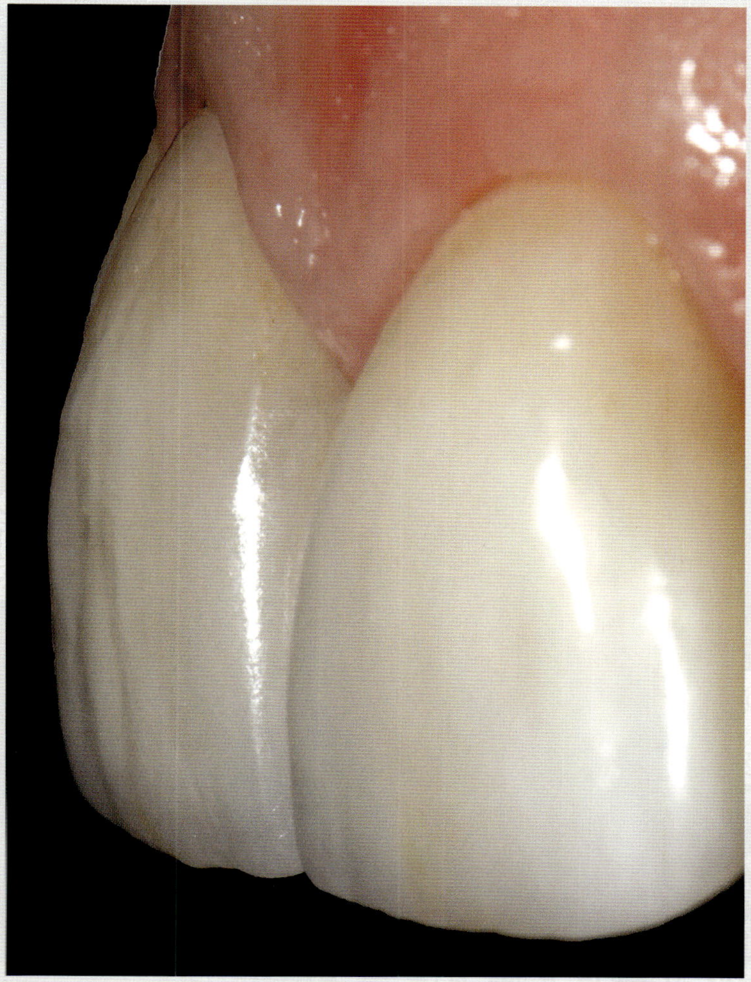

Fig 8-4y
Close-up of the beautiful surface of the veneers.

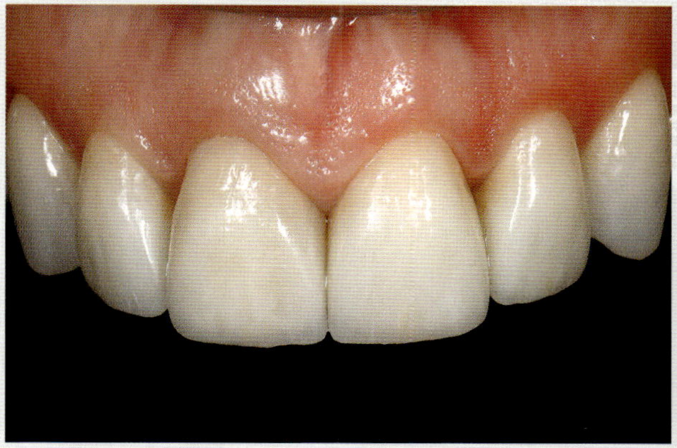

Fig 8-4w
Clinical situation a few weeks after veneer cementation on teeth 12–22.

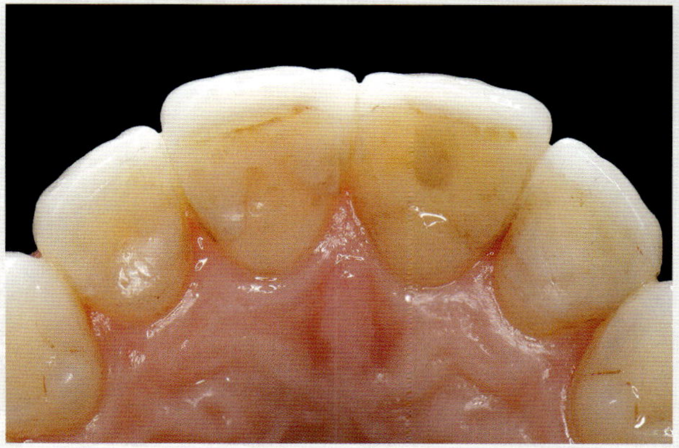

Fig 8-4x
The clinical situation with cemented veneers – palatal view.

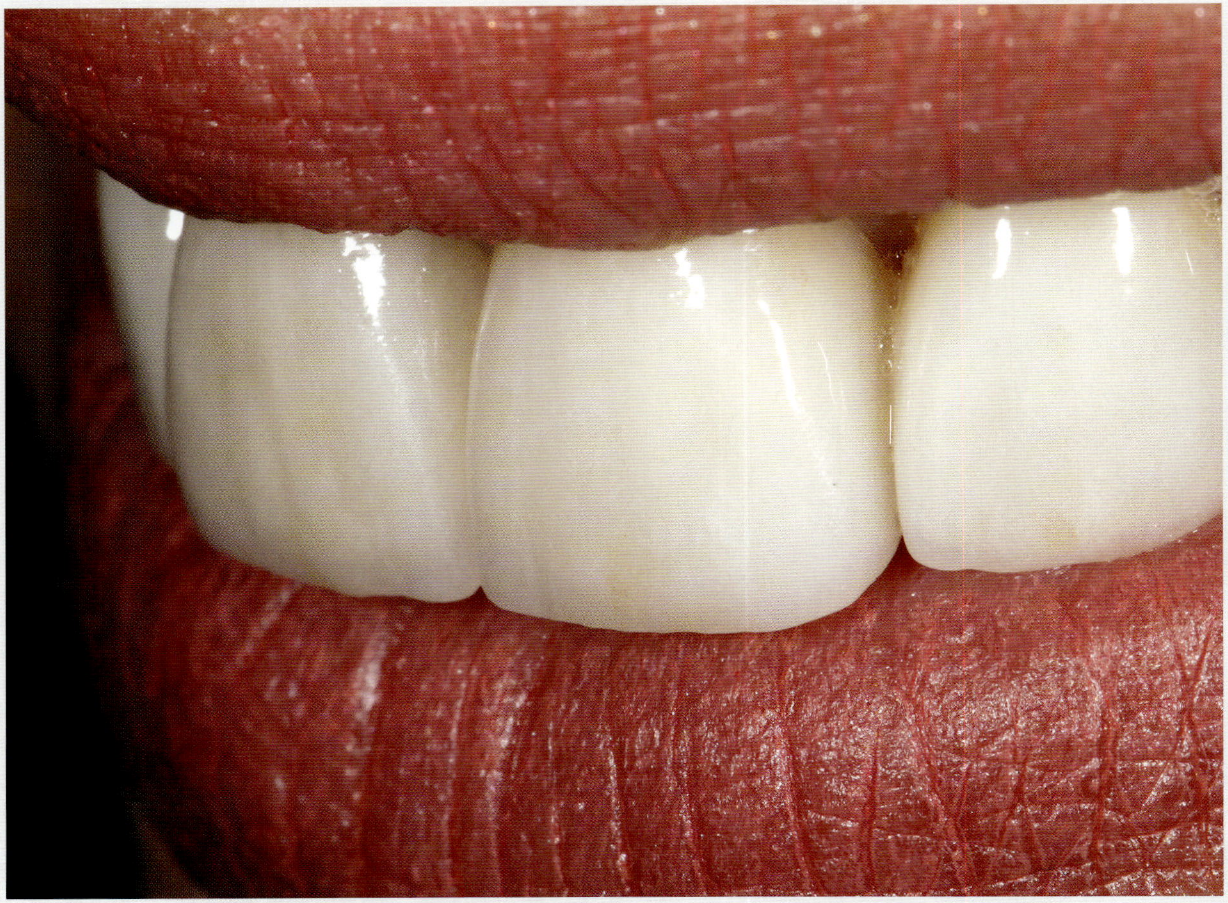

Fig 8-4z
Patient's smile with new porcelain veneers.

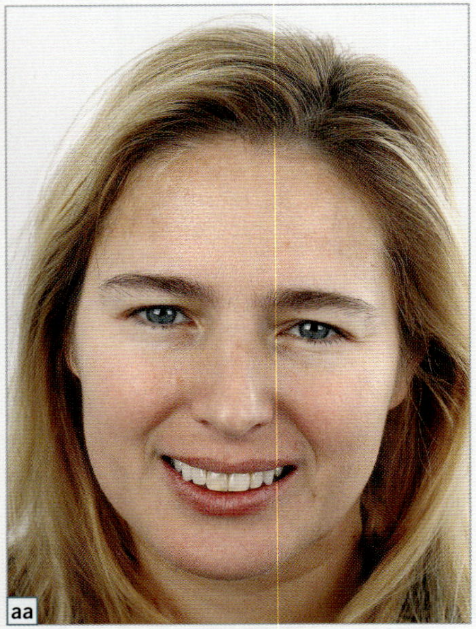

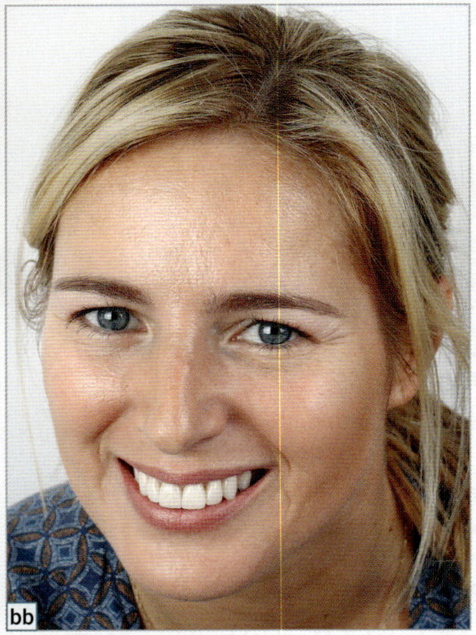

Figs 8-4aa and 8-4bb
The situations (aa) before and (bb) after four veneers cementation on teeth 12–22.

VENEERS AND OCCLUSAL PROBLEMS

If we plan esthetic treatment with veneers, and the medical history and oral cavity examination raise doubts about the occlusion, it is worth carrying out a functional analysis.

In many dental practices, in the world of advanced dental diagnostics, deprogramming of the stomatognathic system will dispel all doubts. The most well-proven deprogramming technique requires 4-week use of a special device introduced into clinical practice by Dr. John Kois.[14–16]

With the deprogrammer, we can:

- "Reset" (deprogram) the muscle memory of the temporomandibular joints
- Diagnose the direction in which the mandible will move after deprogramming and thus confirm the suspicion of a **constricted envelope of function** or **occlusal dysfunction**
- Simplify **the registration of the centric relation** necessary for further treatment planning, including changes in the occlusion (alteration of the vertical dimension)
- Pre-indicate **a new proposed occlusal vertical dimension** by reducing or adding a platform to the deprogrammer
- **Equilibrate**, if necessary, as the deprogrammer can be used as an instrument that controls equilibration (the dentist gradually reduces the platform until premature contacts are identified, which can be gradually eliminated)[17,18]

KOIS DEPROGRAMMER (KD)

Suppose the loading test and the immobilization test are negative (which initially excludes structural problems and indicates muscular problems of the temporomandibular joint). In that case, a KD may be offered to the patient.[19]

To fabricate a conventional KD, impressions should be taken with an alginate impression material (Fig 8-5a). The casts should be poured in the next few hours in the dental office or laboratory (Fig 8-5b). The casts should be trimmed using a model trimmer (Fig 8-5c) and then mounted in the articulator in the position of maximum intercuspation (Fig 8-5d).

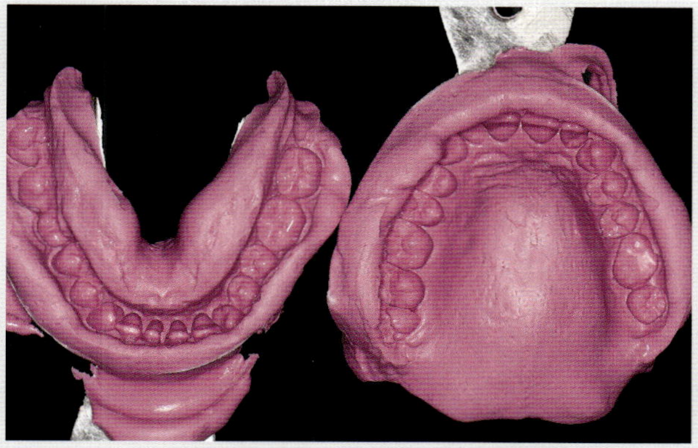

Fig 8-5a
Alginate impressions of the mandibular and maxillary dental arches for the Kois Deprogrammer.

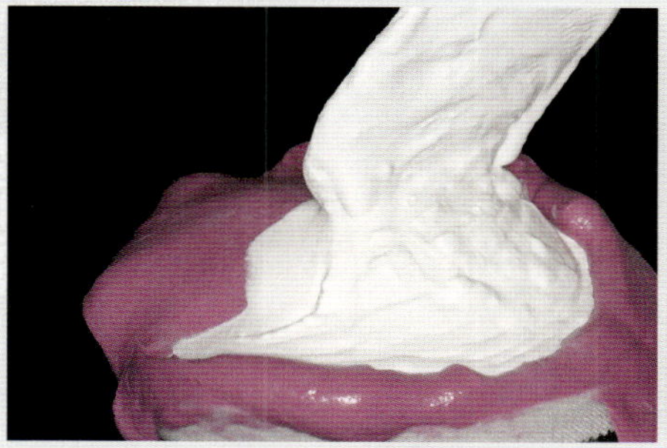

Fig 8-5b
Alginate impressions should be poured within a few hours so they do not deform.

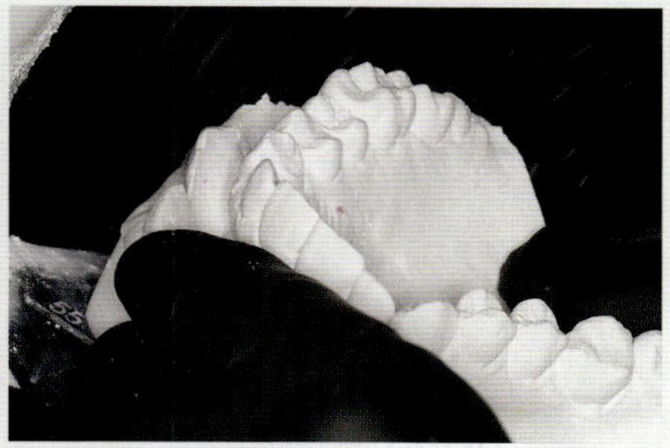

Fig 8-5c
After pouring, dental casts are trimmed in the model trimmer.

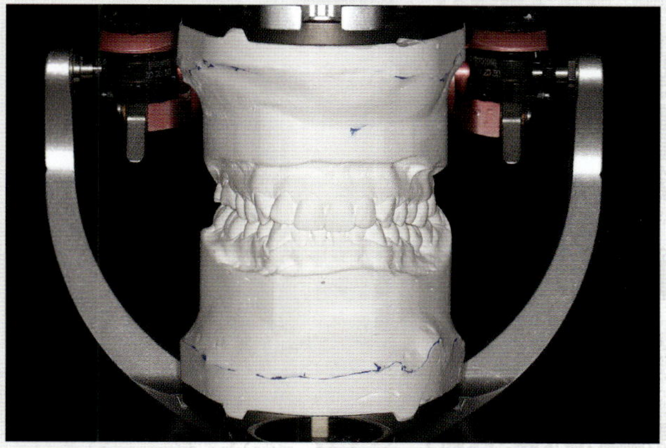

Fig 8-5d
Casts mounted in the articulator.

Next, the dental technician fabricates a labial bow to extend from the most distal tooth on each side of the arch (Fig 8-5e). Then open (horseshoe) palatal coverage with acrylic is made (Fig 8-5f), and an anterior platform is shaped opposing the mandibular central incisors (Fig 8-5g).

The deprogrammer should be polymerized in a high-pressure polymerization device, and the final shaping of the platform and polishing of the deprogrammer takes place after the ultimate polymerization. The platform should slightly disclude all remaining teeth by approximately 1–1.5 mm. The platform should be wide enough in the anterior-posterior dimension, so the patient cannot bite beyond it (Fig 8-5h).

It should also be flat (parallel to the horizontal plane) to allow protrusive and retrusive mandibular movement during muscle deprogramming.[17,18]

Fig 8-5e
Fabricating the labial bow.

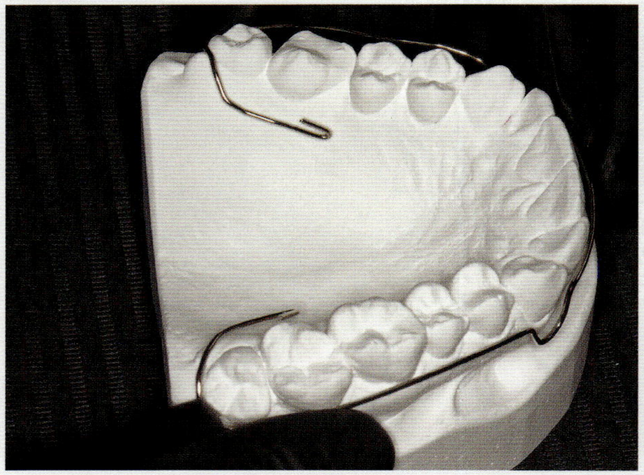

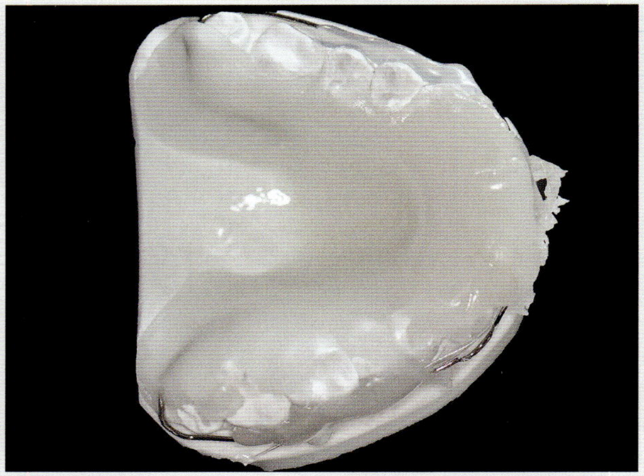

Fig 8-5f
Applying the acrylic resin to form a deprogrammer with an anterior platform.

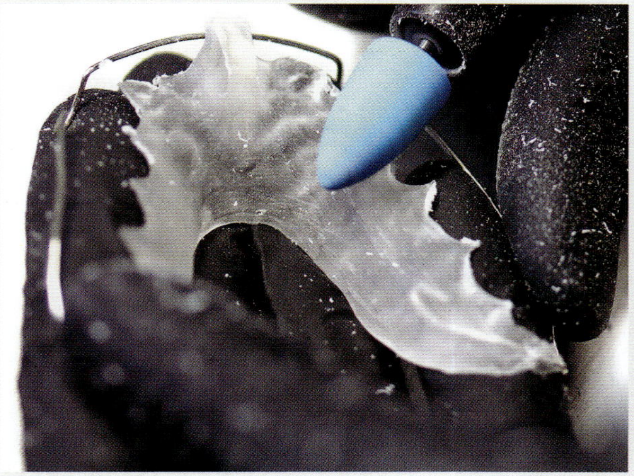

Fig 8-5g
Shaping the deprogrammer's platform after final polymerization in a high-pressure polymerization device.

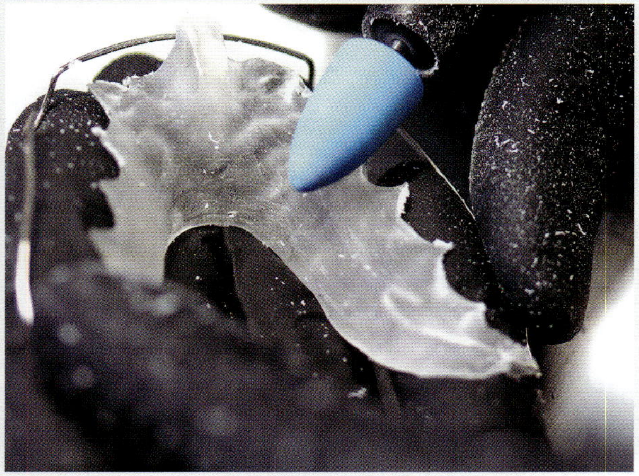

Fig 8-5h
Polished deprogrammer ready to be adjusted in the oral cavity.

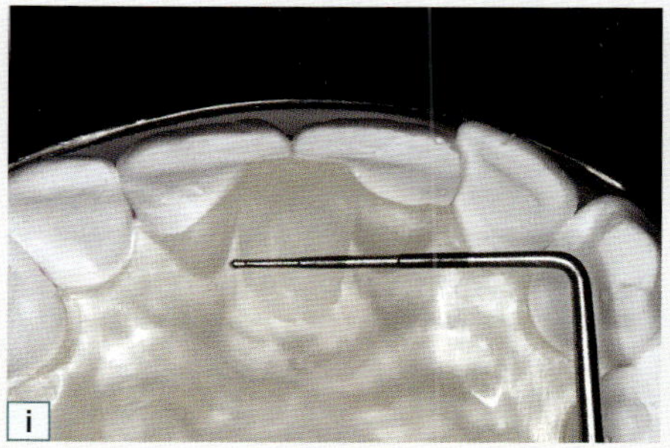

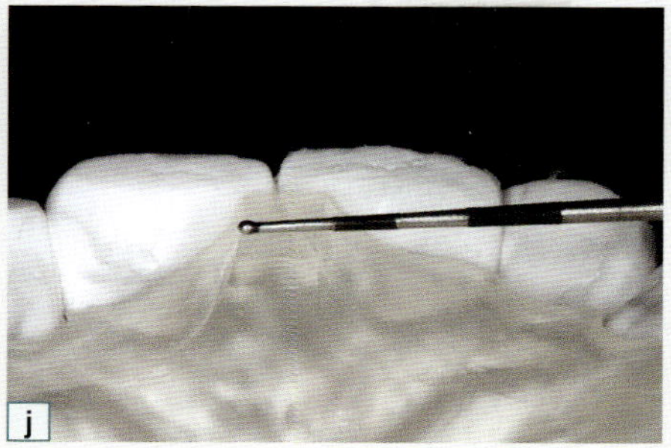

Figs 8-5i and 8-5j
(i) Platform shaped in the dental laboratory is wide enough and should be
(j) Narrowed individually by the dentist to 3–5 mm.

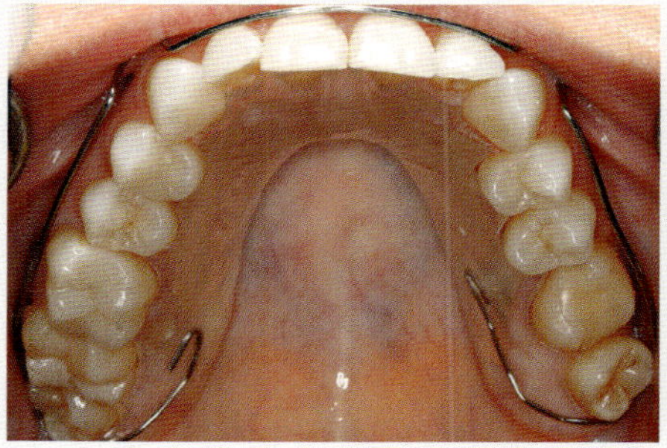

Fig 8-5k
Deprogrammer should be inserted passively and stay in place by accurate fit of the KD plate to the palatal surface of the teeth.

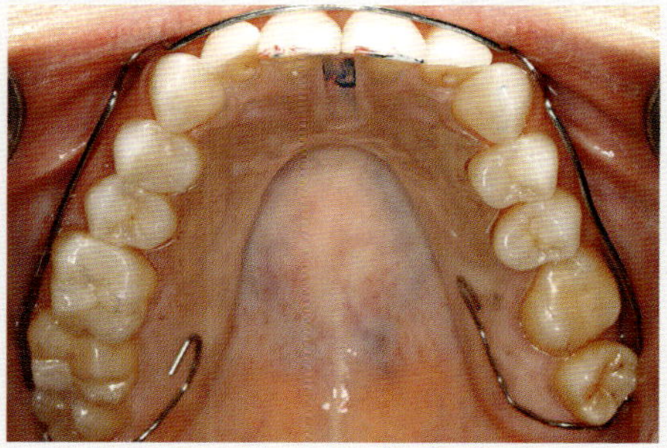

Fig 8-5l
With articulating paper, mark protrusive and retrusive mandibular movements on the deprogrammer's platform.

PROCEDURES WHEN DELIVERING THE DEPROGRAMMER (according to Kois Center, Seattle)[18,19]

1. Confirm that the anterior platform is not wider than 3 mm (Figs 8-5i and 8-5j)
2. The deprogrammer should be inserted passively to avoid any obstacles (Fig 8-5k)
3. Appropriate stabilization is achieved by accurate fitting of the palatal plate and labial bow
4. When the patient has a gag reflex, reduce the palatal plate
5. In the case of a very thick palatal plate, make it thinner, so it does not block the tongue
6. Ask the patient to slide the mandible forward and backward on the appliance (marking with the articulation paper) (Fig 8-5l) and relieve any acrylic thickness, which is palatal to the most retrusive contact on the platform (relieving 3 mm from the most retrusive position) (Fig 8-5m)

Fig 8-5m
Excess of the KD platform should be relieved in the palatal part.

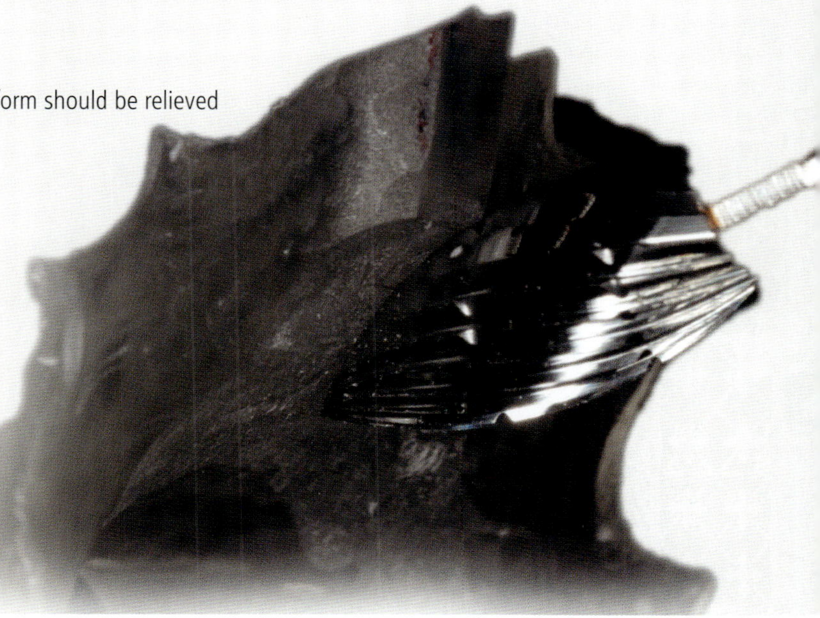

> ### REMEMBER
> The term **deprogramming** is defined as actions aimed at changing a specific way of working the muscles, ie, erasing muscle memory using various methods …

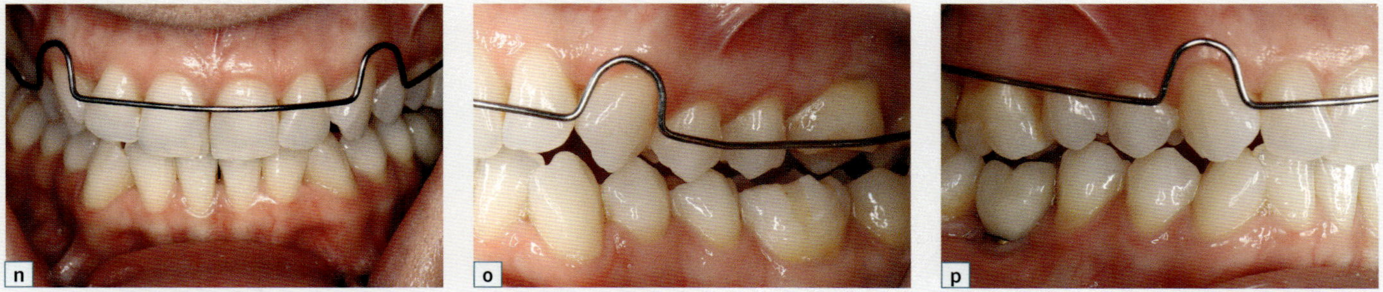

Figs 8-5n to 8-5p
(n) Intraoral photograph of the adjusted deprogrammer; (o, p) disclusion of the posterior teeth due to appropriate shape of the deprogrammer's platform.

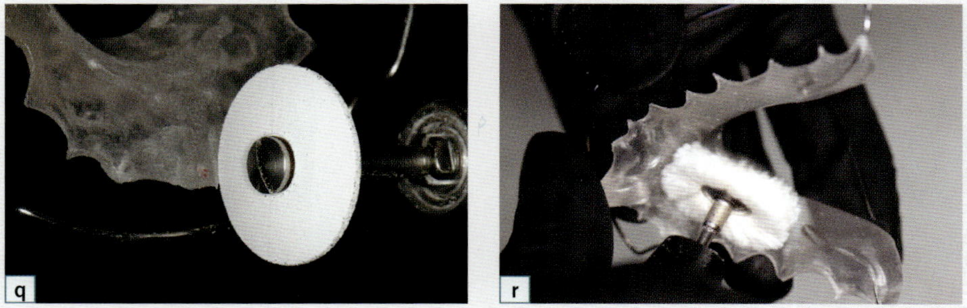

Figs 8-5q and 8-5r
(q) Final reduction of the deprogrammer's platform and (r) final polishing (laboratory work: DT Iwona Domagała).

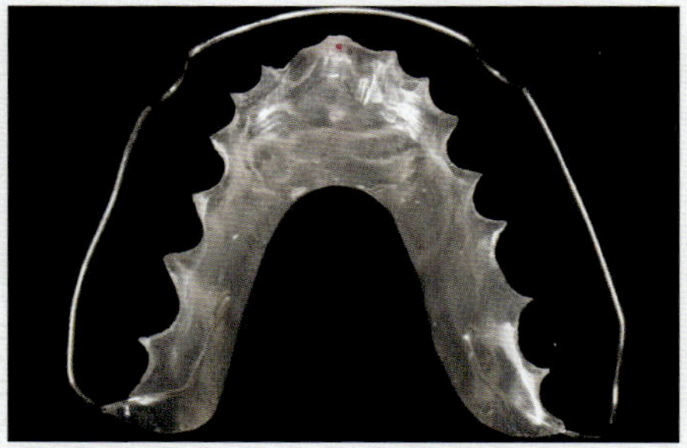

Fig 8-5s
One contact point will guarantee proper disclusion and muscle deprogramming.

7. Reduce the anterior platform to achieve 1–1.5 mm disclusion in the molar region (Figs 8-5n to 8-5p)
8. Reduce the width of the anterior platform until the patient makes one contact point on the platform (Fig 8-5q)
9. Final polishing (Fig 8-5r)
10. When delivering the splint, make sure that there is one contact point (Fig 8-5s) on the platform and disclusion between posterior teeth
11. Patient receives the Kois Deprogrammer for 4 weeks, with a recommendation to use at night and as much as possible during the day to maximize the effect of muscle deprogramming (Fig 8-5t)

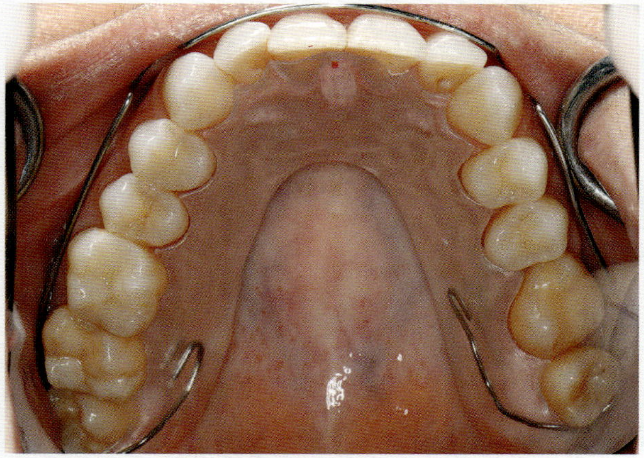

Fig 8-5t
After using the deprogrammer for 4 weeks, confirm that the patient has been correctly deprogrammed – it is achieved when the patient spontaneously adducts the mandible into one certain point of the platform marked with a thin red articulating paper (Parkell 21 μm).

DIAGNOSTICS AFTER DEPROGRAMMING – CENTRIC RELATION (CR) REGISTRATION

Confirmation that the patient has been deprogrammed after 4 weeks of using the KD is achieved when the initial point of contact marked with articulating paper is **single, repeatable, and achieved spontaneously upon closing the patient's mouth, not with any manipulation of the mandible**. Using KD, the CR registration can be executed by confirming one reproducible contact point of the anterior platform and simultaneous bite registration with a hard VPS-based material. For this purpose, self-curing acrylic resin (for example, Pattern Resin, GC) is placed on the deprogrammer's platform. The patient is then asked to close the mandible several times and make sure that they are always biting in the same place (previously premarked with articulating paper). Then, the patient remains in the position that was established on the platform, and the dentist injects the VPS-based material into the space between the posteriors. In this way, the dental technician will receive a bite record of the anterior teeth and a bilateral record of the posterior teeth. **Thanks to appropriate registration with the Kois Deprogrammer** (Fig 8-6), **it is possible to analyze the casts mounted in the articulator in the CR position**, confirm the case diagnosis (constricted envelope of function vs. occlusal dysfunction; Fig 8-7) or study the models in different scenarios when changing vertical dimension of occlusion (VDO).[20–22]

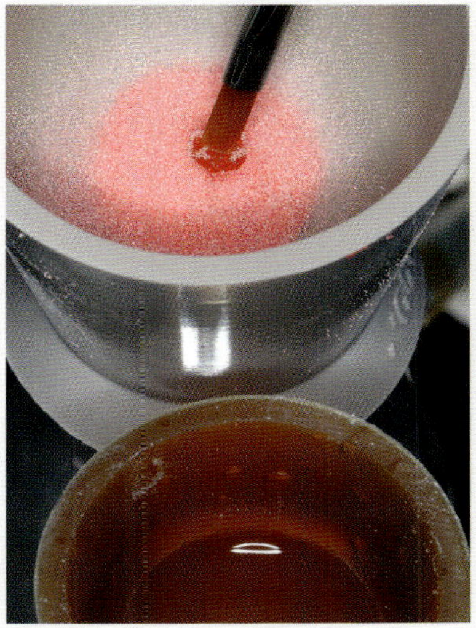

Fig 8-6a
Pattern Resin LS (GC Europe): powder and liquid are gently mixed and transferred with a brush …

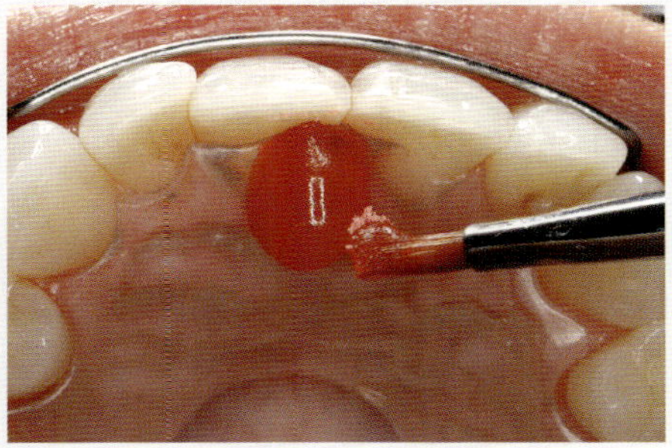

Fig 8-6b
… on the deprogrammer's platform.

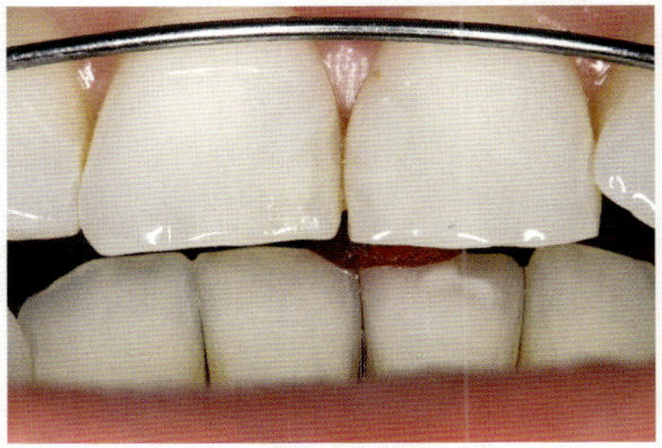

Fig 8-6c
Next, the patient closes their mouth several times, biting on the platform so that the dentist is sure that the position marked on the platform (centric occlusion, CO) is consistent with the CR obtained after the patient's deprogramming.

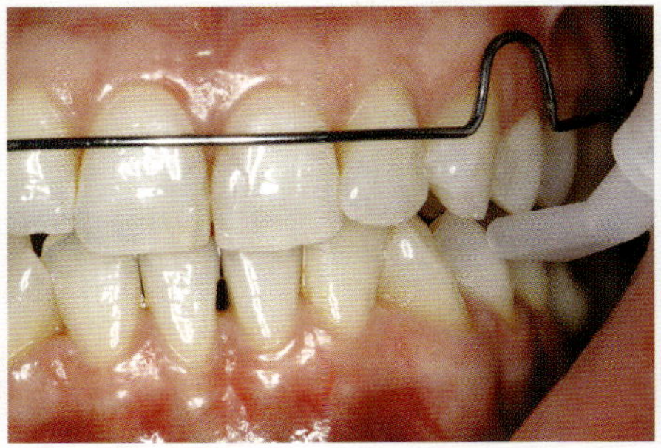

Fig 8-6d
After the material is set on the platform, the dentist places the mixing tip between the posterior teeth …

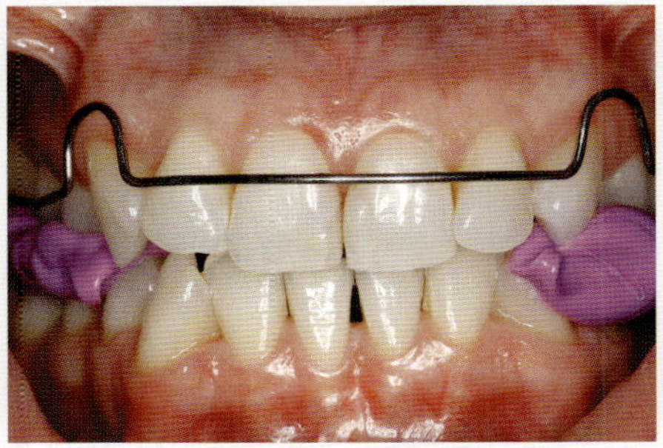

Fig 8-6e
… and injects the silicone mass for occlusal registration on both sides, which will record the relationship between the maxillary and mandibular teeth.

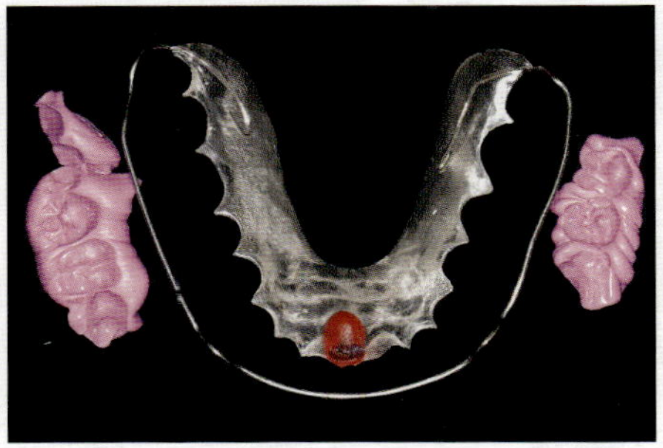

Fig 8-6f
After the impression material is set, we receive three places of registration: in the posterior segment on the left and right sides and on the deprogrammer's platform. Based on this, the dental technician mounts the casts in the articulator.

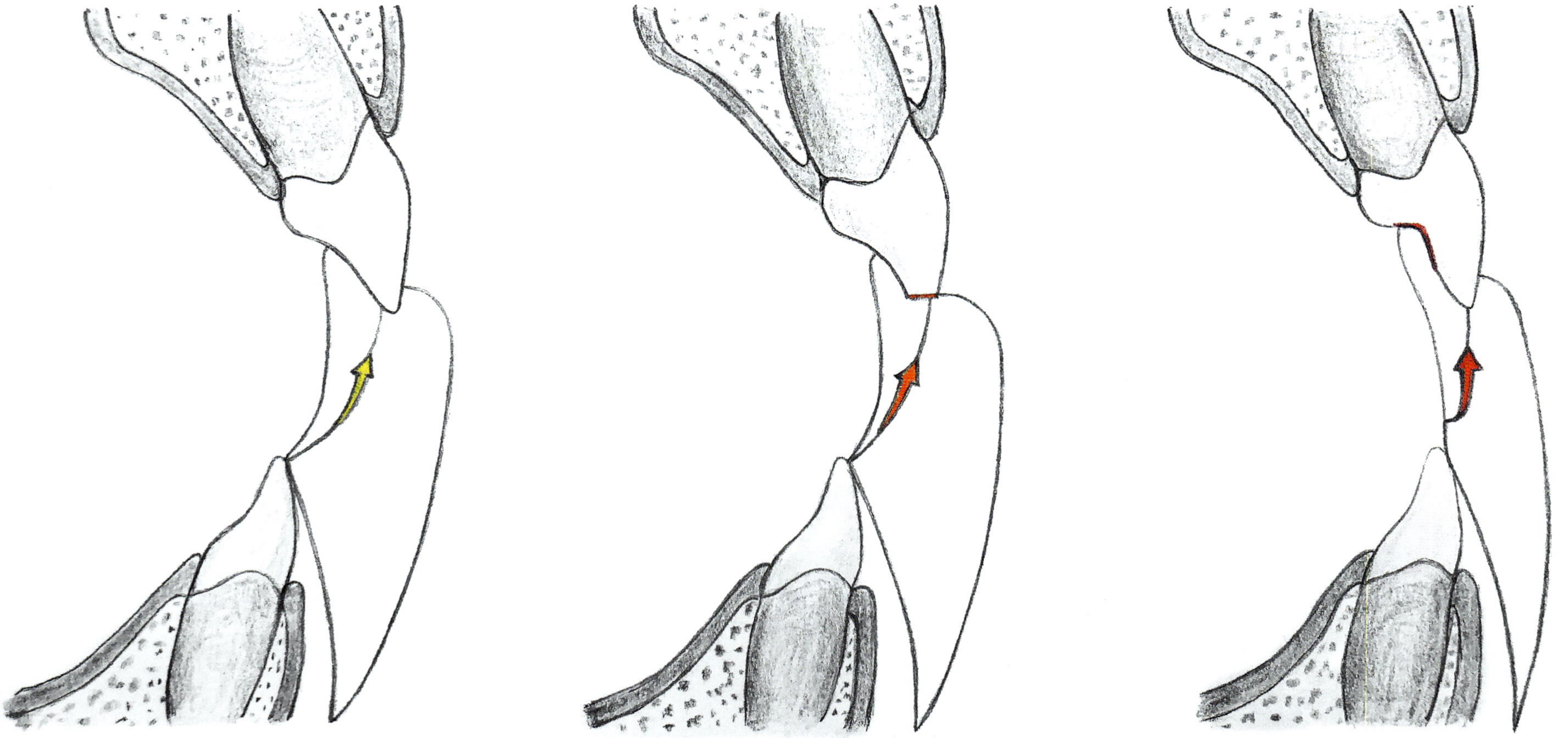

Envelope with an acceptable function

Widened envelope of function

Constricted envelope of function

Fig 8-7
Envelope of mandibular functional movements, the Posselt envelope or envelope of function:

- Left: an envelope with an acceptable function
- Center: widened envelope of function, typical for occlusal dysfunction, often causing a horizontal wear pattern
- Right: constricted envelope of function, often causing a vertical wear pattern

WHY CENTRIC RELATION?

The centric relation (CR) is the mandibular jaw position, in which the condylar processes are situated in the most orthopedically stable position in the fossa of the temporomandibular joints (Fig 8-8).[23,24]

In CR, the condyles articulate with the thinnest avascular portion of their respective discs with the complex in the anterior-superior position against the slopes of the articular eminences. In the past, this position was mainly used when performing complete dentures as a reference point for the relationship between the mandible and the maxilla. Over time, the concept of CR was transferred to fixed prosthodontics, and the validity of this procedure was confirmed using repeatability and studies of muscle function analysis.[25–28]

The starting point for planning comprehensive restorative treatment is to determine a repeatable position of the mandible in relation to the maxilla. There are two positions of the mandible that can meet this condition:

A. Position of maximum intercuspation (habitual position)

This position may be used when dealing with restorative/prosthetic treatment that does not change the occlusal conditions.

B. Centric relation (reference position)

We need this position in restorative treatment as the position "0" for treatment planning (diagnostic wax-up) and for comprehensive restorative treatment. The ultimate goal in restorative therapy is to achieve maximum intercuspation (MIP) in the CR.

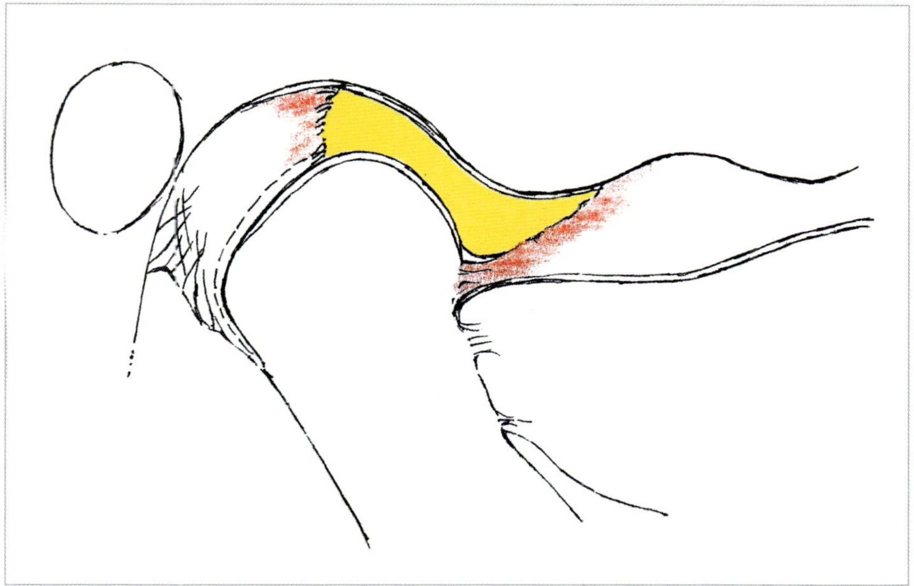

Fig 8-8
In centric relation (CR), the condyles articulate with the thinnest avascular portion of their respective discs with the complex in the anterior-superior position against the slopes of the articular eminences.

CONSTRICTED CHEWING PATTERN (CCP)

If, after deprogramming, the initial contact is located on the anterior teeth, we can diagnose constricted envelope of function (contact points are checked in position at 45 degrees). The 8 μm articulation foil or Shimstock is held between the anterior teeth (or fremitus can be detected). Orthodontic treatment or alteration of the vertical dimension should be considered to relieve the anterior teeth and reduce the risk of failure of future restorations.[29–30] To evaluate and select the appropriate therapy:

- Analyze the casts mounted in CR in the articulator.
- If you are considering alteration of VDO, you can do a test drive with the diagnostic wax-up (assess whether occlusal rehabilitation by means of restorative dentistry will meet the expected goals).
- In the case of a constricted envelope of function, orthodontic treatment should always be considered after appropriate cephalometric analysis. When performing the analysis, the cephalometric reference values should be taken into account and moving the teeth toward the norms should be prioritized when planning the treatment (Table 8-1)[31]:

REMEMBER

Do not plan comprehensive restorative treatment without CR registration. This position should always be considered as a starting point for prosthetic or orthodontic treatment.

Table 8-1 Cephalometric reference values

SNA	82° ± 3°	Horizontal position of the maxilla relative to cranial base
Slope of the maxillary central incisor (U1) relative to the SN	103° ± 6°	Inclination of the maxillary central incisors relative to the anterior cranial base
SNB	79° ± 3°	Horizontal position of the mandible relative to the cranial base using B point as a cephalometric landmark
Slope of the mandibular central incisor (L1) relative to the MP	90° ± 5°	Axial inclination of the mandibular incisors and the inferior border of the mandible
SN–MP	32° ± 5°	It determines the type of growth we are dealing with: vertical (> 32°), horizontal (< 32°)
ANB	3° ± 2°	Occlusal skeleton class: > 5° Class II, <1° Class III
Maxillary anterior facial height (N – ANS) in relation to the mandibular anterior facial height (ANS – Me)	0.8	Defines facial height (< 0.8 defines an elongated anterior mandibular part of the face); an important esthetic parameter when planning to increase the vertical dimension of occlusion
Interincisal angle	135° ± 11°	> 135° indicates the possibility of constricted envelope of function (risk of tooth wear and overloading of the anterior teeth)

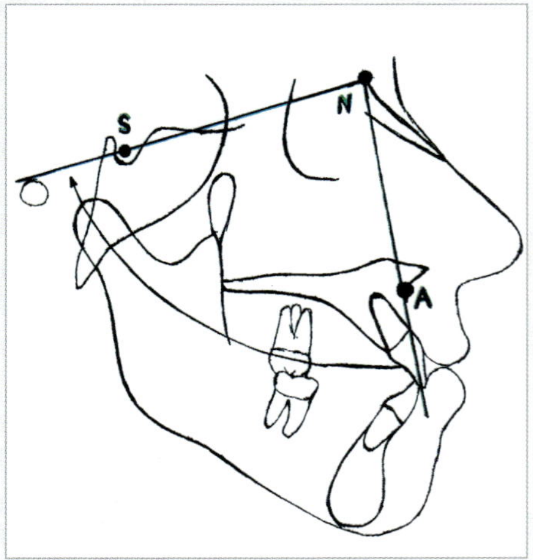

Fig 8-9a
SNA angle (Sella – Nasion – point A) 82° ± 3°.

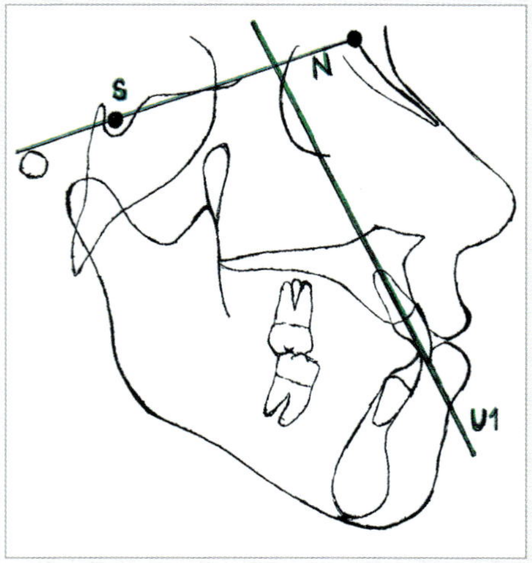

Fig 8-9b
U1 relative to MV: 103° ± 6°.

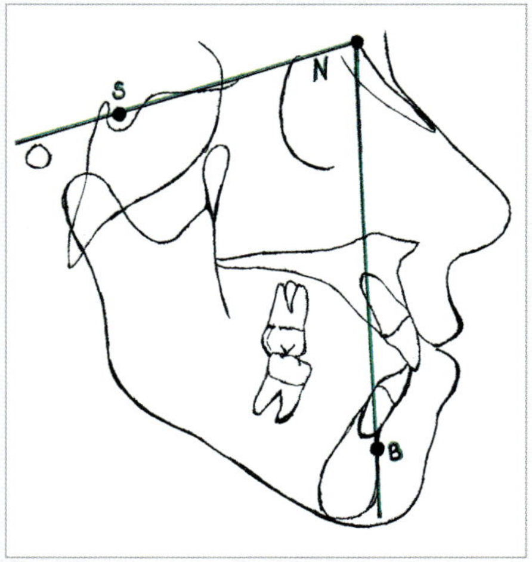

Fig 8-9c
SNB angle (Sella – Nasion – point B): 72° ± 3°.

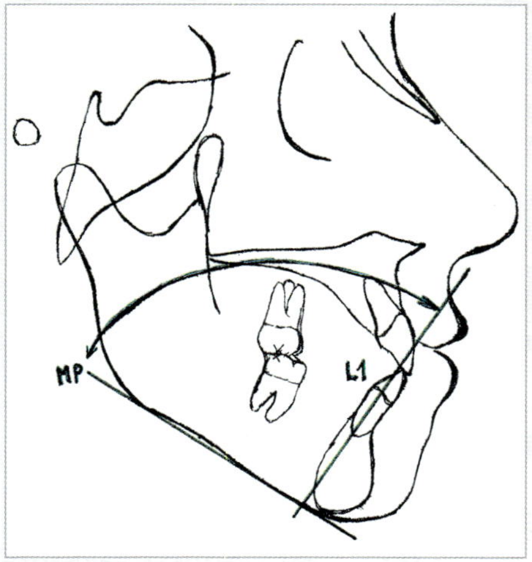

Fig 8-9d
L1 to MP: 90° ± 5°.

Case 5: Constricted envelope of function

A patient presented to the office seeking dental treatment and improved teeth function (Figs 8-10a to 8-10g). While collecting medical history, the following information about functional complaints was obtained:

- In the left temporomandibular joint, gentle popping without pain during mandible opening
- In the past five years, the patient had noticed that his anterior teeth had started to wear down considerably
- The patient noted in the information card that he tends to clench his teeth during the day, which was related to the intensity of his work

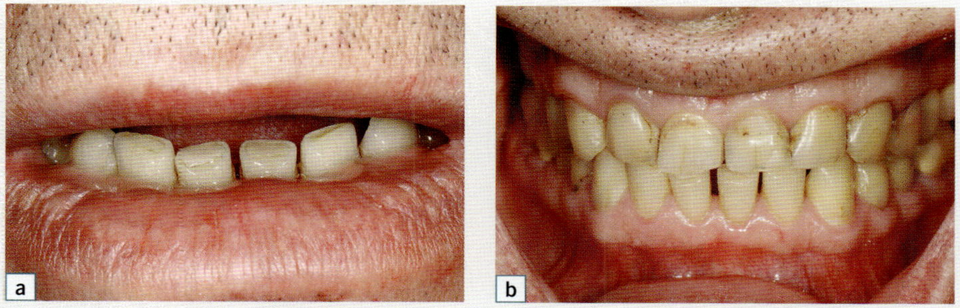

Figs 8-10a and 8-10b
(a) Patient's lips in repose allow us to determine the display of the position of the anterior maxillary teeth in relation to the upper lip. If the teeth do not expose from under the upper lip, when planning esthetic treatment, the length of the maxillary front teeth should be increased. (b) Intraoral photograph: teeth in the maximum intercuspation.

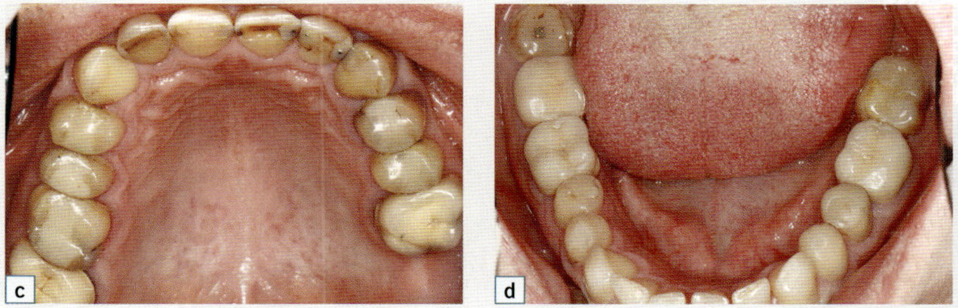

Figs 8-10c and 8-10d
Intraoral photographs of (c) maxillary and (d) mandibular arches.

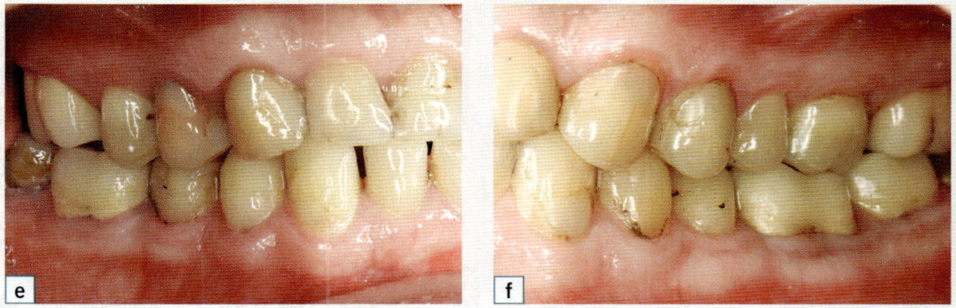

Figs 8-10e and 8-10f
Posterior intraoral photographs in the maximum intercuspation.

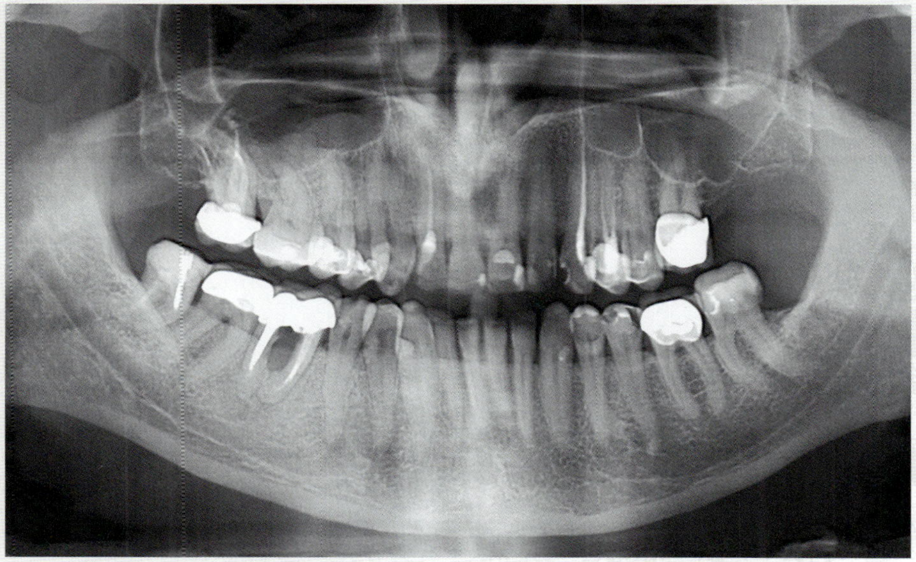

Fig 8-10g
Panoramic radiograph during the patient's first appointment.

The clinical examination revealed many restorations with poor marginal adaptation, several carious cavities, extensive tooth wear – especially in the anterior segment of the maxilla and mandible, and erosion cavities on worn surfaces, partially filled with composite by the previous dentist. Examination of the gingival sulcus depth revealed a third-grade furcation defect in tooth 46. In the initial phase of treatment, the focus was on scaling and root planing, treatment of the cavities and replacement of some restorations (Figs 8-10h to 8-10j). Tooth 46 was planned for extraction, which the patient wanted to avoid at all costs.

Step 1: Esthetic treatment planning

Although the patient did not wish to improve the esthetics of the teeth, it was explained to him that **when thinking about changing the function, the treatment planning should start with the anterior teeth**.

At this stage **Digital Smile Design, DSD** was created (Fig 8-10k), followed by making a wax-up of the anterior maxillary teeth (Fig 8-10l). The patient was also asked to bring his historical photograph, in which the maxillary teeth are visible. This evaluation aimed to understand how the smile changed and how much the maxillary teeth were displayed in the past (Fig 8-10o).

Impressions were taken, the facebow was registered, and, together with photographs, these were all sent to the dental laboratory to be used by the technician during waxing-up. Based on the wax-up, a silicone index was made (Fig 8-10m), followed by a mock-up (Fig 8-10n). Next, the patient was presented with pictures of the expected esthetic plan (Figs 8-10p and 8-10q). The patient and the photographs consultation team accepted the mock-up and, thus, it was possible to proceed **to step 2**.

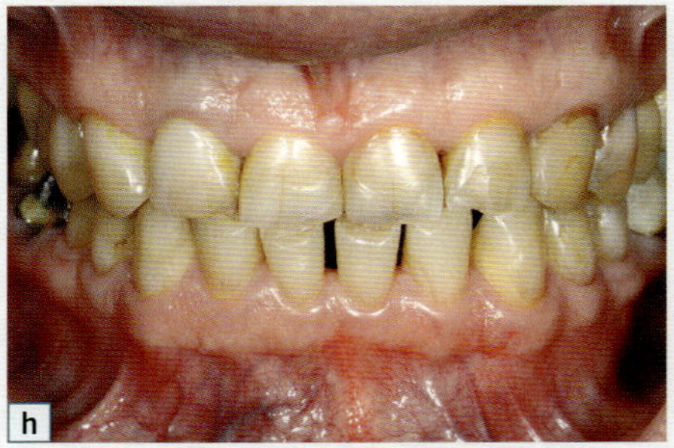

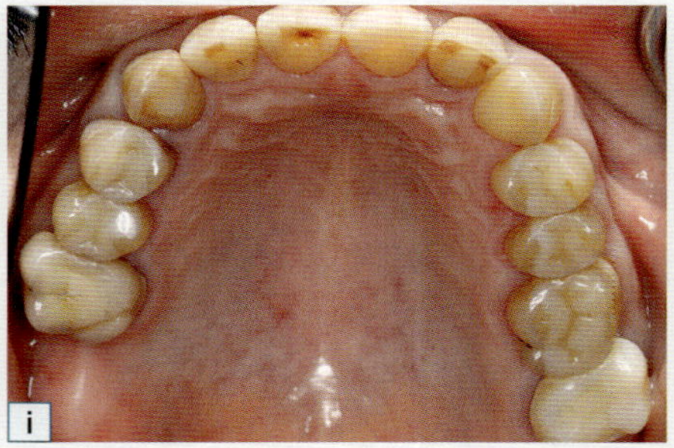

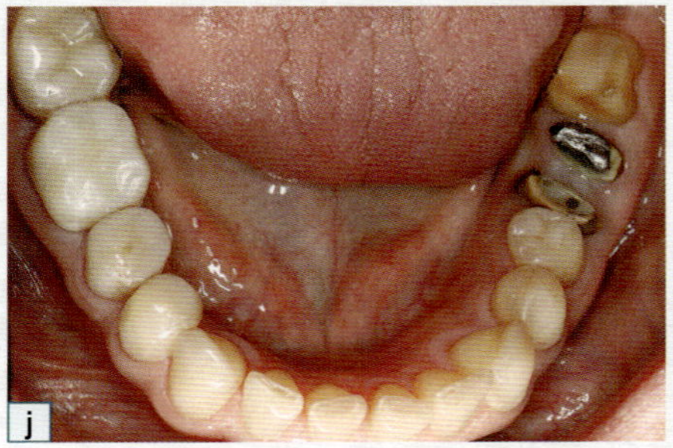

Figs 8-10h to 8-10j
Intraoral photographs after the initial phase of treatment, including scaling and root planing, replacement of failing restorations, and caries treatment.

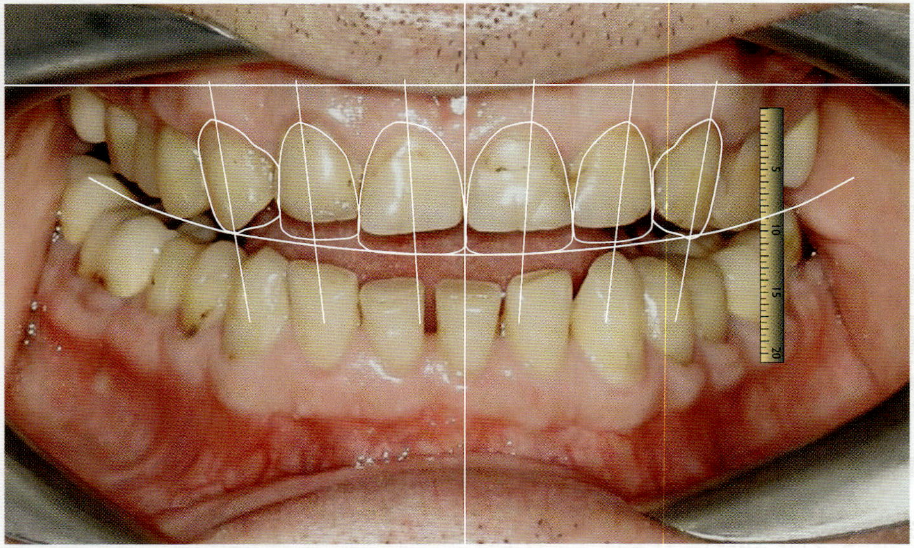

Fig 8-10k
DSD presents an esthetic treatment plan proposition before creating the diagnostic wax-up.

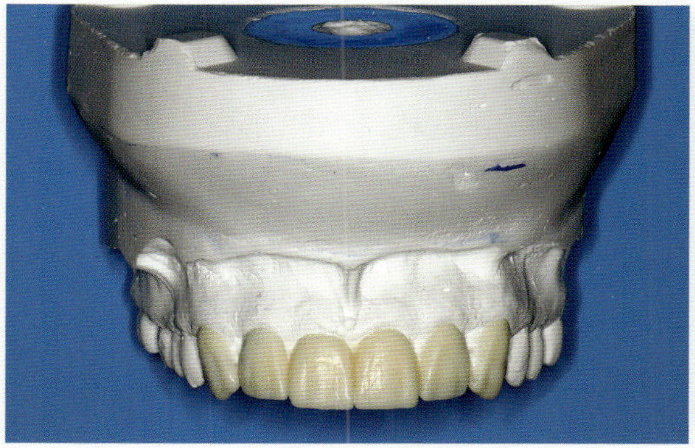

Fig 8-10l
Diagnostic wax-up of the maxillary front teeth made on the basis of DSD.

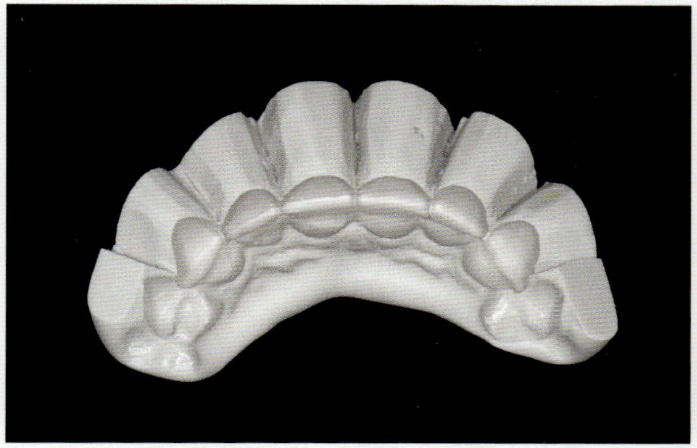

Fig 8-10m
Silicone index was taken from the diagnostic wax-up.

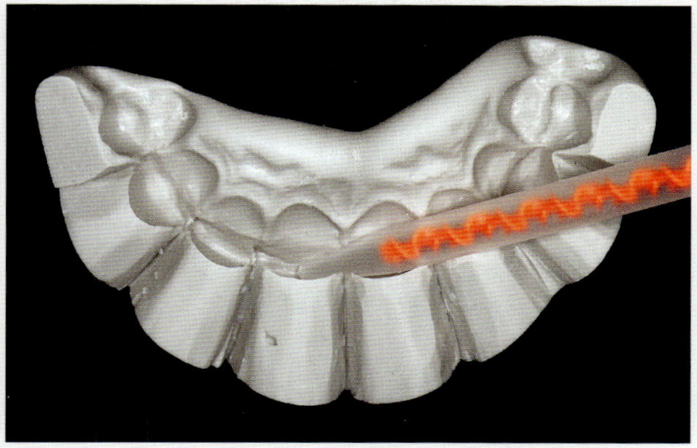

Fig 8-10n
Bis-acrylic composite material (Protemp) is applied to the silicone index to obtain a mock-up.

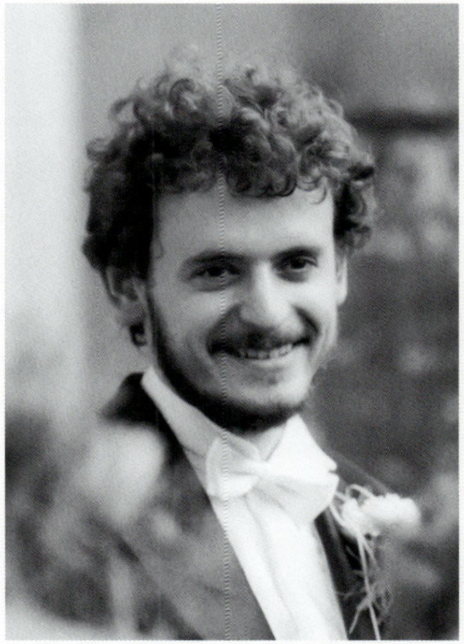

Fig 8-10o
The patient provided a historical photograph to make it easier to plan the future esthetics and visualize how the tooth wear would progress.

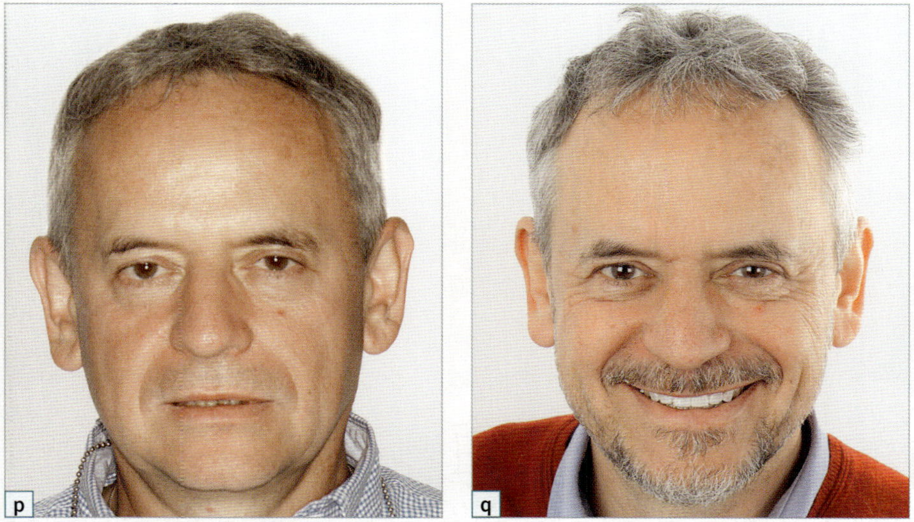

Figs 8-10p and 8-10q
(p) Photograph of the current condition of the patient's teeth and (q) photograph after mock-up.

Step 2: Centric relation (CR)

As the loading and immobilization test revealed negative, the patient was provided with a Kois Deprogrammer, which he had worn for 4 weeks, day and night. The appointment after 4 weeks confirmed the diagnosis of a **constricted chewing pattern (CCP)** because the first contacts without a deprogrammer were found on the anterior teeth. After 4 weeks, the CR was registered, and the bite records were transferred to the dental laboratory, thanks to which the casts were mounted in the articulator in a CR (Fig 8-10r).

Orthodontic treatment to improve incisor inclination was discussed, but the patient expected restorative treatment without orthodontics. For this purpose, functional wax-up of the mandibular arch was obtained to eliminate anterior overload (Fig 8-10s).

Step 3: Functional wax-up

It was analyzed how much the VDO should be increased to avoid occlusal overloading of the newly designed anterior teeth. In this case, increasing VDO with the mandibular arch was obtained. It was decided to increase the vertical dimension of occlusion by waxing-up only the mandibular arch. With the wax-up of the mandibular arch, it was possible to study the visualization of the treatment plan.

Step 4: Restorative treatment

A. Mandibular arch

The patient and the dental team executing the treatment plan wanted the most conservative treatment approach and to minimize or eliminate teeth preparation.

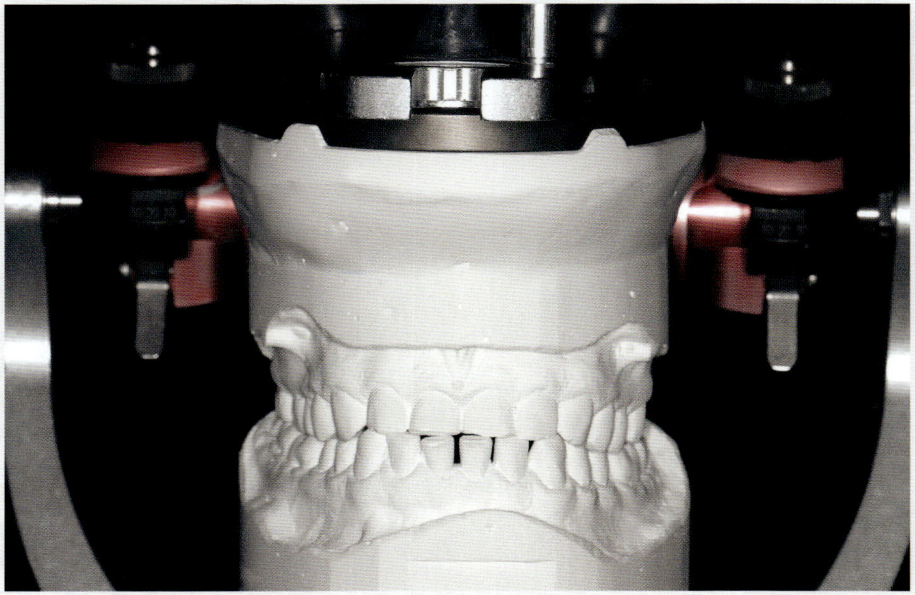

Fig 8-10r
Casts are mounted in centric relation in the articulator.

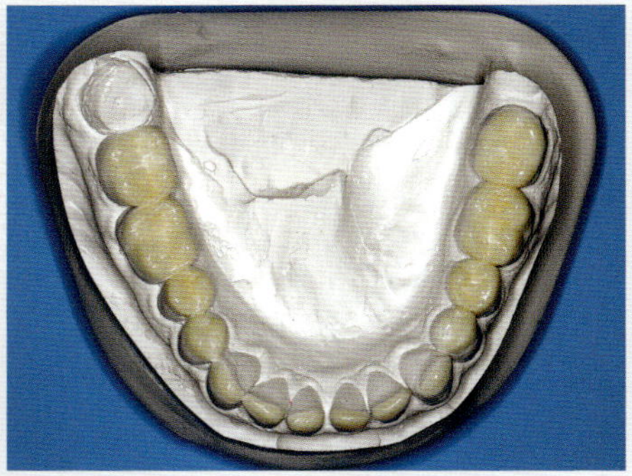

Fig 8-10s
Functional wax-up of the mandibular arch was obtained in order to eliminate anterior overload.

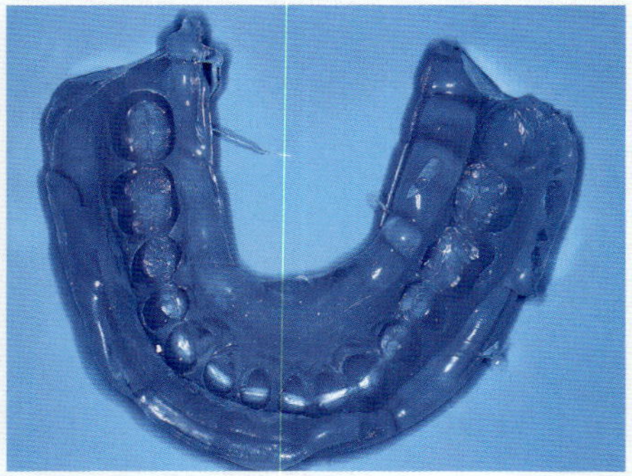

Fig 8-10t
Transparent silicone index made based on functional wax-up.

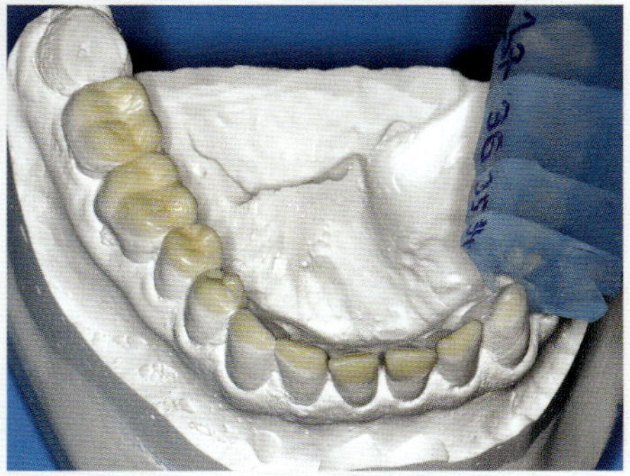

Fig 8-10u
Silicone index was cut tooth by tooth with a surgical blade in order to make direct restorations based on functional wax-up.

To restore the new occlusal surface of the mandibular arch, a transparent silicone index was fabricated (Fig 8-10t), made from the diagnostic wax-up. The index was taken in an impression tray. Then, after removing the silicone part, the index was cut (Fig 8-10u) tooth by tooth to make it possible to place each piece in a stable position on the teeth after isolating them with the rubber dam. The cut was made on the cast in such a way as to enable the removal of excess and to avoid loss of stability when being placed on the teeth. Next, the teeth were isolated with a rubber dam (Fig 8-10v), the tooth surface and the restorations were gently roughened with a diamond bur and air abrasion (Air Abrasion Cavity Prep Unit, Danville) (Fig 8-10w). The occlusal, buccal, and lingual surfaces were etched, and after rinsing with a water spray and dried, the bonding system was applied and cured. Each tooth during the restoration process was isolated from the adjacent teeth with metal strips.

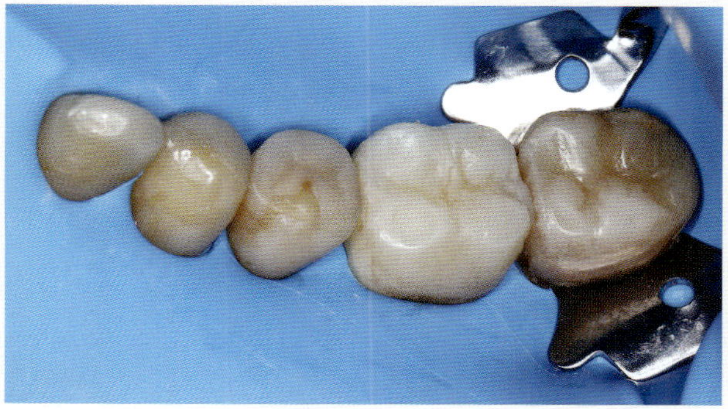

Fig 8-10v
Teeth isolation in the third quadrant with a rubber dam.

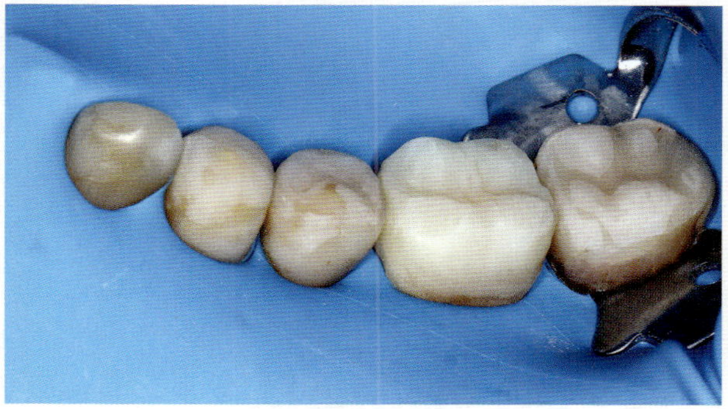

Fig 8-10w
Slight roughening of the tooth surface with a diamond bur and air abrasion will increase the adhesion to the formerly polymerized composite and untouched tooth surface.

Steps of composite application:

- The dentin layer was applied directly on the occlusal surface (Fig 8-11a), then the index was placed on the tooth so the dentin layer would not exceed the planned restoration volume (Fig 8-11b) and light-cured first through the index and then directly after index removal (Fig 8-11c).

- The enamel layer was applied directly to the inner surface of the index and then placed again on the occlusal surface, excess material from the buccal and lingual surface was removed, pre-polymerization was done through the index, and the final polymerization was carried out without silicone index (Fig 8-11d).

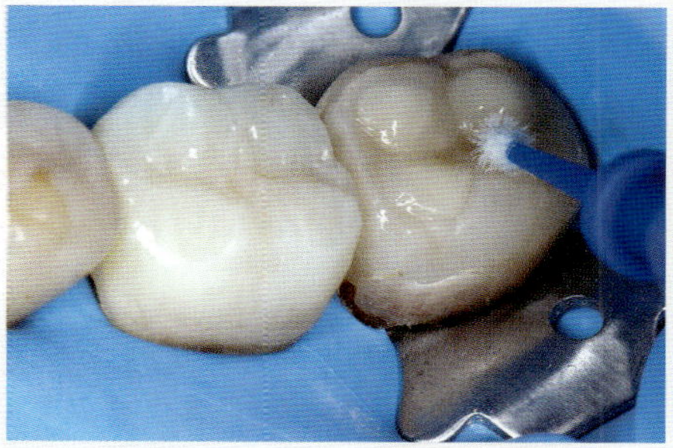

Fig 8-11a
Application of the first layer – dentin composite (Enamel Plus HRi, UD3).

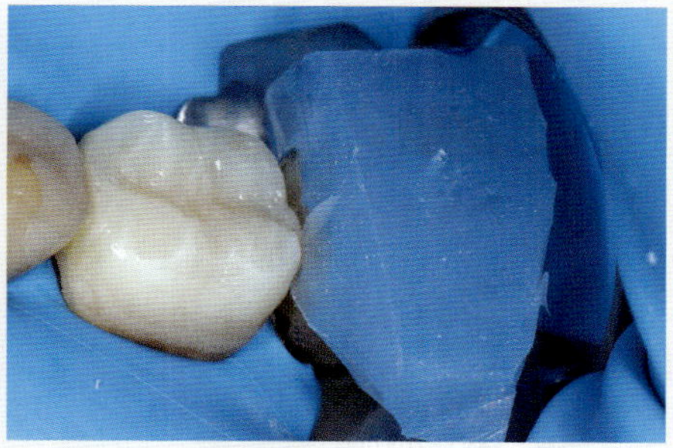

Fig 8-11b
Placing the silicone index before polymerization.

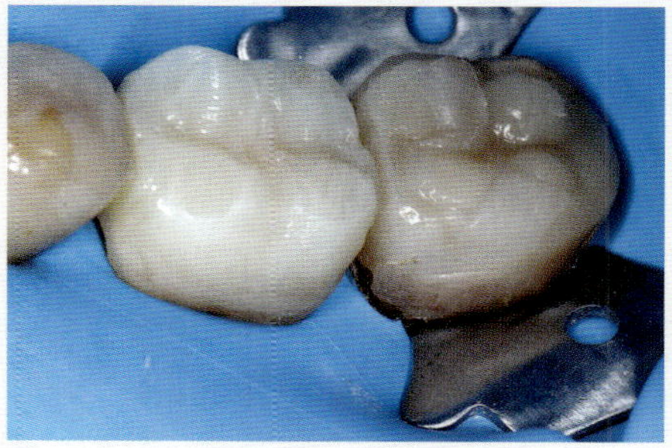

Fig 8-11c
Clinical situation after polymerizing the first dentin layer on tooth 37.

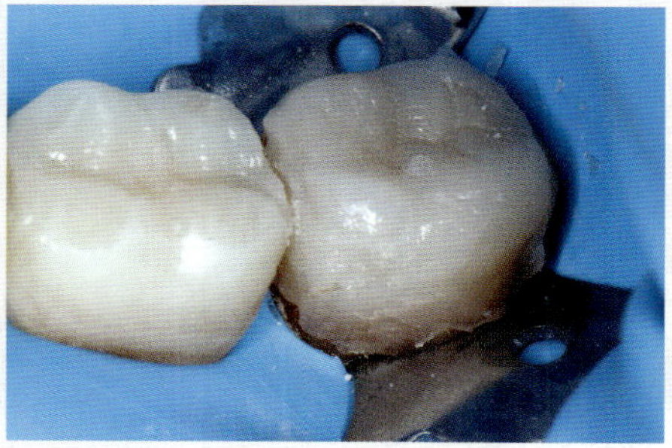

Fig 8-11d
Clinical situation after polymerizing the enamel layer on tooth 37 (Enamel Plus HRi Bio Function BF2, Micerium).

After restoring molars and premolars (Fig 8-11e) in the third and fourth quadrants, an initial equilibration was performed (Fig 8-11f) to balance the achieved bilateral posterior occlusal stability. Next, the restoration of the anterior teeth was performed. For this purpose, the index made from hard laboratory silicone was adjusted in order to restore the lingual surfaces and the incisal edges. The anterior teeth were isolated with a rubber dam (Fig 8-11g), and a slight chamfer and a long bevel were created on the labial surface. The enamel and the dentin were sandblasted and etched (Fig 8-11h) and thoroughly rinsed with a water spray (Fig 8-11i) before the bonding system was applied. The lingual surface was restored with the silicone index (Figs 8-11j and 8-11k) using the resin of enamel shade for this purpose. The proximal surfaces were restored and formed with the same material using the VariStrip matrix (Garrison) (Fig 8-11l). Once the tooth frame was created (Fig 8-11m), the dentin mamelons were applied to secure appropriate space for the enamel layer (thickness < 0.5 mm) (Figs 8-11n and 8-11o). After applying the outer enamel layer (Fig 8-11p), final light-curing was performed.

A Profin handpiece was used to create an anatomical shape, and the labial surface was gently corrected (Fig 8-11q).

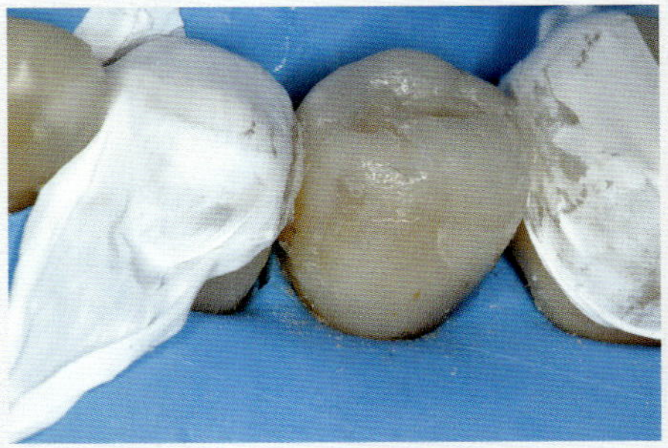

Fig 8-11e
Clinical situation after tooth 35 direct composite restoration with index technique.

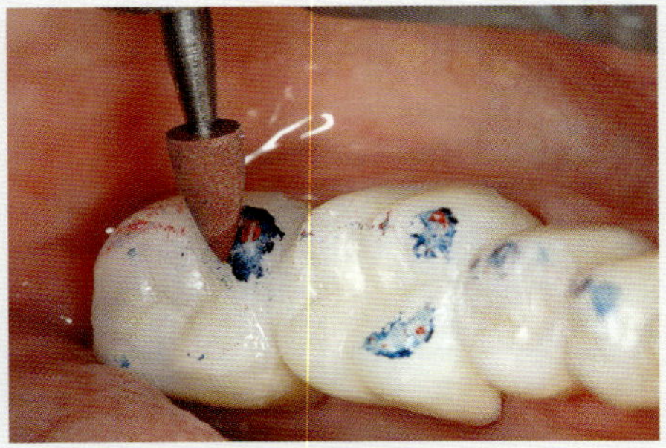

Fig 8-11f
Initial occlusal equilibration to balance out the contacts between the left and right side after posterior teeth direct reconstruction.

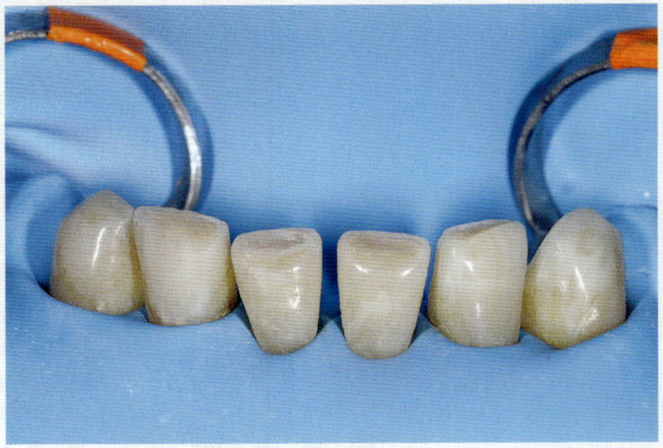

Fig 8-11g
Reconstructing the anterior teeth in the rubber dam isolation.

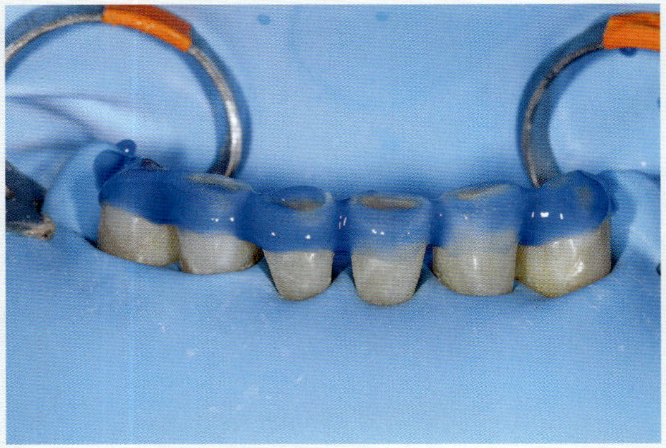

Fig 8-11h
Etching the anterior teeth.

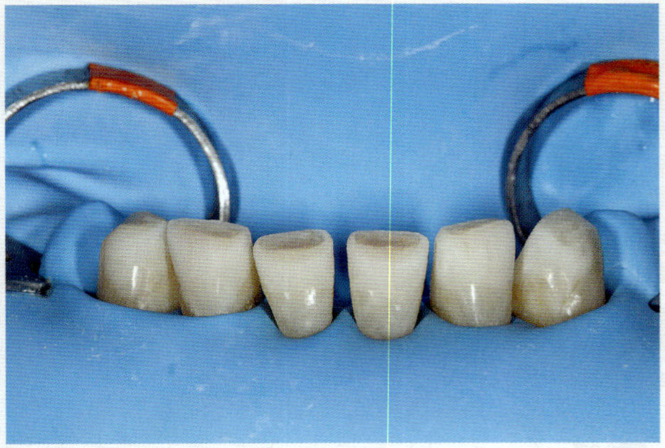

Fig 8-11i
Situation after rinsing the etchant and before applying the bonding agent.

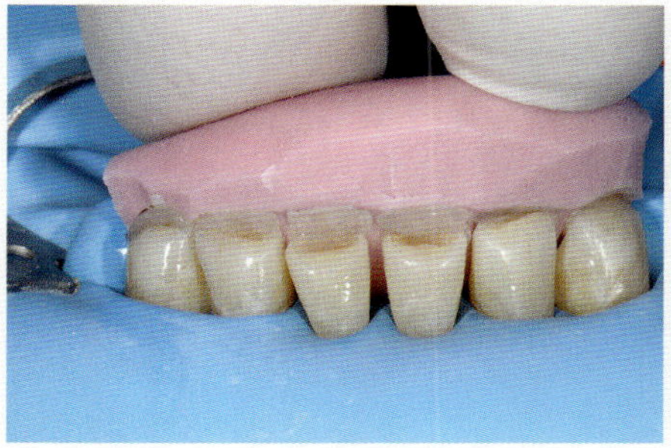

Fig 8-11j
Lingual walls of all restorations were simultaneously restored using an adjusted silicone index.

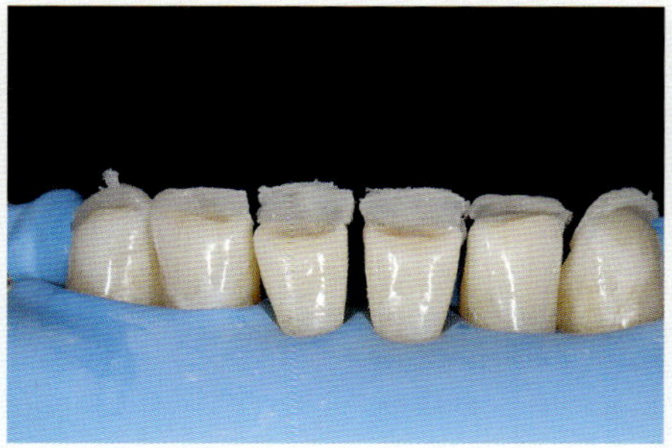

Fig 8-11k
Situation after light-curing the composite resin of the lingual surfaces.

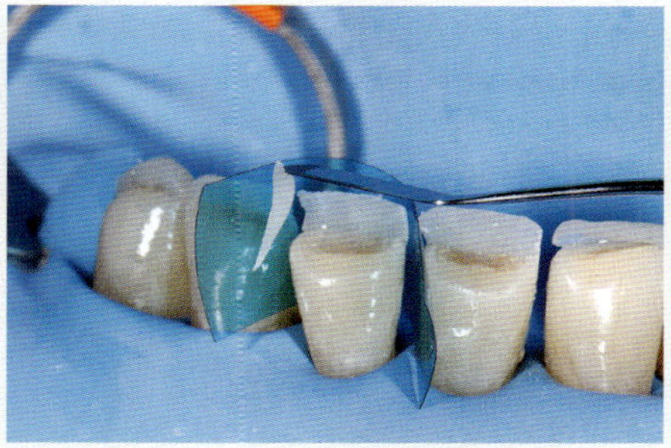

Fig 8-11l
Reconstructing proximal surfaces of the mandible anterior teeth with VariStrip (Garrison). The composite resin was applied with a flexible and thin spatula (Applica, LM Arte, Style Italiano).

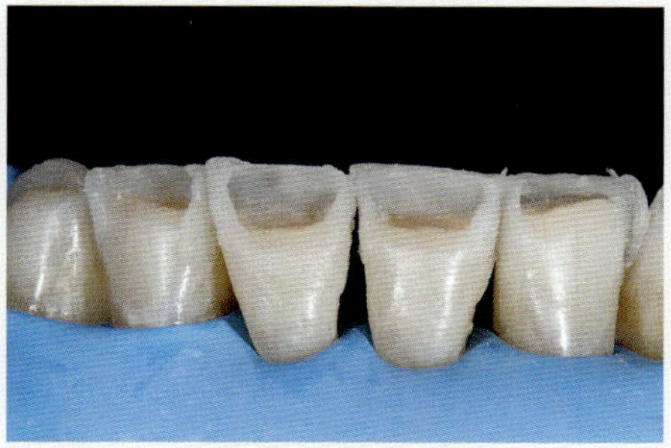

Fig 8-11m
Situation after reconstructing the tooth frames from the lingual and proximal surface (Enamel Plus HRi Bio Function BF2).

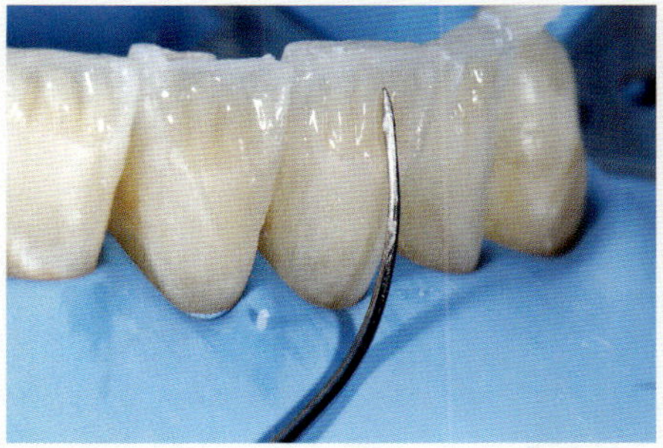

Fig 8-11n
Dentin mamelons (Enamel Plus HRi, UD3) are shaped using the Fissura instrument (LM Arte).

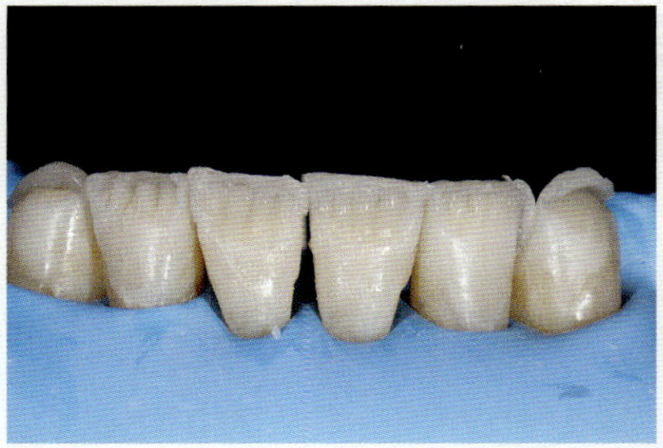

Fig 8-11o
Situation after light-curing of the dentin layer.

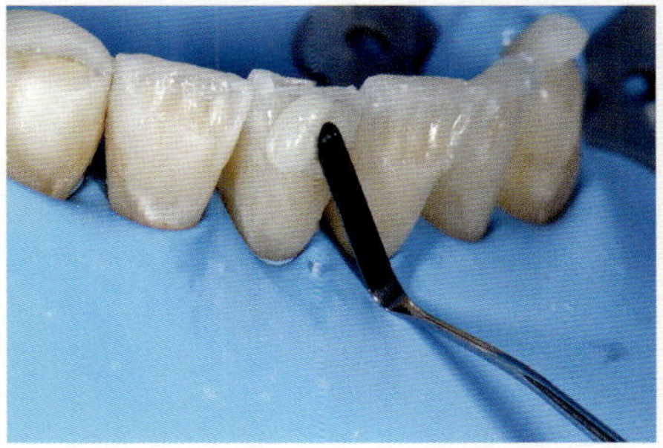

Fig 8-11p
Application of the final enamel layer (Enamel Plus HRi Bio Function BF2) with the Applica spatula (LM Arte).

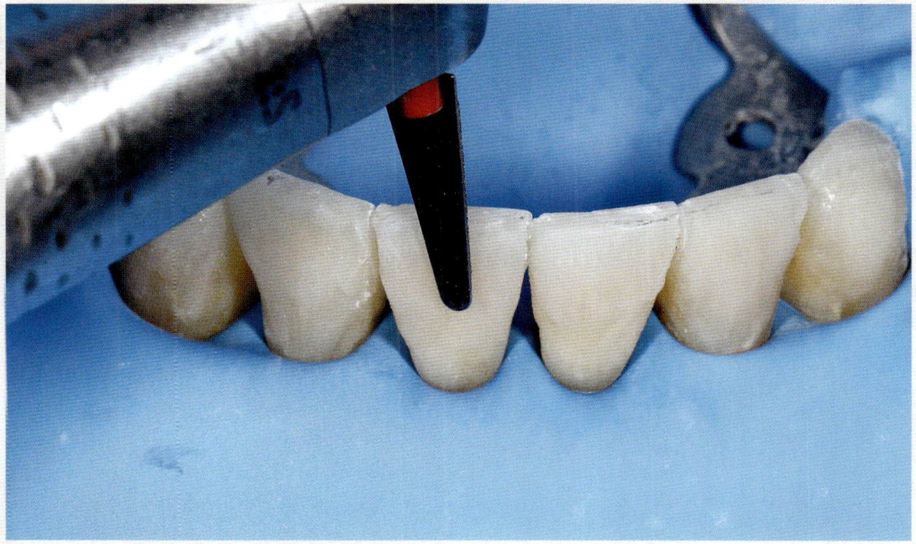

Fig 8-11q
Creating an anatomical structure with a Profin handpiece.

After removing the rubber dam, the functional corrections of the anterior composite restorations were carried out **(equilibration)** (Figs 8-11r and 8-11s). All composite areas heavily marked with a 200 μm blue horseshoe articulating paper (after **Kois chewing test**) were eliminated. At the end of the equilibration, bilateral contacts points were obtained in the posterior segments from the canines to the second molars (Fig 8-11t). At the next appointments, an implant-supported crown was performed on the previously placed implant 46, and a prosthetic crown was replaced on tooth 47 (Figs 8-11u and 8-11v). The situation after reconstructing the entire mandibular arch is shown in Fig 8-11w.

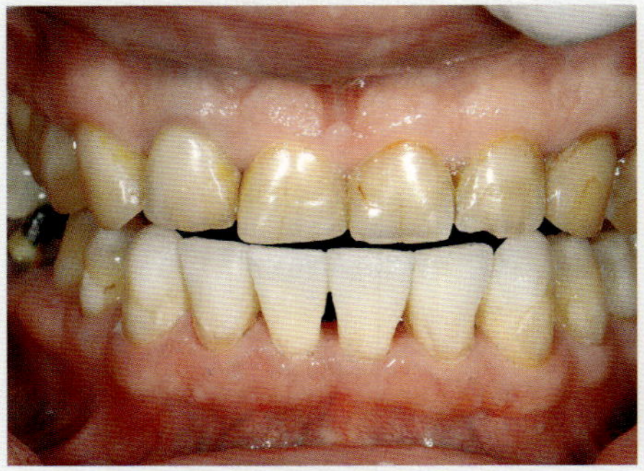

Fig 8-11r
Clinical situation after final reconstruction of the mandibular arch with direct restorations.

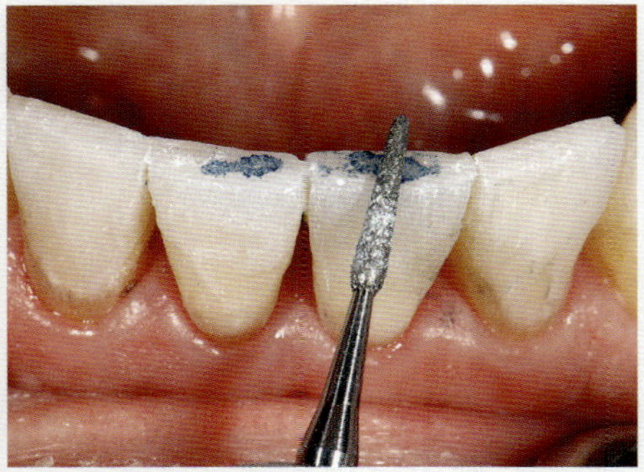

Fig 8-11s
Functional shaping of the anatomy of the mandible anterior restorations after the Kois chewing test.

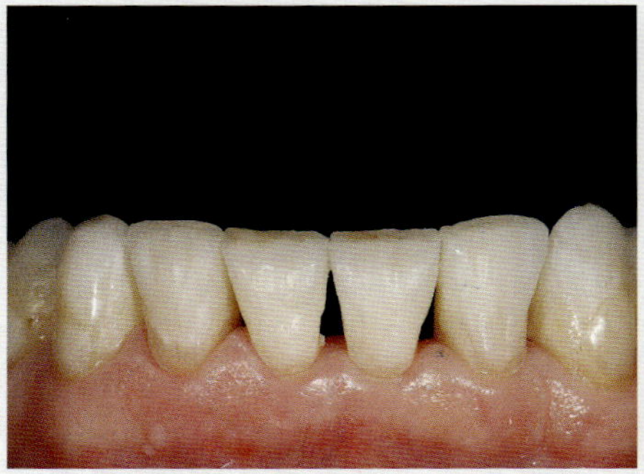

Fig 8-11t
The clinical situation immediately after performing restorations.

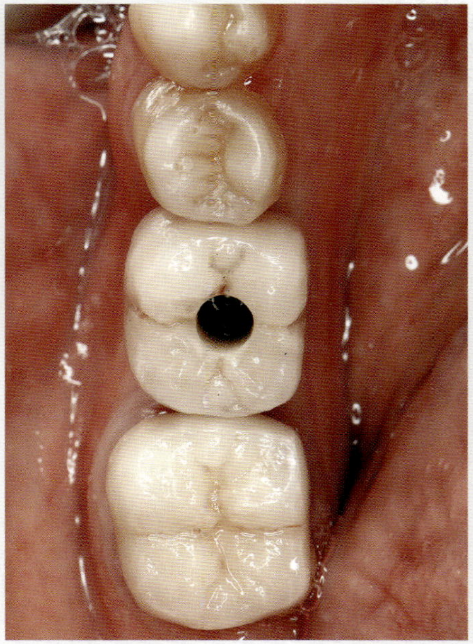

Fig 8-11u
Dental implant reconstruction in place of tooth 46 and prosthetic crown on tooth 47.

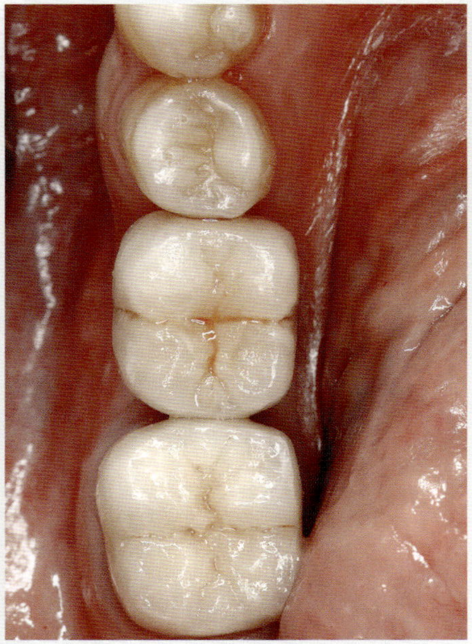

Fig 8-11v
Clinical situation after placing the composite into the access of the screw-retained crown.

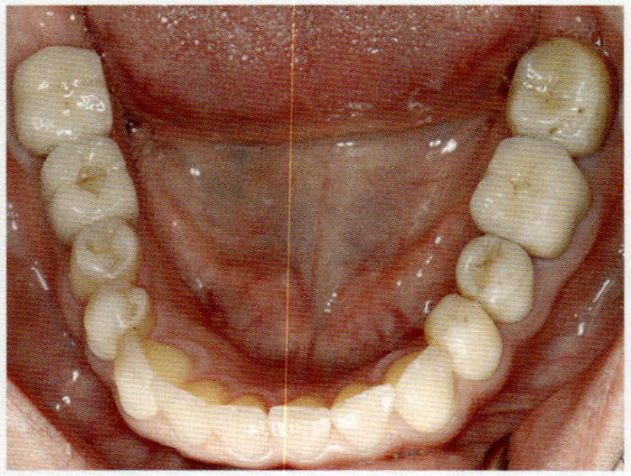

Fig 8-11w
Mandibular arch after restorative treatment.

B. Maxillary arch

Increasing the VDO with direct composite restorations in the mandibular posterior teeth creates a space for previously planned esthetic restorations (porcelain veneers) in the maxillary arch (Figs 8-12a to 8-12s). The quintessence of complex treatment planning was wax-up performed at step 1 (Fig 8-10l). Now, the mock-up created of temporary resin was reapplied. After gaining the patient's approval, the preparation through the mock-up was carried out. The postoperative view is shown in Figs 8-12t to 8-12cc.

FROM THE LITERATURE REVIEW

Increasing the VDO is a biocompatible treatment (it reduces the amount of tissue preparation). In addition, it improves dental and facial esthetics and the proportions of the vertical dimension of the face, and is also a part of the TMJ treatment.[22]

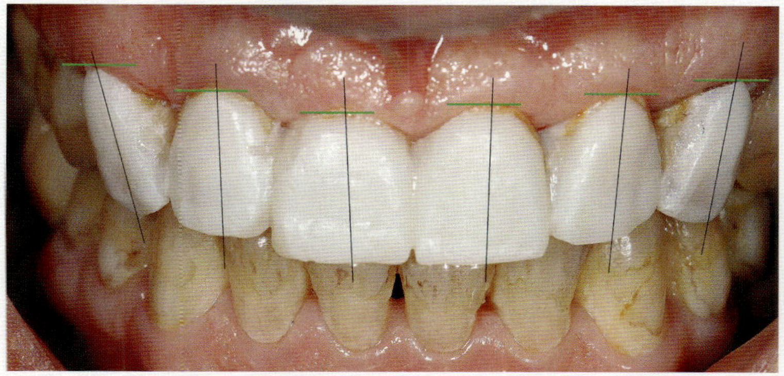

Fig 8-12a
Mock-up created on the basis of the diagnostic wax-up: the location of the zenith of the gingival margin was analyzed, and a cauterization procedure was performed to balance out the symmetry of the gingival line.

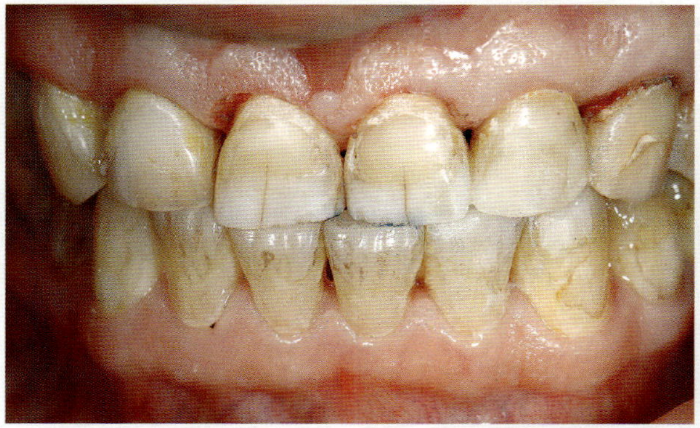

Fig 8-12b
The clinical situation immediately after electrosurgery of the gingiva on teeth 11, 21, and 23.

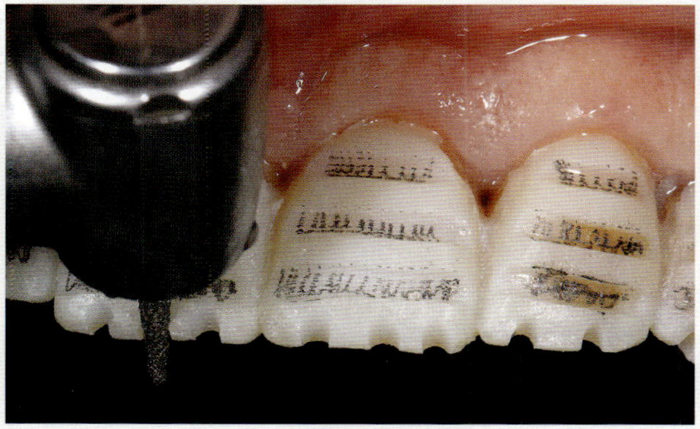

Fig 8-12c
Porcelain veneer preparation was started from the mock-up level, reducing the risk of dentin exposure during preparation.

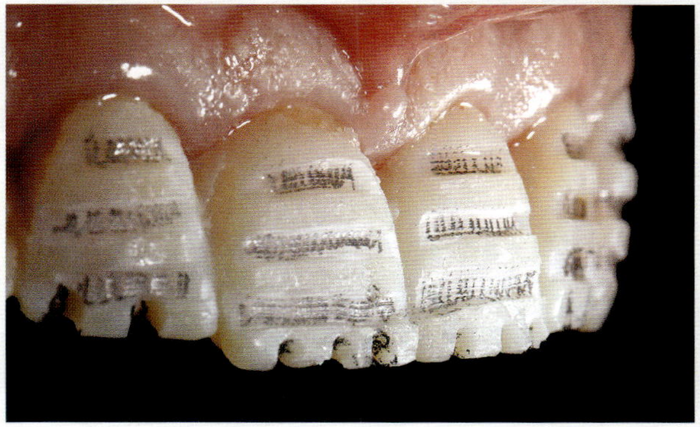

Fig 8-12d
Depth grooves performed on mock-up.

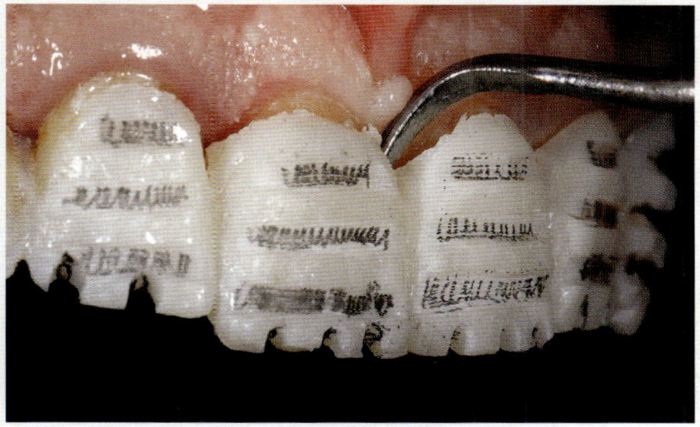

Fig 8-12e
After performing the depth grooves and marking them with a pencil, the mock-up was removed with a curette.

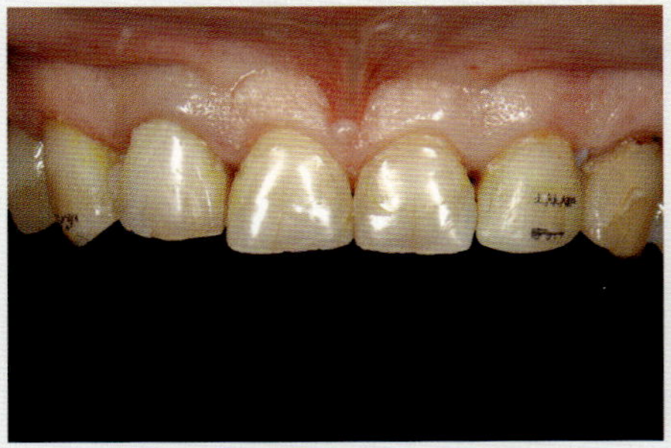

Fig 8-12f
Clinical situation after removing the mock-up: visible, marked depth grooves only on teeth 22 and 13, there is no trace of preparation on the other teeth.

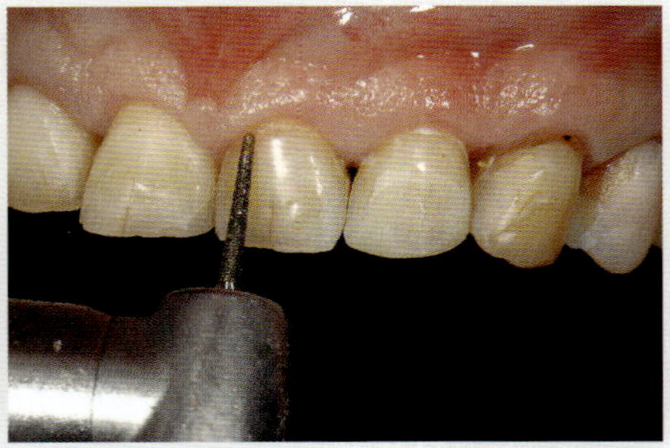

Fig 8-12g
The next step is making the preparation margin, which will be visible for the dental technician and prov de a "stopping point" while cementing veneers.

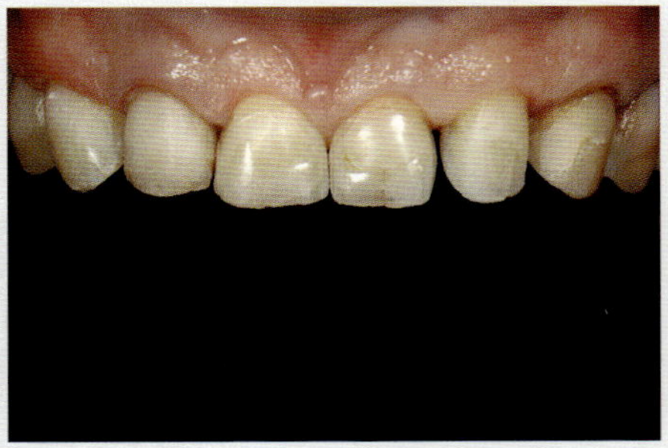

Fig 8-12h
Final minimally invasive veneer preparation.

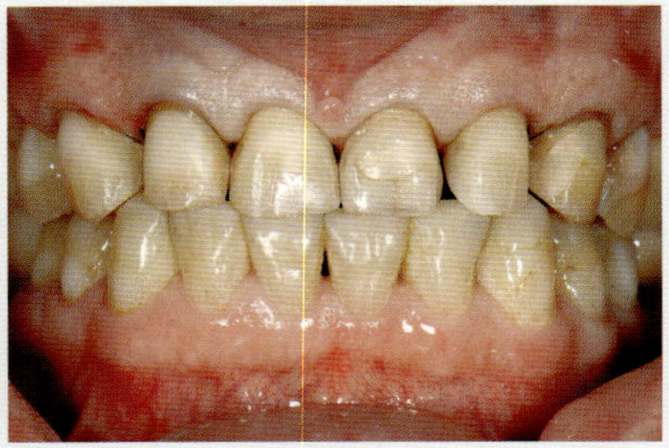

Fig 8-12i
Control of the teeth preparation in maximum intercuspation.

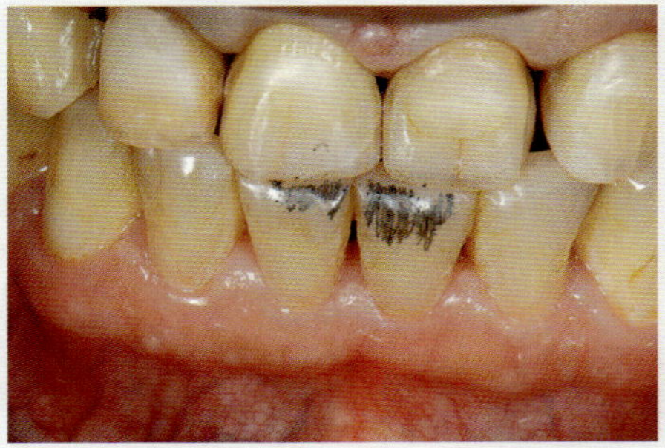

Fig 8-12j
As the mandible teeth have been restored with composite, it is possible to correct them. Hence, the porcelain veneers have enough space, and there is no need to reduce other tissues of the maxillary teeth. Therefore, the reconstruction of the mandibular arch with composite is practical and easy to correct (the photograph shows the area marked with the pencil that needs to be reduced).

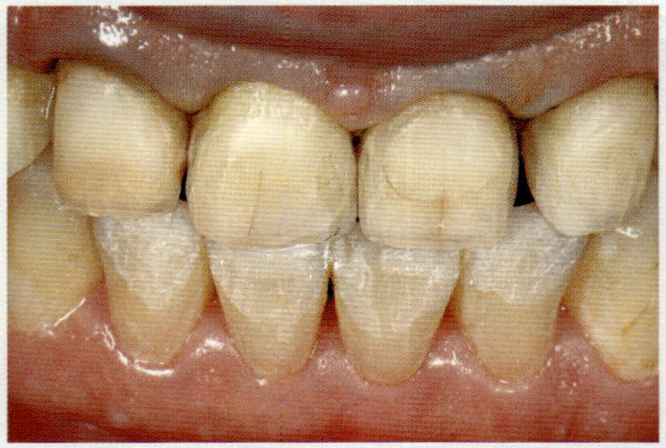

Fig 8-12k
Clinical situation after adjusting the mandibular teeth.

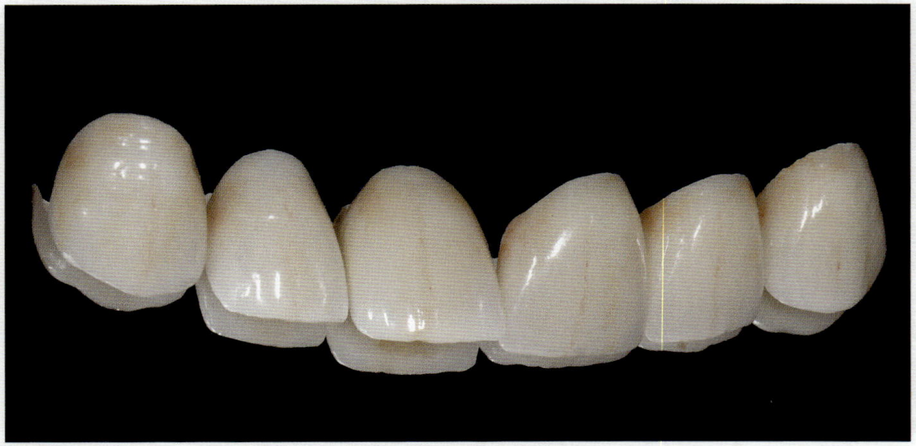

Fig 8-12l
Feldspathic porcelain veneers (IPS InLine, Ivoclar), ready for adhesive preparation and cementation in the oral cavity (laboratory work: DT Artur Nyga).

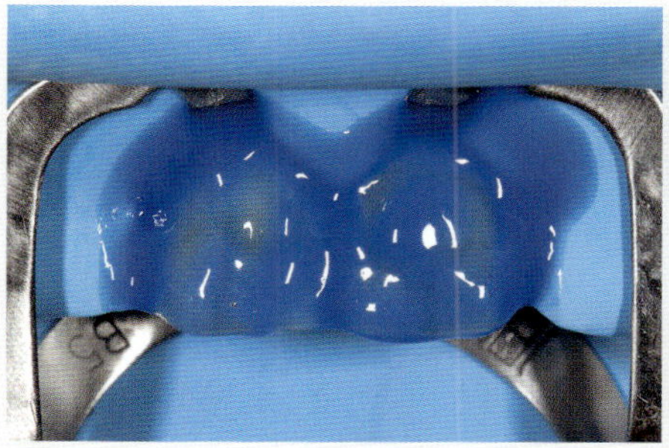

Fig 8-12m
Rubber dam isolation of two central incisors; under local anesthesia, the tooth structure was sandblasted and then etched with orthophosphoric acid for 20 seconds.

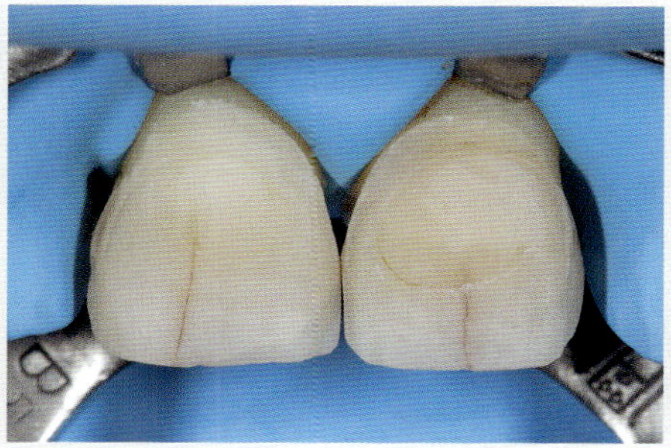

Fig 8-12n
Clinical situation after thorough rinsing of the phosphoric acid …

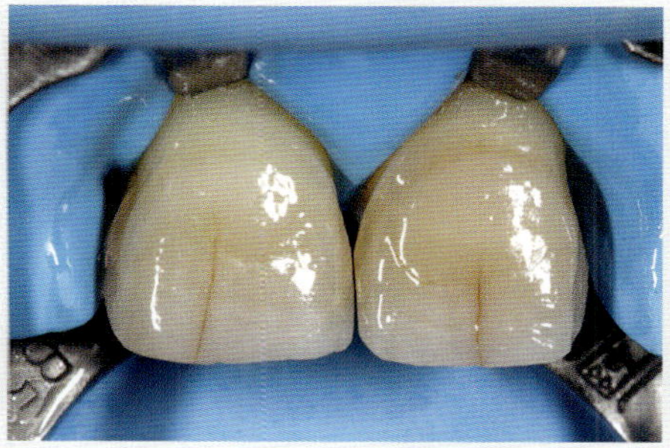

Fig 8-12o
… and after applying the adhesive system.

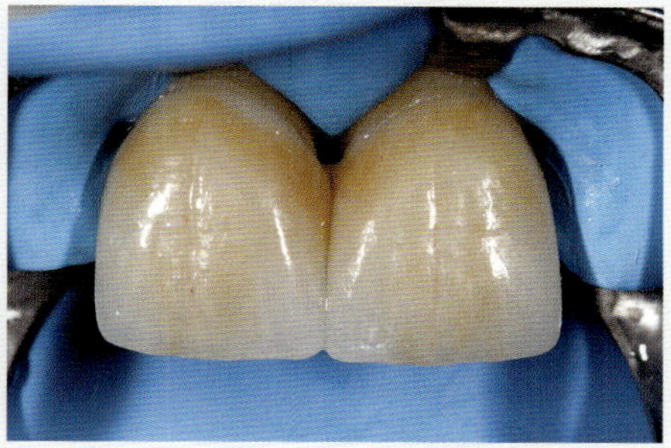

Fig 8-12p
Porcelain veneers were cemented symmetrically in pairs; due to very thin veneers (less than 0.4 mm), Variolink Esthetic LC was used for cementation.

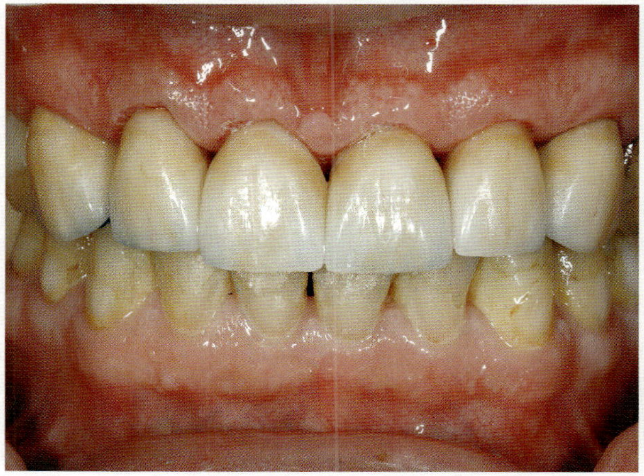

Fig 8-12q
Porcelain veneers on teeth 13–23 immediately after cementing and removing the rubber dam.

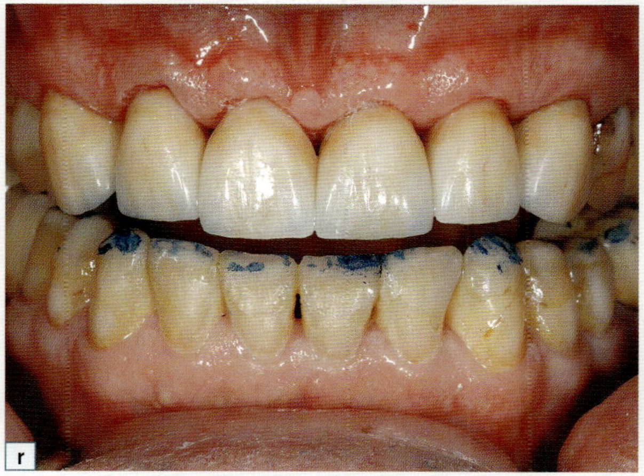

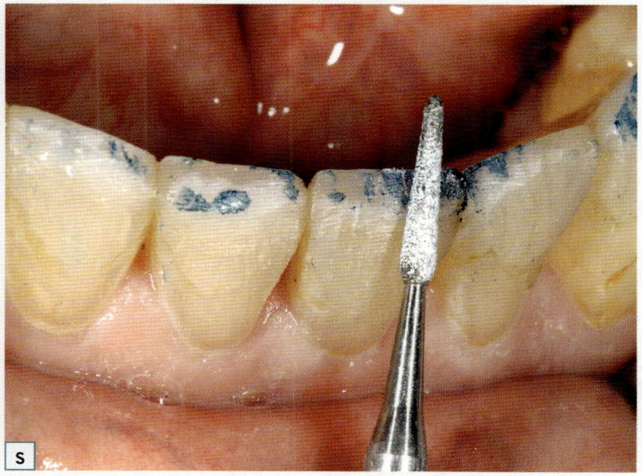

Figs 8-12r and 8-12s
Marking the occlusal-articulation contacts according to the Kois chewing test (200 μm horseshoe articulating paper) and adjust ng in order to eliminate the risk of possible fr ction observed between maxillary and mandibular front teeth.

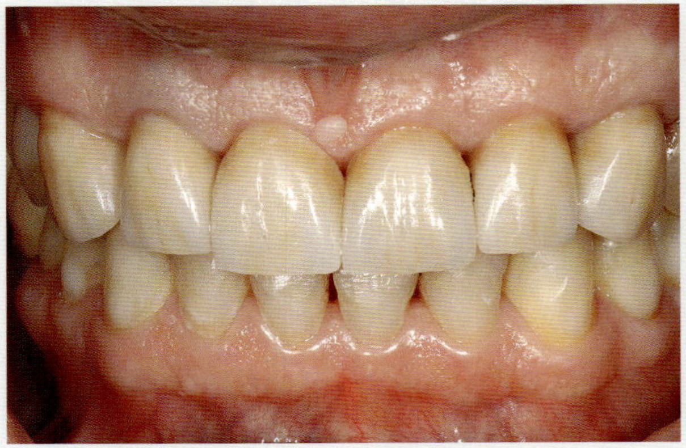

Fig 8-12t
Clinical situation a few weeks after cemetation of porcelain veneers on teeth 13–23.

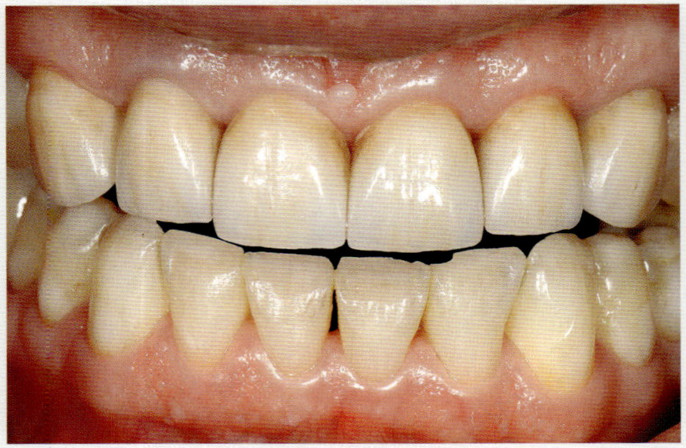

Fig 8-12u
Clinical situation 12 months after restoration. The mandibular arch shows minor chipping of the composite resin in tooth 32, which is considered as an adaptation of the current envelope of function. Chipping of the composite restoration can always be easily restored or polished.

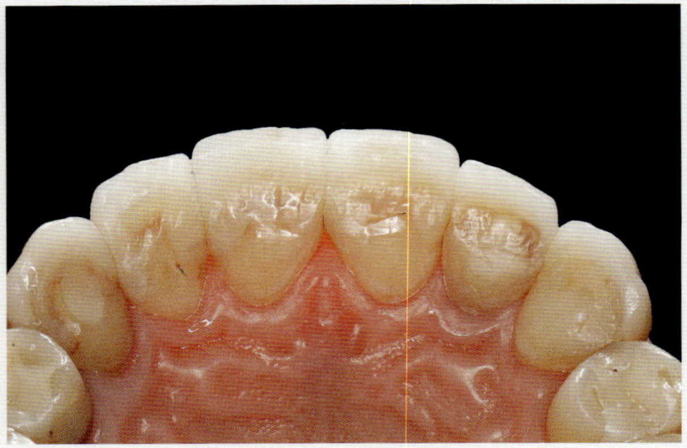

Fig 8-12v
Maxillary arch after reconstruction with porcelain veneers.

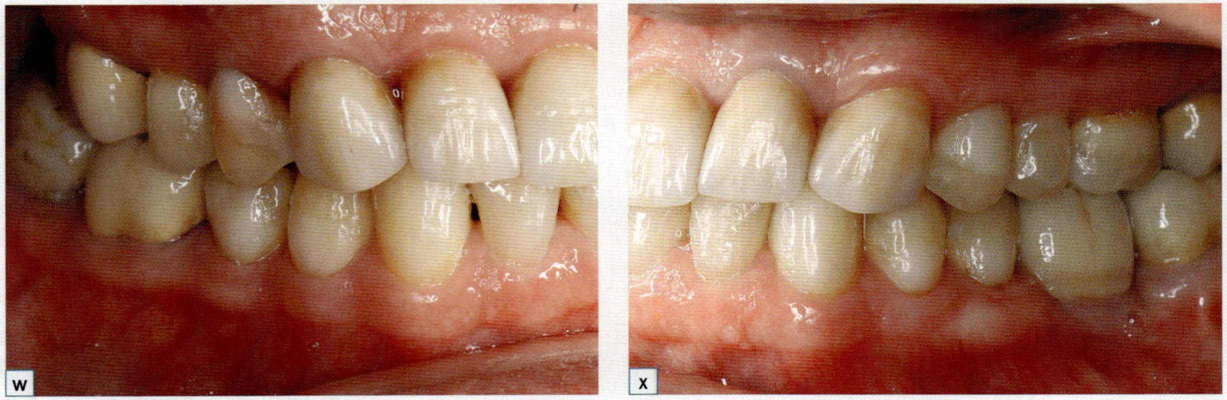

Figs 8-12w and 8-12x
Maxillary and mandibular arches in the maximum intercuspation – view (w) from the right and (x) from the left side.

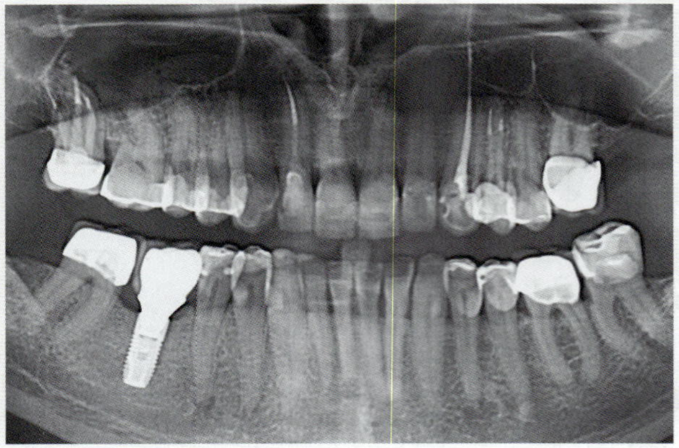

Fig 8-12y
Pantomographic radiograph after complex treatment (teeth 12 and 24 after root canal retreatment; implant in place of tooth 46).

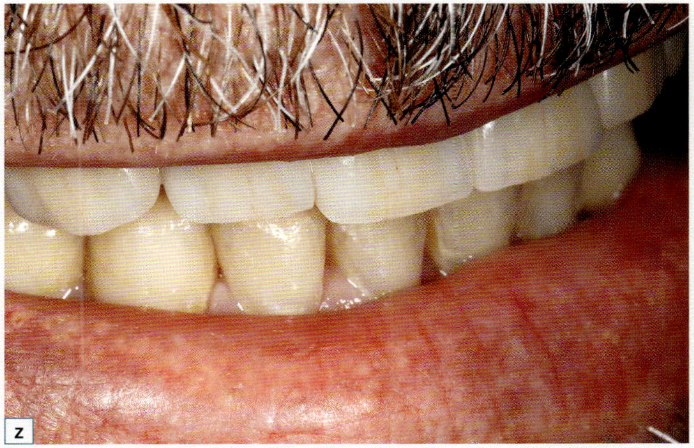

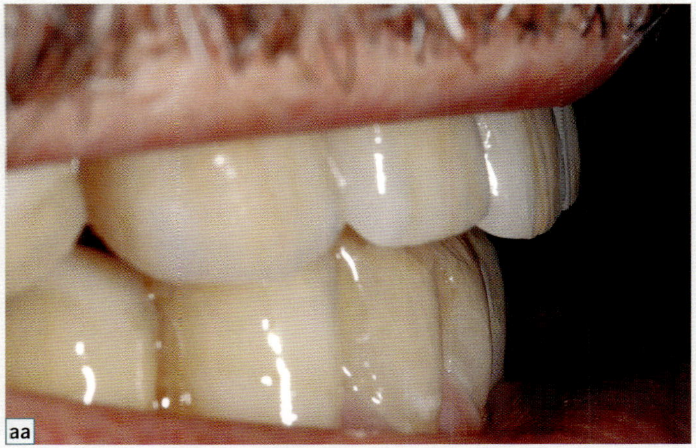

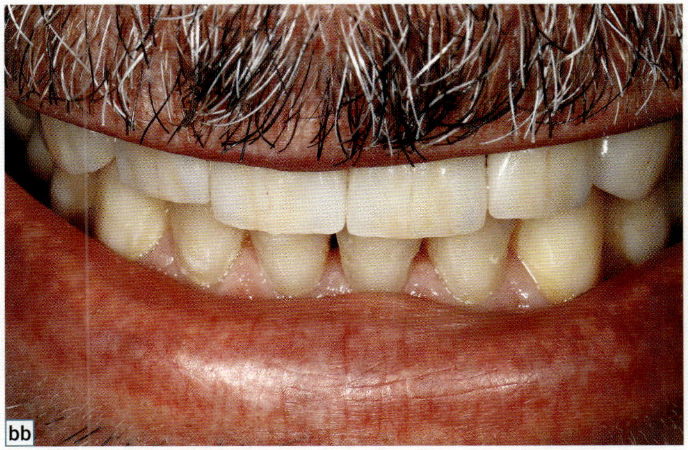

Figs 8-12z to 8-12bb
Photographs of the patient's smile from (z, aa) semi-profile and (bb) en face after treatment.

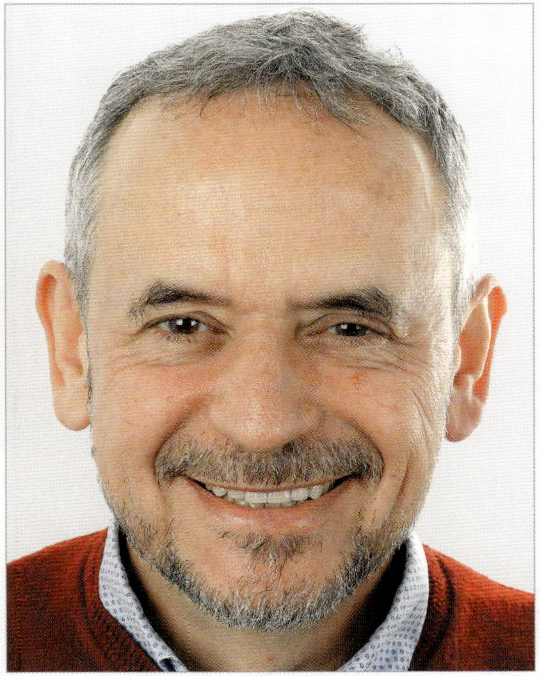

Fig 8-12cc
Photograph of the patient's face with a new smile after treatment.

OCCLUSAL DYSFUNCTION

If, after deprogramming the patient, in centric relation (CR) position, the mandible draws back and the first contact points appear on the posterior teeth, we can talk about occlusal dysfunction. In the process of avoiding premature contacts, the patient looks for a new, most comfortable position while grinding the other teeth, most often generating a horizontal wear pattern.[16,32–36]

A typical symptom of occlusal dysfunction is, for example, when the third molar of the maxilla is overerupted and represents a significant premature contact, which, bypassed by the lower jaw, wears other teeth. Another cause of occlusal dysfunction is the lack of the first molars, which causes the adjacent molars to incline, and the consequence is the lack of simultaneous bilateral support on the posterior teeth. In such a clinical situation, the patient's central nervous system begins to look for another, more comfortable position to bite the teeth while wearing the teeth.

Depending on the level of the tooth wear, treatment may include:

- Removal of premature contacts and equilibration of the occlusion (ie, achieving bilateral balanced occlusal contacts in the posterior segment)
- Reconstruction of the new occlusal surfaces in both arches or one of them in order to obtain bilateral balanced occlusal contact points in the posterior segment

Premature occlusal contacts

Premature contact occurs during jaw closure (when the conduces in CR) before achieving maximum intercuspation. The presence of interference can lead to temporomandibular joint (TMJ) overload and its pathology. The articular disc can change its position and lead to a huge overload of the TMJ anatomical structures.

Case 6: Occlusal dysfunction

A 54-year-old patient presented to the dental office to improve the esthetics of the anterior teeth (Figs 8-13a to 8-13f). Relevant information for treatment planning was obtained while collecting medical history:

- Generalized tooth wear had intensified, especially in the last 5 years, proving that the anterior segment's tooth wear process had accelerated.
- The patient did not have equal simultaneous bilateral contacts while biting the teeth and had difficulties fitting the mandibular and maxillary dental arches against each other.
- In the past, he had noticed clenching of his teeth during the day, which he associated with a stressful lifestyle.

The TMJ loading and immobilization tests were negative; the patient did not indicate any symptoms related to TMJ. The clinical examination revealed symptoms of anterior teeth overloading – fremitus was detected while mandible closing to the maximum intercuspation. The left lateral incisor had a gingival pocket with a depth of 5.5 mm, which was related to anterior overload. In the anterior teeth, a horizontal wear pattern was found. Additionally, the erosion problem was overlapping (Figs 8-13g and 8-13h). The patient was referred to the dental hygienist for routine scaling and root planing, oral hygiene instruction was given, and information was provided about the effect of diet on teeth (erosions).

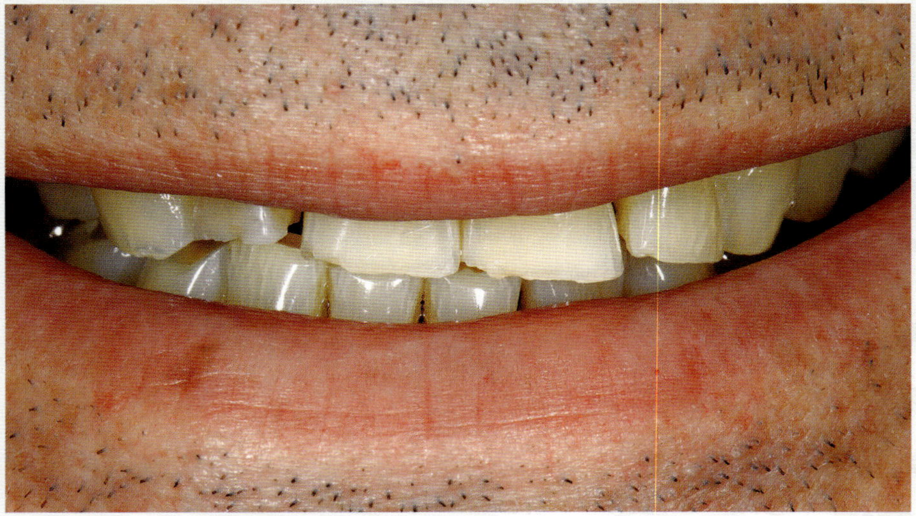

Fig 8-13a
A patient presented to the dental office because of visible tooth wear in the anterior segment. He noticed that the tooth wear had become more visible in the last 5 years.

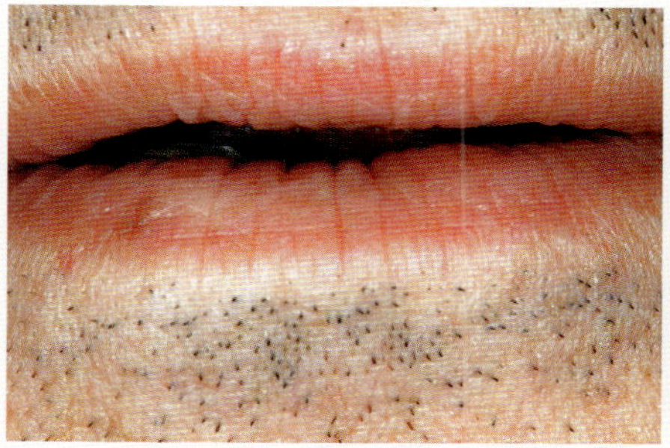

Fig 8-13b
Lips in repose: the lack of maxillary incisors display indicates that elongation of the anterior maxillary teeth should be considered when planning the treatment.

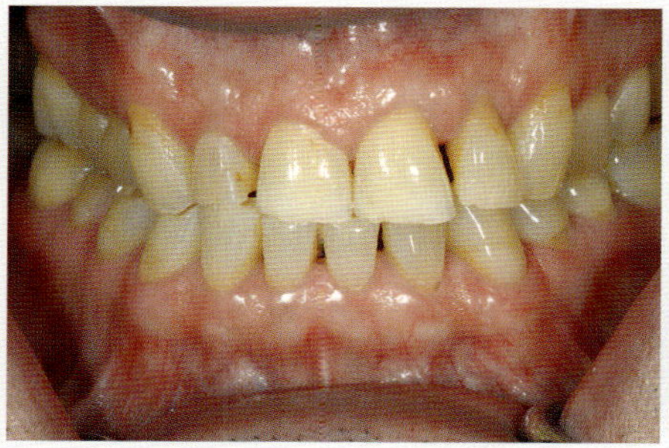

Fig 8-13c
Intraoral photograph of the teeth in the maximum intercuspation.

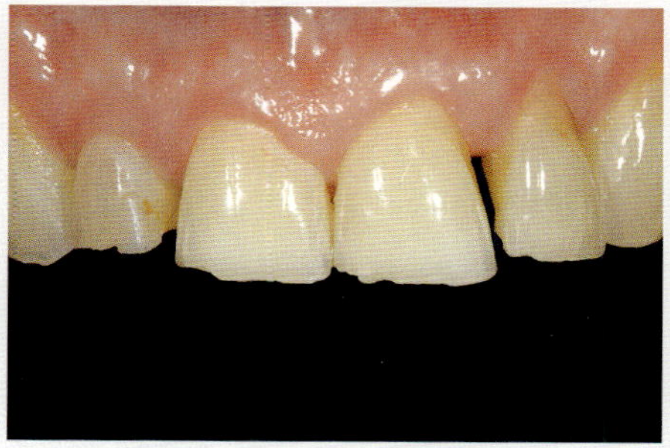

Fig 8-13d
A photograph of the anterior maxillary teeth shows the level of the teeth wear.

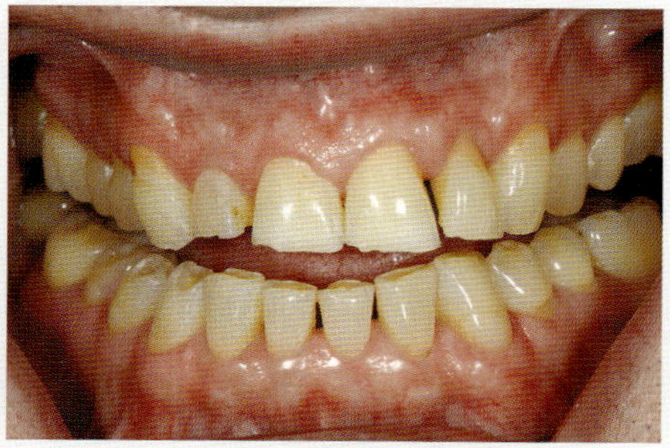

Fig 8-13e
The intraoral photograph shows the extend of wear in the maxillary and mandibular arches.

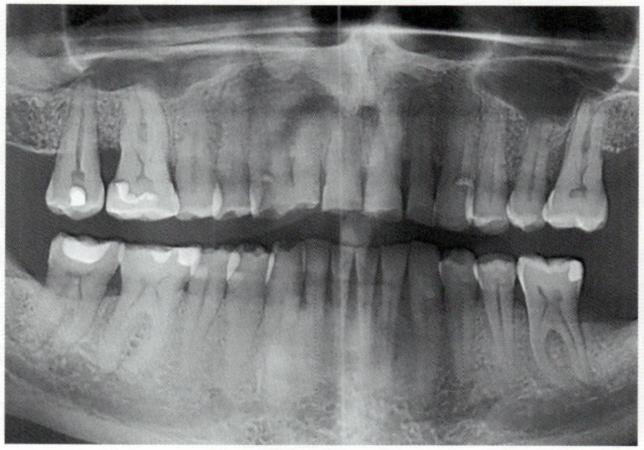

Fig 8-13f
Pantomographic radiograph – visible atrophic periodontal changes in the anterior segment, especially around tooth 22 (due to overload). Relieving the anterior segment by increasing the VDO and obtaining bilateral balanced occlusal contacts will also have a therapeutic goal for the periodontium.

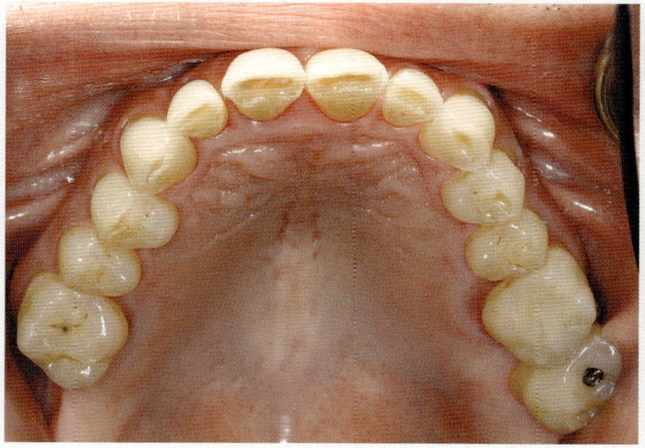

Fig 8-13g
Maxillary arch – visible facets of wear with overlapping erosions.

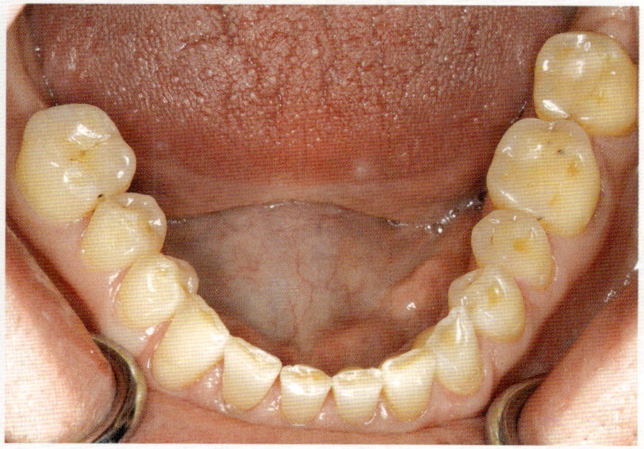

Fig 8-13h
Mandibular arch – visible facets of wear with horizontal pattern and overlapping erosions.

Step 1: Esthetic treatment planning

Digital Smile Design (DSD) was performed to prepare the diagnostic wax-up (Fig 8-13i). Impressions and facebow registration were transferred to the dental laboratory along with photographic documentation. Next, the dental technician created an esthetic wax-up (Fig 8-13j) of six anterior maxillary teeth which, after the dentist's approval, was used to create a silicone index and a mock-up (Fig 8-13k). Thanks to the mock-up, the esthetic treatment plan was explained to the patient. The patient and the consultation team accepted the mock-up, and thus it was possible to proceed to step 2.

Step 2: Centric relation (CR)

As the TMJ load test was negative, a Kois Deprogrammer was fabricated, which the patient used for four weeks during the day and at night. The appointment after 4 weeks confirmed the suspected diagnosis of occlusal dysfunction, as the first contact points without the deprogrammer were observed in the posterior segment. The centric relation was registered, and the bite registration was transferred to the dental laboratory, thanks to which the models were mounted in the articulator in a CR (Fig 8-13l). The models were carefully studied in the articulator to understand the range of vertical dimension of occlusion (VDO) alteration that will relieve new.

Step 3: Functional wax-up

As there was no need to significantly increase the VDO to realize an esthetic treatment plan, it was decided to restore only the occlusal surfaces of the mandibular arch (Fig 8-13m). The wax-up visualized the treatment plan and served as a matrix for direct restorations assembly in the posterior segment.

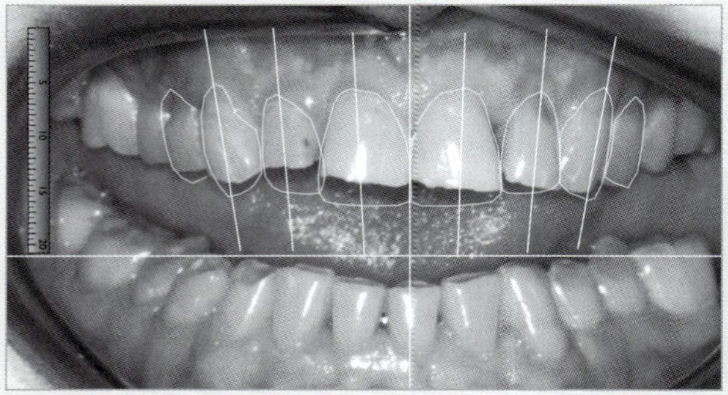

Fig 8-13i
Digital Smile Design (DSD).

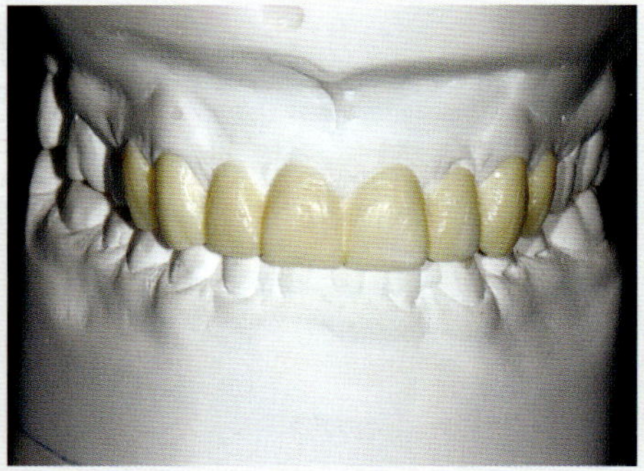

Fig 8-13j
Initial esthetic wax-up of maxillary anteriors in order to visualize the treatment plan.

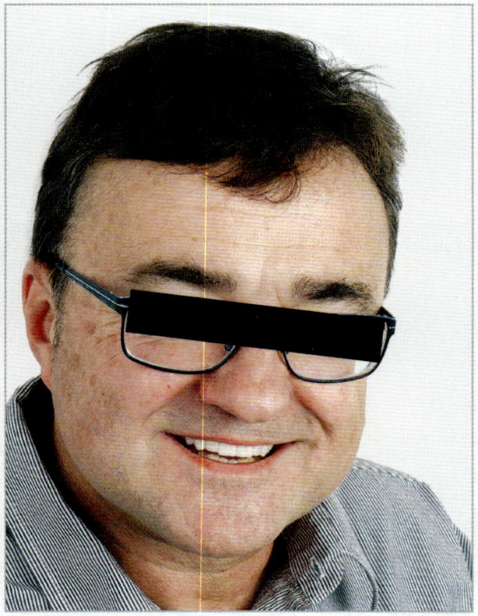

Fig 8-13k
Mock-up (Protemp) created with a silicone index taken from the diagnostic wax-up.

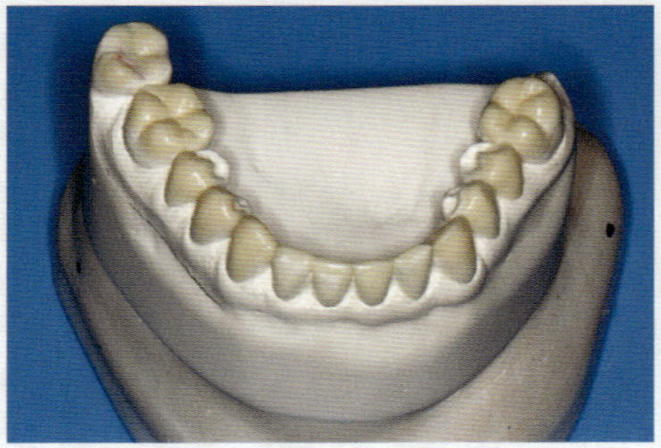

Fig 8-13l
Functional wax-up of the posterior segment created after mounting the models in the articulator in a CR.

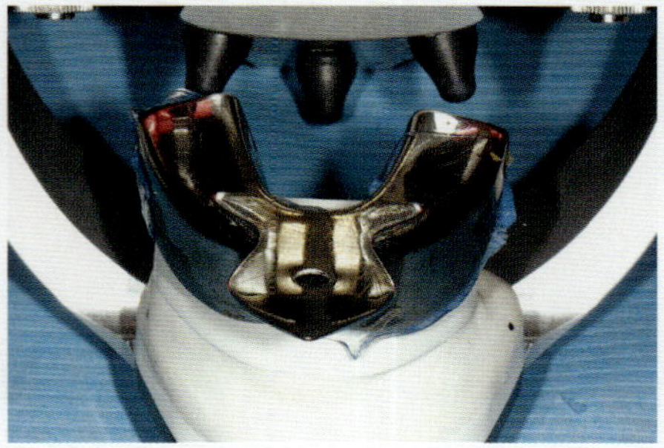

Fig 8-13m
Taking a transparent silicone index from the wax-up of the mandibular arch.
Note: before taking the impression, you need to put vaseline on the model!

Step 4: Restorative treatment

A. Direct restorations – no preparation

A transparent silicone index taken from the diagnostic wax-up (Fig 8-13n) was cut into segments corresponding to individual teeth. The fit was checked on the models and in the oral cavity. After rubber dam isolation (Fig 8-13o), the adhesive addition of the composite resin was obtained (Figs 8-13p to 8-13z) in the same way as shown in Fig 8-11. After restoring the posterior teeth, direct restoration of the front teeth was performed (Figs 8-13aa to 8-13nn). The final result of the direct restoration of the mandibular arch is shown in Figs 8-13oo and 8-11pp.

As the maxillary anteriors showed significant tooth wear, they were restored with direct composite during the same visit. For this purpose, an index made of hard laboratory silicone was used; first the palatal and the proximal surfaces were created. Then, step by step, the dentin layer followed by an enamel layer was applied (Fig 8-14). In the case of maxillary teeth, the reconstructions were considered as provisional, as porcelain veneers were planned.

PRACTITIONER'S ADVICE

The silicone index should be at least 1 cm thick above the occlusal surface to ensure the stiffness of the segment during reconstruction with the composite resin.

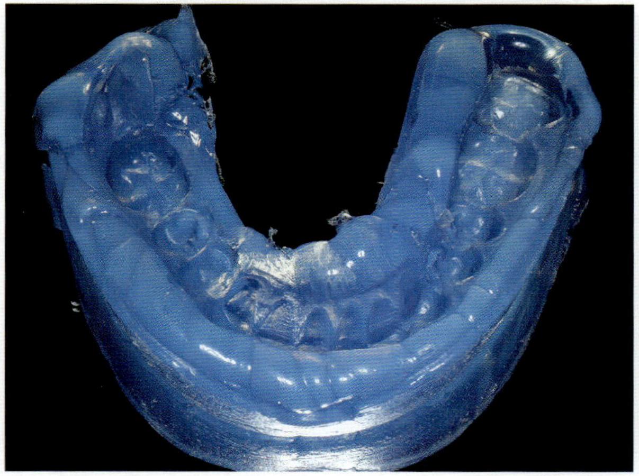

Fig 8-13n
Transparent silicone index (Memosil 2, Kulzer) ready for segmentation (the index should be at least 1 cm thick above the occlusal surface to ensure adequate rigidity while performing the restoration). The right choice of material helps to maintain rigidity after cutting into segments.

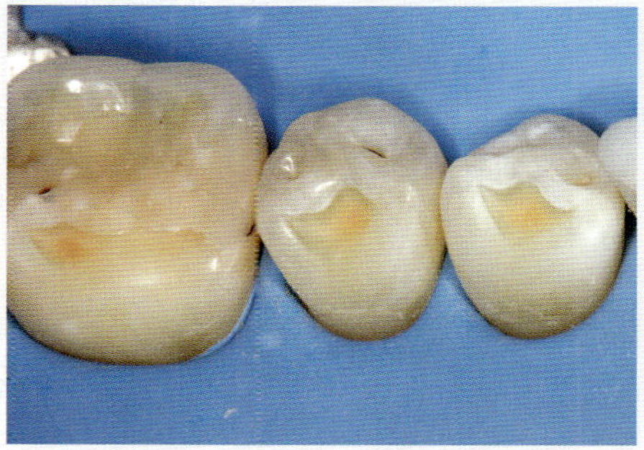

Fig 8-13o
Posterior teeth isolated with a rubber dam.

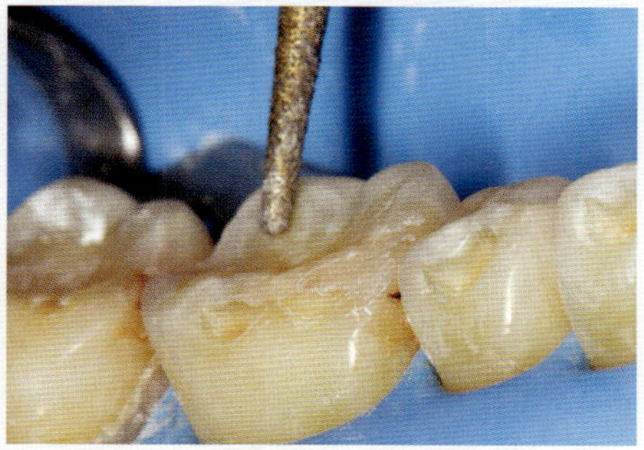

Fig 8-13p
Roughening the occlusal surface of the posterior teeth with a diamond bur before reconstruction.

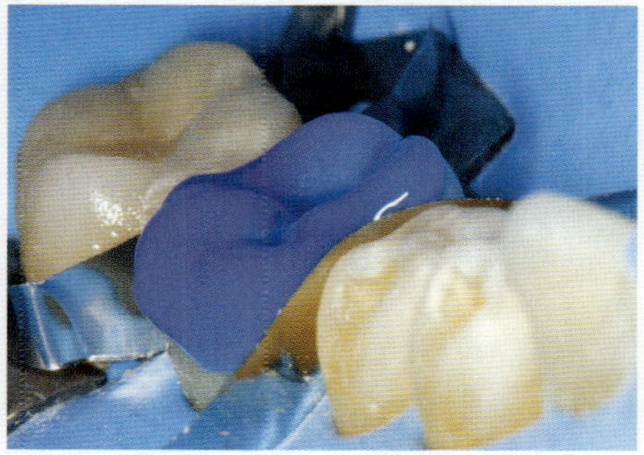

Fig 8-13q
Etching the tooth surfaces with orthophosphoric acid (20 seconds). Care should be taken to separate the adjacent teeth with metal strips.

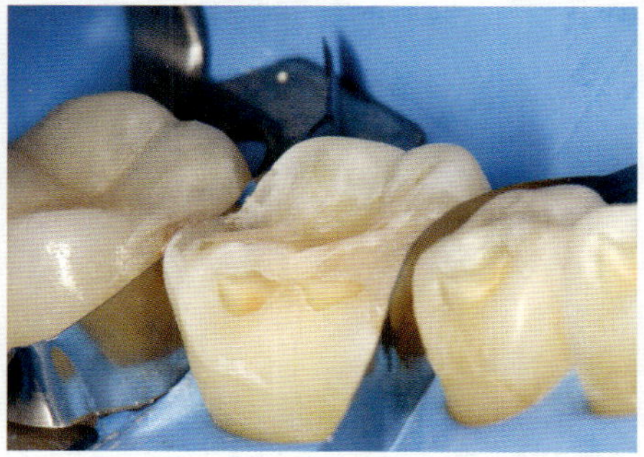

Fig 8-13r
Clinical situation after rinsing the orthophosphoric acid and gentle drying of the tooth surface.

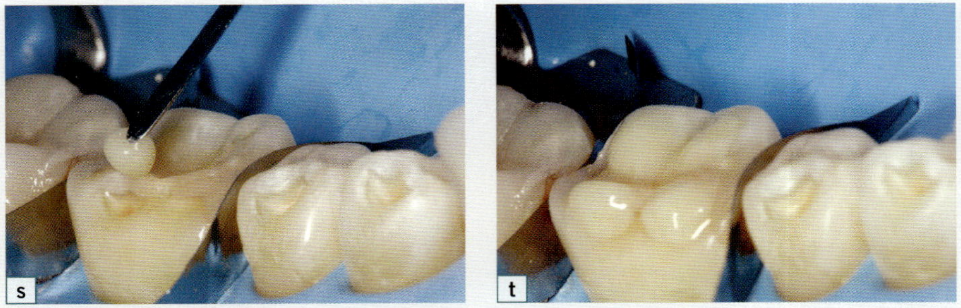

Figs 8-13s and 8-13t
After application and light-curing of the bonding system, the dentin layer was applied in four portions on each of the tooth cusps ...

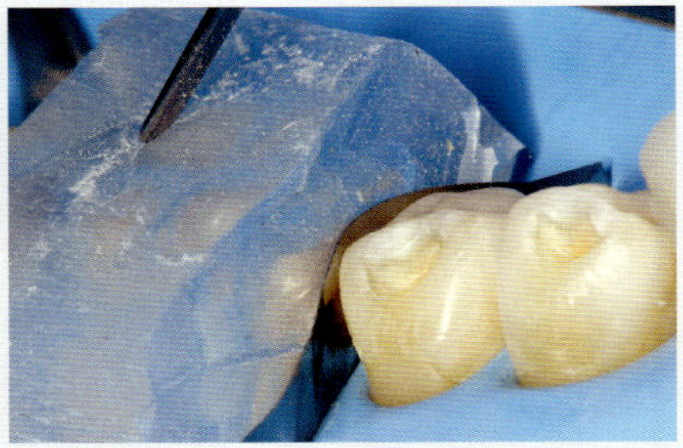

Fig 8-13u
... then, the silicone index was placed on the tooth, so the dentin layer would not exceed the planned tooth volume.

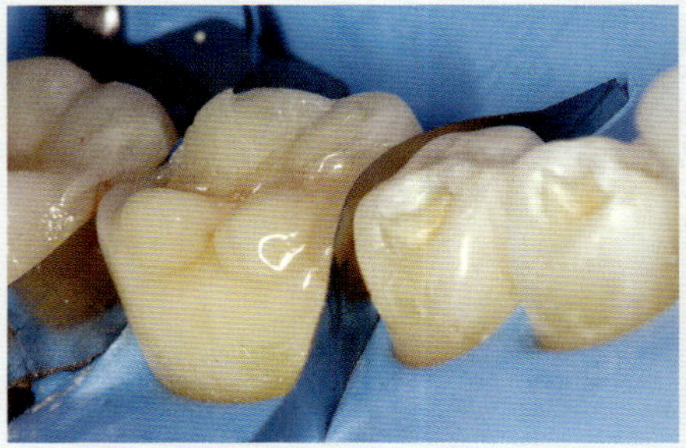

Fig 8-13v
Polymerization through the index and additional curing after index removal.

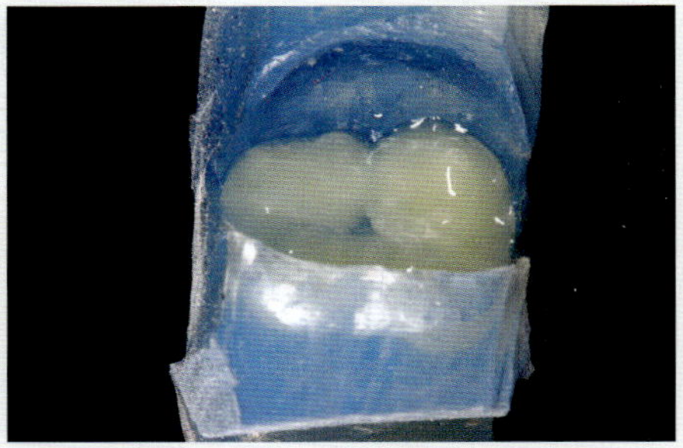

Fig 8-13w
The outer enamel layer applied in the index was then positioned on the tooth surface. Final polymerization was carried out through the index, and then directly without the index ...

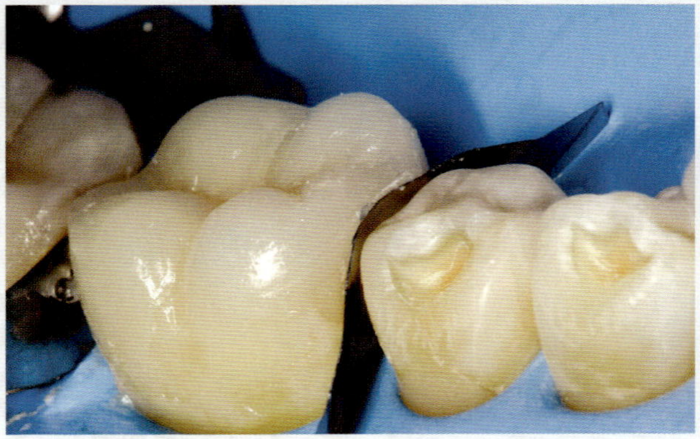

Fig 8-13x
... a final anatomical result was achieved corresponding to the previous wax-up.

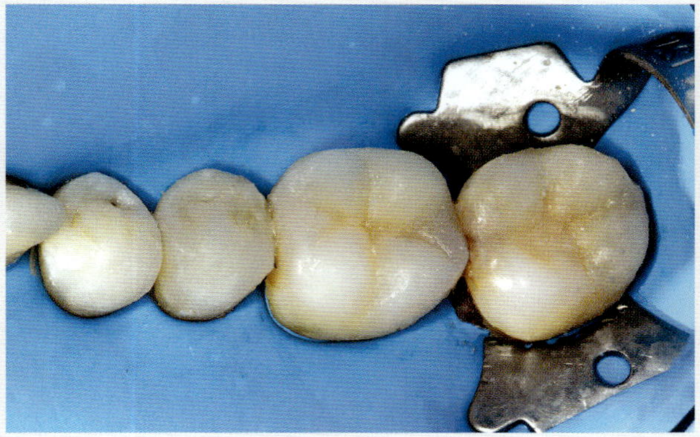

Fig 8-13y
Final outcome after reconstructing one mandibular quadrant ...

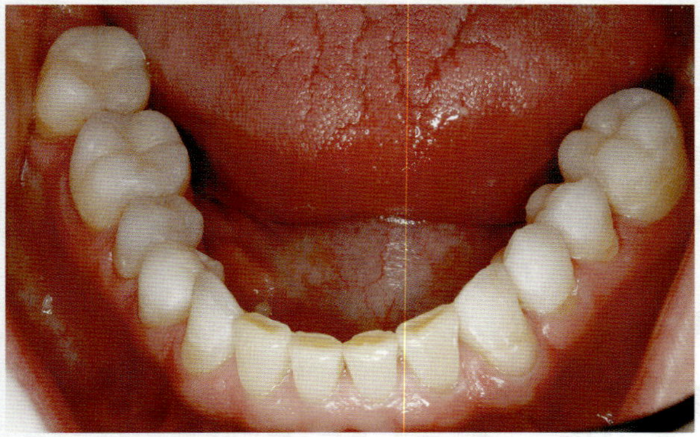

Fig 8-13z
... and after reconstructing two lateral quadrants.

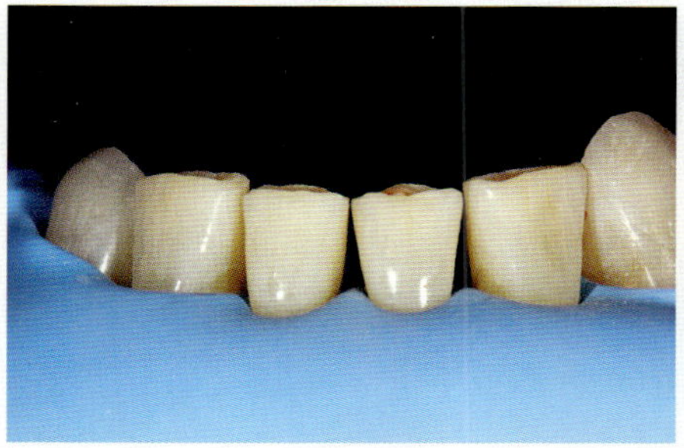

Fig 8-13aa
Isolation of the anterior teeth before direct composite restorations.

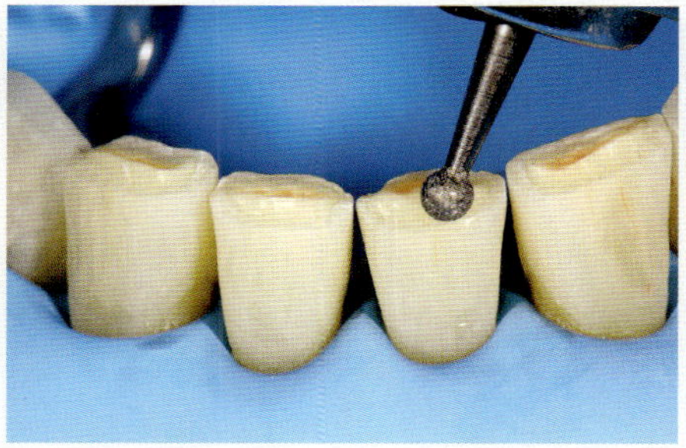

Fig 8-13bb
Chamfer was performed with a ball-shaped diamond bur no. 12.

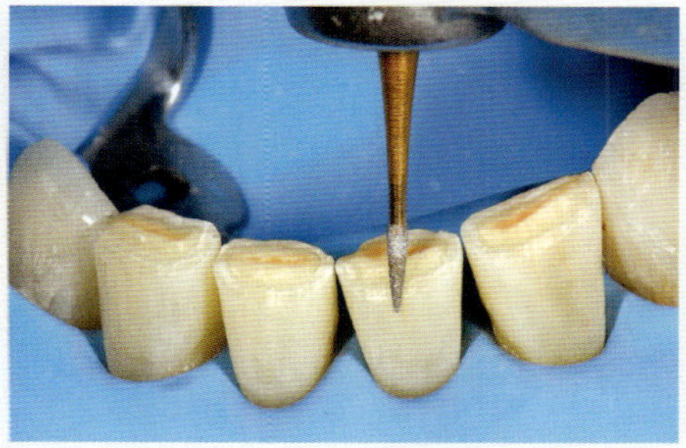

Fig 8-13cc
Extending the chamfer with a bevel. Chamfer and bevel are obtained to enlarge the adhesive marginal adaptation surface and facilitate an esthetic transition between the composite and the tooth surfaces.

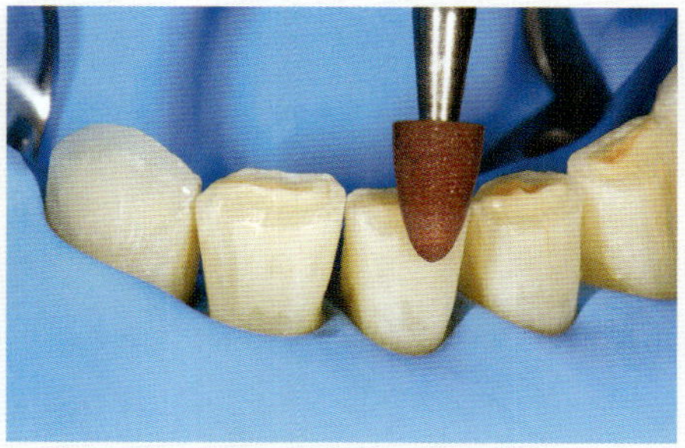

Fig 8-13dd
Polishing the bevels to improve the final composite restorations (Brownie Polisher).

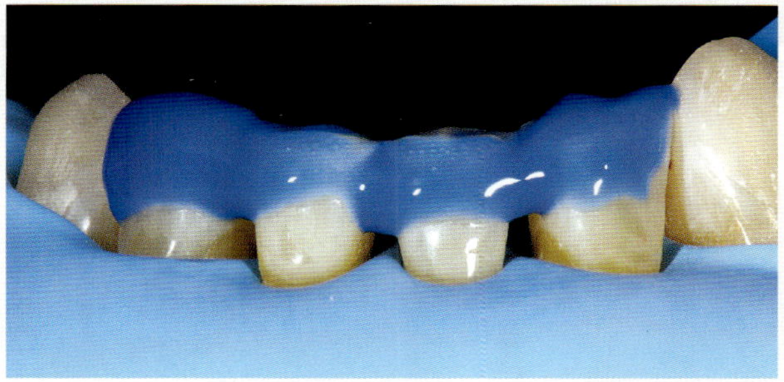

Fig 8-13ee
Etching the hard tissues with orthophosphoric acid.

PRACTITIONER'S ADVICE

A chamfer and a bevel on the labial surface of the mandibular teeth enhance the adhesion of the restoration, reduce the risk of chipping, and improve the color merge of the anterior restoration.

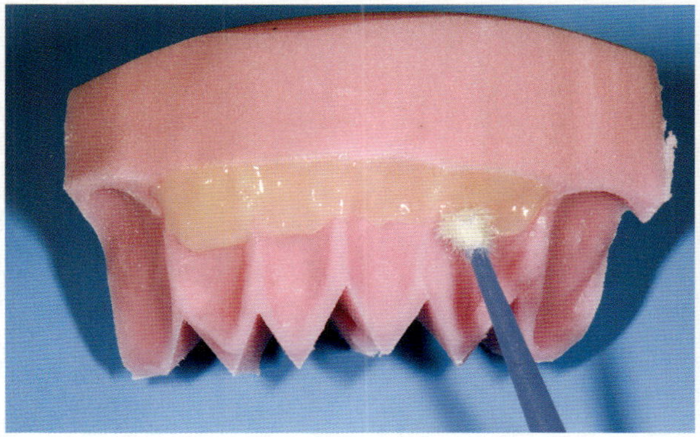

Fig 8-13ff
Application of the enamel composite resin to reconstruct the lingual surfaces (Essentia LE, GC).

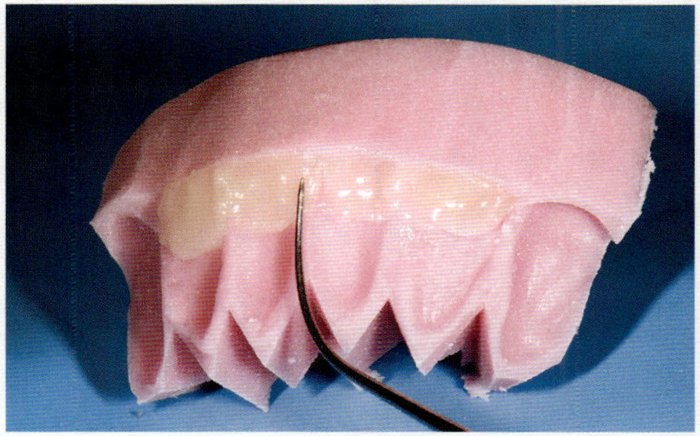

Fig 8-13gg
Composite resin excess removal with the Fissura instrument (LM Arte) to avoid the risk of teeth splinting.

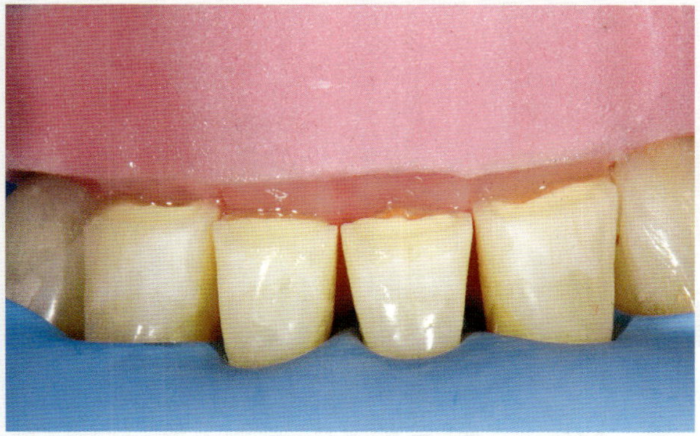

Fig 8-13hh
Silicone index with the composite resin placed in the correct position.

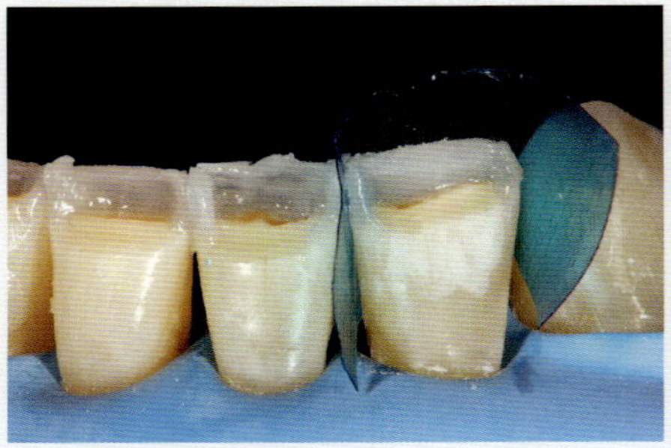

Fig 8-13ii
The proximal surfaces were created with the Varistrip matrix. In this way, the enamel frame of the restoration (Essentia LE, GC) was obtained to facilitate further resin application.

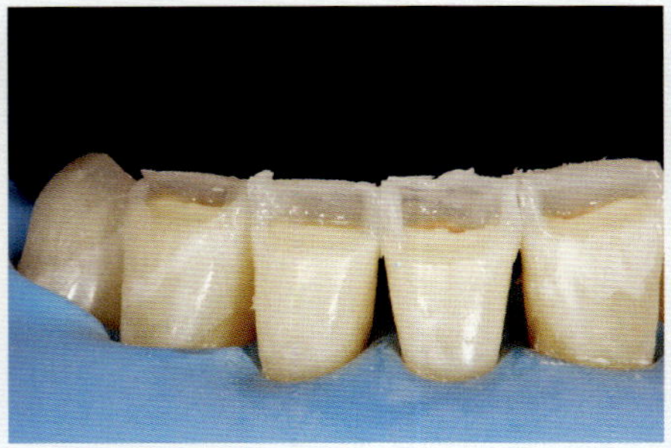

Fig 8-13jj
All lower anterior teeth have been transformed into frames ...

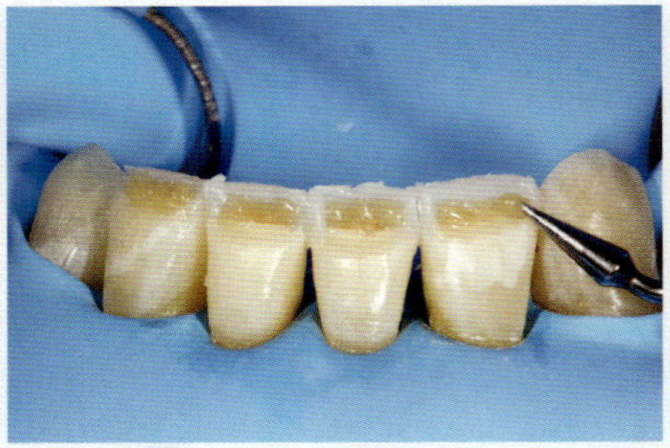

Fig 8-13kk
... the dentin layer was applied ...

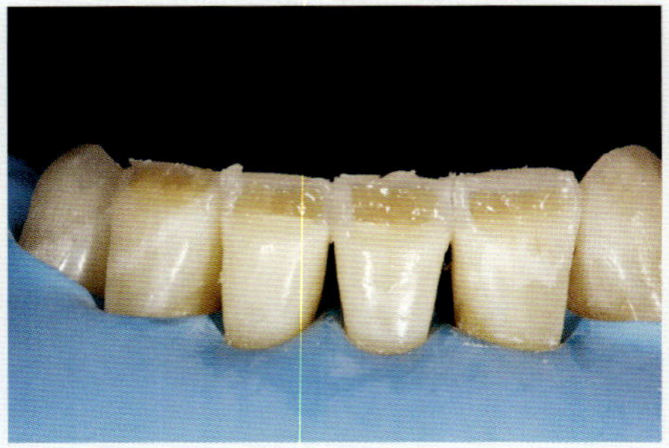

Fig 8-13ll
... and, after making sure that there was enough space for the outer enamel composite, the dentin layer (Essentia MD, GC) was polymerized.

Fig 8-13mm
After the enamel layer (Essentia DE, GC) was applied and finally cured, the surface characterization was obtained by means of a pencil (to draw the transition lines) and a bur no. 831-204-012.

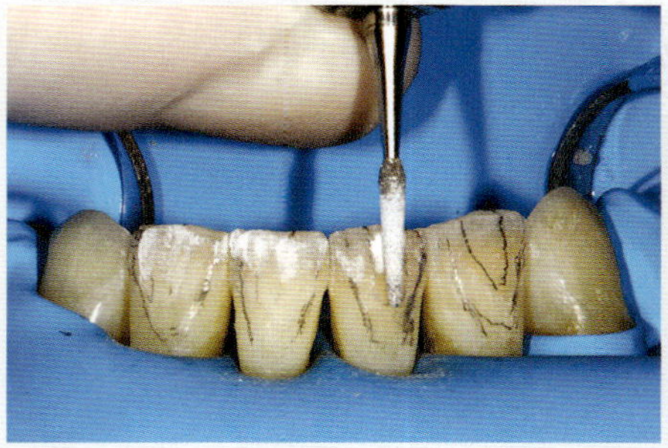

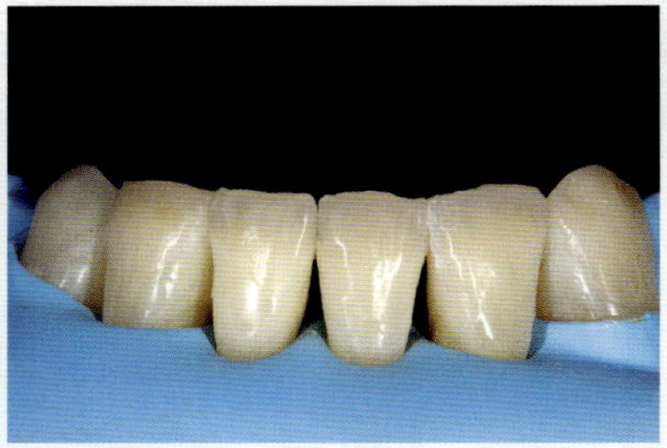

Fig 8-13nn
Clinical situation after direct composite restorations and initial characterization of mandibular incisors.

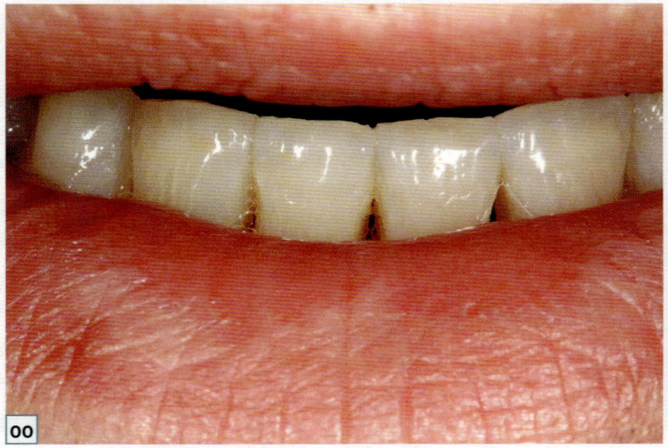

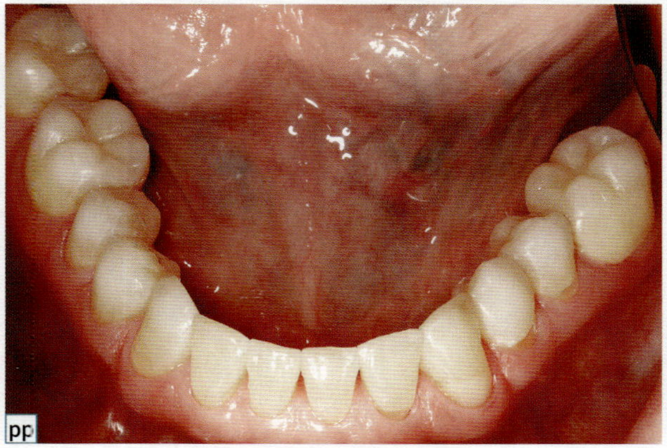

PRACTITIONER'S ADVICE

Creating a frame while restoring the anterior tooth facilitates achieving both the desired tooth shape and adequate color.

Figs 8-13oo and 8-13pp
(oo) Postoperative view of the mandibular incisors after removing the rubber dam. (pp) Mandibular arch after direct composite restoration.

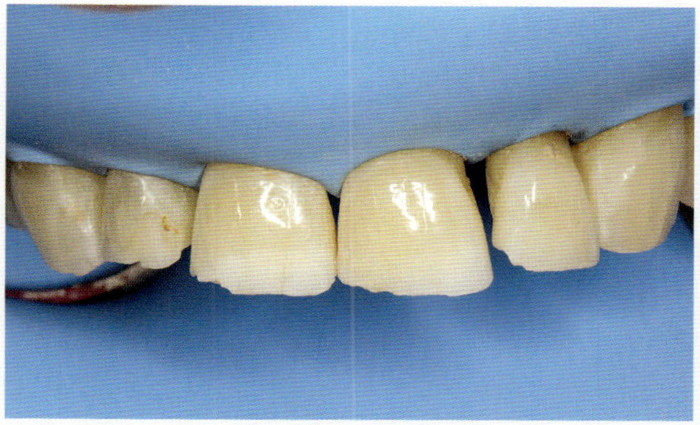

Fig 8-14a
Rubber dam isolation of the maxillary incisors before starting the reconstruction.

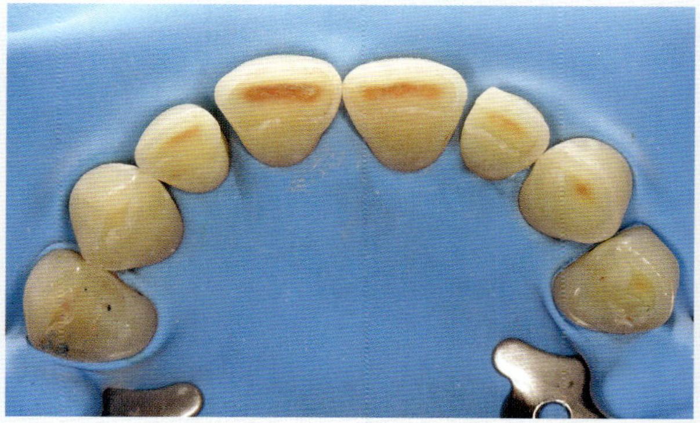

Fig 8-14b
View from the incisal edge after air abrasion with aluminum oxide (50 μm).

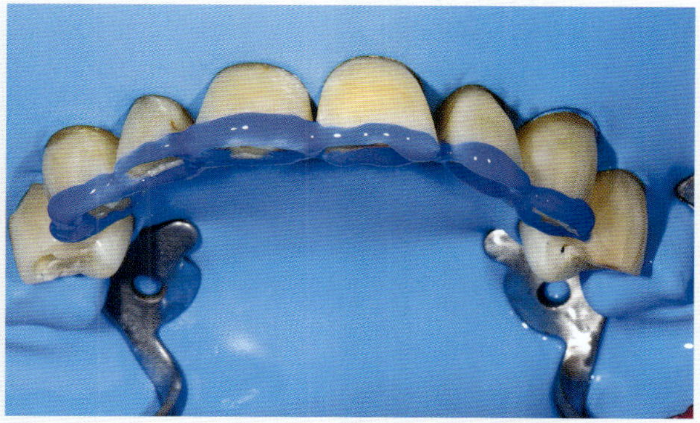

Fig 8-14c
Etching the tooth surface with orthophosphoric acid.

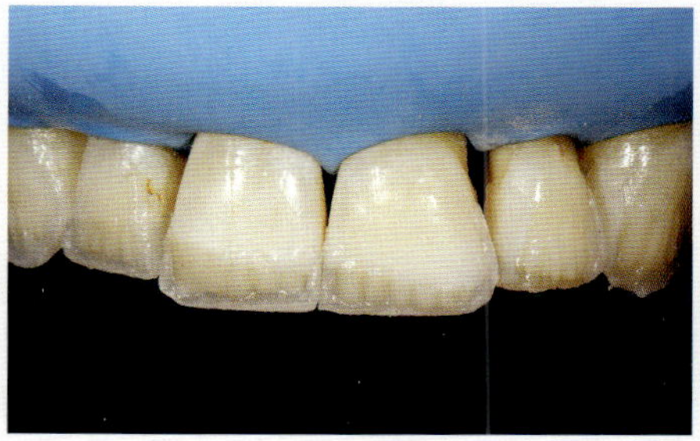

Fig 8-14d
The palatal surface fabrication with enamel composite resin, creating the enamel frame and then application of the mamelons with dentin composite resin.

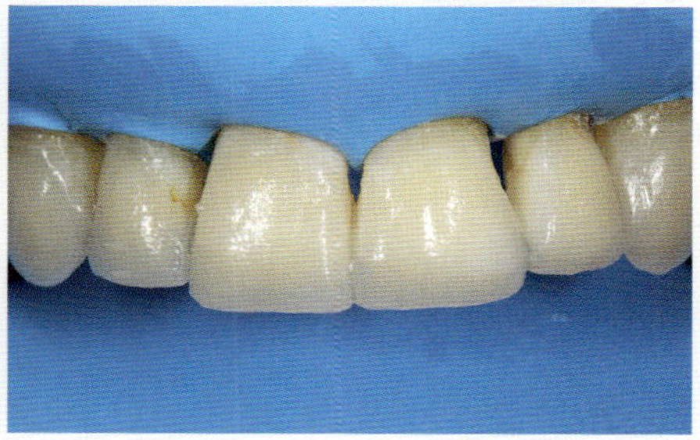

Fig 8-14e
Clinical situation after the direct restoration of the maxillary incisors with composite resin.

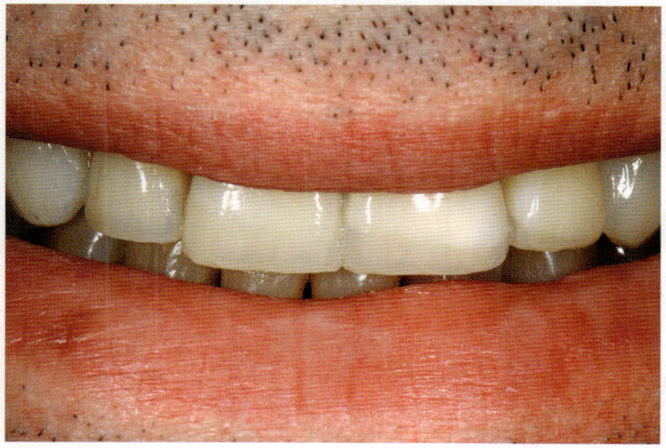

Fig 8-14f
Patient's smile after full occlusal rehabilitation with direct composite resin in one day (maxillary incisors will be covered with porcelain veneers).

B. Porcelain veneers

At the next appointment, the esthetic plan was finalized (see Figs 8-13i to 8-13k). Direct restorations performed in the maxillary anteriors were considered as mock-up, and tooth preparation was controlled constantly by the silicone index (Figs 8-15a to 8-15c) to minimize the removal of the enamel. In order to improve tooth axis lines and close the interdental spaces, tooth preparation involved the contact surfaces (teeth such us 11, 21 and 22; Fig 8-15c). At the next appointment, laboratory-fabricated feldspathic porcelain veneers were tried in and cemented (Fig 8-15d). All adhesive procedures (Figs 8-15e to 8-15j), including veneer cementation, were performed in rubber dam isolation. The immediate esthetic effect is shown in Fig 8-15k. A few days later, the symmetry of anterior guidance (Fig 8-15l) and the lateral guidance through the canines (Figs 8-15m and 8-15n) was verified.

At the follow-up visits, equilibration was performed with the aim to achieve the multiple, bilateral occlusal contact points in the posterior teeth (Fig 8-15o; Parkell articulating paper 21 μm), and the free passage of 8 μm articulating paper between the anterior teeth. Next, the chewing test (according to Dr. John Kois) was performed (Fig 8-15p; 200 μm horseshoe articulating paper). Intensively marked anterior surfaces were eliminated step by step to minimize the interferences while chewing. A Profin handpiece transformed intensive marks into delicate anterior guidance lines (Fig 8-15q). The final result after 24 months is presented in Fig 8-15r. In order to close the "buccal smile corridors" located in the corners of the mouth, non-prep direct composite veneers were also performed on teeth 15, 14, 24, and 25. The result of the five-year clinical follow-up after full occlusal rehabilitation is shown in Figs 8-15s to 8-15u.

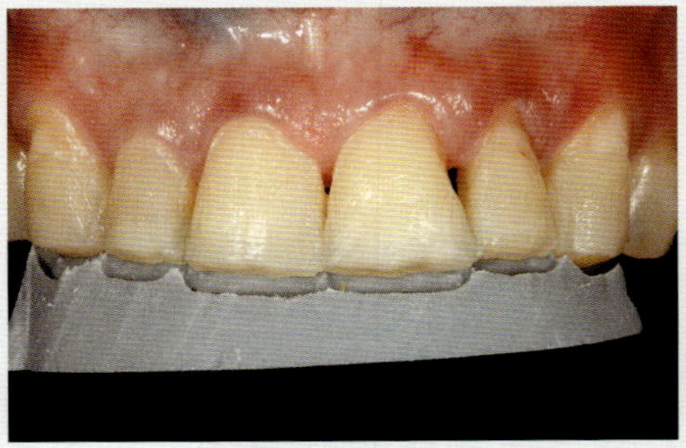

Fig 8-15a
Veneer preparation from the direct composite level. Restorations were done during the previous visit, and they served as a mock-up; the preparation was controlled with a silicone index.

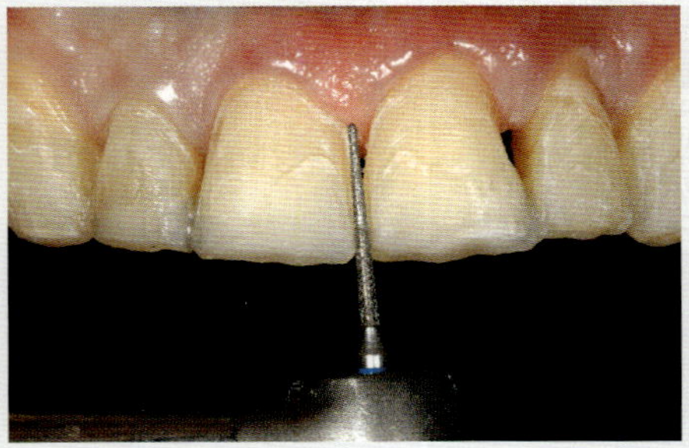

Fig 8-15b
When the axis of the tooth had to be changed or the interdental spaces had to be closed, the contact surfaces were included in the veneer preparation, so the dental technician could obtain the correct symmetry or close the space with porcelain.

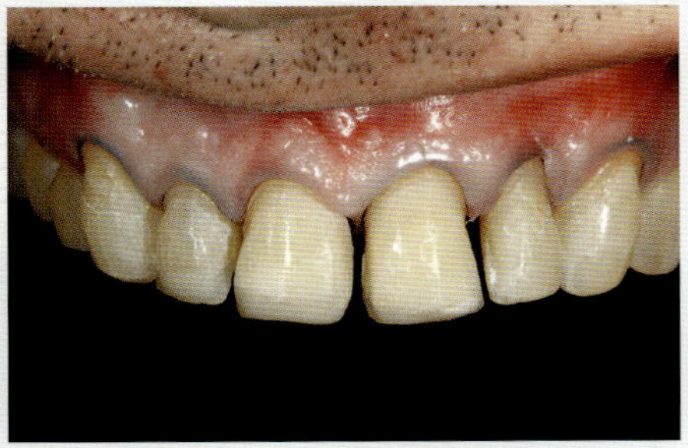

Fig 8-15c
Final preparation for six indirect veneers on teeth 13–23. Pay attention to the proximal surfaces in the veneer preparation on teeth 11, 21, and 22.

PRACTITIONER'S ADVICE

If you intend to change the long axes of the teeth with veneers, extend the veneer preparation on the proximal surfaces!

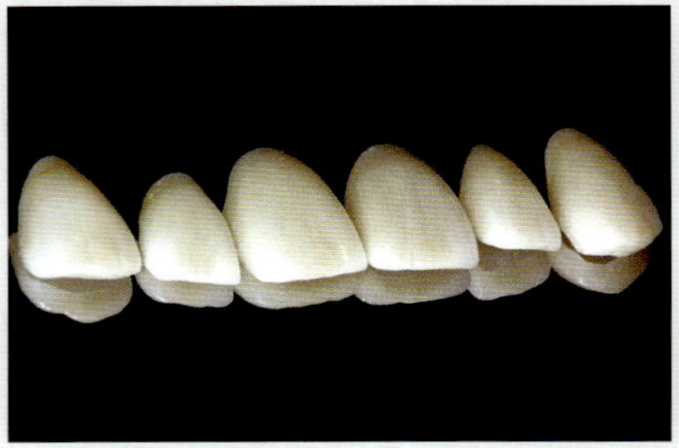

Fig 8-15d
Six feldspathic porcelain veneers are ready to be cemented in the oral cavity (laboratory work: DT Artur Nyga).

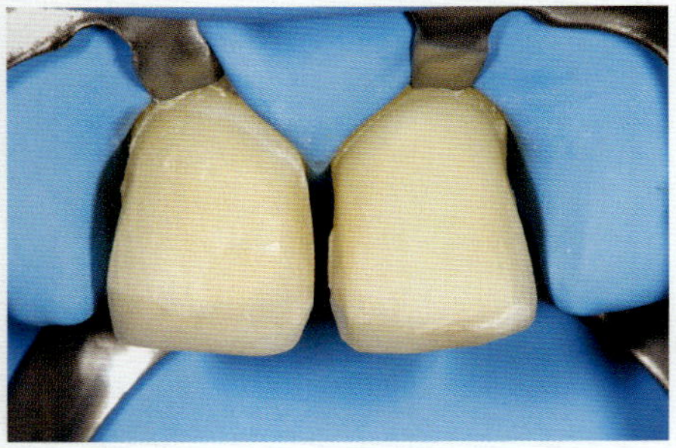

Fig 8-15e
Isolation of two central incisors for the simultaneous and symmetrical placing of two veneers.

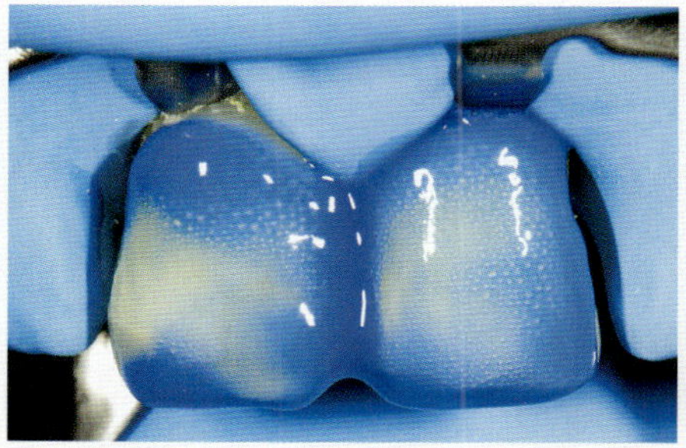

Fig 8-15f
Etching with orthophosphoric acid (20 seconds) . . .

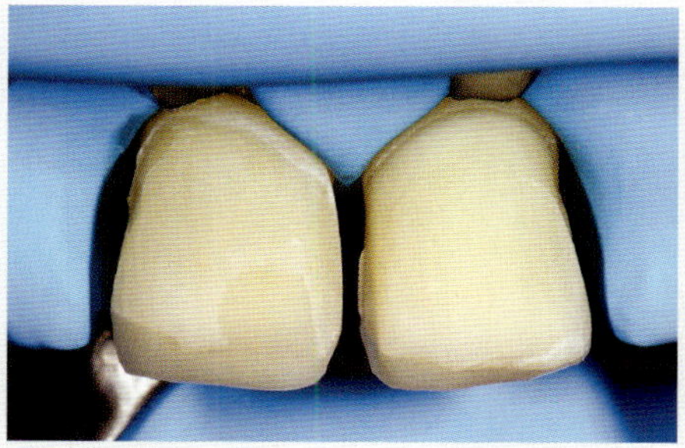

Fig 8-15g
. . . then rinsing for 20 seconds before the tooth tissues were gently dried.

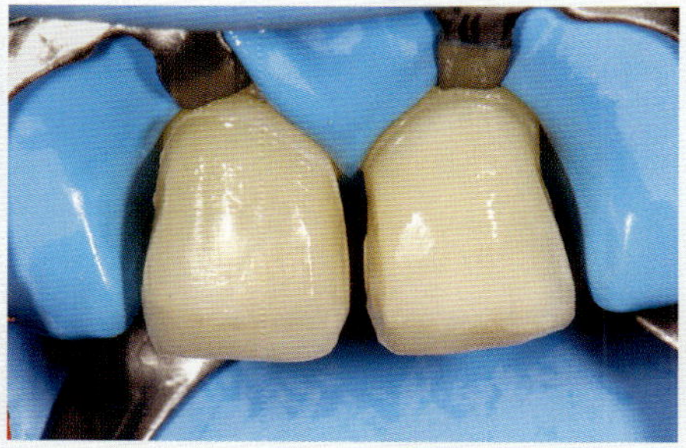

Fig 8-15h
Application of the bonding system in two layers (Ena Bond, Micerium), simultaneous thinning of the system with air spray and light-curing for 20 seconds.

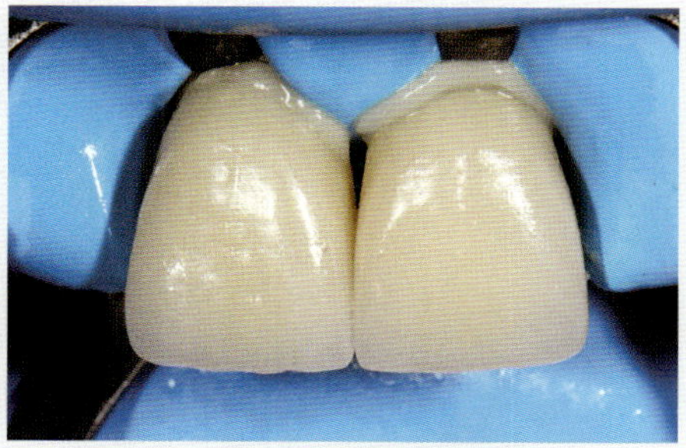

Fig 8-15i
Cementing veneers with the pre-heated Enamel Plus composite (UD3 dentin). The excess material was removed, and the veneers were polymerized for 60 seconds on each side: cervical, mesial, and incisal (palatal). Polymerization was performed after the application of glycerin gel along the preparation margin.

PRACTITIONER'S ADVICE

When cementing the veneer with a heated composite resin, ensure that the composite flows adequately and that the veneer thickness is appropriate (> 0.5 mm) for this type of cementation.

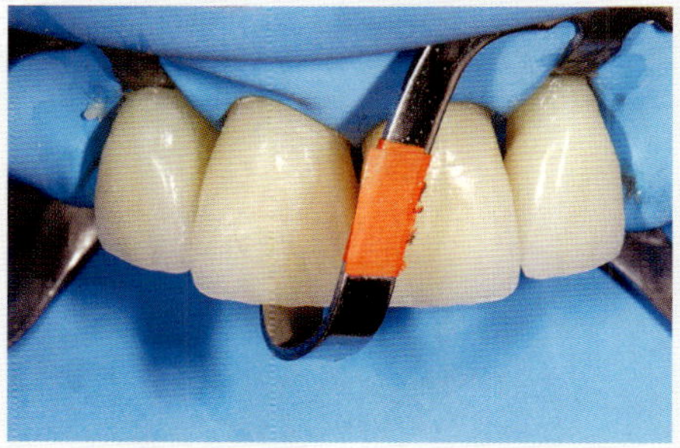

Fig 8-15j
Next, the isolation of the teeth was changed to four anterior teeth, and the lateral incisors were conditioned for adhesive cementation, and two more veneers were placed.

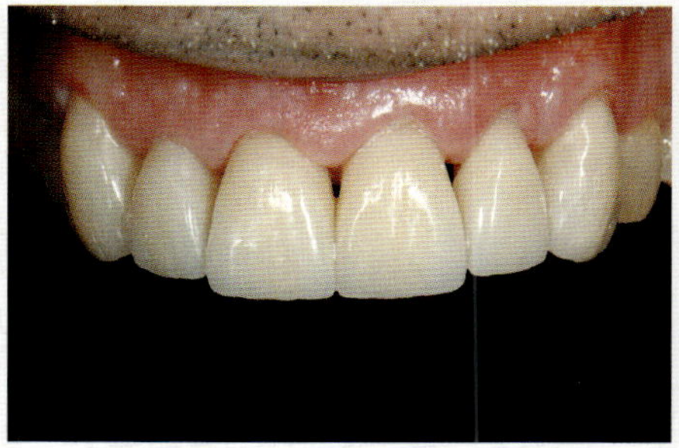

Fig 8-15k
The clinical situation immediately after cementation of six veneers.

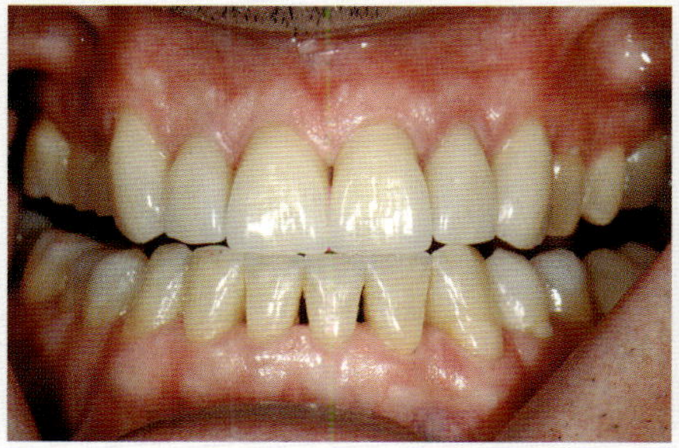

Fig 8-15l
Checking the anterior guidance a few days after cementation of the veneers.

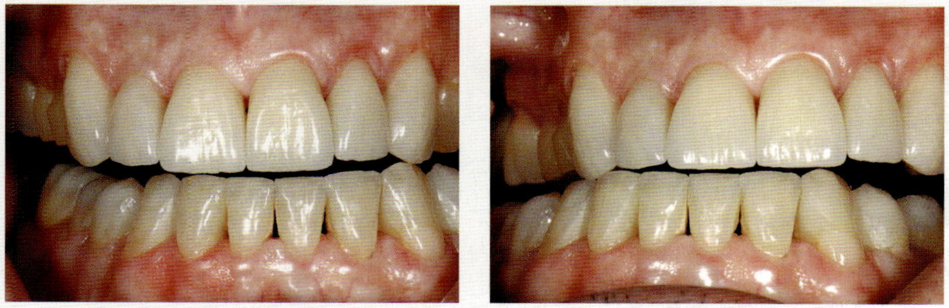

Figs 8-15m and 8-15n
Checking the canine guidance on the (m) left and on (n) right side.

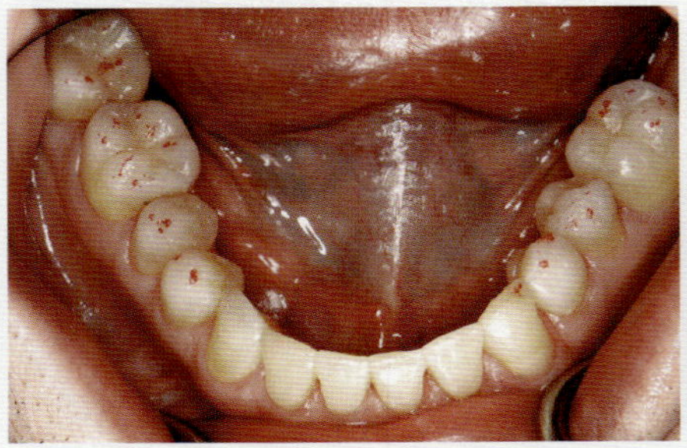

Fig 8-15o
Bilateral balanced occlusal contact points in maximum intercuspation (contact points marked with 21 μm Parkell articulating paper).

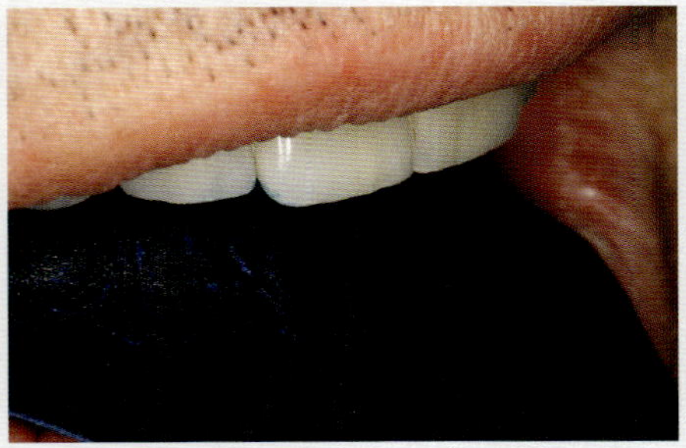

Fig 8-15p
Kois chewing test with the use of horseshoe articulating paper (200 μm), aimed at marking the friction surfaces between two dental arches.

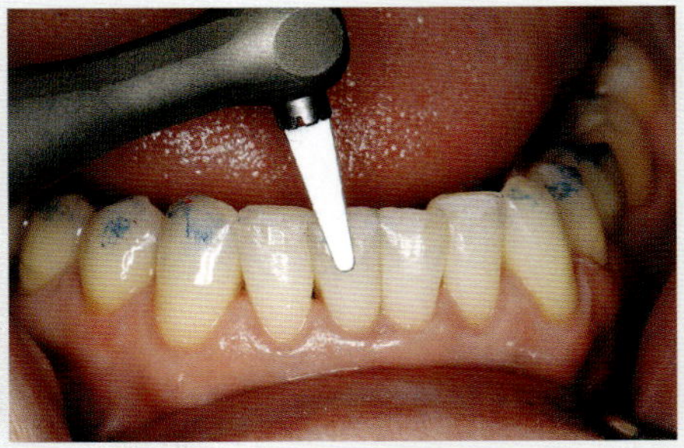

Fig 8-15q
Reducing the marked surfaces on the mandibular incisors restored with direct composite resin. The occlusal corrections are relatively easy, especially when doing it in composite resin.

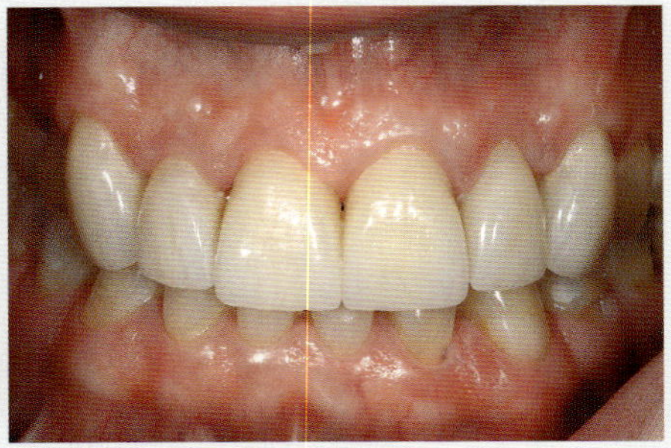

Fig 8-15r
Follow-up visit 24 months after treatment – final result of occlusal rehabilitation.

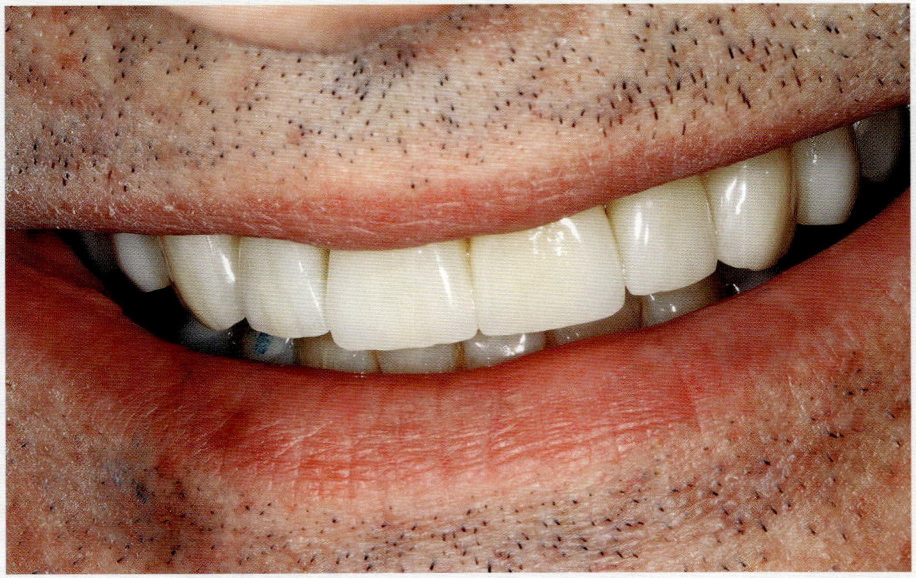

Fig 8-15s
Patient's smile 5 years after treatment (premolars were restored with non-prep direct composite veneers, in order to close the buccal smile corridors).

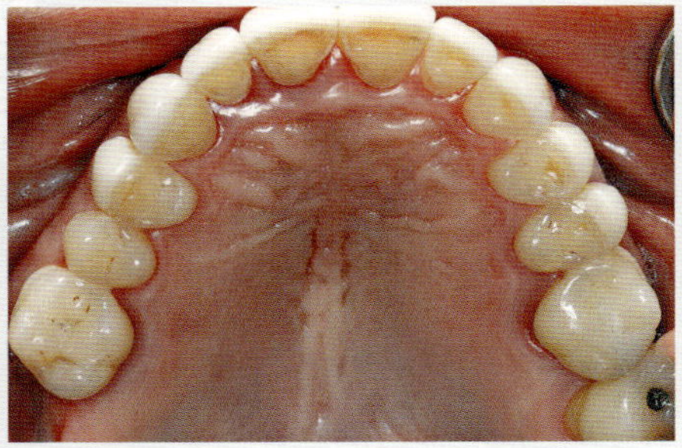

Fig 8-15t
Maxillary arch – recall 5 years after porcelain veneers cementation.

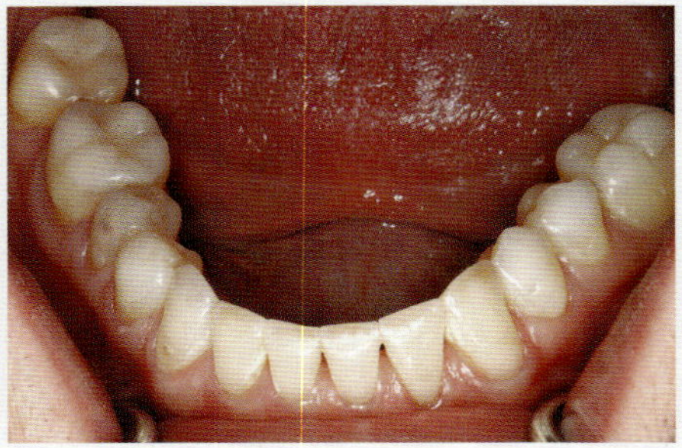

Fig 8-15u
Mandibular arch – recall 5 years after direct transparent index technique.

PRACTITIONER'S ADVICE

In order to minimize the risk of restoration damage, the Kois chewing test should be performed and the friction surfaces (marked with the occlusal paper), particularly those on the palatal surface of the veneers, should be eliminated!

ESTHETICS AND FUNCTION: A, B, C, D OF RESTORATIVE STRATEGY

A. Esthetic treatment planning – esthetic wax-up (Fig 8-16a)

You should always start with esthetic planning by gaining information while collecting medical history, taking extraoral and intraoral photographs, obtaining information about the patient's expectations, and determining whether the patient expects esthetic change. Information about changing the shape or length of the teeth is transferred to the dental laboratory for appropriate wax-up.[38–42] Based on the data obtained from the dentist, the dental technician creates an esthetic wax-up on a cast mounted according to the facebow. Next, using the silicone index taken from the diagnostic wax-up, the dentist performs a mock-up, followed by corrections if needed, and evaluates the esthetics (photographs of the patient's face with mock-up).

Thanks to the mock-up, you can:

- Evaluate the patient's expectations
- Check the validity of the esthetic treatment plan
- Verify that the patient is psychologically prepared for treatment
- Motivate the patient by visualizing what can be achieved at the end of the treatment (sometimes treatment takes too long, and the patient loses motivation without knowing how the final result will look)
- Motivate the dentist and the dental team by creating a personal commitment to the final esthetic results

A mock-up can confirm that the planned esthetics are valid, and from that moment on, we know where we are heading. But it can also reveal that the patient is not psychologically ready or denies the sense of the entire esthetic transformation. If the mock-up is successful and the dentist and patient are happy with it, you can proceed to step B.

B. Finding the centric relation (CR) (Fig 8-16b)

Once the initial treatment plan has been presented to the patient, it is time **to find the CR as a starting point for treatment planning and comprehensive restorative rehabilitation.**[22–28] It should be emphasized that the Kois Deprogrammer described in this chapter is not the only way to find and record CR, but it is the method preferred by the author.

After CR confirmation and registration, the dental technician mounts the casts in the articulator in accordance with the CR for further planning and possible further wax-up of the posterior teeth. Thanks to this, **functional planning will be added to previous esthetic treatment planning**.

> **TIP**
>
> Direct or indirect mock-up with photographs is the key for planning the esthetics!

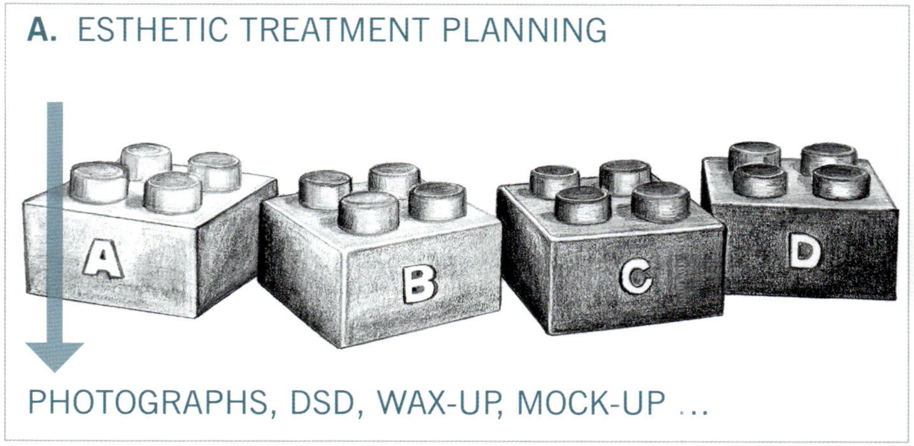

Fig 8-16a
The first stage of comprehensive restorative treatment should always start with esthetic treatment planning.

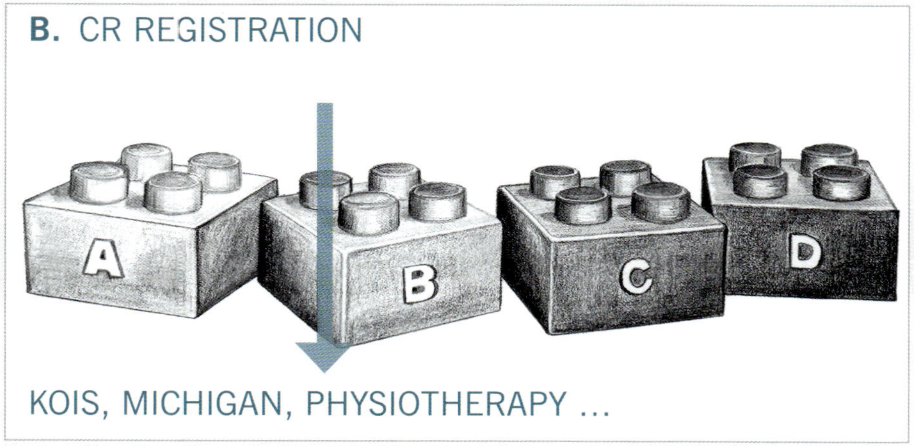

Fig 8-16b
The second stage of comprehensive restorative treatment relies on finding and registering the appropriate CR as a starting point for further treatment planning.

C. Functional planning – functional wax-up (Fig 8-16c)

When the dental technician has casts registered in the CR, the appropriate VDO should be selected to realize a new dimension of maxillary anteriors (tested in step 1).

The wax-up of the posterior teeth occlusal surface will **achieve a bilateral balanced occlusion**.

At this point, a question always arises: **How much to increase the VDO?**

The answer is simple: the vertical dimension of occlusion should be increased to the extent that it will:

- First: **achieve the planned esthetic treatment**
- Second: **have enough space for the chosen restorative material** and minimize the tooth preparation (or assuming that there will be no preparation, only adding)
- Third: **achieve the functional goals** by relieving the anterior teeth and obtaining **bilateral multi posterior contact points (from canines to molars)**[42–45]

The treatment plan can be executed through:

- Reconstruction of the mandibular and maxillary dental arch
- Reconstruction of only the mandibular dental arch
- Reconstruction of only the maxillary dental arch

The decision to choose one of the three methods should be made individually and **depends on factors such as:**

- **Level of tooth wear in the posterior segment** (is the tooth wear so significant that the occlusal surface needs to be restored in both arches?)
- **Range of increasing the vertical dimension of occlusion** (if to a small extent, it may be enough to increase the VDO in only one dental arch)
- **Esthetic factors** (sometimes the "buccal smile corridor" needs to be closed, so we decide to restore the maxillary dental arch)

Once the wax-up of the posterior teeth is complete, the dentist should evaluate it, approve it, and proceed to the restorative stage.

D. Restorative treatment (Fig 8-16d)

A restorative treatment plan determined by the wax-up can be achieved through direct or indirect restorations.

When performing direct restorations, impressions are taken from the waxed model using transparent silicone. Then, with the previously described index technique, the reconstruction of the posterior segment is performed.[46,47] In the case of partial indirect restorations, the mock-up procedure is performed using a temporary resin material (for example, Protemp). The next step is mock-up through preparation for composite or porcelain onlays, similar to the veneer preparation.[48–51]

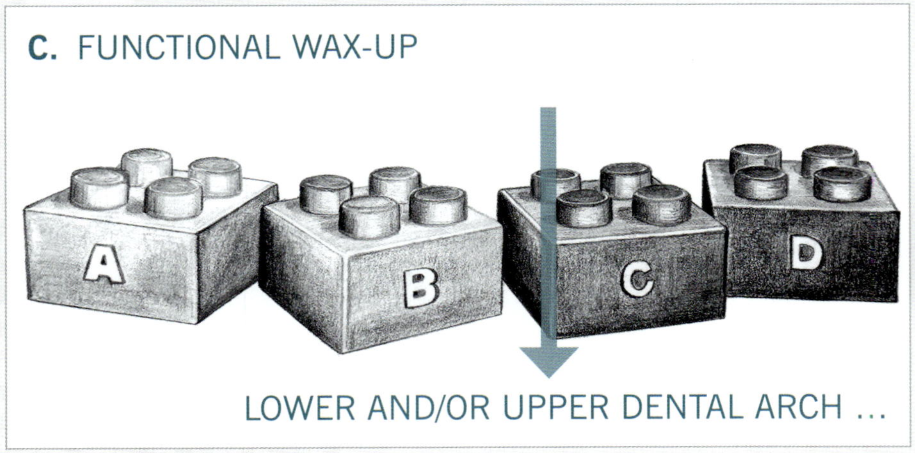

Fig 8-16c
The third step of comprehensive restorative treatment is determining whether to increase the VDO, how much it should be increased, and whether it should be done through the mandibular, maxillary, or both dental arches. Wax-up should be performed according to the treatment plan.

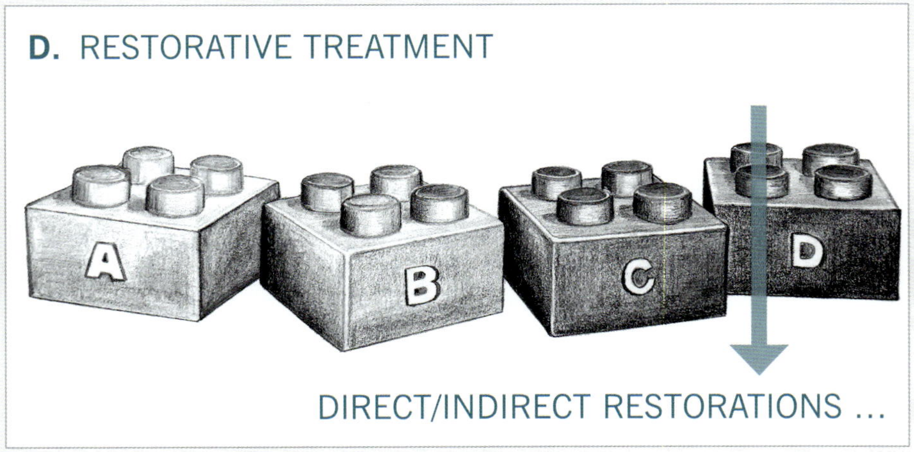

Fig 8-16d
The fourth step of comprehensive restorative treatment is implementing the plan (wax-up) in the oral cavity in the form of direct or indirect restorations.

VENEERS: CHANGING THE TOOTH SHAPE

An excellent indication for porcelain veneers is a significant change in the tooth shape. It is much easier to enlarge the teeth than to reduce their size. When enlarging, the treatment is less invasive, and enamel reduction is usually minimized or reduced to zero.[3,6]

A typical example of such a procedure is enlarging the crown of the peg lateral incisor. Conversely, it will be much more difficult and the tooth preparation will be more invasive if we want to transform the canines into the lateral incisors.

Based on the next two clinical cases, the procedure of changing the tooth shape will be illustrated.

Case 7: Enlargement of the lateral incisor, the transformation of the canine into incisor

A female patient presented to the dental office with a wish to improve the esthetics of the peg lateral crown of tooth 12 and canine 23, which was located in the place of the maxillary left lateral incisor (Fig 8-17a). When the patient smiled, there was a lack of tooth symmetry (Fig 8-17b) and significant black spaces on both sides (Figs 8-17c and 8-17d). The treatment plan included whitening the maxillary and mandibular arches and performing two porcelain veneers, which will provide the teeth with distinct features of lateral incisors. The test-drive of the clinical situation was presented with the mock-up; both the patient and the consultation team approved the treatment plan.

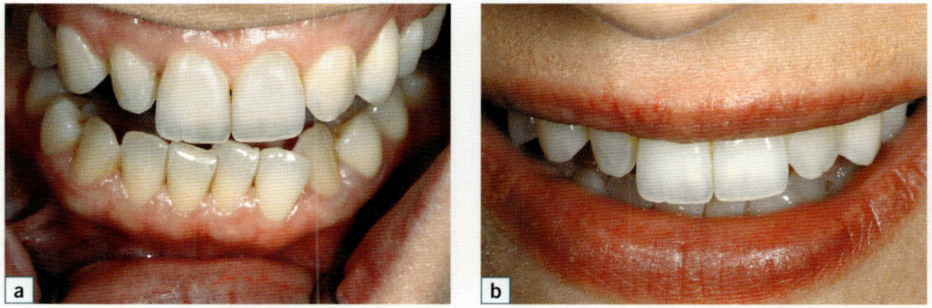

Figs 8-17a and 8-17b
(a) Photograph of the patient who presented to the dental office to improve the esthetic disorder caused by the peg maxillary right lateral incisor and the position of the left canine in the place of tooth 22. (b) Visible lack of symmetry between the right and left side while smiling.

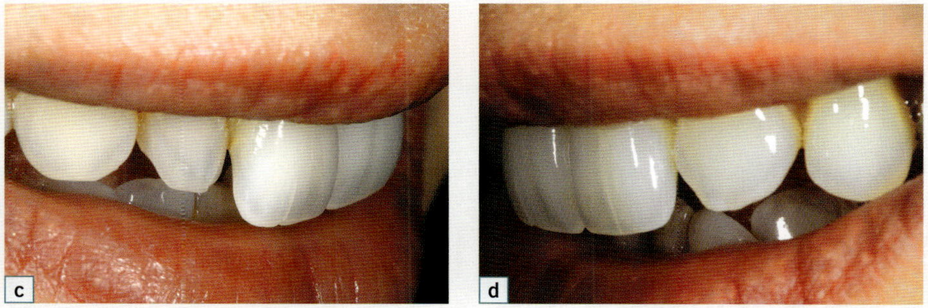

Figs 8-17c and 8-17d
The patient's smile was affected by black spaces between the maxillary incisors.

At the next appointment, teeth 12 and 23 were transformed again to lateral incisors with mock-up (Fig 8-17e), followed by veneer preparation. Orientation grooves were performed (Fig 8-17f) and the temporary resin was removed. It was possible to see how minimal the tooth preparation is within the hard tissues (Figs 8-17g and 8-17h).

Tooth preparation was monitored by the silicone index (Figs 8-17i and 8-17j) and the final preparation is shown in Fig 8-17k. Impressions were taken (Fig 8-17l), and two feldspathic porcelain veneers (IPS InLine, Ivoclar) were fabricated in the dental laboratory (Fig 8-17m).

During the next appointment, provisional restorations were removed (Fig 8-17n) and veneers were tried in. After approval, the tooth surface was conditioned for adhesive cementation (Figs 8-17o to 8-17r). The veneers were etched with hydrofluoric acid and thoroughly rinsed in an ultrasonic cleaner by applying the silane and bonding system. Veneers were cemented with a heated light-cured composite (Figs 8-17s to 8-17v), composite resin excess was removed, and the veneer/tooth margin was gently polished. At the next appointment, intraoral photographs were taken (Figs 8-17w to 8-17z), as well as photographs of the patient's smile (Figs 8-17aa to 8-17cc) and the patient's face (Fig 8-17dd).

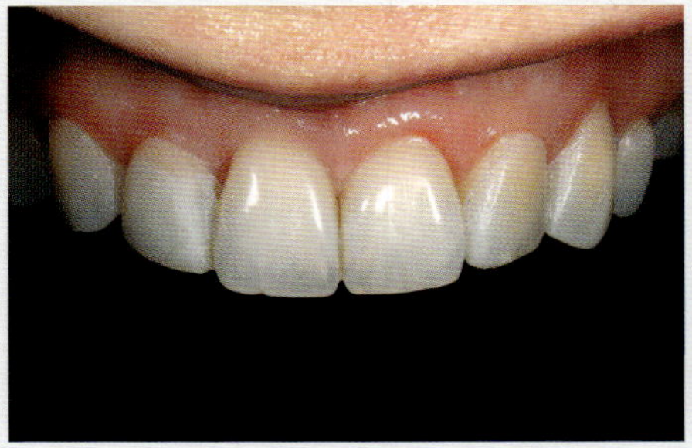

Fig 8-17e
Mock-up made of temporary resin.

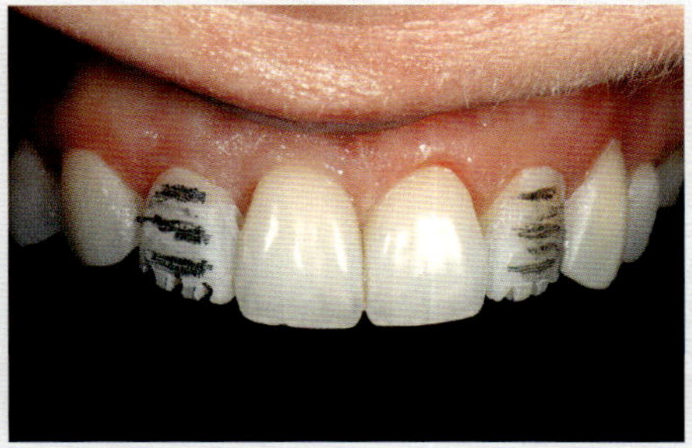

Fig 8-17f
Porcelain veneer preparation from the mock-up level.

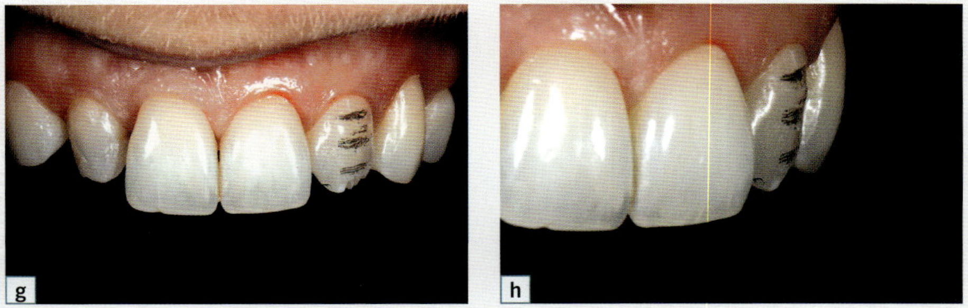

Figs 8-17g and 8-17h
After removing the mock-up, it can be seen that tooth 12 has not been touched at all and tooth 23 had minimal preparation.

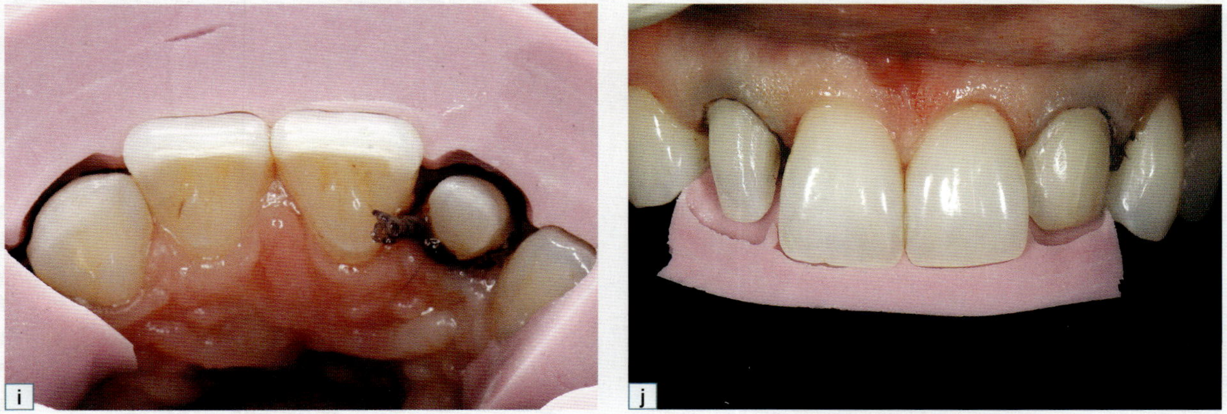

Figs 8-17i and 8-17j
Controlling the space for porcelain veneers with a silicone index cut in the horizontal and vertical plane (the index was taken from the diagnostic wax-up).

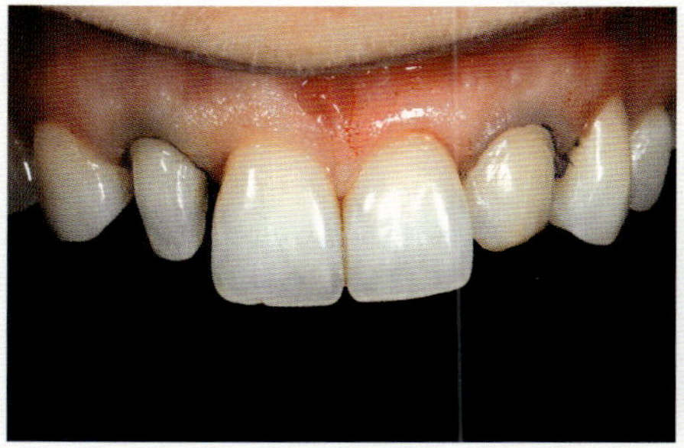

Fig 8-17k
Final veneer preparation with retraction cords inserted.

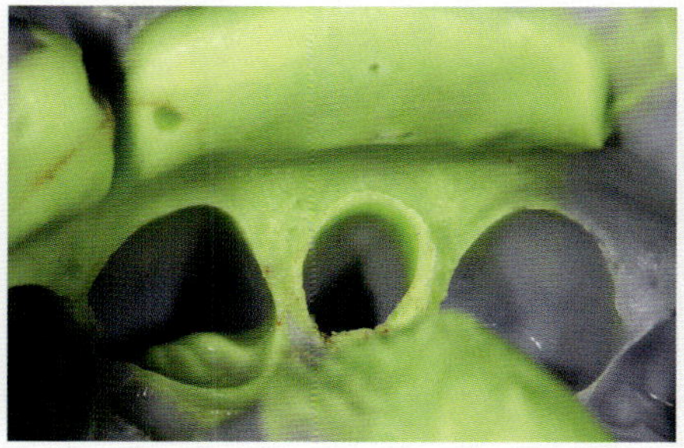

Fig 8-17l
Impression is taken with a polyvinyl siloxane material – visible, delicate preparation margin in the juxtagingival area.

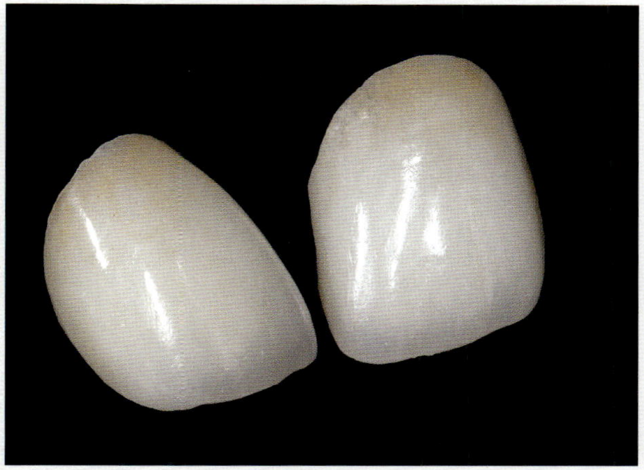

Fig 8-17m
Veneers made of feldspathic porcelain (IPS InLine, Ivoclar) ready for cementation (laboratory work: DT Artur Nyga).

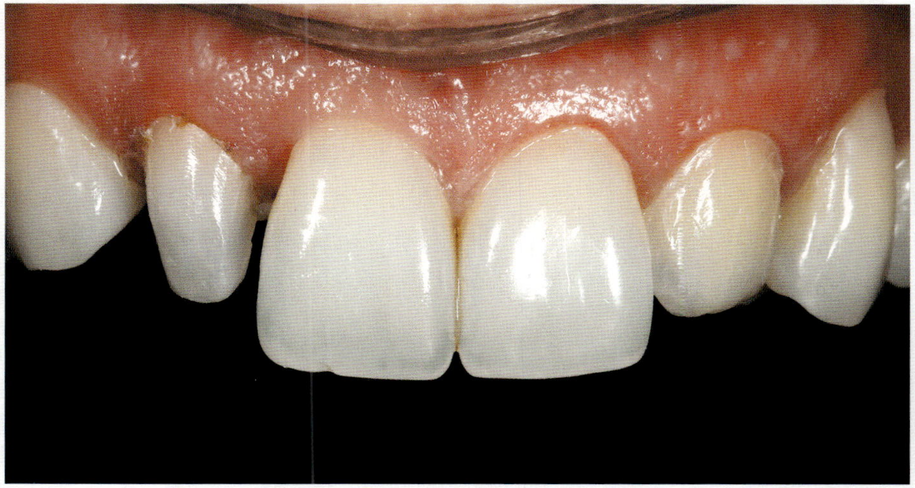

Fig 8-17n
Clinical situation after removing the provisional restorations.

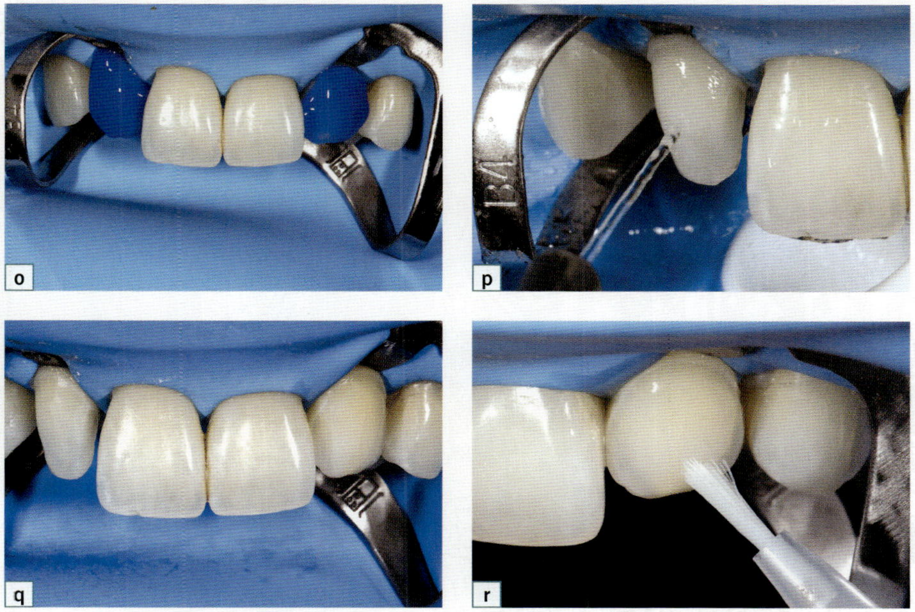

Figs 8-17o to 8-17r
Preparing the tooth surface for adhesive cementation in rubber dam isolation: (o) etching, (p) rinsing the etchant thoroughly, (q) drying the tooth surface, and (r) applying the bonding system.

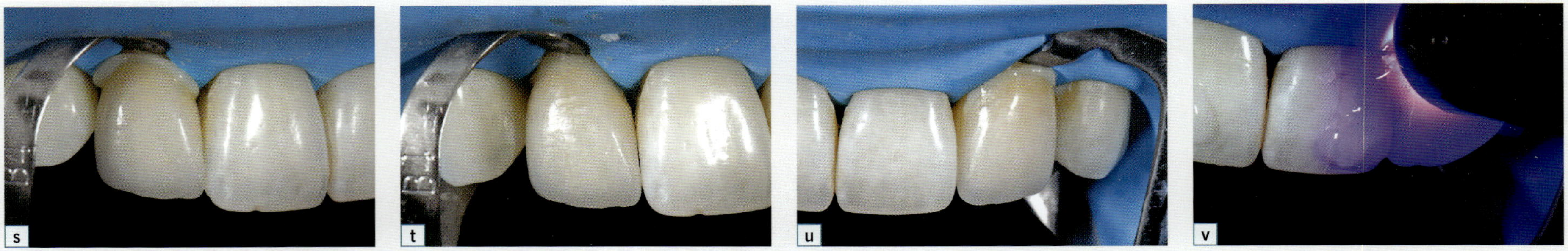

Figs 8-17s to 8-17v
(s to u) Veneer cementation with a heated light-cured composite (Enamel Plus, Micerium), (v) polymerization, removal of composite resin excess and polishing the veneer/tooth margin.

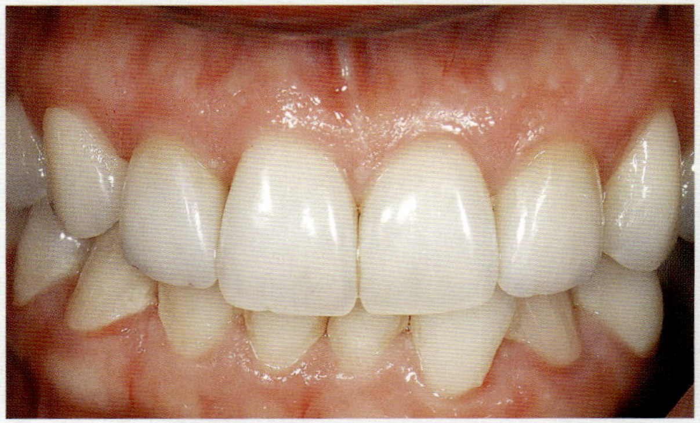

Fig 8-17w
Intraoral photograph a few weeks after veneers' cementation.

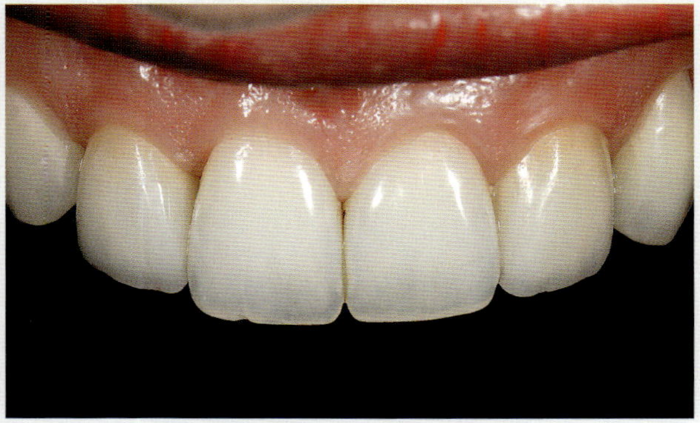

Fig 8-17x
Intraoral photograph of the maxillary arch on a black background.

PRACTITIONER'S ADVICE

Do not use the maximum intensity of the light-curing device immediately when cementing. Start with low power, for example, by polymerizing for the first few seconds further away from the veneer.

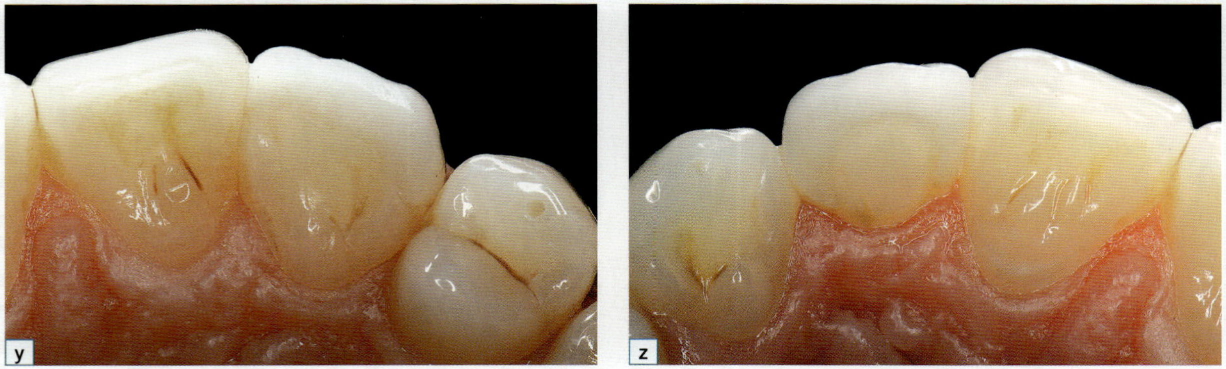

Figs 8-17y and 8-17z
Teeth 12 and 23 with cemented veneers – palatal view.

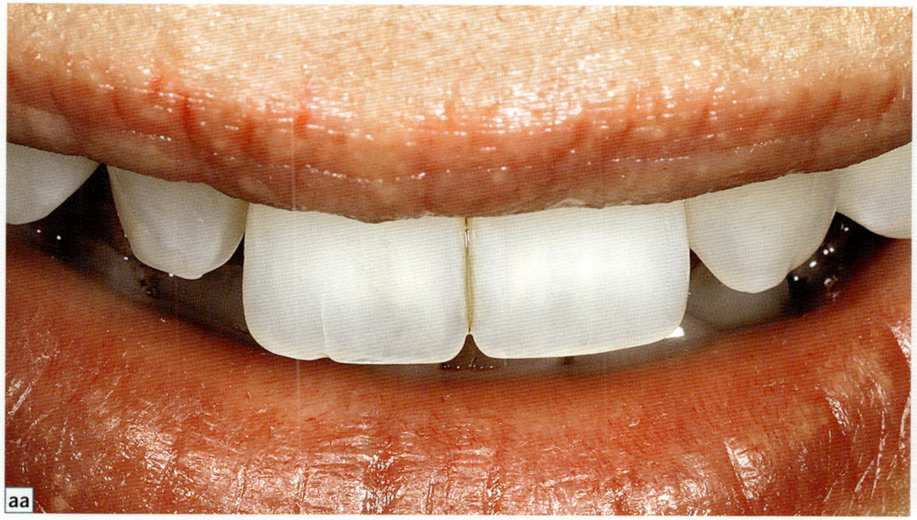

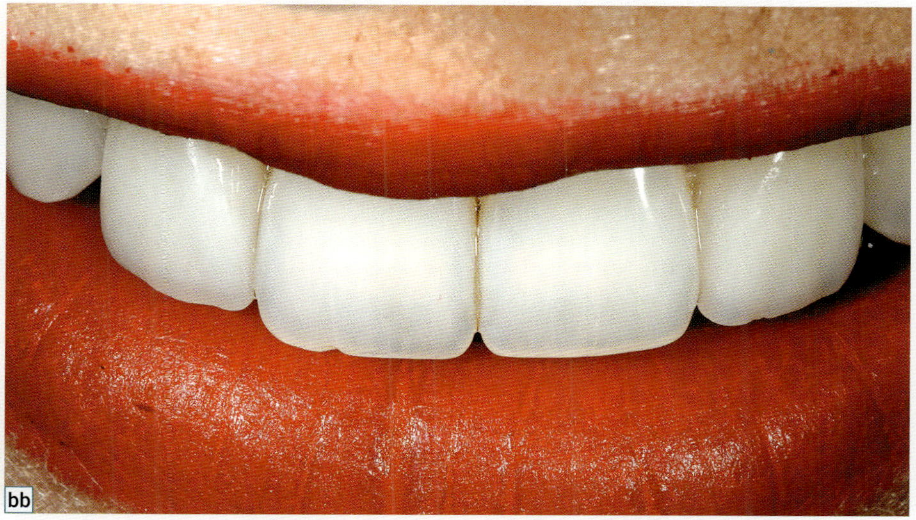

Figs 8-17aa and 8-17bb
Photographs of the patient's smile (aa) before and (bb) after treatment.

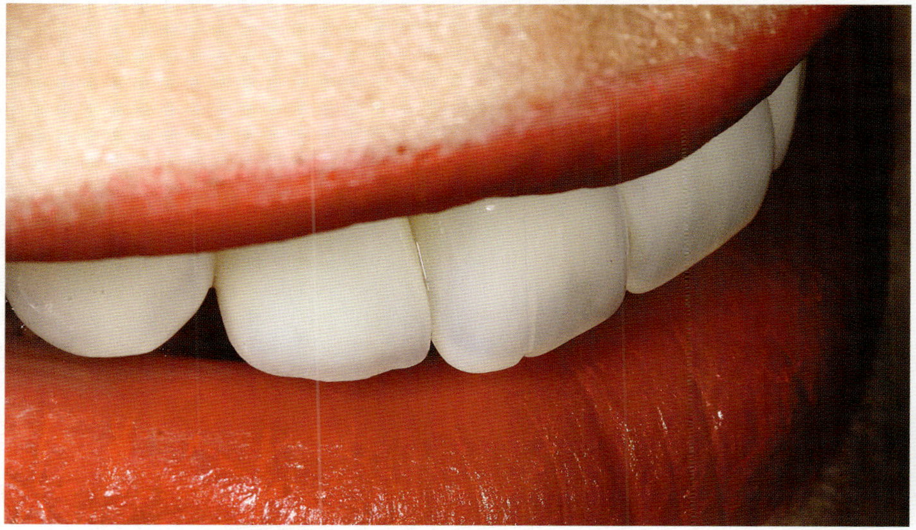

Fig 8-17cc
At the next appointment, photographs of the smile …

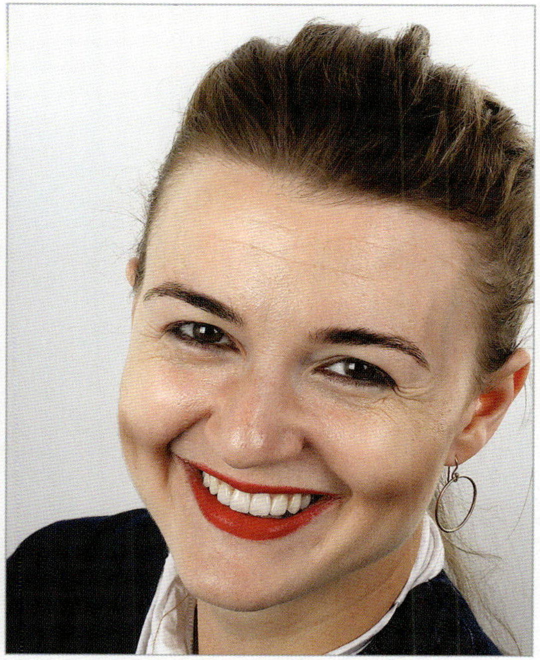

Fig 8-17dd
… and the patient's face were taken.

Case 8: Enlargement of the lateral incisor, the transformation of the canine into incisor, and the lateral incisor into canine

A female patient presented to the dental office during orthodontic treatment with a request to undertake esthetic treatment after completing orthodontic therapy (Figs 8-18a and 8-18b). The orthodontist was asked to slightly correct the position of the teeth in order to easily achieve final symmetry with the porcelain veneers.

After completing the orthodontic treatment, the maxillary and mandibular arches were bleached (Figs 8-18c to 8-18e), a mock-up was created to assess possible changes and, after its approval, five veneers were planned on teeth 12–23. At the next appointment, the mock-up was performed again (Fig 8-18f), and the veneer preparation was started by creating depth grooves through the mock-up (Fig 8-18g). After that, the mock-up was removed (Fig 8-18h), and the preparation was completed (Fig 8-18i) under the control of the silicone index. Then impressions were taken and provisional veneers were performed.

At the next appointment, the porcelain veneers fabricated in the dental laboratory (Fig 8-18j) were checked for their marginal integrity and esthetics, and cemented in rubber dam isolation (Figs 8-18k to 8-18r). Intraoral and extraoral control photographs of the patient's smile are shown in Figs 8-18s to 8-18w.

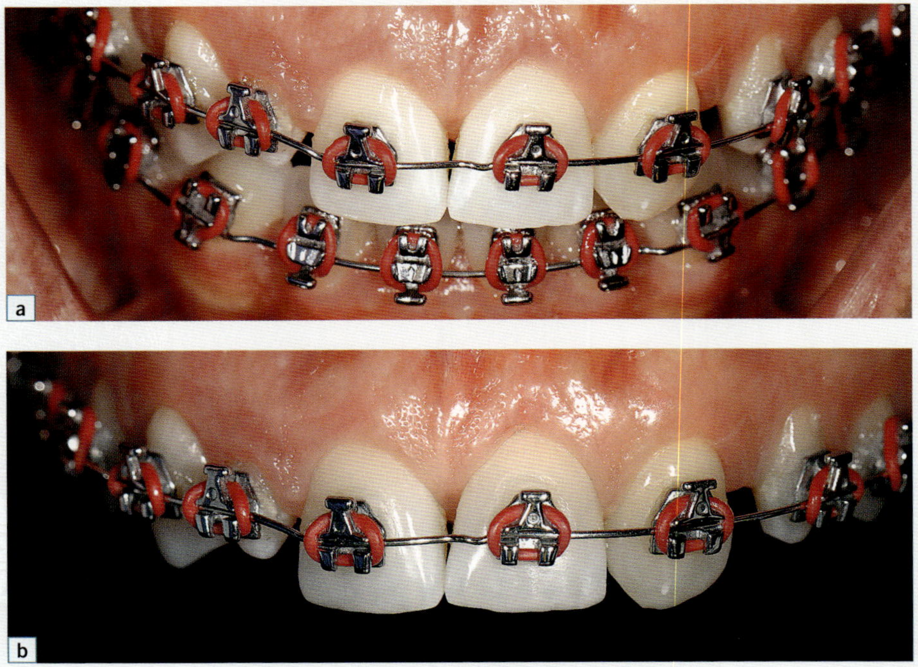

Figs 8-18a and 8-18b
While undergoing orthodontic treatment, a patient presented to the dental office with a request to undertake esthetic treatment after completing orthodontic therapy.

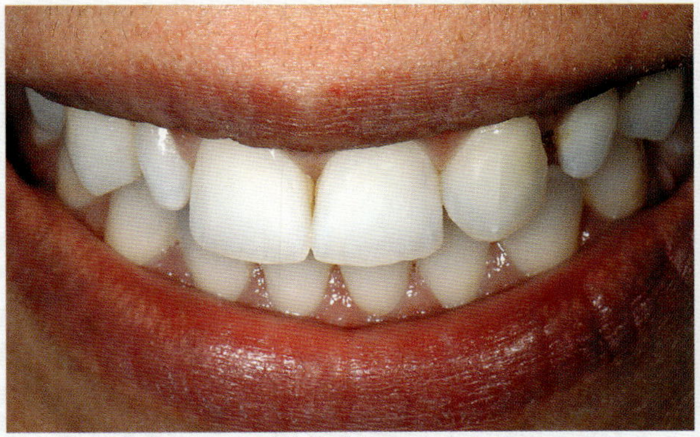

Fig 8-18c
Patient's smile after completing orthodontic treatment.

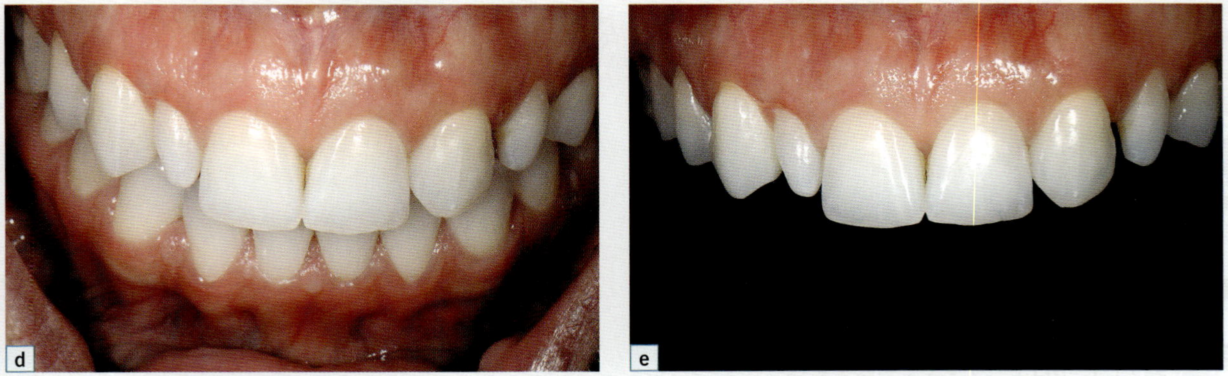

Figs 8-18d and 8-18e
The patient wanted to balance the symmetry between the right and left sides; it was decided to perform five porcelain veneers on teeth 12–23.

Fig 8-18f
A mock-up made of temporary resin material (Protemp, 3M) was approved by the patient and the consultation team.

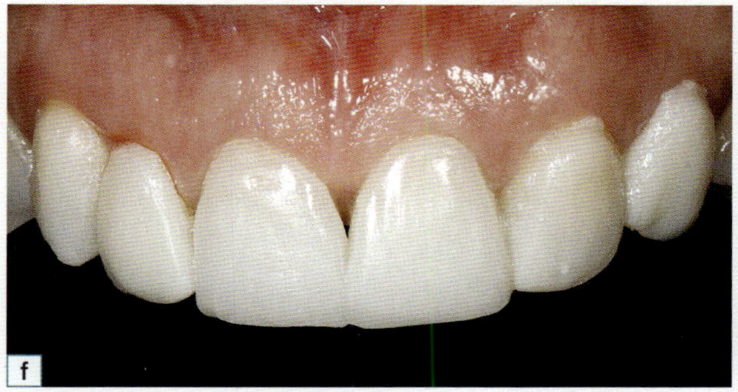

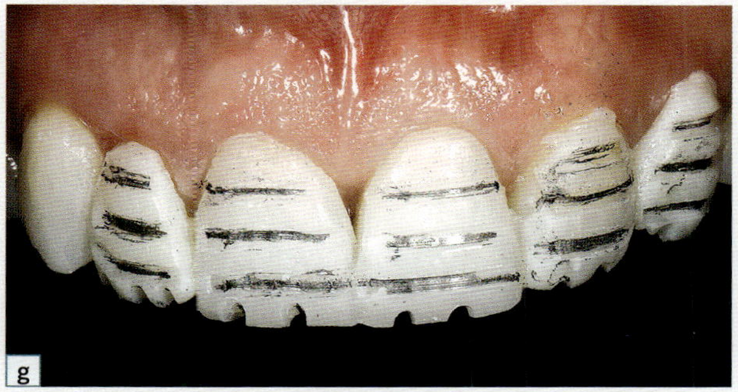

Fig 8-18g
Mock-up through preparation for the veneers, depth grooves.

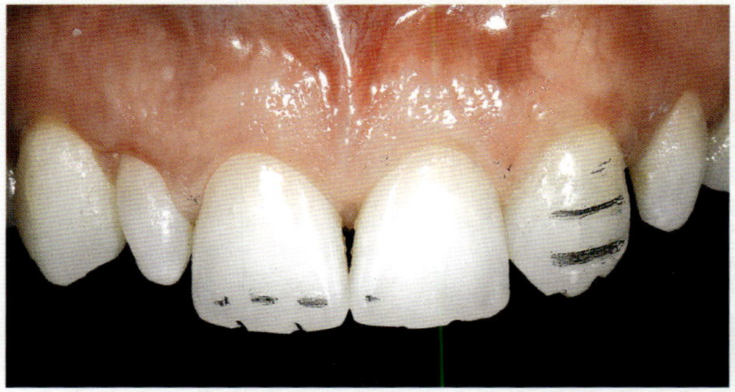

Fig 8-18h
Situation after removing the mock-up.

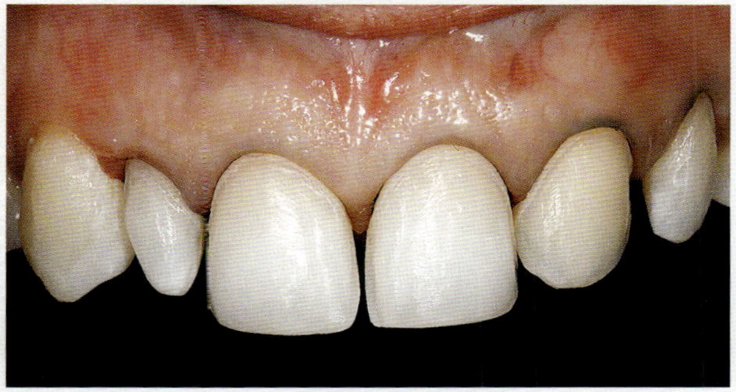

Fig 8-18i
Five teeth after minimal invasive veneer preparation.

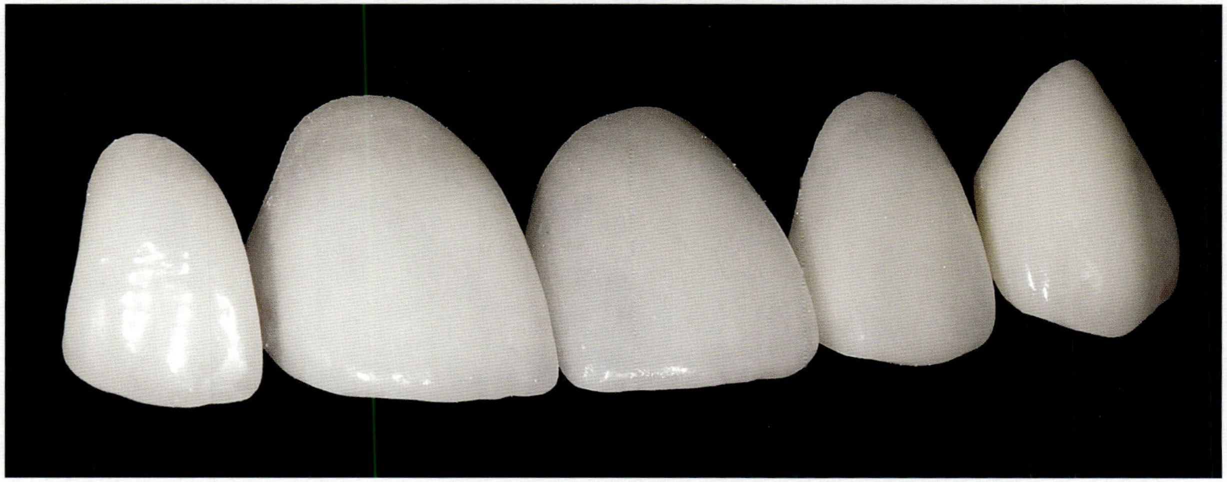

Fig 8-18j
Feldspathic porcelain veneers (IPS InLine, Ivoclar) fabricated in the dental laboratory, ready for cementation (laboratory work: DT Artur Nyga).

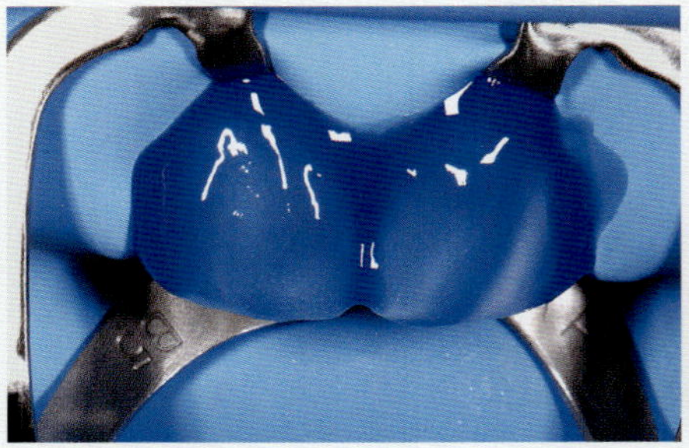

Fig 8-18k
Teeth 11 and 21: etching with the orthophosphoric acid for 20 seconds.

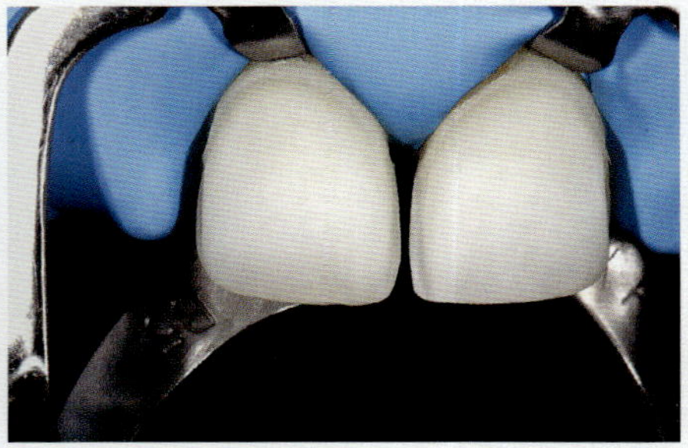

Fig 8-18l
Situation after etching, rinsing, gentle drying of the tooth surface …

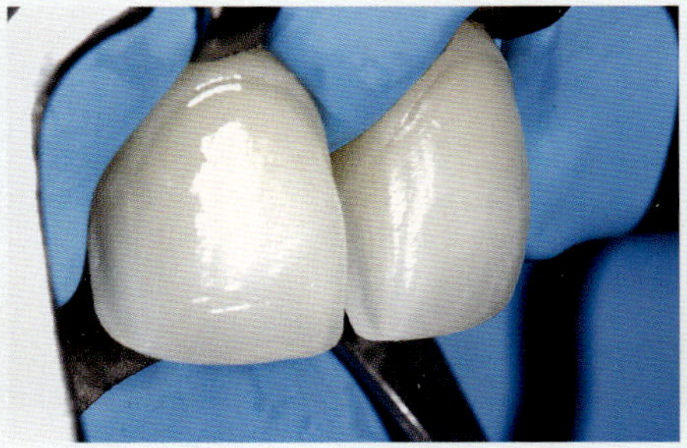

Fig 8-18m
… and after application and polymerization of the bonding system.

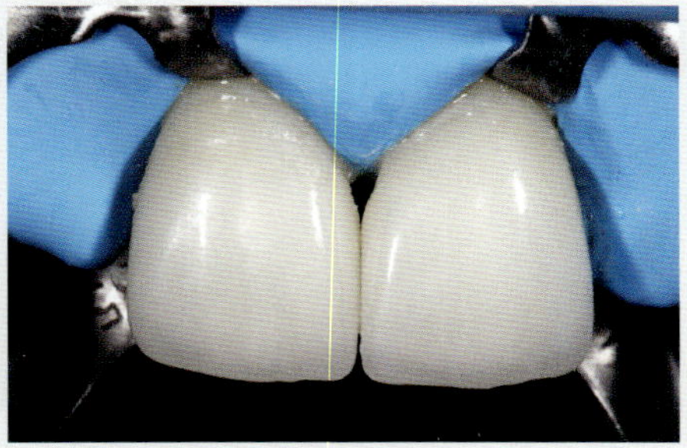

Fig 8-18n
Veneers were cemented with a heated light-cured composite (Enamel Plus, Micerium).

Fig 8-18o
After initial short polymerization (five seconds) and removal of the composite resin excess, glycerin gel was applied to the preparation margins and the final polymerization was carried out.

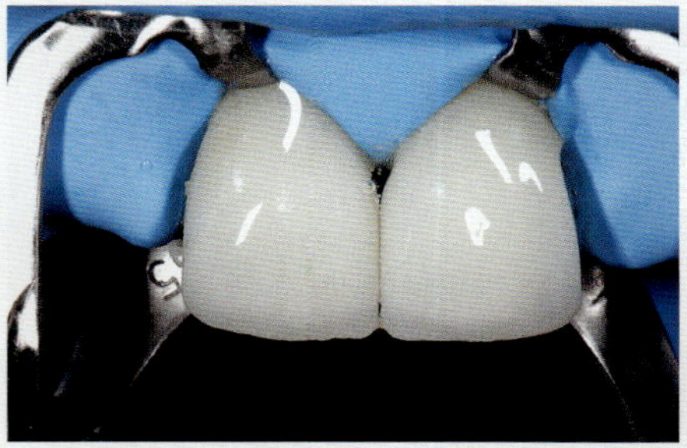

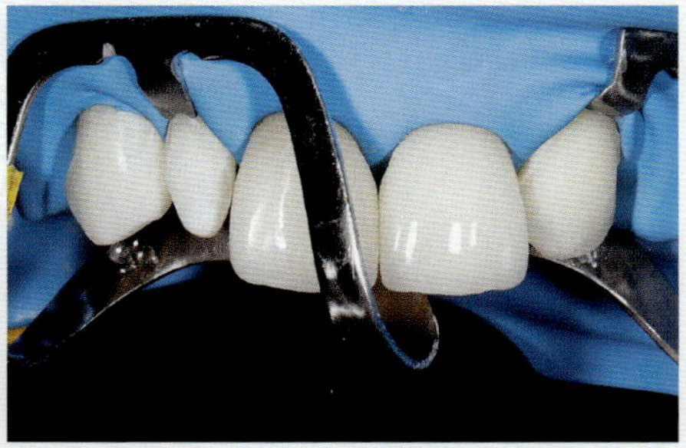

Fig 8-18p
Cementation of following veneers in rubber dam isolation.

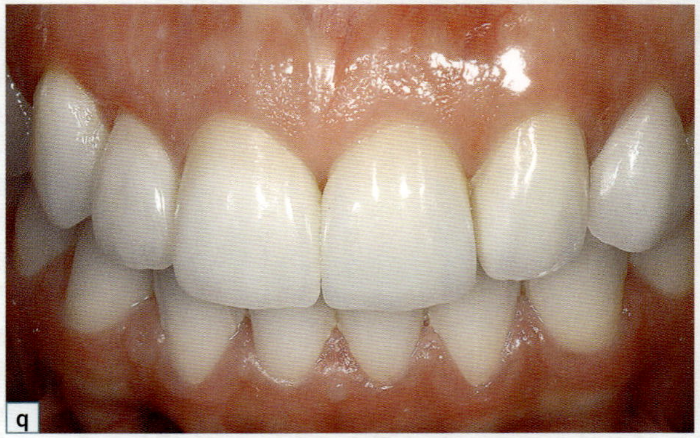

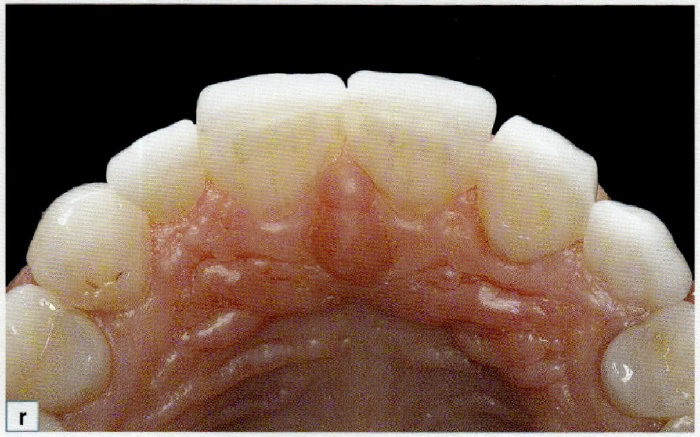

Figs 8-18q and 8-18r
Clinical situation after cementing five porcelain veneers.

PRACTITIONER'S ADVICE

The bonding system applied on the tooth surface must be carefully thinned with an air spray prior to polymerization!

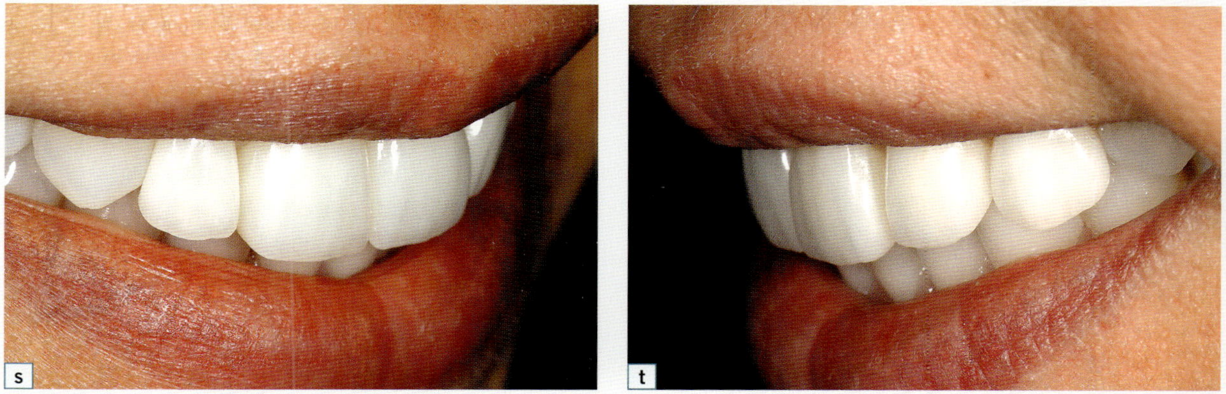

Figs 8-18s and 8-18t
Patient's smile with porcelain veneers (s) from the right and (t) left semi-profile.

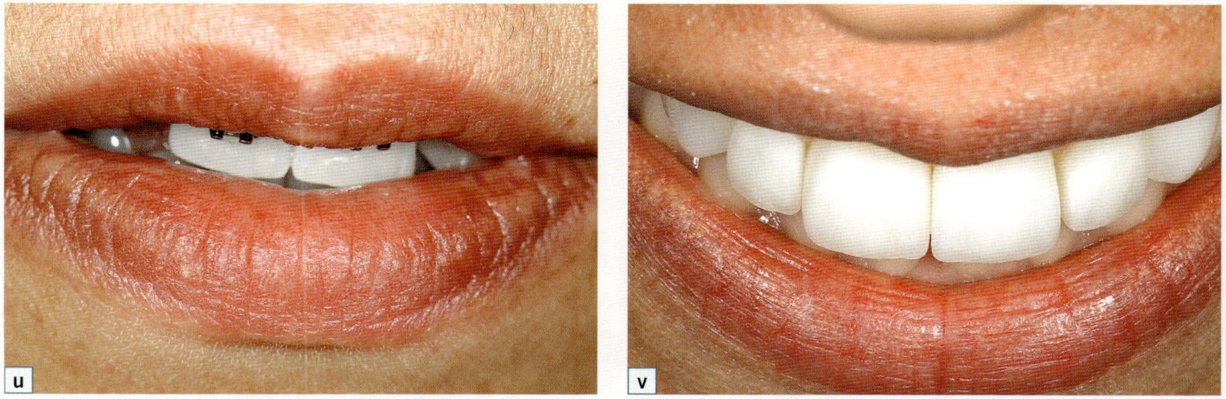

Figs 8-18u and 8-18v
Photographs of the patient (u) before and (v) after treatment.

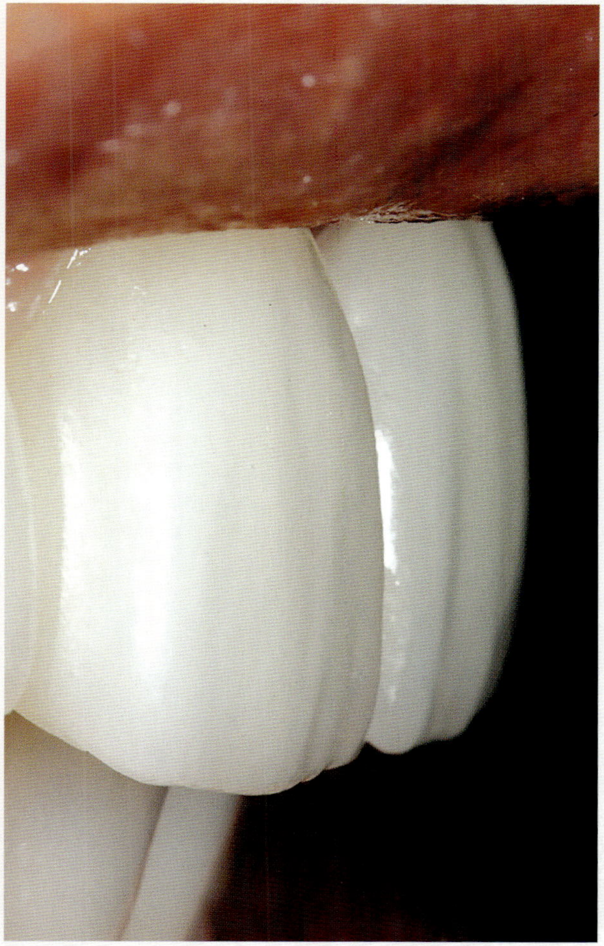

Fig 8-18w
Close-up on the beautiful veneers (laboratory work: DT Artur Nyga).

VENEERS: DIASTEMA CLOSURE

Against all appearances, closing the diastema is a responsible esthetic treatment. When planning, some important aspects have to be considered, including:[52–54]

- **Psychological aspects:** Is the patient and their closest family ready to close the diastema, which from the point of view of changing the appearance can be a bold decision and requires thorough analysis. The author of the chapter remembers a situation where, after closing the diastema with veneers, the patient demanded to return to the initial situation. Therefore, any such change requires a test drive (mock-up) and absolute confidence that the patient wants to undertake the treatment
- **Esthetic aspects:**
  - Will diastema closure improve the esthetic?
  - After closing the diastema, will the teeth not be too square?
  - Will the width of the tooth not exceed its length?
  - When closing the diastema and increasing the width of the teeth, do you not have to change their length and the entire composition of the anterior teeth?
- **The aspect of the restorative material:** Is a direct composite enough to close the diastema, or will the diastema closure be a more comprehensive procedure (Need to change the length of the teeth? Do the teeth have many restorations? Changing other parameters of the tooth shape?) and require indirect veneers?
- **Gingival aspect:** Will the diastema closure and the emergence profile of the new restoration allow for proper cleaning and maintaining healthy soft tissues?

Case 9: Diastema reduction

A patient presented to the dental office to improve the esthetics of the anterior teeth (Figs 8-19a to 8-19e). The medical history revealed that, apart from the esthetics of the anterior teeth, the patient was concerned about increasing tooth wear, especially noticeable in the anterior segment of the maxillary and mandibular arches.

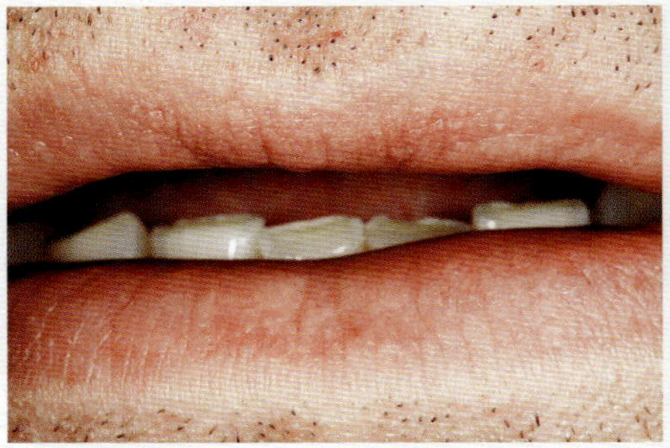

Fig 8-19a
Extraoral photograph of the patient's lips in repose. He presented to the dental office in order to improve the esthetics; there is no maxillary incisors display and greater exposure of worn mandibular incisors.

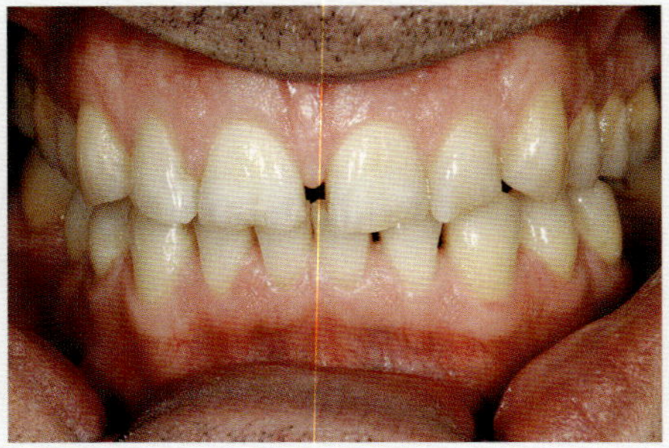

Fig 8-19b
Intraoral photograph in the position of maximum intercuspation.

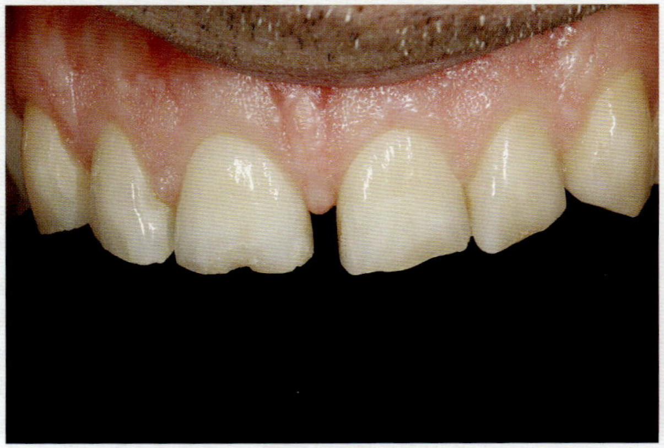

Fig 8-19c
Intraoral photograph of the anterior maxillary teeth.

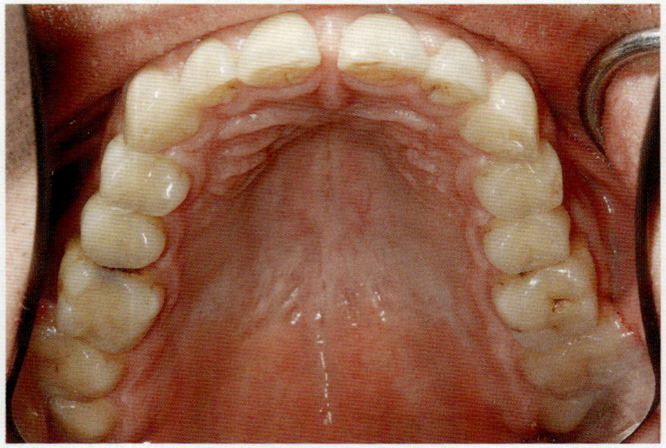

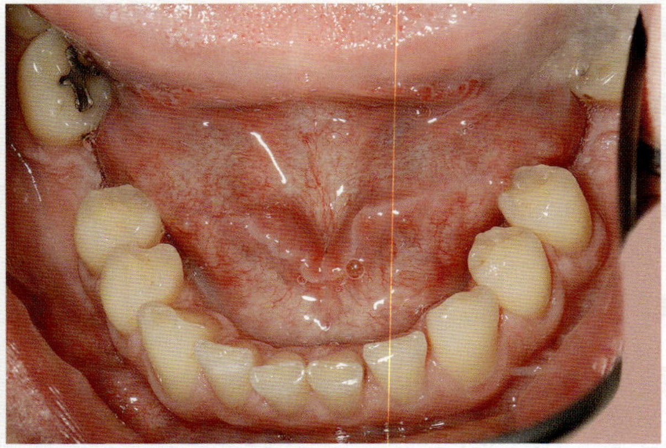

Figs 8-19d and 8-19e
Intraoral photographs of (d) maxillary and (e) mandibular arches.

Step 1: Esthetic treatment planning

A wax-up was performed, and various methods of diastema closure were tested by mock-up. Despite the ambition of the consultation team to close the diastema completely, the patient and his closest family were not ready for such a big change, and it was decided to close the diastema only partially. Since it was found that extending the central incisors and reconstructing the smile line would be necessary, a decision was made to perform porcelain veneers. However, to obtain a space for safe reconstruction of the new teeth shape, increasing the vertical dimension of occlusion (VDO) was necessary.

Step 2: Centric relation (CR)

As the temporomandibular joint (TMJ) loading test was negative, a Kois Deprogrammer was fabricated, and the patient used it for 4 weeks during the day and night. After 4 weeks, the CR registration was performed, the casts were mounted in the articulator accordingly to the bite registration.

Step 3: Functional wax-up

Wax-up of the mandibular arch was performed (Fig 8-19f), which allowed the dentist to achieve the goal of creating appropriate space for porcelain veneers in the maxillary anteriors.

Step 4: Restorative treatment

A. Mandibular arch – no preparation

Direct composite restorations were performed using the index technique without any tooth preparation (Figs 8-19g to 8-19k) – the method was already described in Cases 5 and 6.

B. Partial diastema closure with veneers

In the anterior segment of the maxilla, the palatal surfaces were first reconstructed with direct composite resin (Fig 8-19l), followed by veneer treatment (Figs 8-19m and 8-19n). Preparation for six porcelain veneers was obtained (Figs 8-19o and 8-19p). Special attention was paid during proximal surface preparation, to enable the dental technician to build an appropriate emergence profile that met the esthetic expectations discussed with the patient (Figs 8-19q and 8-19r).

Feldspathic porcelain veneers were fabricated (Fig 8-19s) in such a way as to optically reduce the diastema by decreasing the space between the maxillary central incisors and also by teeth lengthening, thanks to which a good proportion between the length and width was obtained. Veneers were cemented in the rubber dam isolation – and the intended esthetic result of a discreet diastema "closure" was achieved without excessive interference in the patient's psychological zone (Figs 8-19t to 8-19ee).

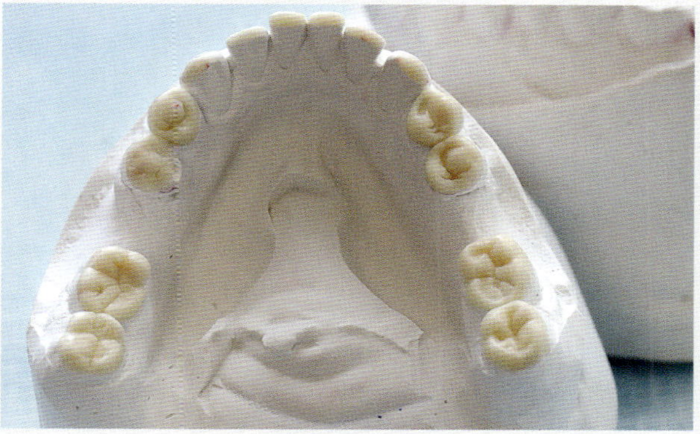

Fig 8-19f
Wax-up of the mandibular arch (functional wax-up), to increase the VDO and create space for esthetic restorations in the anterior segment.

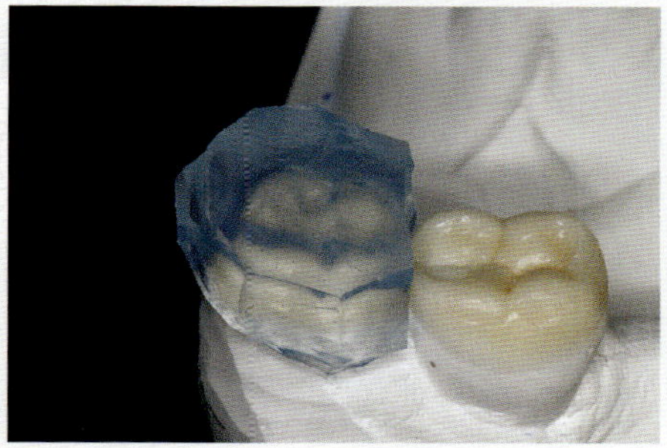

Fig 8-19g
Try in of the silicone index segments on the wax-up model.

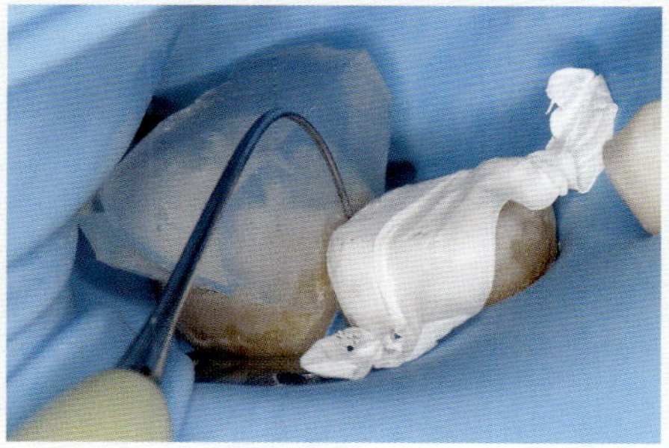

Fig 8-19h
Direct composite restorations performed using the index technique.

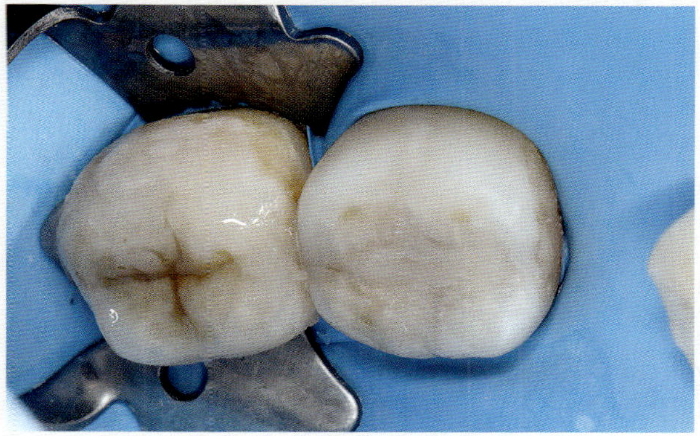

Fig 8-19i
Finished direct restoration in tooth 47 after final polymerization.

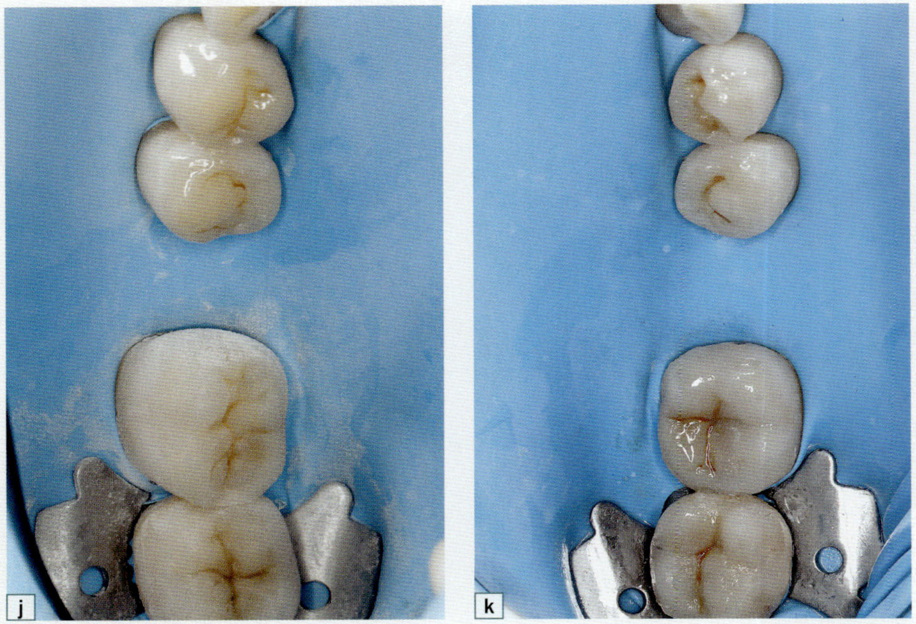

Figs 8-19j and 8-19k
Direct composite restorations in the posterior teeth of the mandible performed using the index technique.

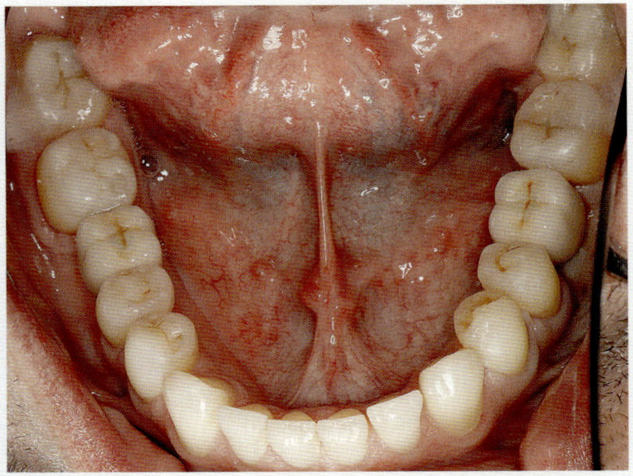

Fig 8-19l
Mandibular arch reconstructed with direct composite resin using the index technique. In the positions of teeth 36 and 46, implants were placed, and screw-retained implant crowns were performed.

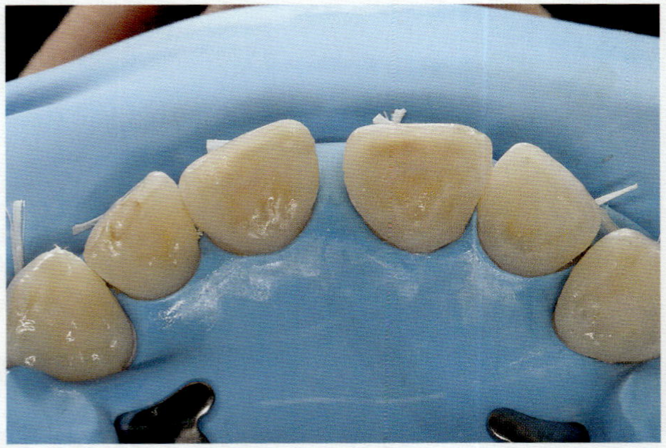

Fig 8-19m
Direct composite resin restorations on the palatal surfaces of anterior maxillary teeth were performed in rubber dam isolation.

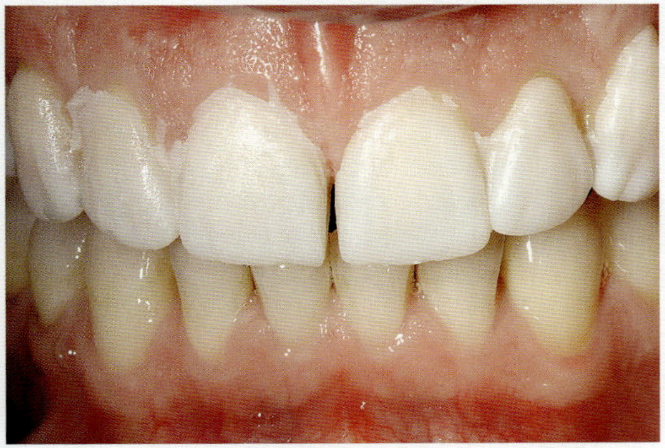

Fig 8-19n
Mock-up created of temporary resin prior to veneer preparation.

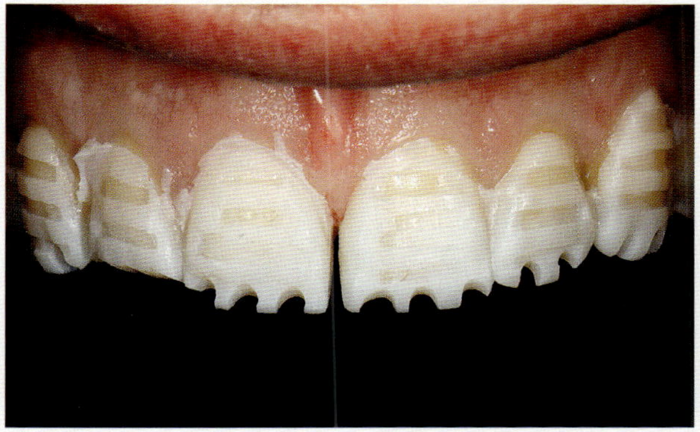

Fig 8-19o
Veneer preparation from the mock-up level.

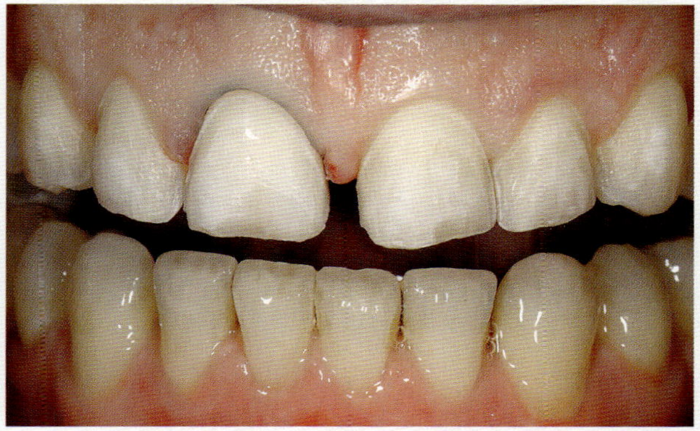

Fig 8-19p
Veneer preparation of teeth 13–23 prior to final polishing.

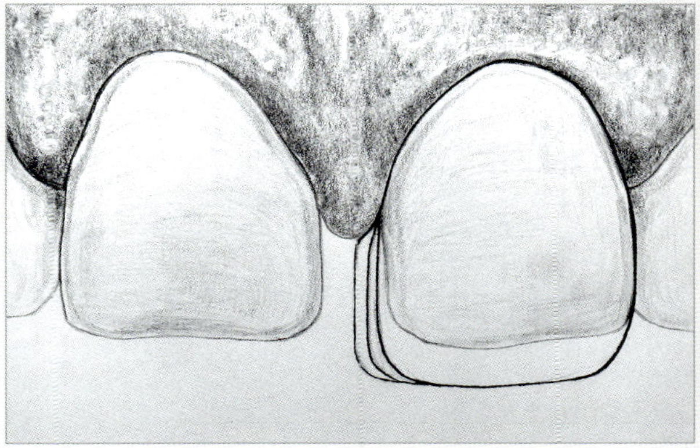

Fig 8-19q
Appropriate preparation gives the dental technician the possibility to close the diastema in different scenarios.

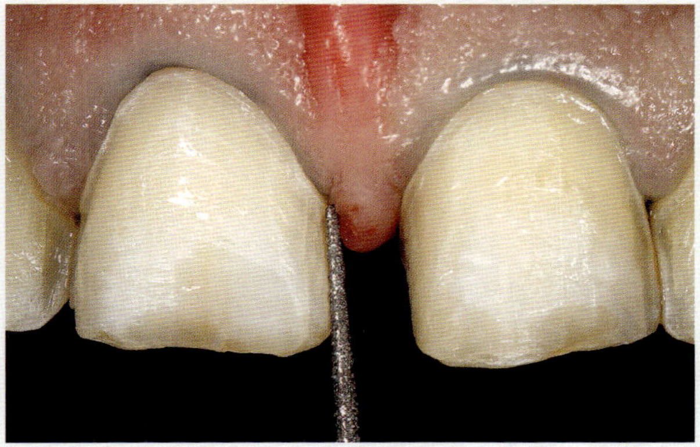

Fig 8-19r
The key to proper diastema closure is proximal surface preparation. The juxtagingival margin must be located below the gingival papilla so that the dental technician can create a proper emergence profile. In some cases, this is necessary for complete diastema closure (in this case, the diastema was not closed completely, but such a preparation technique gives more options for possible corrections).

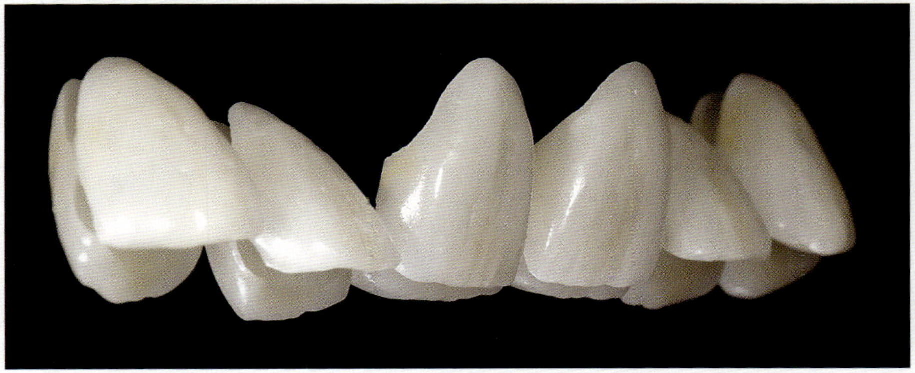

Fig 8-19s
Feldspathic porcelain veneers ready for cementation (laboratory work: DT Artur Nyga).

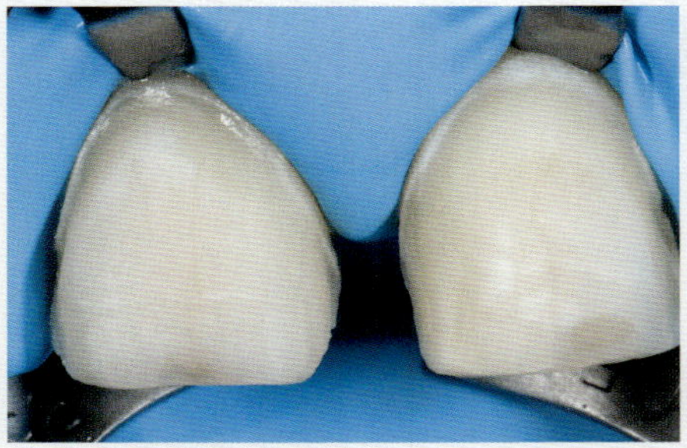

Fig 8-19t
Teeth 11 and 21 after etching, thorough rinsing with water spray, gentle drying …

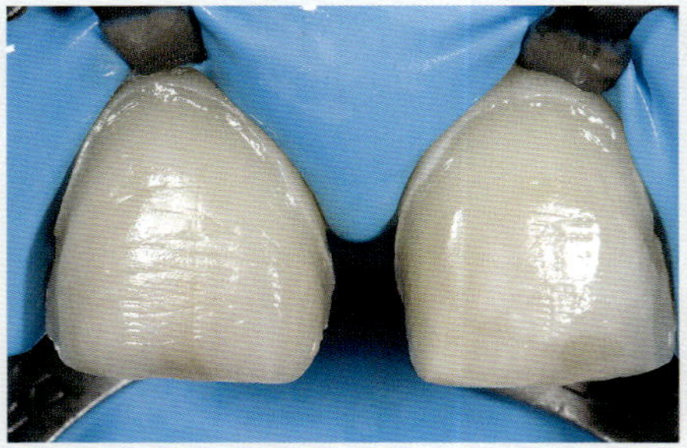

Fig 8-19u
… and after applying the bonding system.

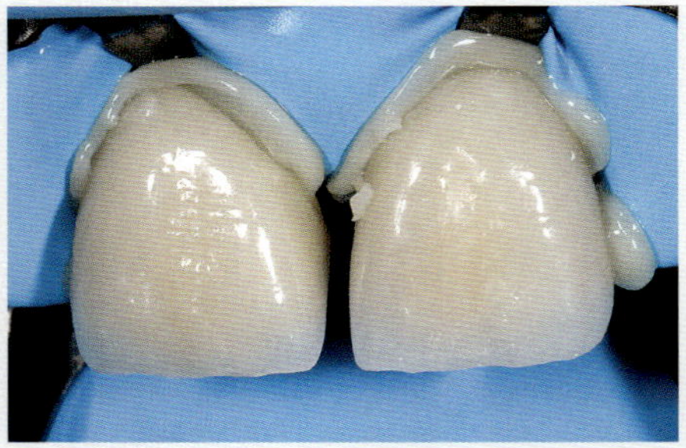

Fig 8-19v
Cementing veneers with a heated composite resin (Enamel Plus HRi, Micerium), before removing the resin excess.

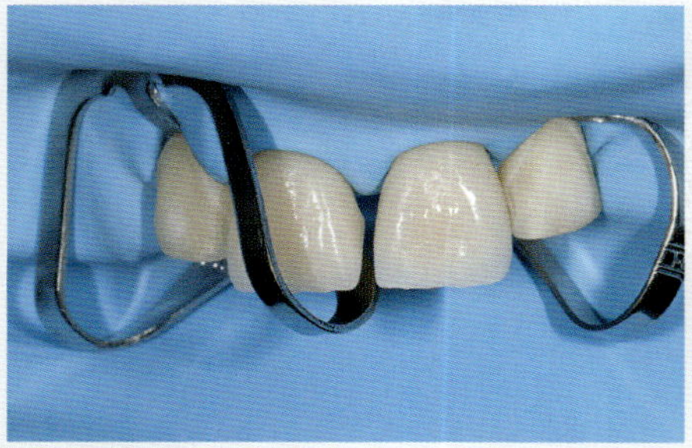

Fig 8-19w
Rubber dam isolation and cementing subsequent veneers on teeth 12 and 22.

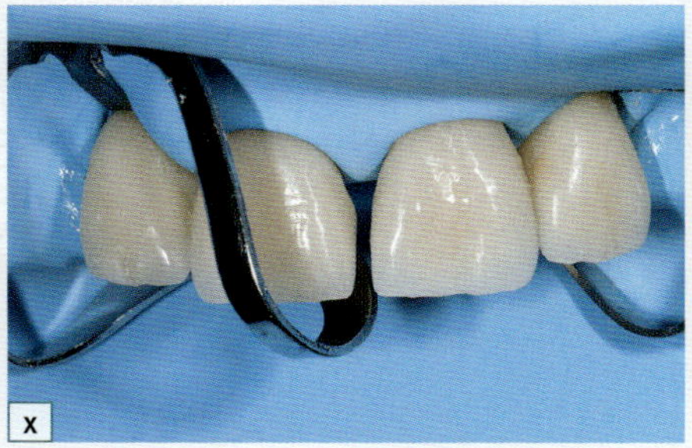

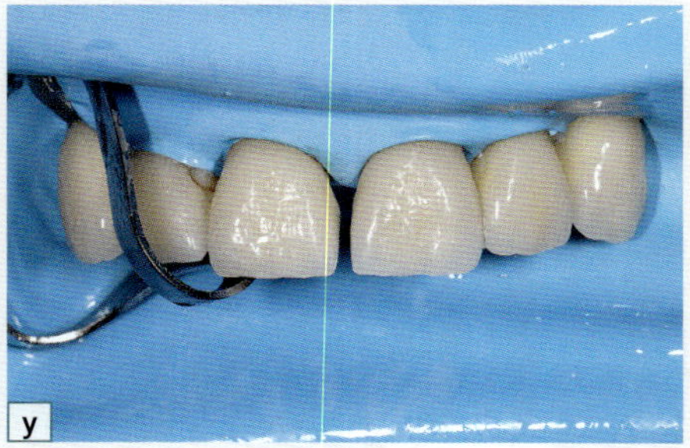

Figs 8-19x and 8-19y
Situation after cementing veneers (x) on teeth 12 and 22 and (y) on teeth 13 and 23.

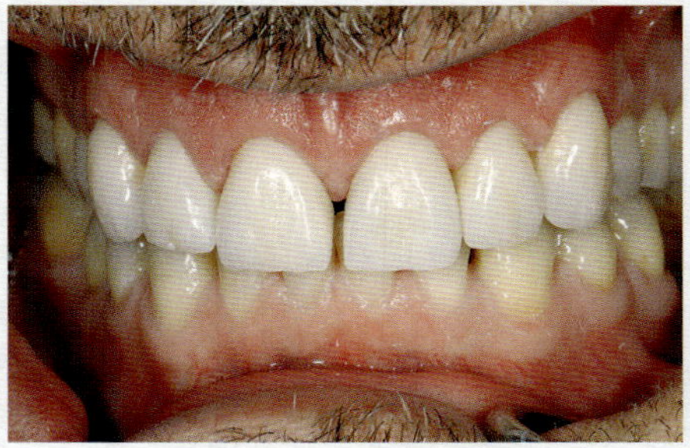

Fig 8-19z
Situation after cementing veneers on teeth 13–23, immediately after removing the rubber dam.

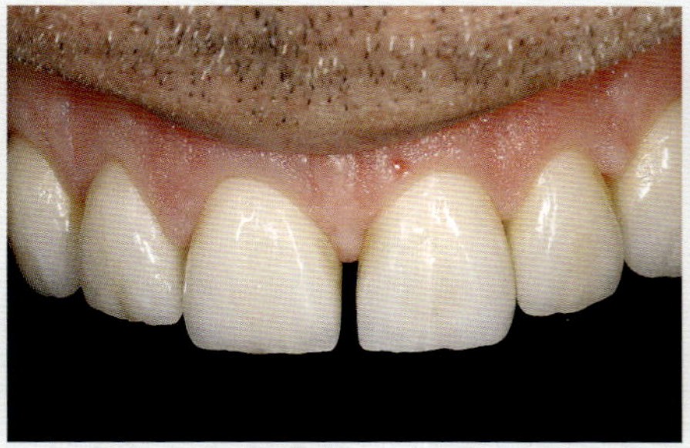

Fig 8-19aa
Porcelain veneers on teeth 13–23 a few weeks after cementation.

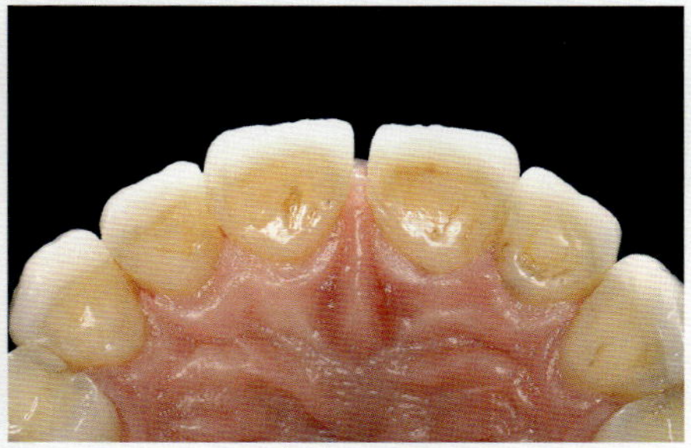

Fig 8-19bb
Veneers on teeth 13–23: palatal view.

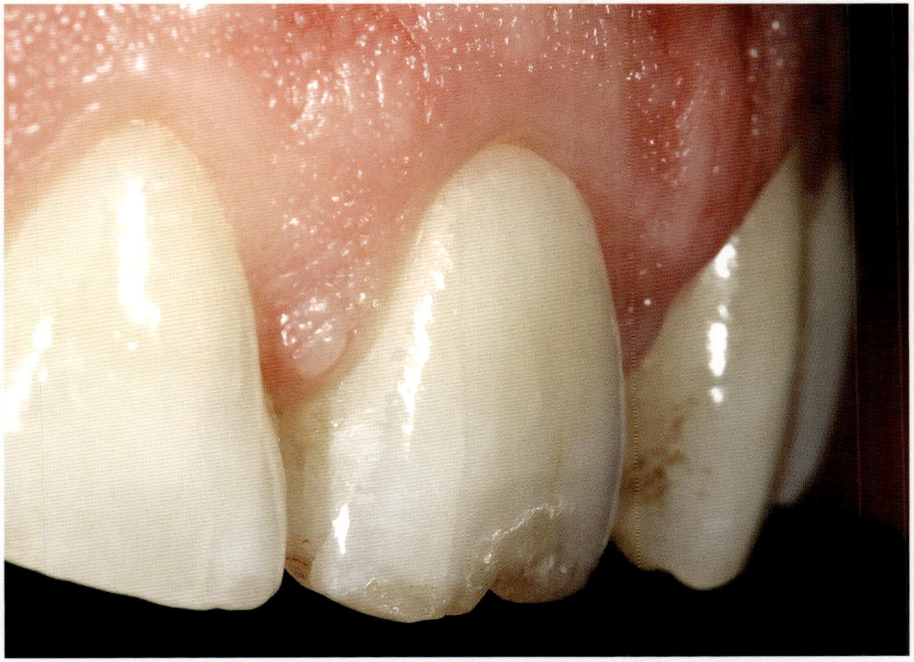

Fig 8-19cc
Initial situation before starting the treatment.

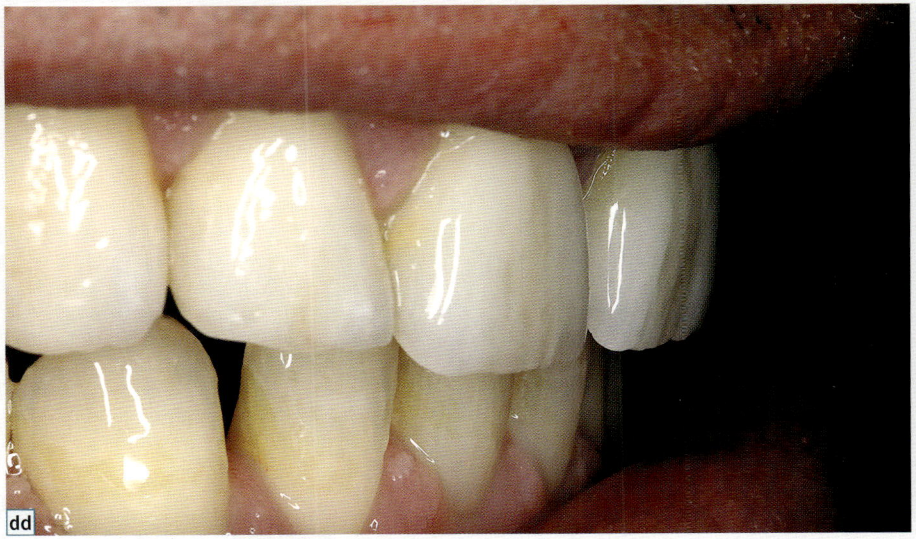

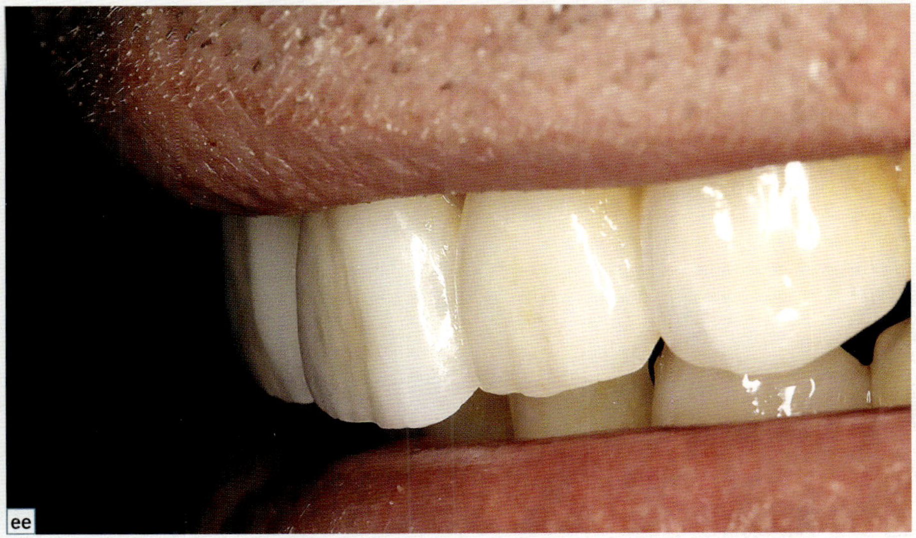

Figs 8-19dd and 9-19ee
Clinical situation after the treatment is completed.

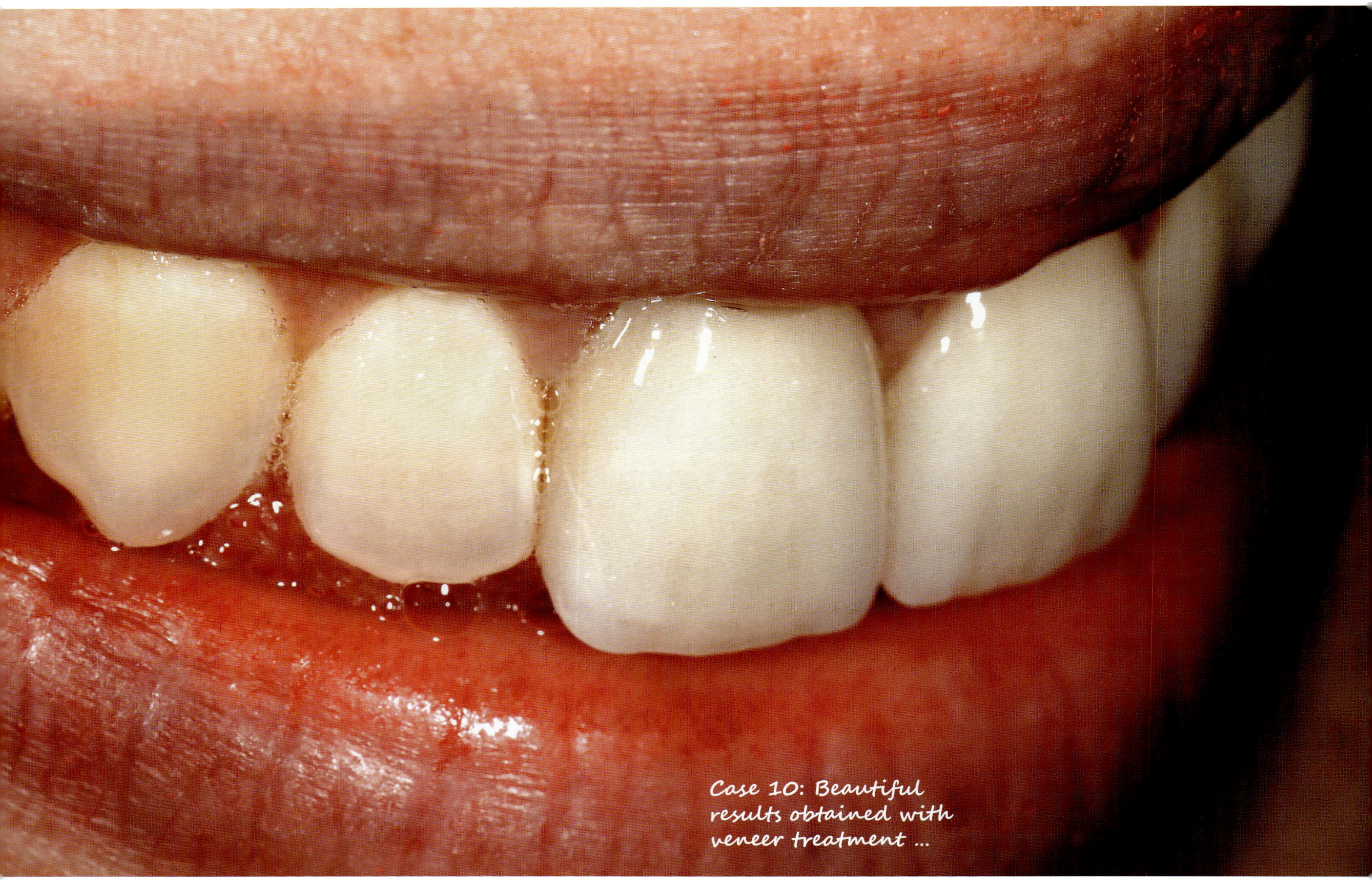

Case 10: Beautiful results obtained with veneer treatment ...

Case 10: Complete diastema closure

Unlike in the previous case, in many clinical situations complete diastema closure can be beneficial from an esthetic and psychological point of view. It is very important to perform a mock-up and confirm the diastema closure concept with the patient and the consultation team.

In this case (Figs 8-20), not only the procedure of diastema closure was performed, but also the discoloration of tooth 11 after root canal treatment was masked, as internal bleaching was contraindicated.

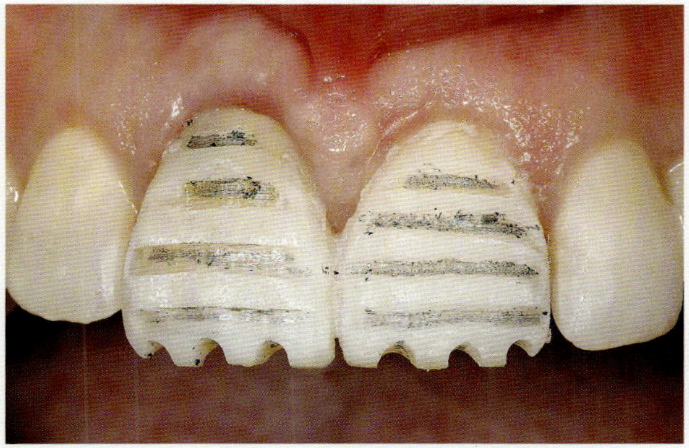

Fig 8-20d
After approving the mock-up simulating diastema closure, veneer preparation was performed from the mock-up level.

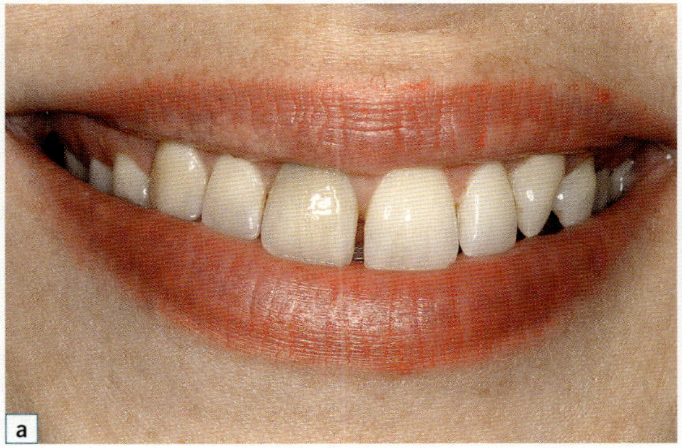

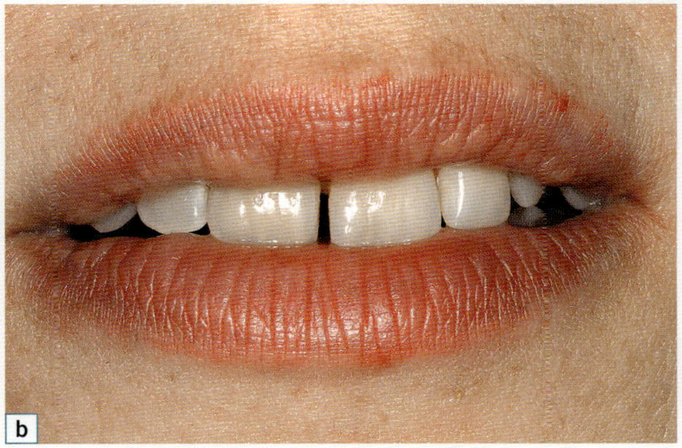

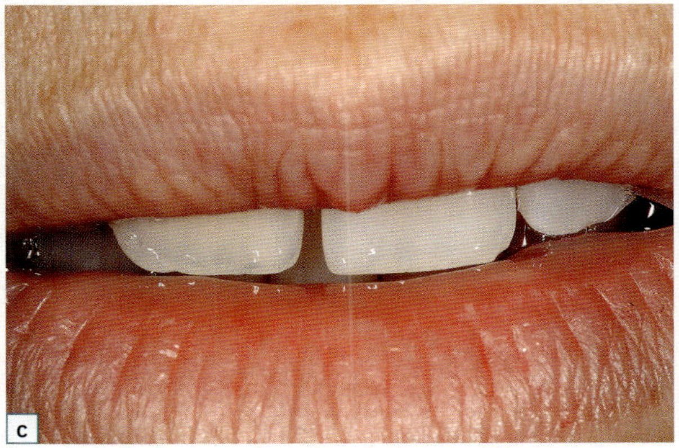

Figs 8-20a to 8-20c
A female patient presented to the dental office with an esthetic problem related to the discoloration of tooth 11; the tooth underwent root canal treatment. Due to the perforation formed in the past during the root canal treatment, the possibility of internal bleaching was excluded, and a decision was taken to perform a veneer while closing the diastema by performing a symmetrical veneer on tooth 21.

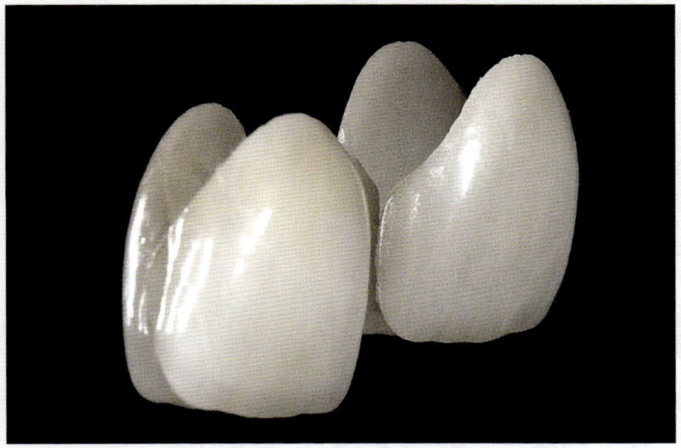

Fig 8-20e
Lithium disilicate porcelain veneers were fabricated in the dental laboratory (E.max) (laboratory work: DT Artur Nyga).

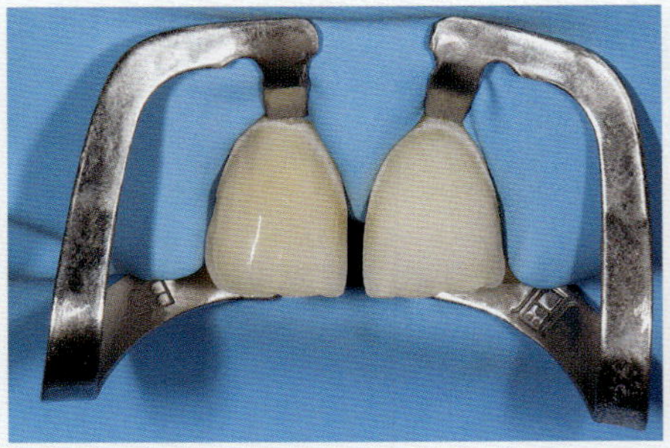

Fig 8-20f
After accepting the esthetics, cementation in rubber dam isolation was performed.

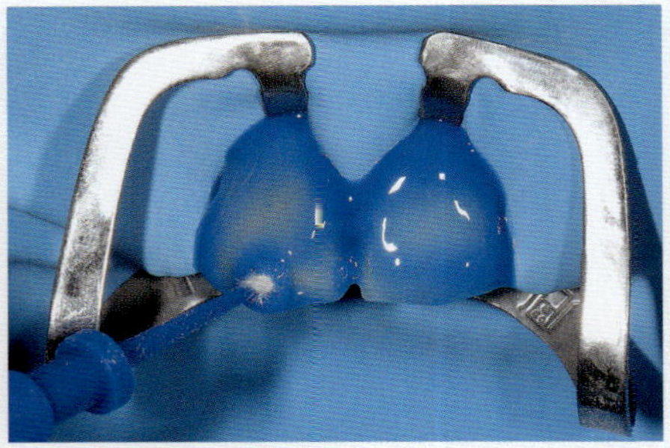

Fig 8-20g
The tooth surface was etched with orthophosphoric acid for 20 seconds . . .

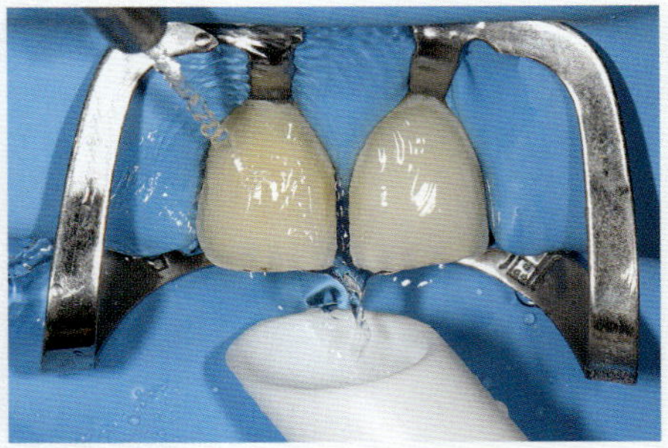

Fig 8-20h
. . . next, the acid was thoroughly rinsed with a water spray . . .

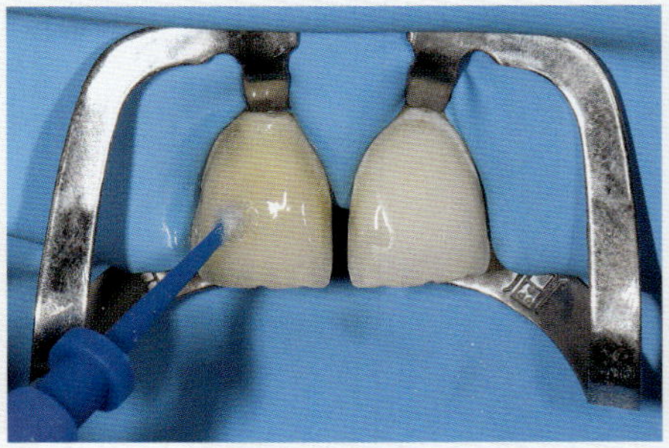

Fig 8-20i
. . . and gently dried, and the bonding system was applied in two layers.

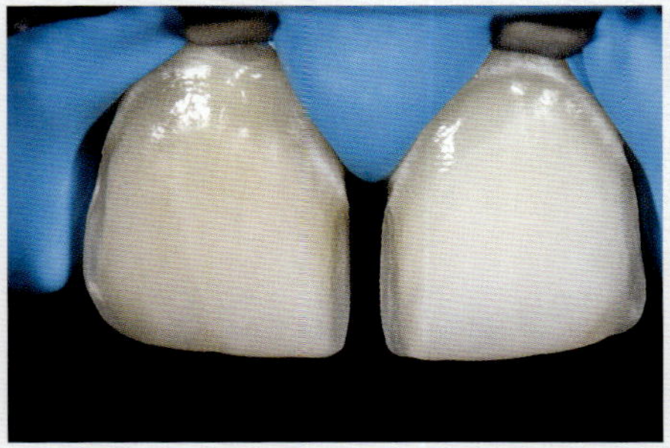

Fig 8-20j
A layer of bonding system was thinned with an air spray and then thoroughly polymerized.

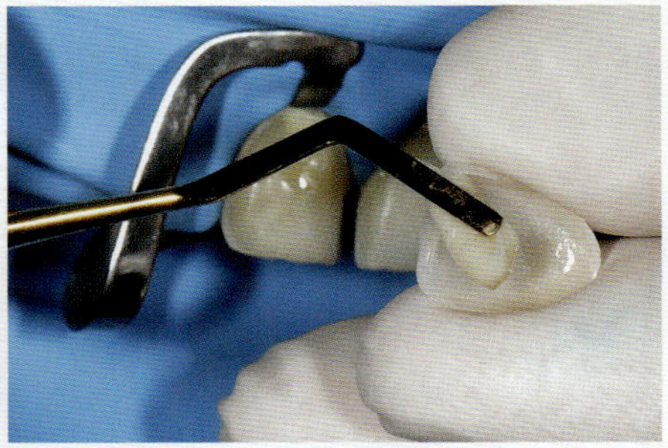

Fig 8-20k
Application of the heated light-cured composite resin.

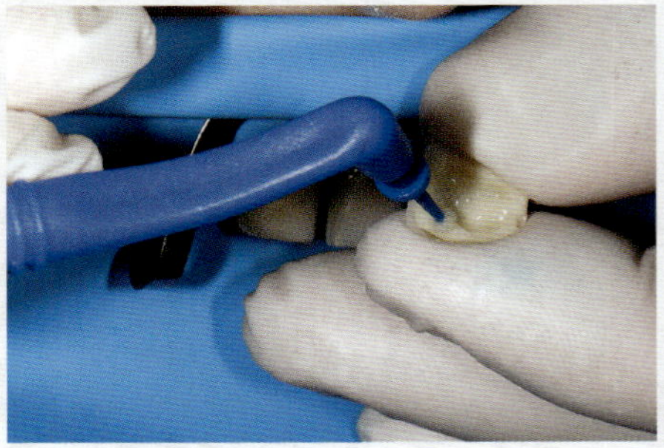

Fig 8-20l
Composite was thoroughly spread with a disposable applicator.

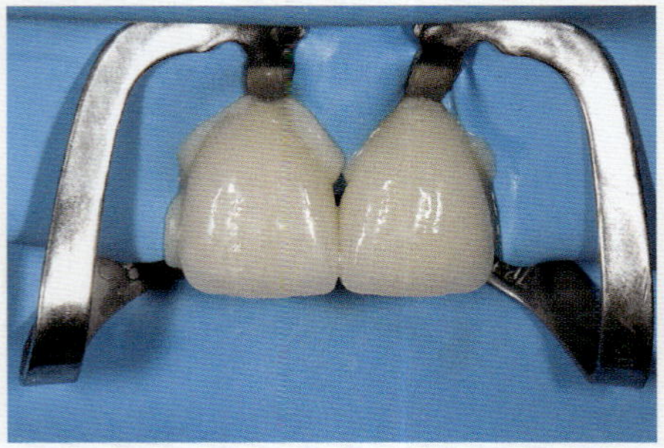

Fig 8-20m
Two veneers were cemented, and excess composite was removed before polymerization.

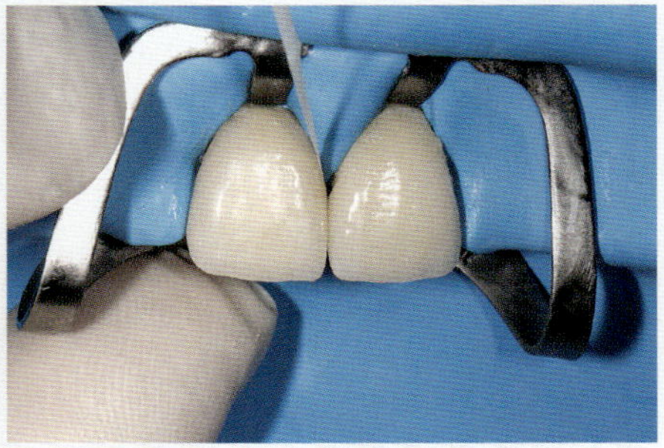

Fig 8-20n
The excess composite was removed with dental floss from the interdental spaces.

NO-PREP VENEERS PARTIAL VENEERS

In recent years, there has been much discussion about no-prep porcelain veneers and about partial veneers that change the shape of the tooth or restore the missing part of the tooth. Even though this concept might sound great and fashionable to the patient, it does come with some limitations:

- **Esthetics:** It is not always possible to increase the volume to make it esthetically acceptable without preparation.
- **Emergence profile:** Excessive enlargement of the emergence profile can create a problem for gingival health.
- **Cementation:** Cementing no-prep porcelain veneers can be problematic, because the dentist does not see the preparation margin and does not know whether the veneer has reached its margin or whether they should still "press" it into place. Consequently, the veneer may not be cemented in the correct position.
- **Risk of fracture:** A no-prep veneer is very thin by definition (especially in the gingival area). As a consequence, there is a risk of porcelain fracture when it is pressed with too much force against the tooth during cementation.
- **Positioning:** Positioning and relocating the partial veneers is a challenge due to their small size and difficulty with handling.

To sum up, certain conditions related to the current shape of the tooth and the possibility of its enlargement without major esthetic compromise, should be met when performing no-prep veneers.

Case 11: No-prep veneers

A female patient presented to the dental office to improve the esthetics of the maxillary arch. She was unsatisfied with the lack of symmetry between the left and right sides (Figs 8-21a and 8-21b). The patient was offered orthodontic treatment, which she definitely rejected: she wanted the least invasive solution, so she was initially offered composite restorations. However, after taking photographs and analyzing the casts, it was decided that the patient would be an ideal candidate for no-prep porcelain veneers. A mock-up simulating the treatment outcome was performed, and the patient and the consultation team approved the preliminary result of the proposed tooth shape change (Figs 8-21c and 8-21d). During the next appointment, impressions were taken with polyvinyl siloxane material, and two veneers were fabricated: a no-prep veneer for tooth 22 and a partial veneer for tooth 23 (Fig 8-21e).

A week later, after adhesive conditioning of the tooth surface and the porcelain veneers, the restorations were tried in and cemented in a rubber dam isolation (Figs 8-21f to 8-21p). The final result of the treatment is presented in Figs 8-21q to 8-21s.

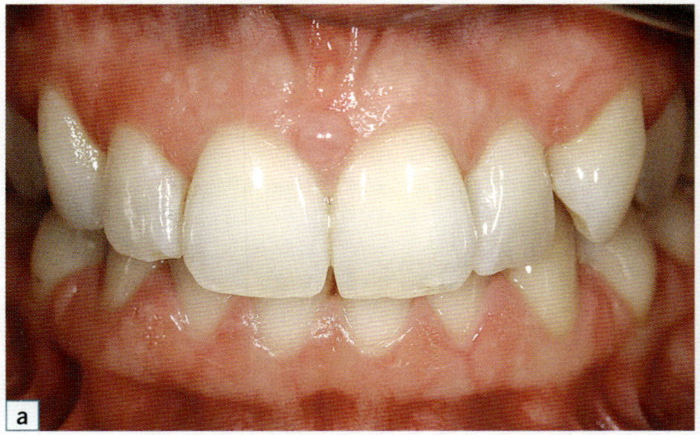

a

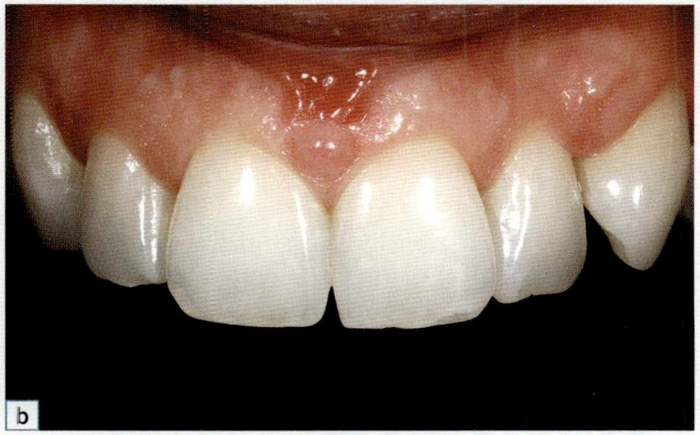

b

Figs 8-21a and 8-21b
Patient's intraoral photographs after she presented at the dental office with a wish of improving esthetics: patient insisted on a symmetrical smile without orthodontic treatment.

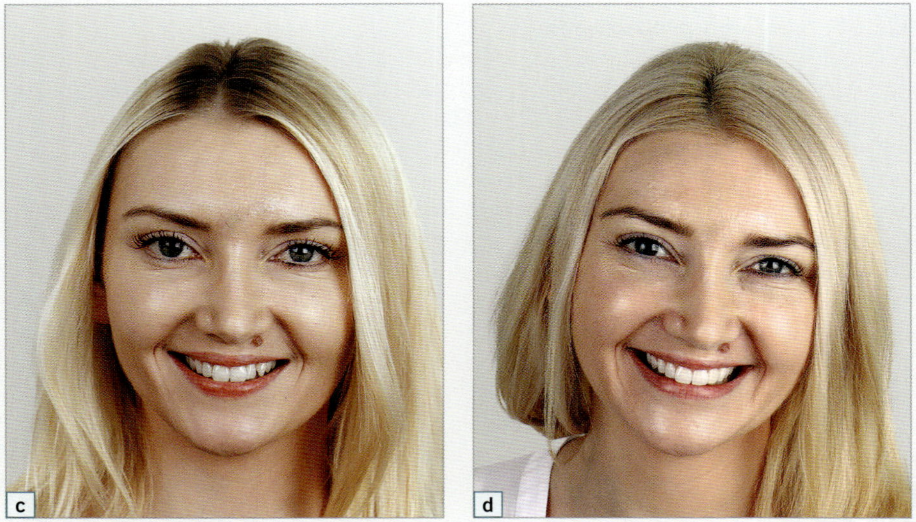

Figs 8-21c and 8-21d
Situation (c) before treatment and (d) after mock-up, showed that non-invasive addition of restorative material could significantly improve the esthetics of the smile.

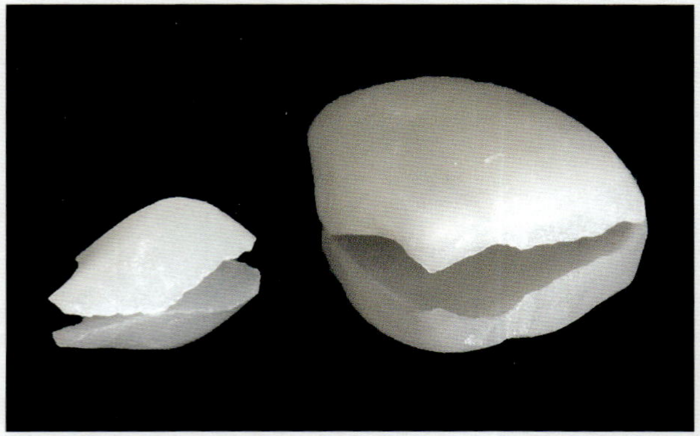

Fig 8-21e
Porcelain veneers fabricated in the laboratory ready for cementation (laboratory work: DT Artur Nyga).

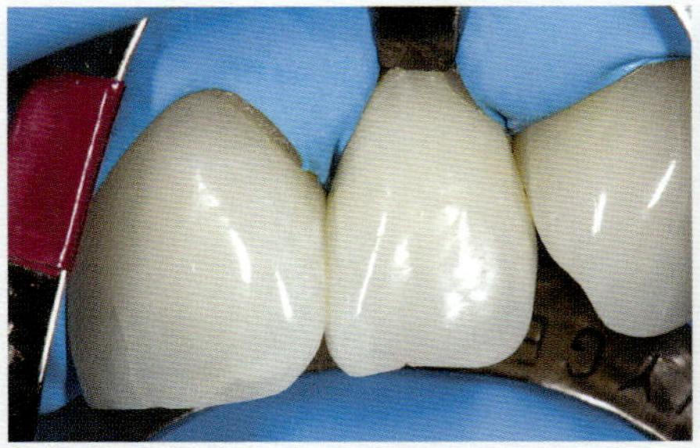

Fig 8-21f
Teeth 22 and 23 were isolated with a rubber dam before veneer cementation. Trying veneers to ensure that the rubber dam clamp does not interfere with the correct veneer placement.

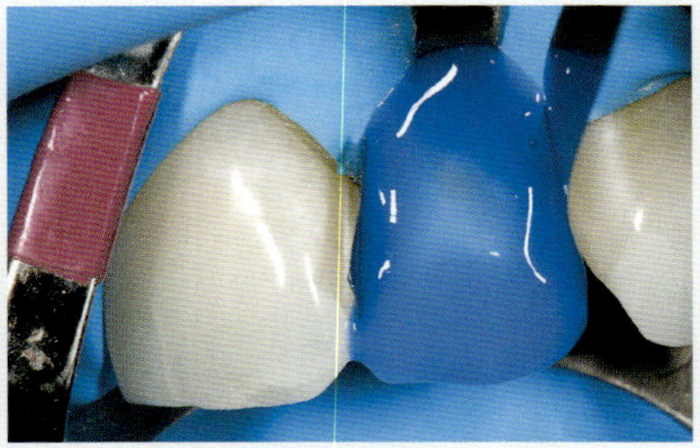

Fig 8-21g
After air abrasion of the surface of tooth 22, etching with orthophosphoric acid was performed ...

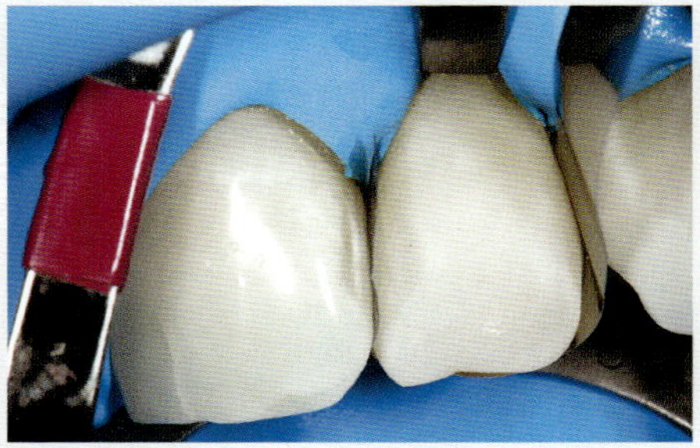

Fig 8-21h
... next, rinsing and gentle drying were carried out ...

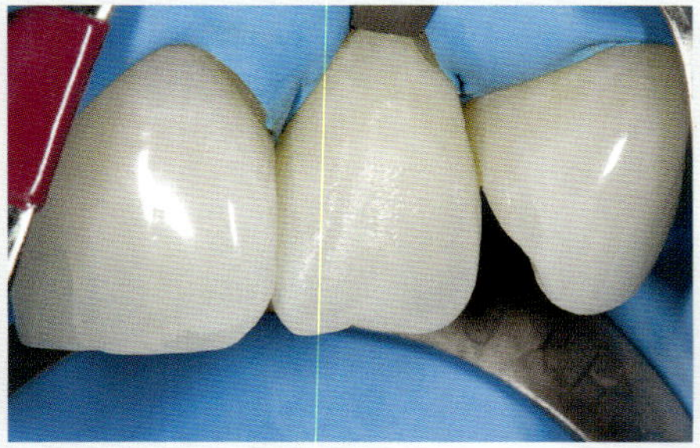

Fig 8-21i
... and the bonding system was applied twice, which was thoroughly air-blown and light-cured.

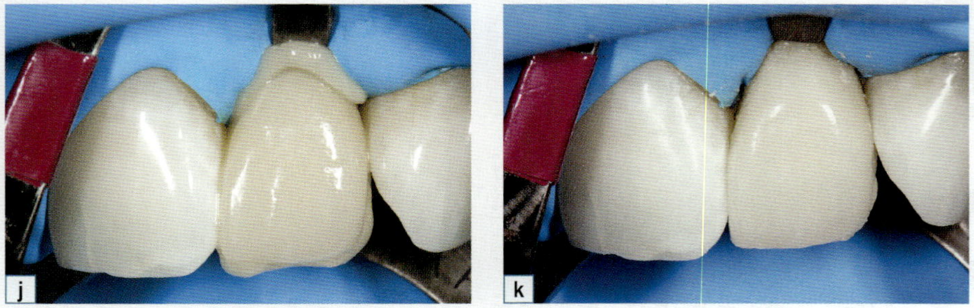

Figs 8-21j and 8-21k
(j) Cementing veneer with light-cure luting cement. (k) Luting cement excess was thoroughly removed prior to polymerization.

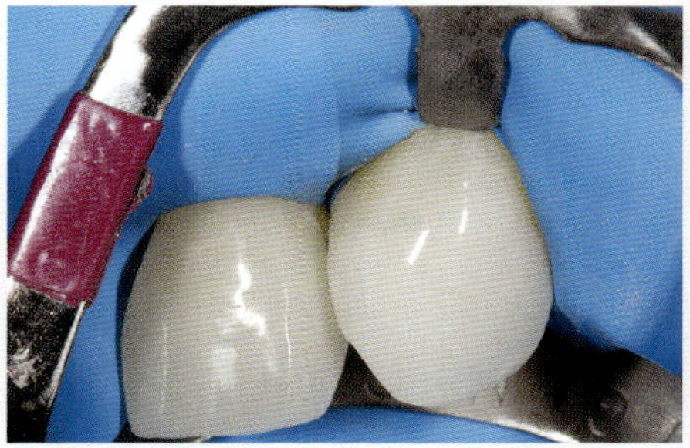

Fig 8-21l
In the next step, the partial veneer was cemented on tooth 23.

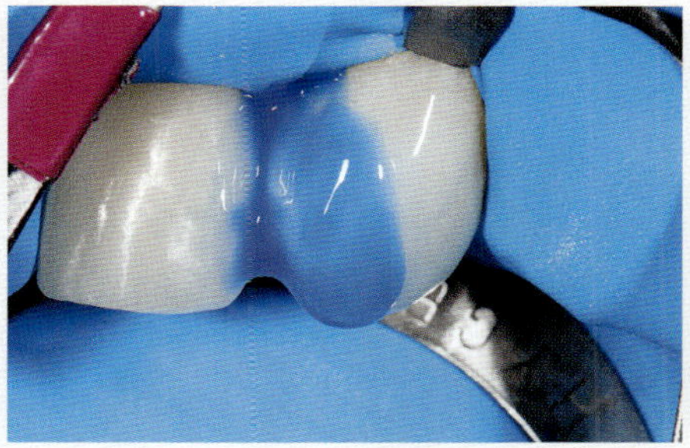

Fig 8-21m
First, the surface of tooth 23 was thoroughly etched with orthophosphoric acid ...

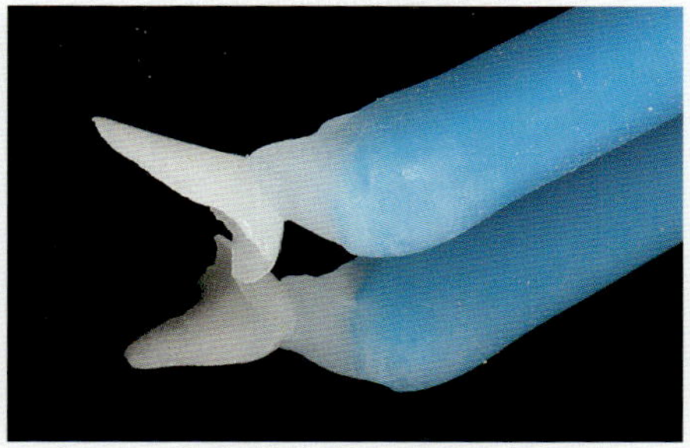

Fig 8-21n
... then, the veneer was placed on the PickUp Stick (Hager & Werken) ...

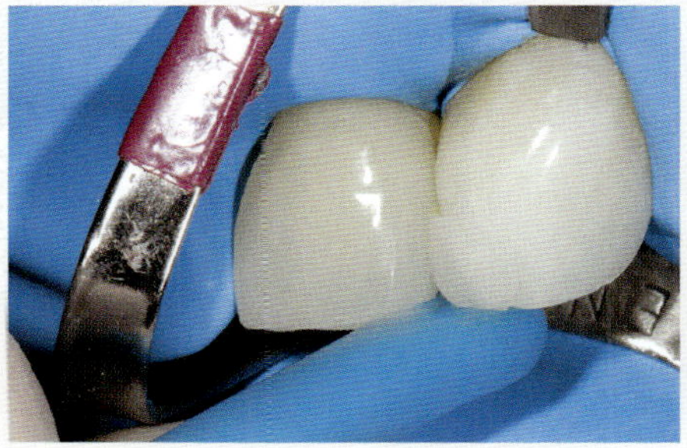

Fig 8-21o
... placing the veneer in the appropriate position was trained ...

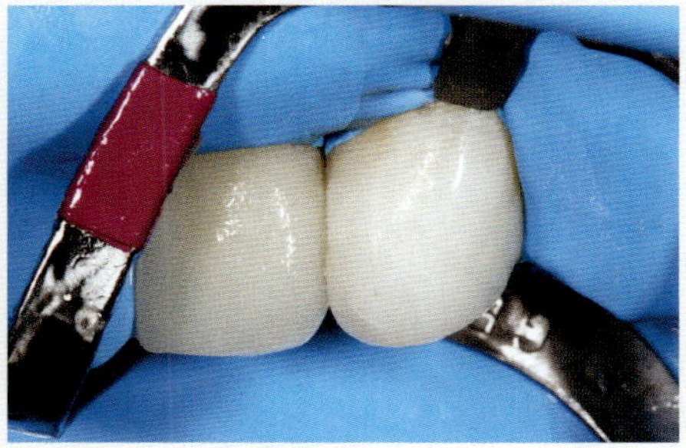

Fig 8-21p
... and finally cemented with light-cure luting cement.

PRACTITIONER'S ADVICE

When cementing thin no-prep veneers, use a light-cure luting cement or a flowable composite (to read more: see Chapter 7).

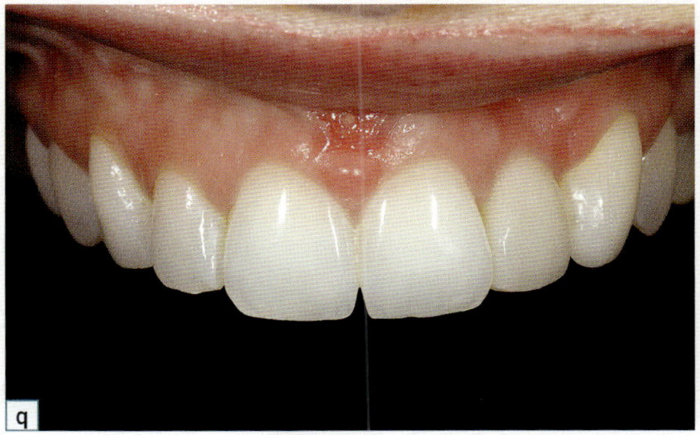

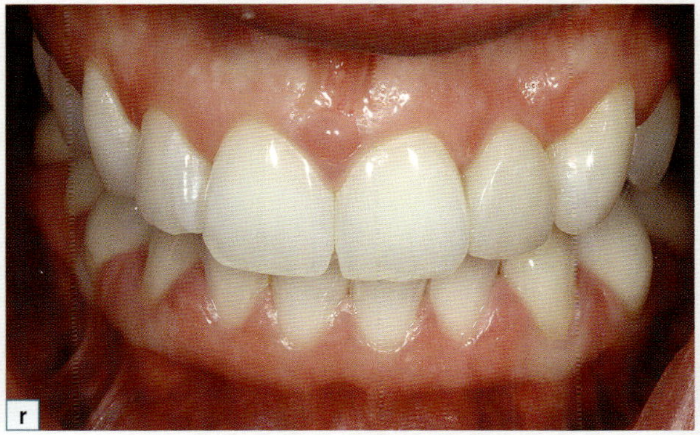

Figs 8-21q and 8-21r
Intraoral photographs show the clinical result a few weeks after cementing veneers on teeth 22 and 23.

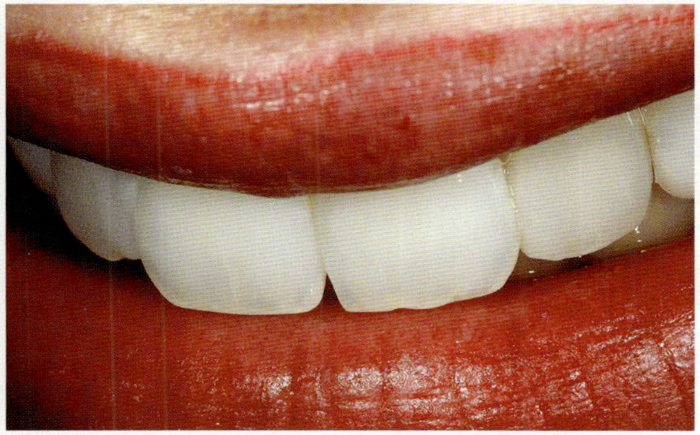

Fig 8-21s
Patient's smile after treatment.

VENEERS: CREATING SYMMETRY WITH THE PROSTHETIC CROWN

In restorative dentistry, there are many clinical situations where there is a need to replace an old crown with a new, more esthetic one. In the patient's mind, it may often seem that replacing one crown will solve the problem of an unesthetic smile. In fact, a single prosthetic crown will pose many problems, such as:

- **Color:** A single crown will usually differ from the rest of the teeth in terms of color, if not in daylight, then in artificial light (sometimes the color of porcelain is perfectly matched to the adjacent natural teeth in daylight, but in artificial light, one-sided porcelain restoration can be a problem for a demanding patient)
- **Size and shape:** If there is asymmetry in the size of the left and right crown of the central incisors, a single crown will not solve the esthetic problem
- **Midline off-center:** When the midline is off-center (between the contact surfaces of the central incisors), it is usually not possible to correct misalignment with one crown

In conclusion, performing a single prosthetic crown carries a big esthetic risk, which can lead to the patient's dissatisfaction, especially when expectations are high. Nowadays, it is possible to fabricate a lithium disilicate crown and a veneer from the same material, which greatly facilitates the work of dental technicians. By working with the same material on the crown and the veneer at the same time, the dental technician can achieve the same color, shape, and characterization so that the restorations will look identical, even under different types of light.

Case 12: Prosthetic crown and veneer

A female patient presented to the dental office in order to replace the old, unesthetic crown on tooth 21 (Figs 8-22a to 8-22c). The patient was disturbed by the color of the crown, which differed from the adjacent teeth, as well as by the exposed dark root in the cervical part of the tooth. The tooth underwent root canal treatment in the past, and a metal post and core were placed. It was also proposed in the past to remove the old post and core and, during the current consultation, the patient asked about this treatment option. A radiograph of tooth 21 was taken (Fig 8-22d). The condition of the periapical tissues was satisfactory. The procedure related to removing the post and core was discouraged due to structural risk (risk of damaging the tooth core while removing the metal post).

Instead of removing the post and core, the focus was on masking the metal post with an opaque composite material.[55] Covering the metal post with an opaque composite allowed a lithium disilicate crown to be performed. The patient was also given an explanation of the purpose of performing two porcelain restorations: a new prosthetic crown in place of the old one on tooth 21 and a porcelain veneer on tooth 11. As a result of this treatment, there was a chance to make two restorations from the same material, improving the symmetry between the central incisors and correcting the midline (Figs 8-22e and 8-22f).

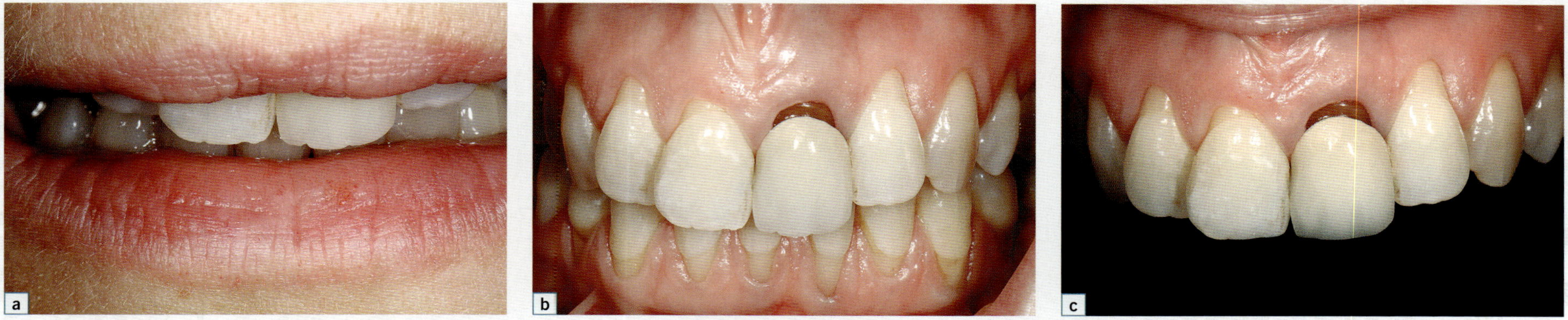

Figs 8-22a to 8-22c
Initial situation: the patient presented to the dental office to improve the esthetics of the anterior teeth. Tooth 21 was covered with an old metal-ceramic crown, and the patient was upset by the dark, exposed root.

After the initial approval of the treatment plan, shown and explained with the mock-up, a request was sent to the dental laboratory to fabricate a provisional shell acrylic crown (Fig 8-22g), and the maxillary and mandibular arches were whitened. Two weeks later, the old crown was removed (Figs 8-22h and 8-22i) and the metal post was covered with a flowable opaque composite resin (Figs 8-22j and 8-22k). Next, the provisional crown was relined with self-curing acrylic (Fig 8-22l), excess material was removed (Fig 8-22m), and the finished and polished resin crown was fitted with temporary cement (Fig 8-22n).

At the next appointment, the crown preparation was modified on tooth 21. A minimally invasive veneer preparation was performed on tooth 11, all the time controlling the preparation depth with a silicone index (Figs 8-22o and 8-22p). Using intraoral photographs (Figs 8-22q and 8-22r), it was checked whether the preparation was sufficient to obtain symmetrical restorations. Impressions were taken and lithium disilicate porcelain restorations were fabricated in the dental laboratory (Fig 8-22s). At the next appointment, the color, shape, symmetry, and the course of the midline created by the proximal surfaces of the restorations were analyzed. The veneer was cemented in rubber dam isolation, and after removing the excess material and re-checking the fit of the proximal surface, the porcelain crown was cemented on tooth 21 (Figs 8-22t and 8-22u). A comparison of the situation before and after treatment is presented in Figs 8-22v and 8-22w.

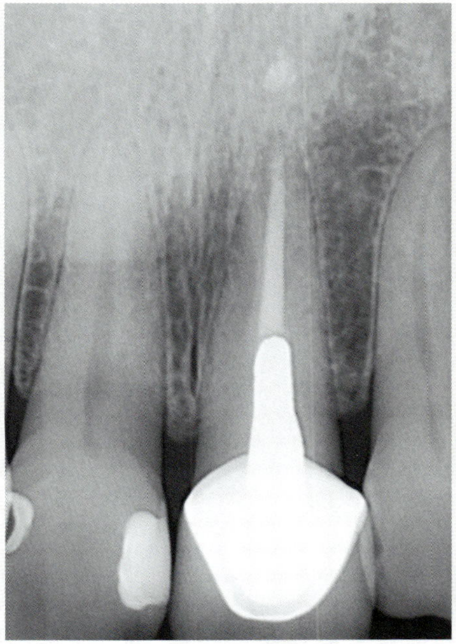

Fig 8-22d
Radiograph: tooth 21 underwent root canal treatment, and a cast metal post was cemented. The radiograph did not show any changes in the periapical tissues; there were no indications for the post and core removal, and to undertake this would risk tooth structural damage.

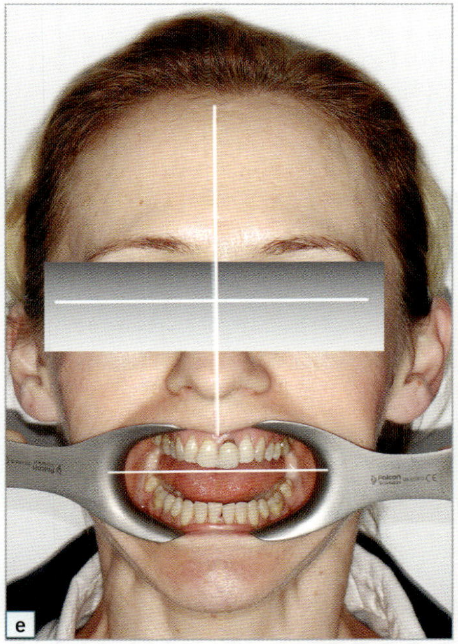

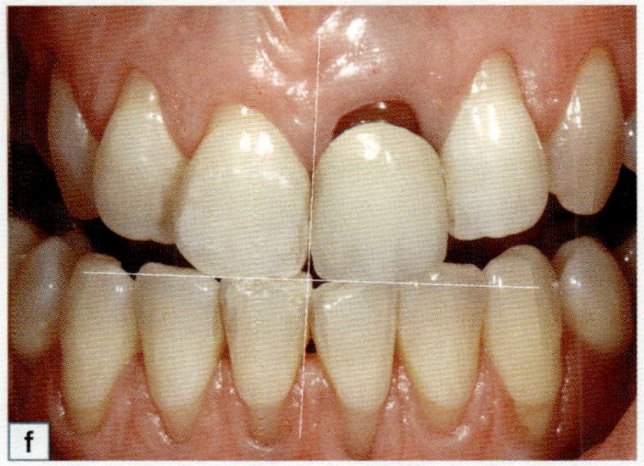

Figs 8-22e and 8-22f
Photograph of the patient with the buccal retractors, allowing control of the midline and the incisal line in relation to the pupillary line (as a reference line in the horizontal plane). This photograph is very helpful in planning restorations and in proper tooth preparation.

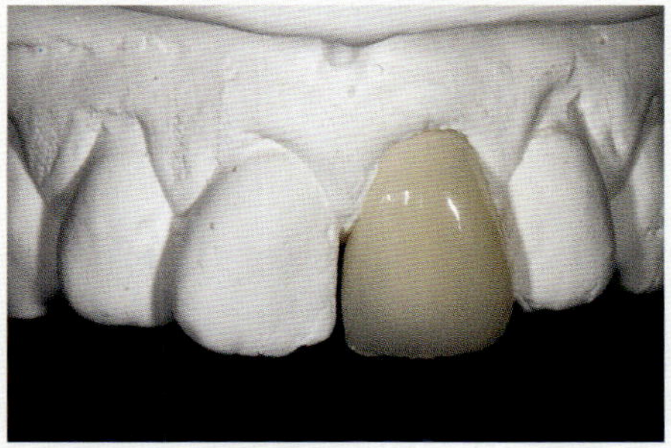

Fig 8-22g
A provisional shell crown made of acrylic was fabricated in the dental laboratory (crown requires relining).

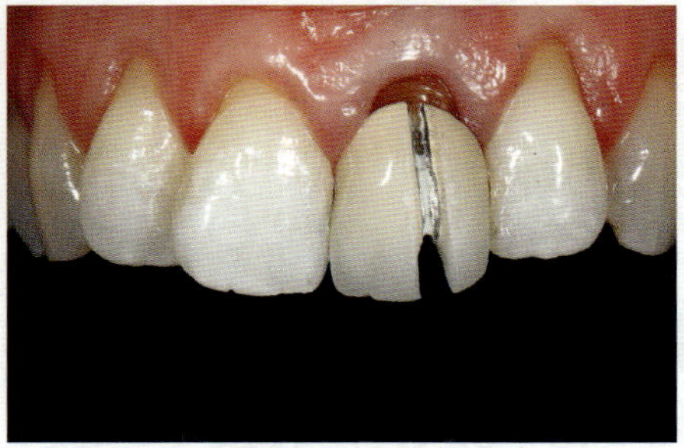

Fig 8-22h
Cutting the crown along the tooth axis from the labial and palatal surface usually enables its removal.

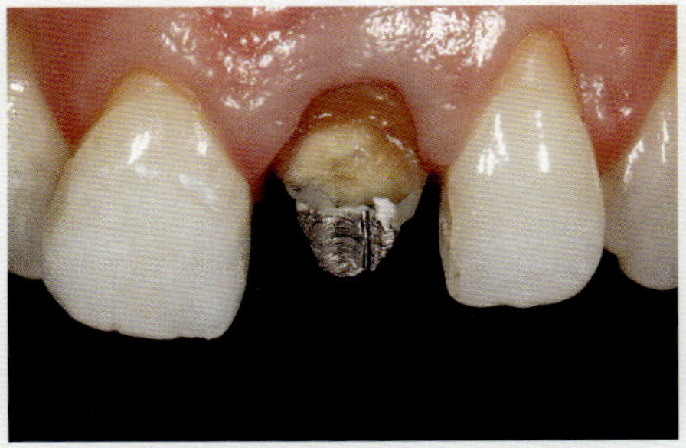

Fig 8-22i
The old cast metal post in tooth 21 after removing the old prosthetic crown.

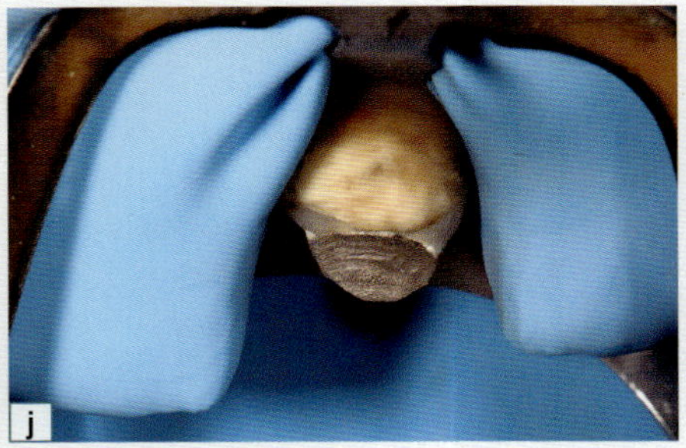

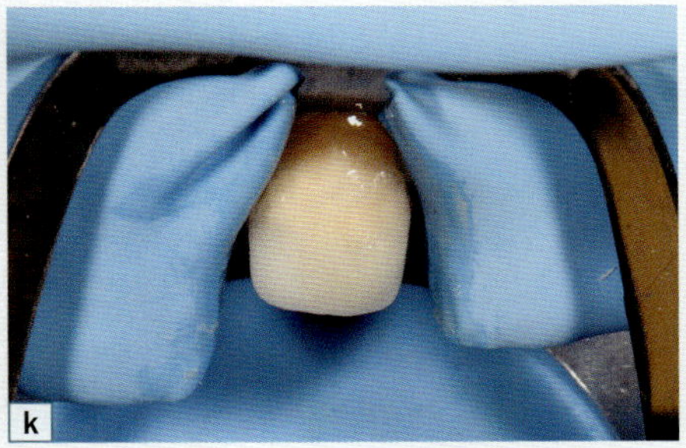

Figs 8-22j and 8-22k
(j) In rubber dam isolation, the core of the tooth with the post was airborne-particle abraded with aluminum oxide particles (50 μm in diameter), a bonding system containing MDP (G-Premio Bond, GC), was applied (k), and the metal was masked with a flowable opaque composite (Essentia ML, GC) that had been thoroughly polymerized.

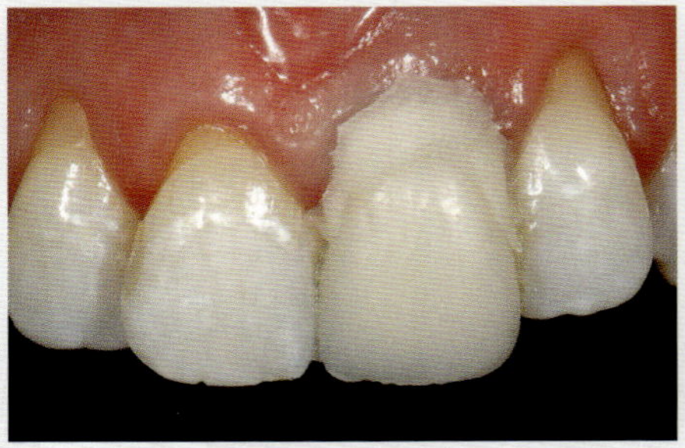

Fig 8-22l
The provisional shell crown was relined with acrylic …

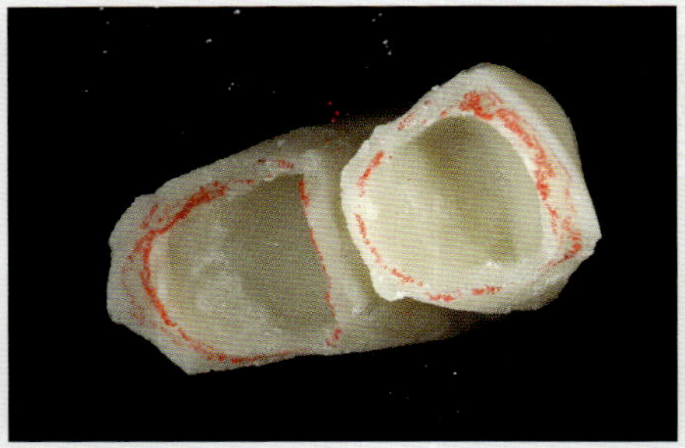

Fig 8-22m
… next, the preparation margin was marked with a red pencil, the excess material beyond the red line was removed, and the outer surface of the crown was polished.

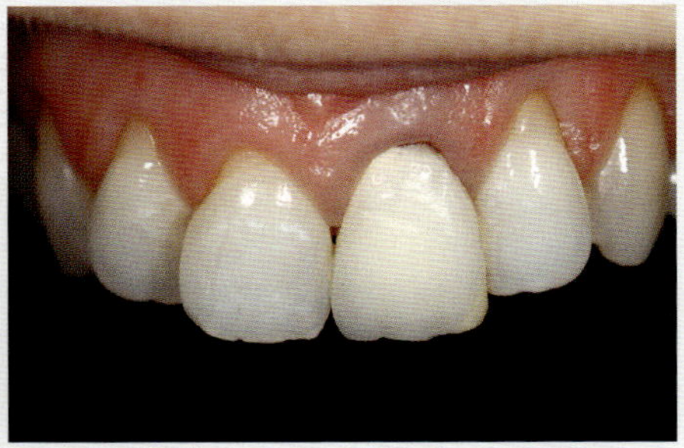

Fig 8-22n
The provisional crown was placed using temporary cement.

Fig 8-22o
During the next appointment, veneer preparation on tooth 11 and crown preparation on tooth 21 were performed. The preparation was controlled with an adjusted silicone index …

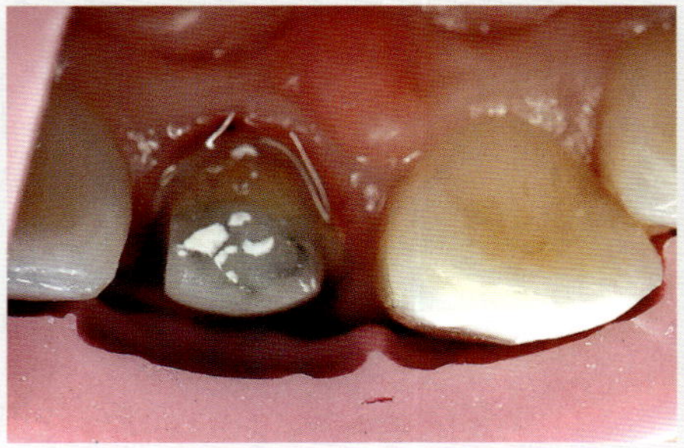

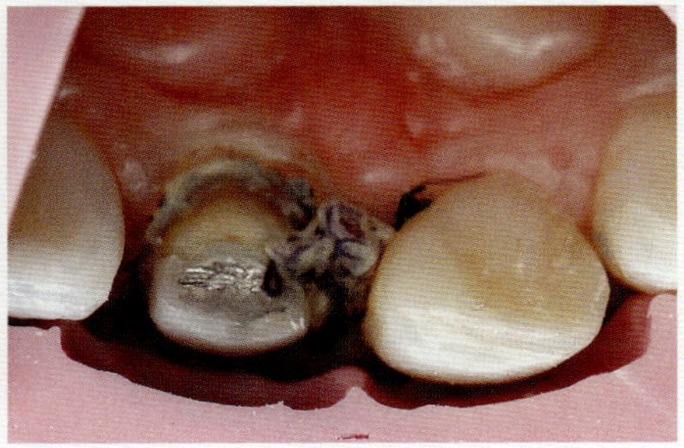

Fig 8-22p
… and adequately corrected.

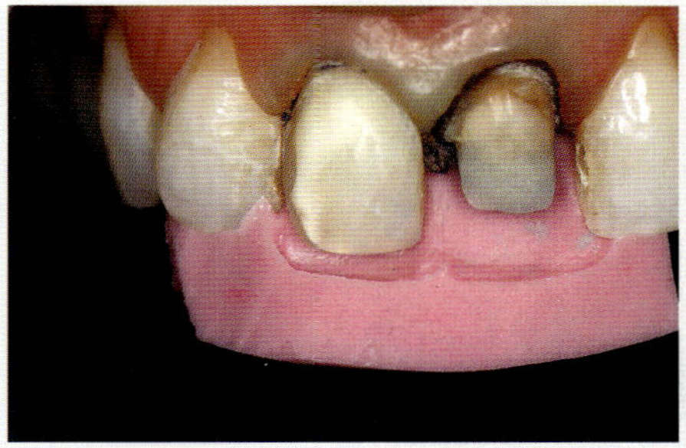

Fig 8-22q
Verifying the location of the incisal edge with a silicone index cut in the frontal (coronal) plane.

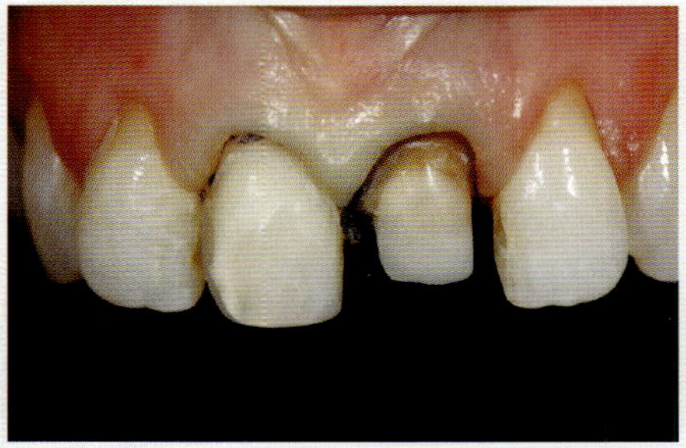

Fig 8-22r
Intraoral photograph taken at the preparation stage to check if the dental technician would have appropriate conditions to change the midline between the proximal surfaces of the central incisors and to obtain symmetrical restorations.

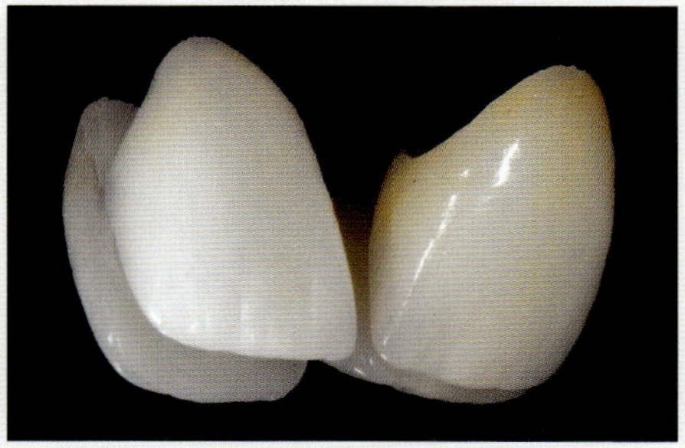

Fig 8-22s
Lithium disilicate restorations fabricated in the dental laboratory: veneer for tooth 11 and crown for tooth 21 (laboratory work: DT Artur Nyga).

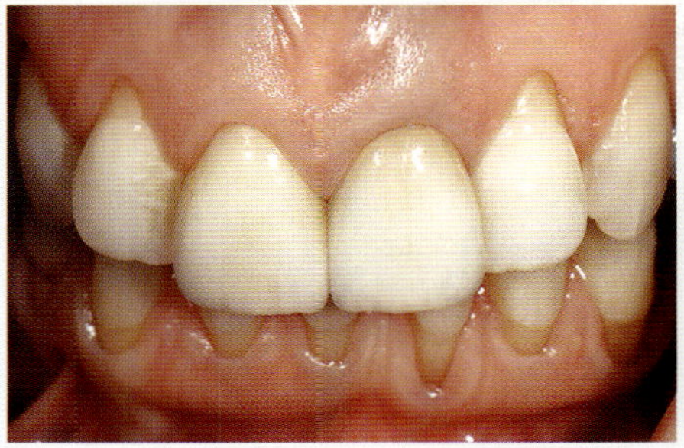

Fig 8-22t
The clinical situation after cementation of the veneer of tooth 11 and crown of tooth 21.

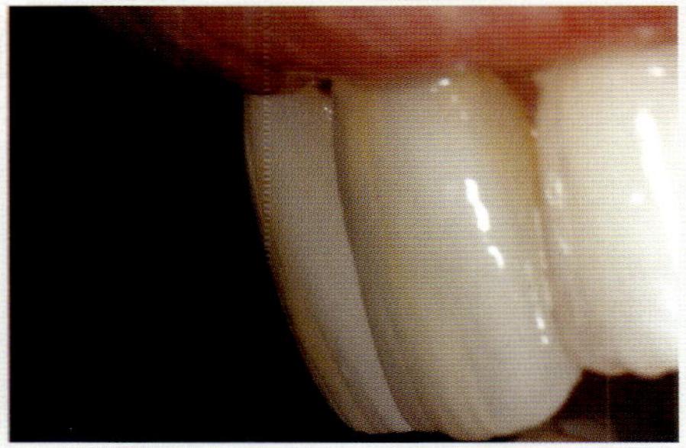

Fig 8-22u
Final clinical outcome.

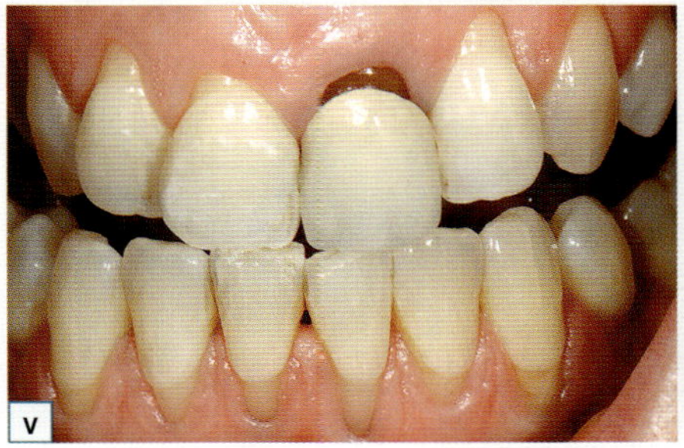

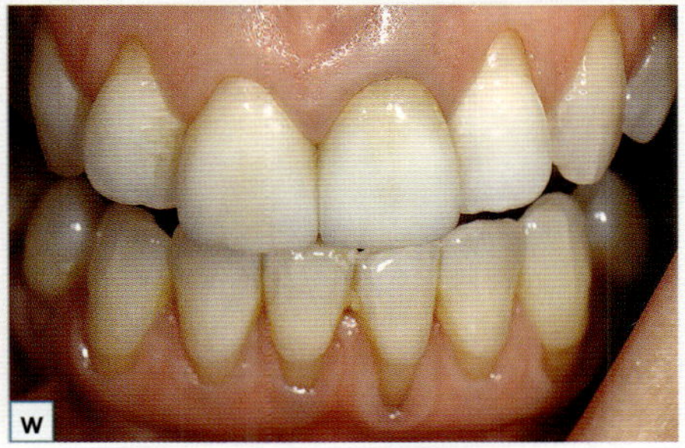

Figs 8-22v and 8-22w
Photographs (v) before and (w) after treatment with lithium disilicate restorations were performed on teeth 11 (veneer) and 21 (crown).

VENEERS: CREATING SYMMETRY WITH THE IMPLANT-SUPPORTED CROWN

Currently, implant restorations have become a dentist's daily practice. Even when we do not engage in implantation, we see patients with implant restorations on a daily basis. Patients with planned or existing anterior implants pose a considerable challenge for restorative dentistry. The three-dimensional position of the implant, the gingival architecture, its biotype, alveolar ridge dimensions and the color and shape of the implant restoration will impact the overall esthetic perception. When performing a single implant crown in the location of the central incisor, it is extremely important to understand the shape of the tooth, which is to be achieved at the end of treatment.[56,57]

The main esthetic goal of a single implant restoration in the location of the central incisor is to obtain the most symmetrically similar restoration to the adjacent tooth, especially in the gingival area. The literature emphasizes that esthetic success in implant-prosthetic restorations is often associated with the presence of teeth characterized by a square shape. Due to the shape of the crown, the incisors were divided into triangular, square/tapered, and square (Fig 8-23).

The tooth's shape is determined by the relationship between the length of the tooth crown (crown length, CL) and the proximal contact surface (CS). In the case of triangular teeth, there is a short contact surface and a long papilla that fills the space below CS.[58]

As Tarnow noted, if the distance between the alveolar ridge and the CS is 5 mm or less, the gingival papilla is almost always present. If this distance is equal or greater than 7 mm, the papilla is usually missing and a black triangle disliked by patients appears.[57]

The above observations show that, in the case of triangular-shaped teeth, the gingival papilla will almost always be missing or will not completely fill the space below the contact surfaces. A few minutes after extraction of one of the two central incisors, there is an immediate papilla recession, which will have implications in reconstructing esthetic restoration.[59] Since there is no predictable regeneration of the gingival papilla, the only option is to reshape the adjacent central incisor to obtain two symmetrical restorations with the goals of:

- Extending the length of the contact point in the incisal-gingival dimension
- Reducing the space for the gingival papilla height
- Shortening the distance between the contact point and the alveolar ridge

These steps will reduce the risk of black triangles.[57]

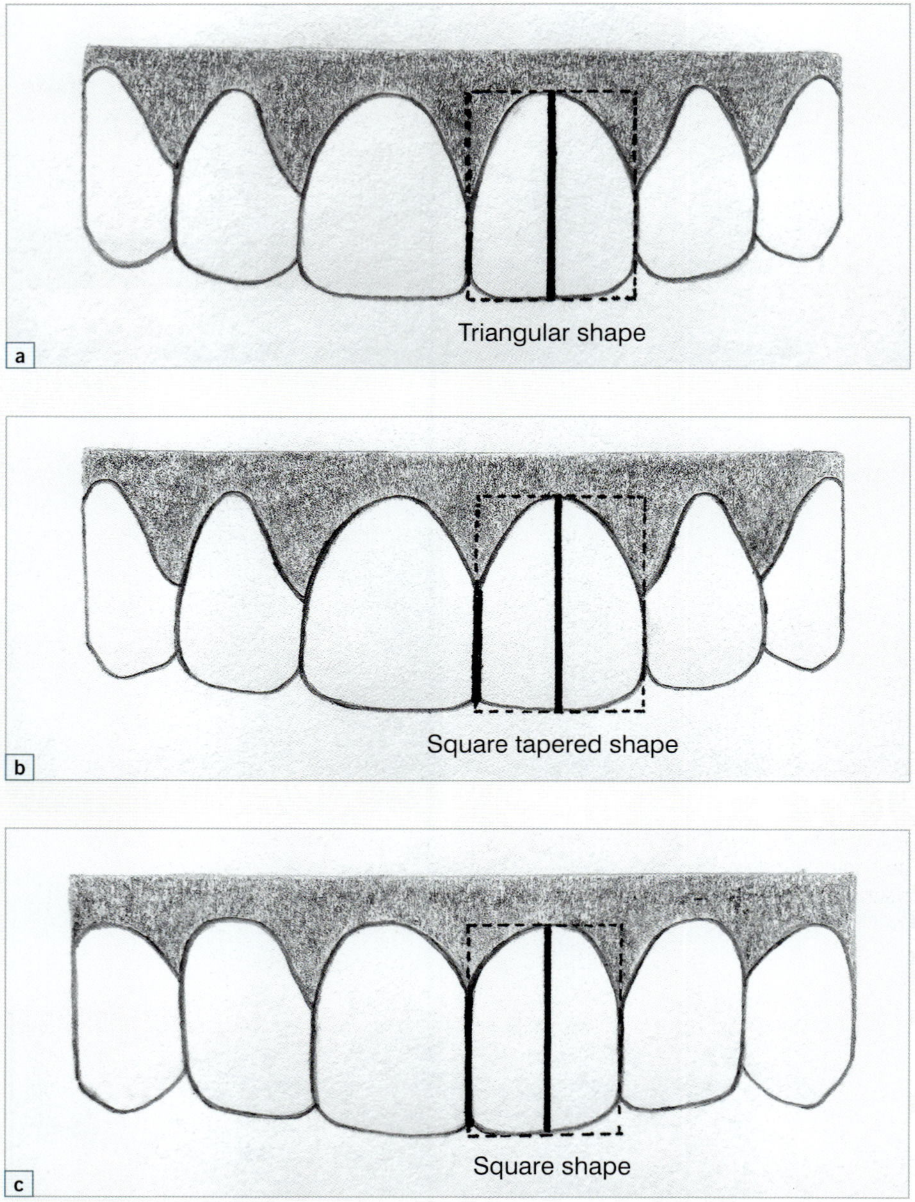

Fig 8-23
Crown shape classification of maxillary central incisors, essential when planning prosthetic restorations on implants.

Case 13: Veneer – creating symmetry with the implant-supported crown

A female patient presented to the dental office for the first time for a routine dental check-up (Fig 8-24a). A control radiograph revealed an external cervical resorption of tooth 21 (Fig 8-24b). The extent of the lesions was confirmed with a cone-beam computed tomography (CBCT) radiograph. Extraction of the maxillary left central incisor was planned, and placing an implant in its location. A standard mock-up visualization of the treatment plan was performed. It revealed that the patient would like a more comprehensive esthetic treatment to improve the appearance of the anterior maxillary teeth while smiling. Tooth 21 was extracted (Figs 8-24c and 8-24d), and an immediate adhesive bridge was fabricated (Fig 8-24e), so no gingival recession occurred immediately after tooth extraction. Two months later, the implant was placed (Fig 8-24f).

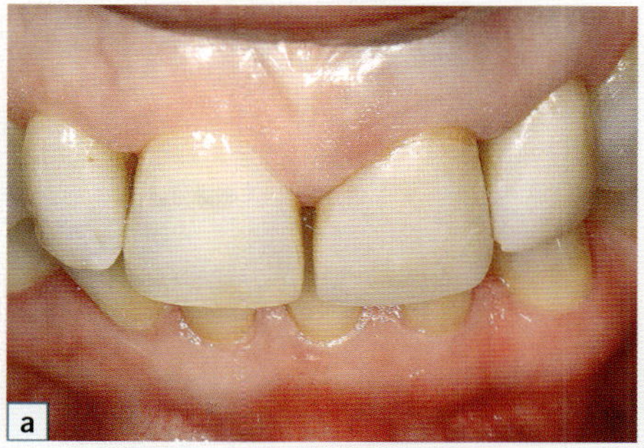

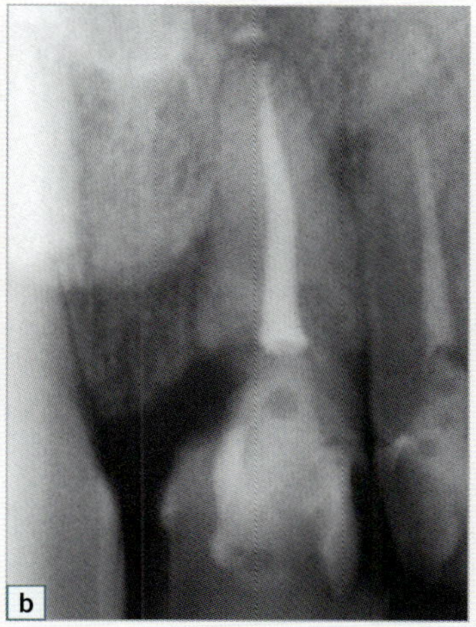

Figs 8-24a and 8-24b
(a) A female patient presented to the dental office for a routine check-up. (b) The radiograph revealed external cervical resorption of tooth 21.

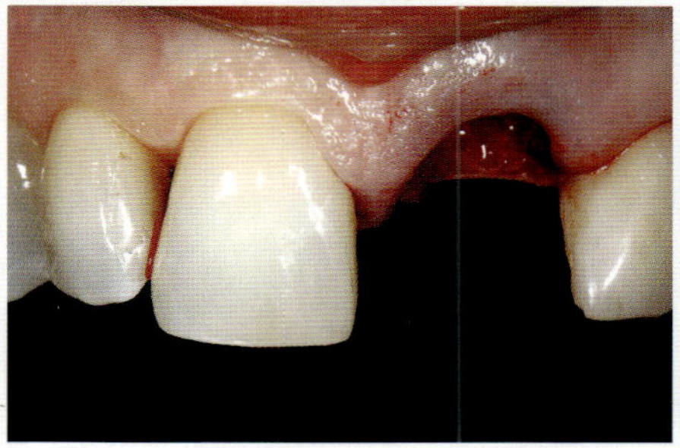

Fig 8-24c
It was planned to extract the tooth, place an implant, and perform comprehensive treatment to relieve the anterior teeth and improve their esthetics.

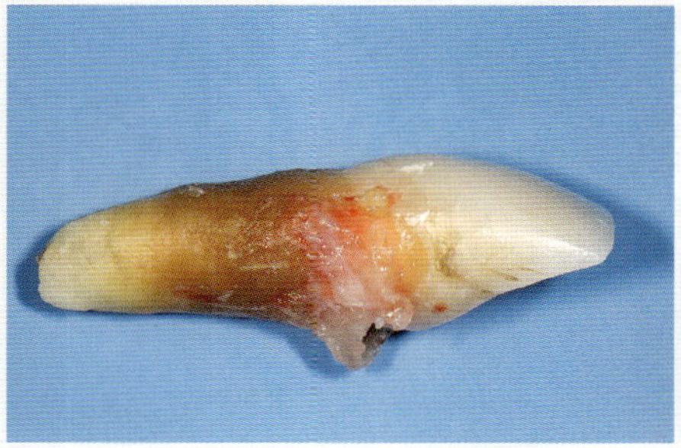

Fig 8-24d
Tooth 21 after extraction, visible extensive resorption of the root surface.

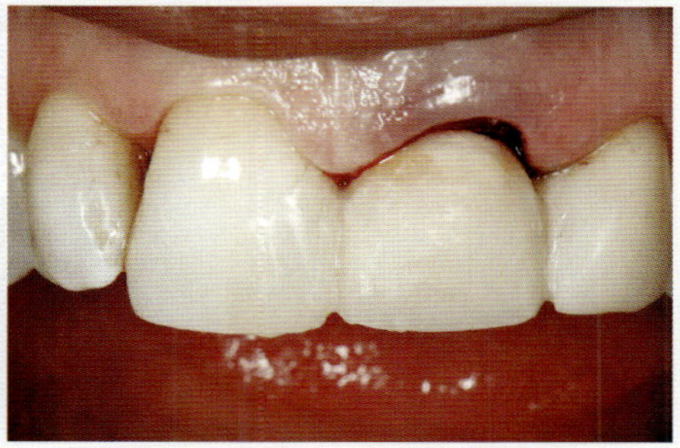

Fig 8-24e
Immediately after extraction, a direct fiberglass-reinforced composite bridge was cemented with an oval-shaped pontic from the gingival surface.

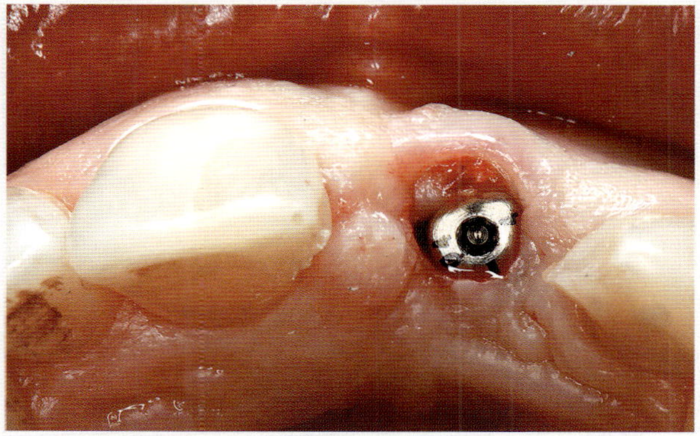

Fig 8-24f
Two months after extraction, the implant was placed (implantation: Dr. Nicolas Hahn).

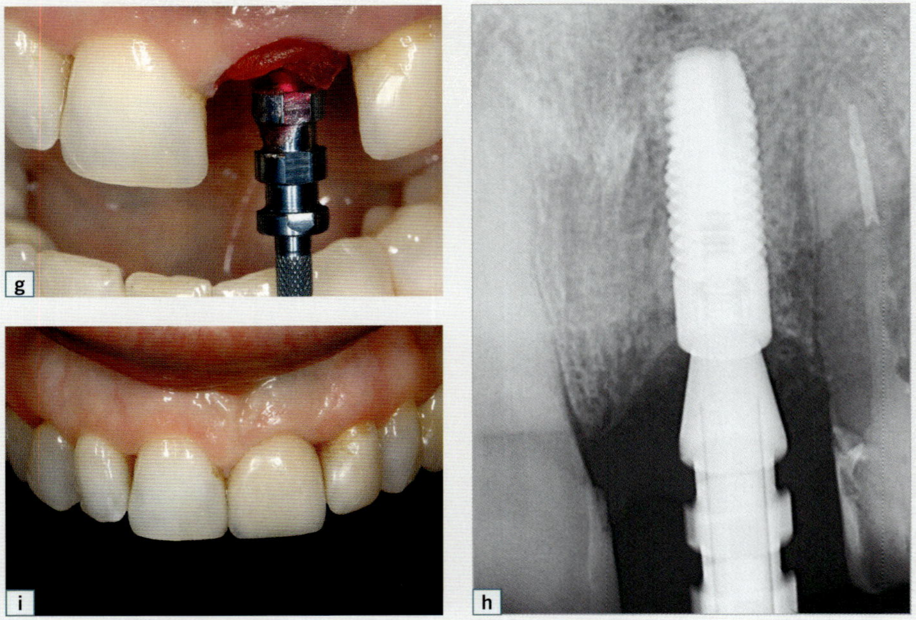

Figs 8-24g to 8-24i
In the next step, a provisional screw-retained implant crown was made.

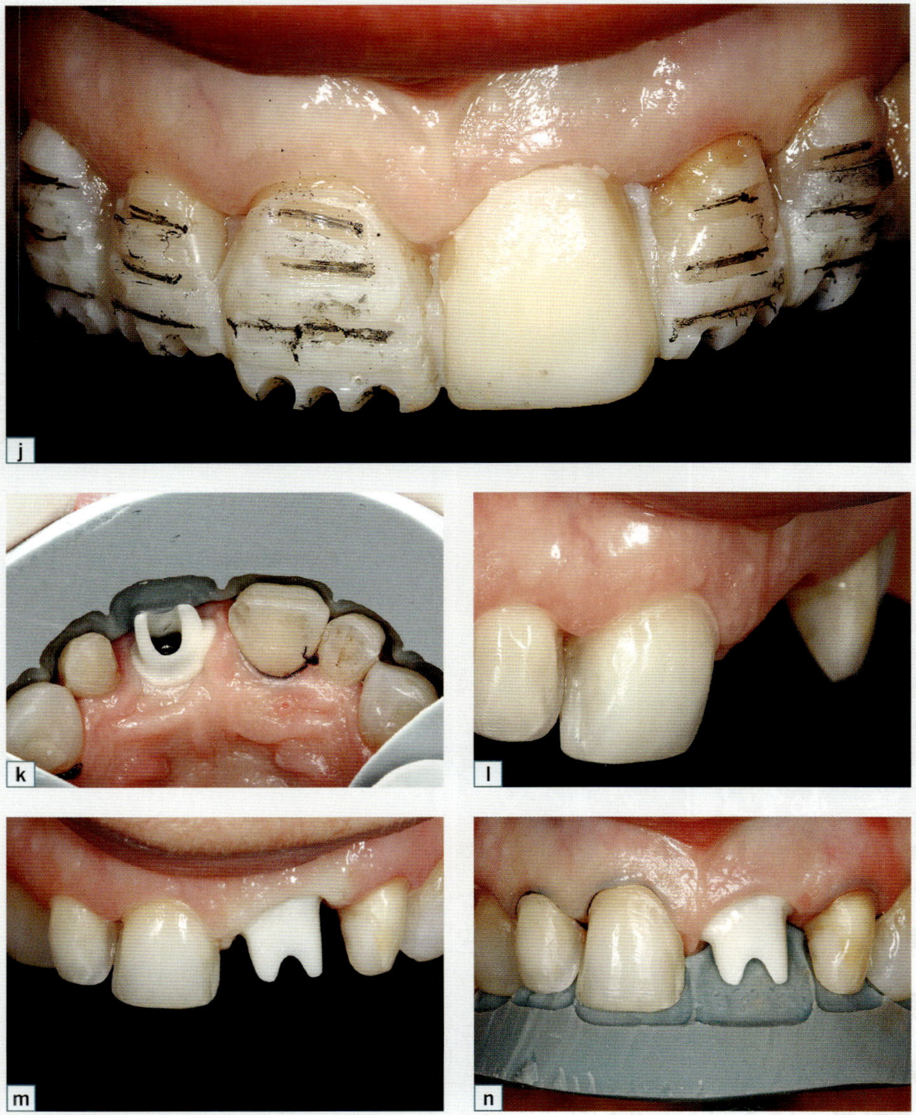

Figs 8-24j to 8-24n
After several months of stabilizing the gingival margin around the implant, an individual abutment was fabricated, and a veneer preparation was performed from the mock-up level. The preparation was performed with silicone index control.

The inserted implant was temporarily restored with a provisional screw-retained implant crown (Figs 8-24g to 8-24i).

After a few months – when it was found that the gingival margin around the implant had stabilized – the definitive esthetic treatment was finalized. The final impression was taken for the individual zirconium abutment (Atlantis, Dentsply Sirona) and, after its fabrication, veneer preparation on teeth 13, 12, 11, 22, and 23 was performed from the mock-up level (Fig 8-24j) to minimize tooth structure loss. Preparation was controlled with silicone index (Figs 8-24k to 8-24n). Porcelain restorations made of lithium disilicate were fabricated in the dental laboratory. The clinical result is presented in Figs 8-24o to 8-24r.

PRACTITIONER'S ADVICE

The most important parameter when planning the contact surfaces of the restorations is the assessment of the distance from the alveolar prccess (4–5 mm), in order to avoid black triangles when performing implants.

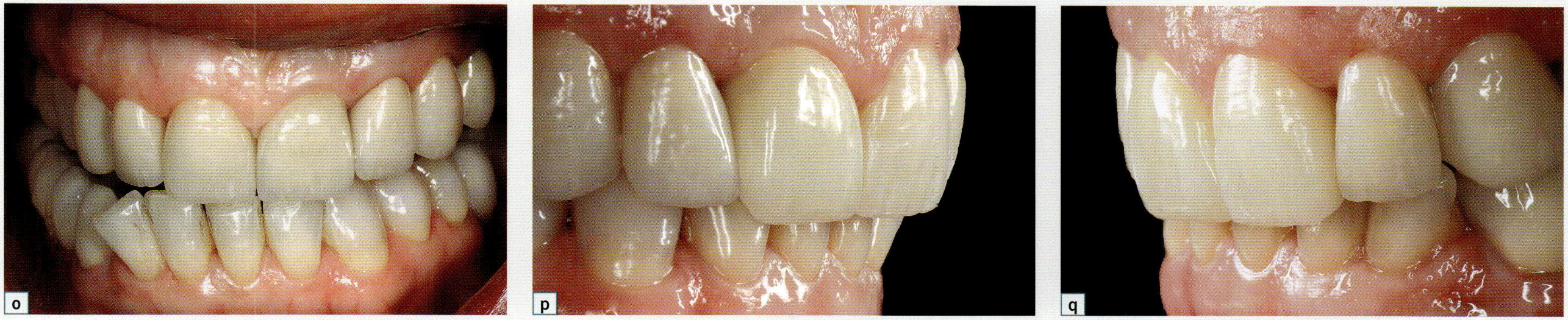

Figs 8-24o to 8-24q
Intraoral photographs after treatment (crown on implant 21 and veneers on teeth 13, 12, 11, 22, and 23).

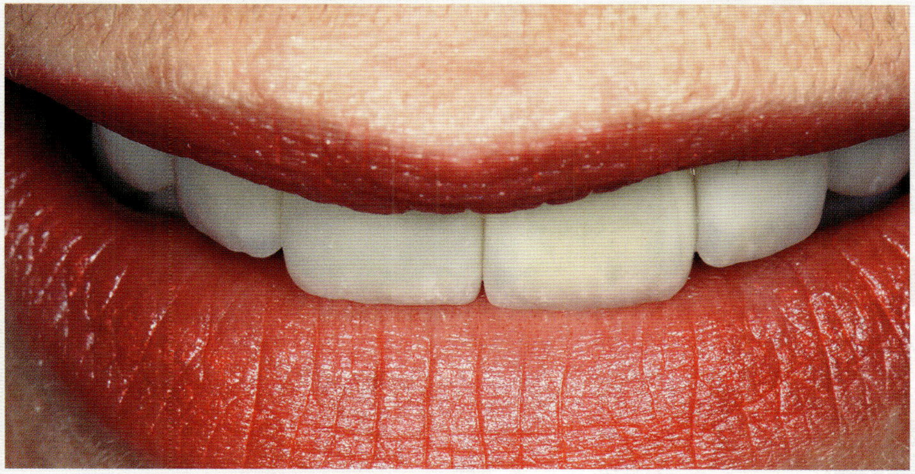

Fig 8-24r
Patient's smile after treatment.

VENEER REPLACEMENT

Can veneers be replaced with new ones? Veneers performed in a minimally invasive way can be replaced with new ones in the future.

Veneers bind with the tooth surface, achieving an extremely durable bond under ideal conditions (rubber dam and properly used adhesive systems) – so stable that removing them is not much different from the preparation of a healthy tooth structure. Problems arise when the previous veneer preparation has not been carried out conservatively. In this case, it is difficult to predict whether the preparation ends in the enamel or the dentin.[60] Therefore, when attempting to replace veneers made years ago, never promise patients that they will have new ones again. Only after the initial preparation is it possible to assess the current condition and the possibility of re-making the veneer or preparing a restoration based on mechanical retention – a prosthetic crown.

Problems with veneer replacement:

- **Risk of exposing a large amount of dentin** (due to previous preparation)
- **Risk of subgingival preparation** (due to previous preparation) and entering the root cementum zone
- **Risk of presence of the restorations under the old veneers** (they may be leaking, and replacement may be necessary)
- **Risk that the veneers cannot be replaced and therefore prosthetic crowns must be performed**
- **Risk of unknown color of the core after the preparation** (tooth discoloration may be extremely difficult to mask with veneers)
- **Risk associated with the difficulty of distinguishing the veneer from the tooth structure while preparing** (in some cases, preparation of the old veneer without a microscope is very difficult)

TIP

When removing old veneers:

- Use a microscope or high-power loupe
- Dry and moisten the tooth alternately during preparation to be able to see the differences in light reflection between tooth structure and remaining porcelain
- If necessary, place a rubber dam for even better contrast and dryness to enhance the porcelain detection

Case 14: Replacing veneers with new ones

A female patient presented to the dental office with a wish to replace the old veneers with new ones. The previous veneers did not meet the patient's esthetic expectations. In the patient's opinion, they were crooked (the midline was off), they were not symmetrical, and looked "like shovels" from the profile (Figs 8-25a to 8-25d). Their appearance seemed artificial for the patient, and inflamed, bleeding gums around the restorations were a nuisance.

Planning was started with a mock-up that would meet the patient's expectations. Only after creating the second mock-up was a consensus reached for the planned esthetics. The symmetry of the gingival margin between the right and left sides was aligned, and veneer preparation was carried out from the mock-up level at the next appointment (Fig 8-25e). The porcelain was removed very carefully under the microscope (Fig 8-25f).

Restorations that were found to be leaking under the old veneers (Fig 8-25g) were replaced with new ones (Fig 8-25h). Impressions were taken, and veneers were fabricated in the dental laboratory in accordance with the approved design (Fig 8-25i). Although the isolation was not easy due to the subgingival preparation caused by previous restorations, the new veneers were cemented with rubber dam isolation (Fig 8-25j). The result immediately after removing the rubber dam is shown in Fig 8-25k, and a few weeks later (Figs 8-25l to 8-25o).

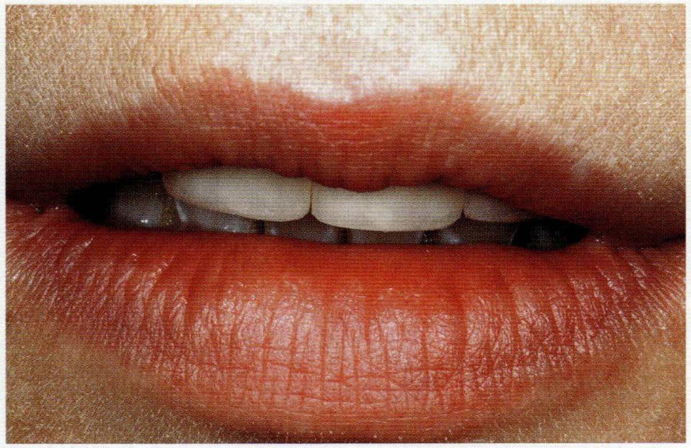

Fig 8-25a
Photograph of the patient's upper and lower lip in repose. The patient presented to the dental office with a request to replace the old veneers with new ones. From under the upper lip, we can see the asymmetrical line of the incisal edges.

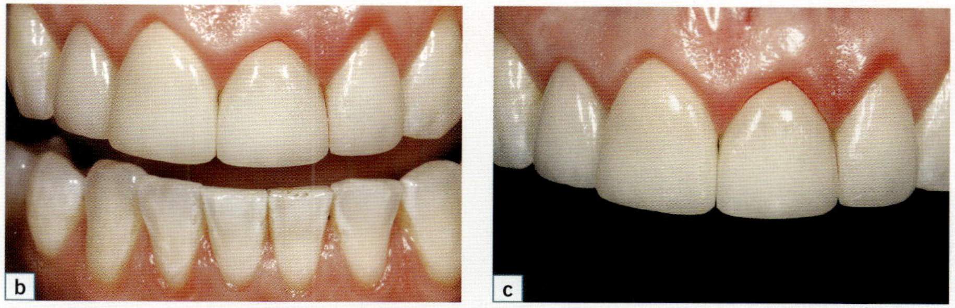

Figs 8-25b and 8-25c
Intraoral photographs of the old veneers. Gingivitis at the teeth 21 and 22, asymmetrical position of the central incisors and asymmetry of the gingival margin between the left and right side.

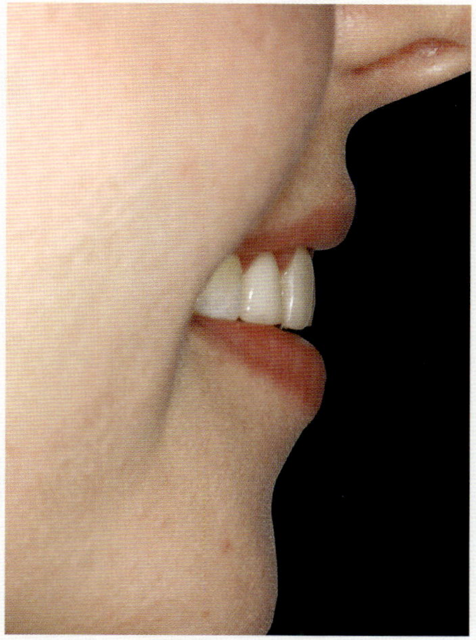

Fig 8-25d
Profile of the veneers: the patient did not like the shape of the teeth from this view; she considered them artificial.

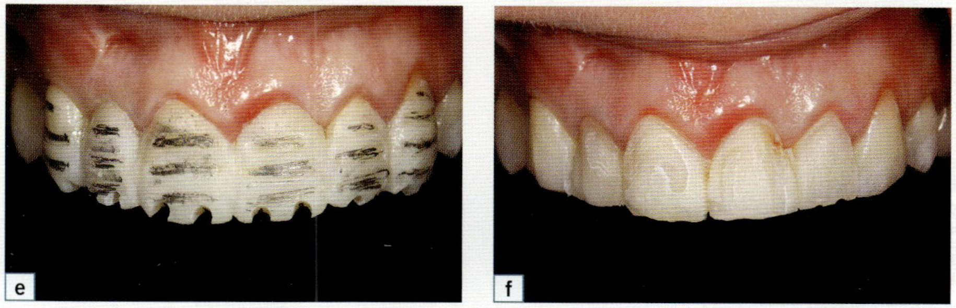

Figs 8-25e and 8-25f
(e) After aligning the symmetry of the gingival margin, at the next appointment veneer preparation was performed from the mock-up level. (f) The porcelain was carefully removed, using a microscope in the final stage. Under the old veneers, there are visible leaking composite restorations, which were qualified for replacement.

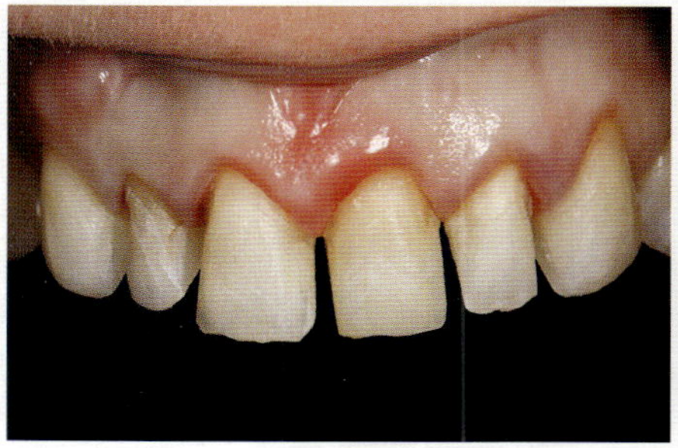

Fig 8-25g
Initial preparation before replacing composite restorations.

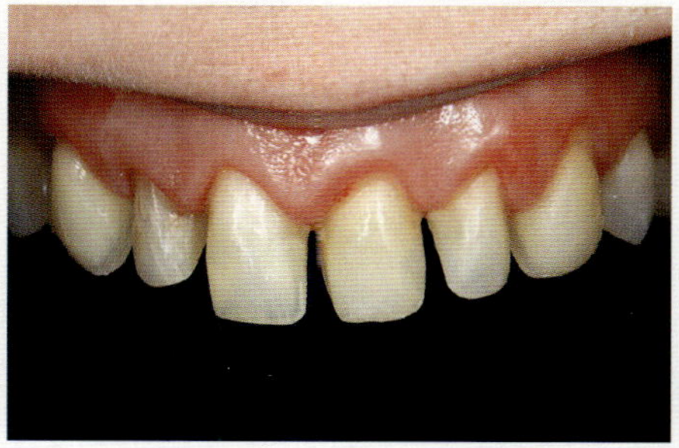

Fig 8-25h
Final tooth preparation after the old veneers removal and replacing the composite restorations with new ones – the subgingival preparation was caused by the old veneers position and the previous preparation.

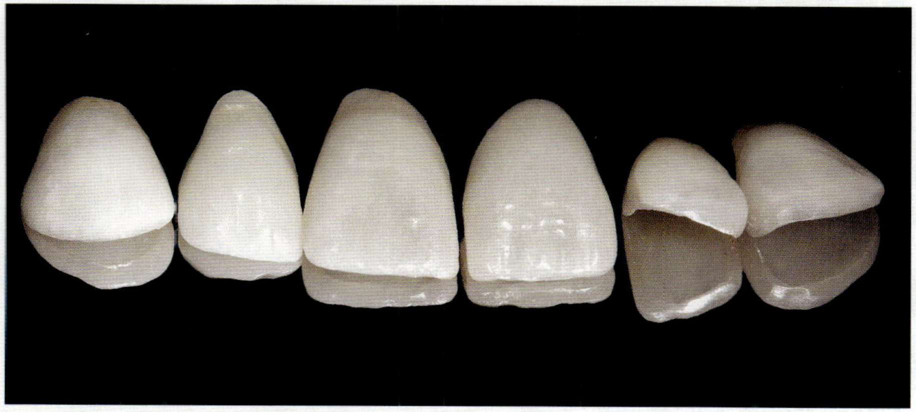

Fig 8-25i
Porcelain veneers ready for cementation (laboratory work: DT Artur Nyga).

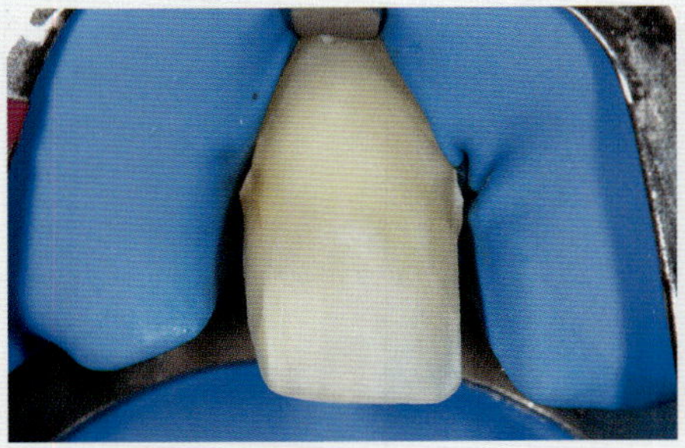

Fig 8-25j
Tooth isolation with a rubber dam during veneer cementation.

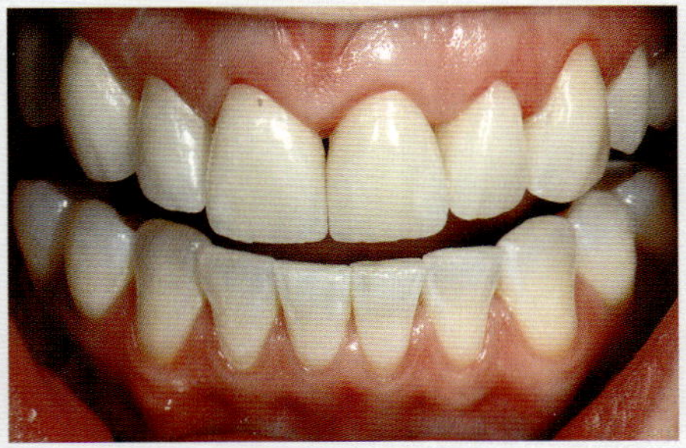

Fig 8-25k
The clinical situation immediately after cementing veneers and removing the rubber dam.

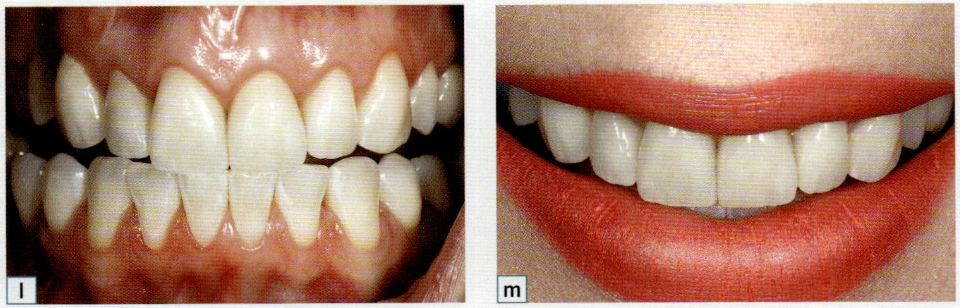

Figs 8-25l and 8-25m
(l) Intraoral photograph and (m) photograph of the patient's smile taken a few weeks after replacing the old veneers with new ones.

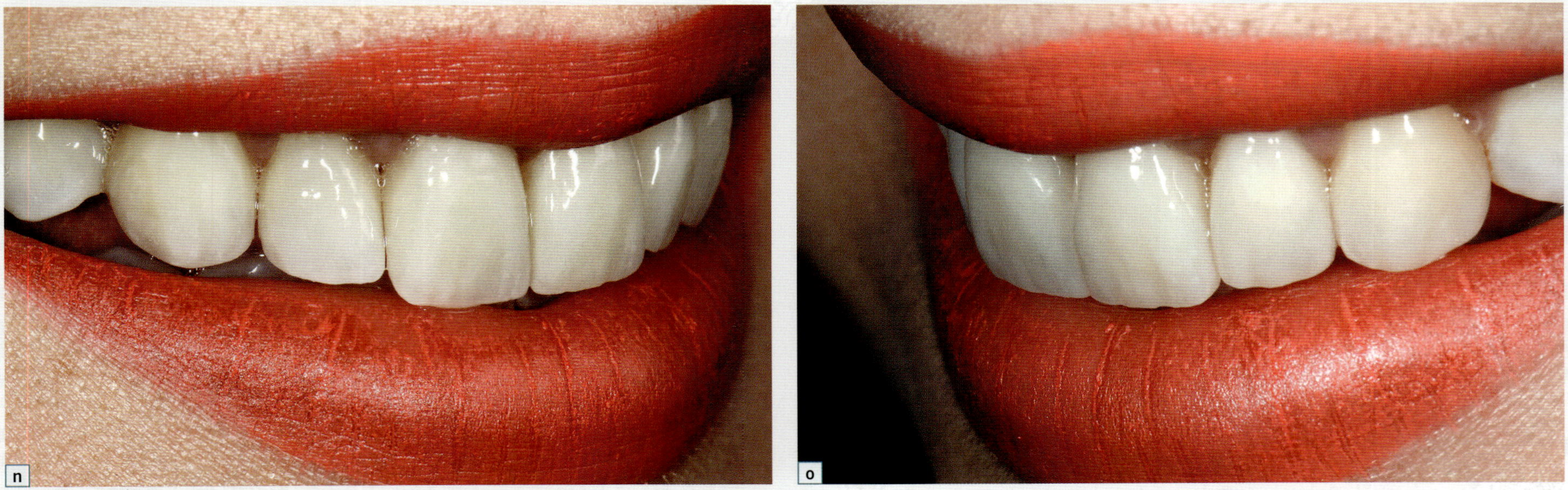

Figs 8-25n and 8-25o
Patient's smile from different views after replacing the veneers with new ones.

REFERENCES

1. Zarow M, D'Arcangelo C, Felippe L A, Paniz G, Paolone G. EndoProsthodontics: A Guide for Practicing Dentists, ed 1. Poland: Quintessence Publishing, 2017.
2. Dumfahrt H, Schäffer H. Porcelain laminate veneers. A retrospective evaluation after 1 to 10 years of service: Part II – clinical results. Int J Prosthodont 2000;13:9–18.
3. D'Arcangelo C, De Angelis F, Vadini M, D'Amario M. Clinical evaluation on porcelain laminate veneers bonded with light-cured composite: results up to 7 years. Clin Oral Investig 2012;16:1071–1079.
4. Burke FJ. Survival rates for porcelain laminate veneers with special reference to the effect of preparation in dentin: a literature review. J Esthet Restor Dent 2012;24:257–265.
5. Gresnigt MM, Kalk W, Özcan M. Clinical longevity of ceramic laminate veneers bonded to teeth with and without existing composite restorations up to 40 months. Clin Oral Investig 2013;17:823–832.
6. Edelhoff D, Prandtner O, Saeidi Pour R, Liebermann A, Stimmelmayr M, Güth JF. Anterior restorations: the performance of ceramic veneers. Quintessence Int 2018;49:89–101.
7. Meyenberg KH. The ideal restoration of endodontically treated teeth – structural and esthetic considerations: a review of the literature and clinical guidelines for the restorative clinician. Eur J Esthet Dent 2013;8:238–268
8. Meyenberg KH. Nonvital teeth and porcelain laminate veneers – a contradiction? Eur J Esthet Dent 2006;1:192–206.
9. Zarow M. Nonvital tooth bleaching: a case discussion for the clinical practice. Compend Contin Educ Dent 2016;37:268–276.
10. Gürel G, Morimoto S, Calamita MA, Coachman C, Sesma N. Clinical performance of porcelain laminate veneers: outcomes of the aesthetic pre-evaluative temporary (APT) technique. Int J Periodontics Restorative Dent 2012;32:625–635
11. Gürel G, Sesma N, Calamita MA, Coachman C, Morimoto S. Influence of enamel preservation on failure rates of porcelain laminate veneers. Int J Periodontics Restorative Dent 2013;33:31–39.
12. Żarow M, Borowska-Sawa J. Licówki porcelanowe na zęby przebarwione po leczeniu endodontycznym. Procedury postępowania na podstawie przeglądu piśmiennictwa oraz przypadku klinicznego [Porcelain veneers for discolored endodontically treated teeth procedures based on the literature review and of the clinical case]. Mag Stom 2010; 7–8:75–83.
13. Zarow M. Contraindicated internal bleaching – what to do? Aesthetic Dentistry Today; 2017/4
14. Kois DE, Kois JC. Comprehensive risk-based diagnostically driven treatment planning: developing sequentially generated treatment. Dent Clin North Am 2015;59:593–608.
15. Seay A. Transitional bonding with the Kois deprogrammer: a conservative treatment approach. Compend Contin Educ Dent 2012;33:758–763.
16. Bynum JH. Clinical case report: testing occlusal management, previewing anterior esthetics, and staging rehabilitation with direct composite and Kois deprogrammer. Compend Contin Educ Dent 2010;31:298–302
17. Hulac S. Porcelain laminate veneers: adjunctive treatment of occlusal disorders. Compend Contin Educ Dent 2013;34:362–366.
18. Zarow M. Finding the Centric Relation – The Kois Deprogrammer. Available at: www.styleitaliano.org/finding-centric-relation-kois-deprogrammer/
19. Kois Course 8 Manual, Functional Occlusion. Seattle, 2019.
20. Seay A. Achieving esthetic and functional objectives with additive equilibration. Compend Contin Educ Dent 2014;35:688–692.
21. Kois JC, Filder BC. Anterior wear: orthodontic and restorative management. Compend Contin Educ Dent 2009;30:420–422, 424, 426–429.
22. Kois JC, Phillips KM. Occlusal vertical dimension: alteration concerns. Compend Contin Educ Dent 1997;18:1169–1174, 1176–1177.
23. Fernandes PR, de Vasconsellos HA, Okeson JP, Bastos RL, Maia ML. The anatomical relationship between the position of the auriculotemporal nerve and mandibular condyle. Cranio 2003;21:165–171.
24. Okeson JP, Hayes DK. Long-term results of treatment for temporomandibular disorders: an evaluation by patients. J Am Dent Assoc 1986;112:473–478.
25. Ramfjord SP. Bruxism, a clinical and electromyographic study. J Am Dent Assoc 1961;62:21–44.
26. Dawson PE. Optimum TMJ condyle position in clinical practice. Int J Periodontics Restorative Dent 1985;5:10–31.
27. Dawson PE. A classification system for occlusions that relates maximal intercuspation to the position and condition of the temporomandibular joints. J Prosthet Dent 1996;75:60–66.
28. Dawson PE. New definition for relating occlusion to varying conditions of the temporomandibular joint. J Prosthet Dent 1995;74:619–627.
29. Huff C. A systematic method for accurate functional diagnosis. Compend Contin Educ Dent 2017;38:308–316.
30. Wilson C. Multidisciplinary treatment of anterior worn dentition: a staged approach. Compend Contin Educ Dent 2015;36:202, 204–207.
31. Kois Symposium Manual. Seattle, 2018.
32. Nishigawa K, Nakano M, Bando E. Study of jaw movement and masticatory muscle activity during unilateral chewing with and without balancing side molar contacts. J Oral Rehabil 1997;24:691–696.
33. Ekfeldt A, Karlsson S. Changes of masticatory movement characteristics after prosthodontic rehabilitation of individuals with extensive tooth wear. Int J Prosthodont 1996;9:539–546.
34. Kumar SN, Patil NP, Guttal SS, Nadiger RK. Full mouth rehabilitation of severely attrited dentition: a case report. N Y State Dent J 2010;76:47–50.
35. Glebocki J. Correction of dysfunctional wear results in esthetic outcome for reluctant patient. Compend Contin Educ Dent 2019;40:302–306.
36. Saeidi Pour R, Engler MLPD, Edelhoff D, Prandtner O, Frei S, Liebermann A. A patient calibrated individual wax-up as an essential tool for planning and creating a patient-oriented treatment concept for pathological tooth wear. Int J Esthet Dent 2018;13:476–492.
37. Devoto W, Saracinelli M, Manauta J. Composite in everyday practice: how to choose the right material and simplify application techniques in the anterior teeth. Eur J Esthet Dent 2010;5:102–124.
38. Spear F. Too much tooth, not enough tooth: making decisions about anterior tooth position. J Am Dent Assoc 2010;141:93–96.

REFERENCES

39. Patil PG. Anterior tooth position. J Am Dent Assoc 2010;141:620.
40. Sabri R. The eight components of a balanced smile. J Clin Orthod 2005;39:155–167.
41. Spear F. The maxillary central incisal edge: a key to esthetic and functional treatment planning. Compend Contin Educ Dent 1999;20:512–516.
42. Calamita MA, Coachman C, Sesma N, Kois J. Occlusal vertical dimension: treatment planning decisions and management considerations. Int J Esthet Dent 2019;14:166–181.
43. Kois JC. Occlusal vertical dimension: what is the controversy? Compend Contin Educ Dent 1997;18:1164.
44. Hellsing G. Functional adaptation to changes in vertical dimension. J Prosthet Dent 1984;52:867–870.
45. Weinberg LA. Vertical dimension: a research and clinical analysis. J Prosthet Dent 1982;47:290–302.
46. Ammannato R, Ferraris F, Marchesi G. The "index technique" in worn dentition: a new and conservative approach. Int J Esthet Dent 2015;10:68–99.
47. Ammannato R, Rondoni D, Ferraris F. Update on the "index technique" in worn dentition: a no-prep restorative approach with a digital workflow. Int J Esthet Dent 2018;13: 516–537.
48. Dietschi D, Argente A. A comprehensive and conservative approach for the restoration of abrasion and erosion. Part I: concepts and clinical rationale for early intervention using adhesive techniques. Eur J Esthet Dent 2011;6:20–33.
49. Koubi S, Gürel G, Margossian P, Massihi R, Tassery H. A simplified approach for restoration of worn dentition using the full mock-up concept: clinical case reports. Int J Periodontics Restorative Dent 2018;38:189–197.
50. Vailati F, Belser UC. Classification and treatment of the anterior maxillary dentition affected by dental erosion: the ACE classification. Int J Periodontics Restorative Dent 2010;30: 559–571.
51. Vailati F, Carciofo S. Treatment planning of adhesive additive rehabilitations: the progressive wax-up of the three-step technique. Int J Esthet Dent 2016;11:356–377.
52. Farias-Neto A, de Medeiros FCD, Vilanova L, Simonetti Chaves M, Freire Batistade Araújo JJ. Tooth preparation for ceramic veneers: when less is more. Int J Esthet Dent 2019;14:156–164.
53. Priest G. Proximal margin modifications for all-ceramic veneers. Pract Proced Aesthet Dent 2004;16:265–272.
54. Calamia V, Pantzis A. Simple case treatment planning: diastema closure. Dent Clin North Am 2015;59:655–664.
55. Zarow M. Metal post and core: how to improve aesthetics. Available at: www.styleitaliano.org/ metal-post-and-core-how-to-improve-aesthetics/
56. Lombardi RE. The principles of visual perception and their clinical application to denture esthetics. J Prosthet Dent 1973;29:358–382.
57. Tarnow DP, Magner AW, Fletcher P. The effect of the distance from the contact point to the crest of bone on the presence or absence of the interproximal dental papilla. J Periodontol 1992;63:995–996.
58. Gobbato L, Paniz G, Mazzocco F, Chierico A, Tsukiyama T, Levi PA Jr, Weisgold AS. Significance of crown shape in the replacement of a central incisor with a single implant-supported crown. Quintessence Int 2013;44:407–413.
59. Tarnow DP, Cho SC, Wallace SS. The effect of interimplant distance on the height of inter-implant bone crest. J Periodontol 2000;71:546–549.
60. Guzmán-Armstrong S, Maia RR. Conservative treatment planning in veneer replacement. J Prosthet Dent 2016;115:393–396.

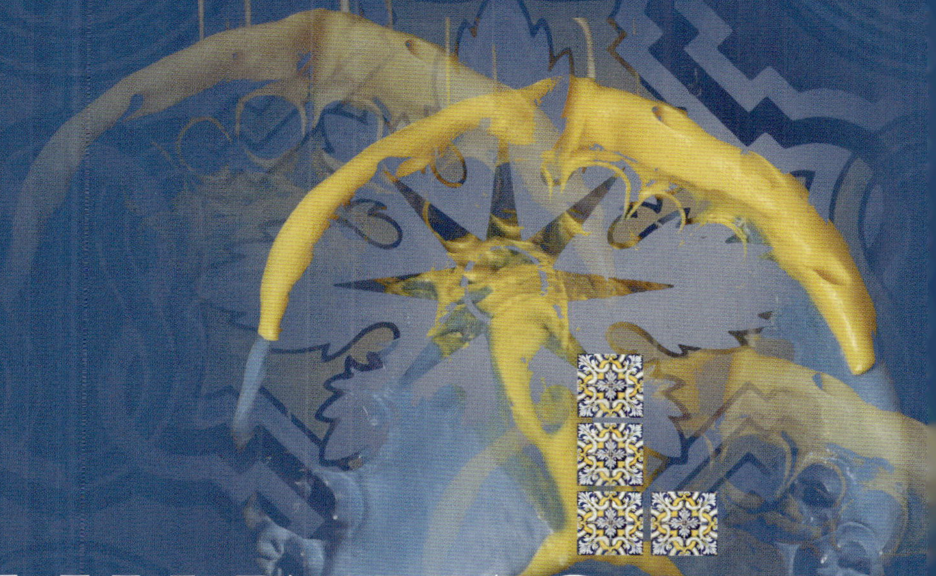

CHAPTER 9

MINIMALLY INVASIVE VENEERS OR NO-PREP VENEERS?

MARCO NICASTRO

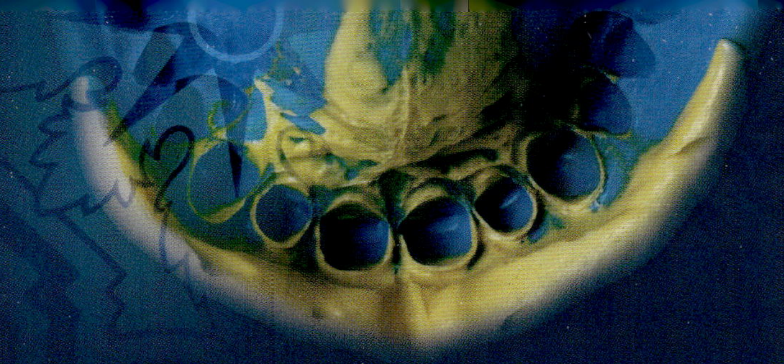

Minimal tooth preparation
and fabrication of thin
veneers is a technique
that not only preserves
the tooth structure,
but is also predictable
when following proper
procedures ...

Minimally invasive veneers or no-prep veneers?

The veneer choice cannot be dictated by what is trendy. Certainly, in recent years the preservation of the enamel and the tooth structure has become an increasingly important issue, but no-prep restorations only give the illusion of being easier to perform than minimally invasive veneers.

PREPARATION TECHNIQUES

In recent years, restorative dentistry has seen a change in the approach to the preparation of the tooth structure toward more conservative methods, including when performing direct and indirect restorations. There has been a gradual reduction of tooth preparation, up to the complete absence of any interference in the tooth structure when creating additive restorations. This became possible thanks to the development of new restorative materials that exhibit greater durability than the materials used earlier. Let's look at the possibilities of restoring teeth in the anterior segment.

Current preparation techniques covering the entire tooth surface at a depth of 0.6–0.7 mm of enamel thickness are no longer preferable. Instead, less invasive methods preserving the enamel are recommenced, even up to the creation of additive restorations with no preparation, ie, no-prep veneers.[1]

TIP

No-prep veneers are not a recent discovery. They appeared in the 1980s as an ultraconservative technique, easy to implement, minimally invasive for the patient and economical.

PREPARATION TECHNIQUES MAY BE CLASSIFIED INTO THE FOLLOWING GROUPS:

A. Full-depth traditional preparation
B. Full-depth preparation with additive diagnostic wax-up
C. Minimally invasive preparation
D. No-prep veneers

First of all, it should be emphasized that the dentist must know all the types of preparation techniques because each of them still has its own specific indications. **The last two techniques belong to the group, which we now call minimally invasive restorations.**

A. FULL-DEPTH TRADITIONAL PREPARATION

Traditional preparation (full-depth) causes a significant reduction of the hard dental tissues.[2,3] It was performed in the 1980s and it assumed the removal of superficial tissues to the thickness of the future restoration. At that time, only feldspathic porcelain was available, and this technique required enamel reduction to a depth of 0.5–0.7 mm.

This technique is perceived as too invasive, during which a large amount of dentin is very often exposed. For these reasons, Magne[4] and Gürel[5,6] proposed a technique with reduced preparation depth due to the wax-up and veneer preparation through the applied mock-up, which avoids dentin exposure. However, the traditional technique may still be necessary if we are restoring a single tooth in the dental arch or as interleaved elements (when we are working in a group of teeth and we need to prepare only some of them, leaving the others without veneer restoration), or when we are performing veneers on only one side of the maxillary arch, as happens after injures. In these situations, due to the esthetics and shape of the restoration, an additive diagnostic wax-up is not possible, as the contours of future restorations would extend beyond the contours of the adjacent teeth, resulting in poor esthetic result in this area. Therefore, we are forced to use a technique that causes the loss of the hard dental tissues to obtain compatibility with the patient's remaining teeth.

Considering the veneer material choice, feldspathic ceramics made on a refractory die or platinum foil are undoubtedly the most appropriate in these cases. They allow the create a restoration with the appropriate color and individual characterization, which integrates well with the natural tissues of the adjacent teeth in the dental arch (Figs 9-1 to 9-4).

Case 1

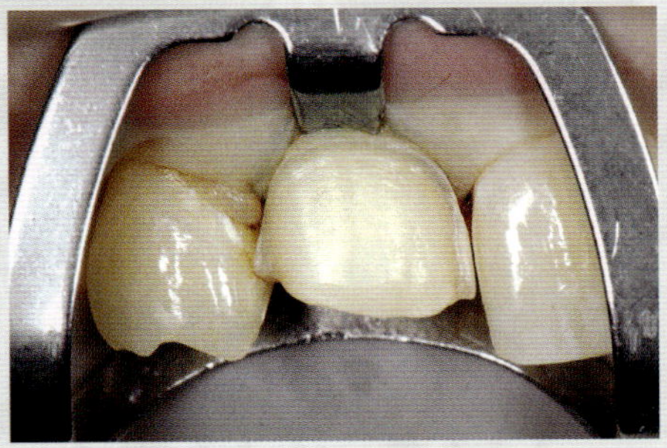

Fig 9-1a
Example of a traditional preparation. Tooth preparation is at a depth of 0.5–0.7 mm to create a space for the restorative material (in this case, feldspathic ceramics was fired on a refractory die).

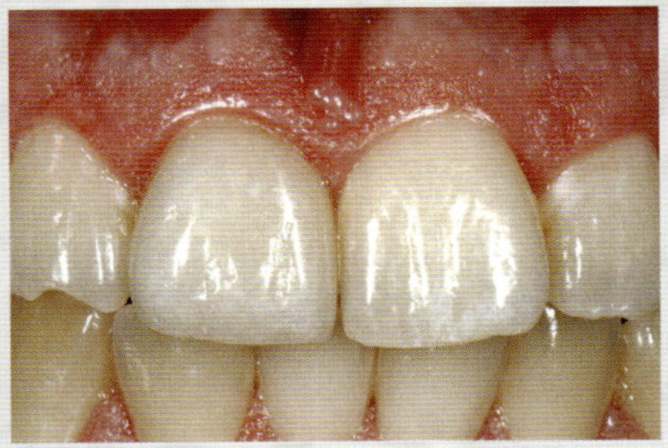

Fig 9-1b
Final result – visible good shape with the restoration color matching the adjacent teeth.

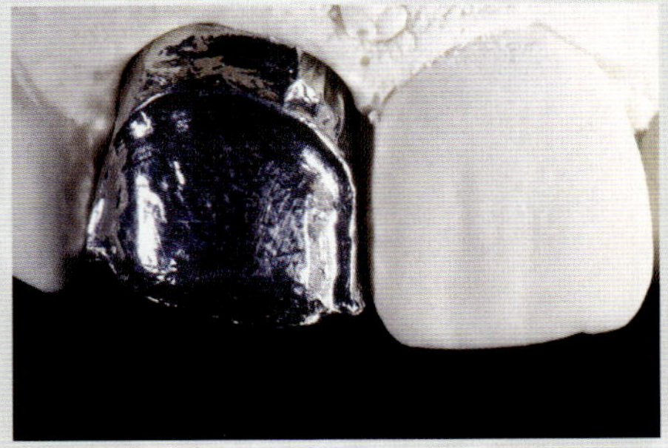

Fig 9-1c
Working cast with the platinum foil ready for firing the feldspathic ceramics.

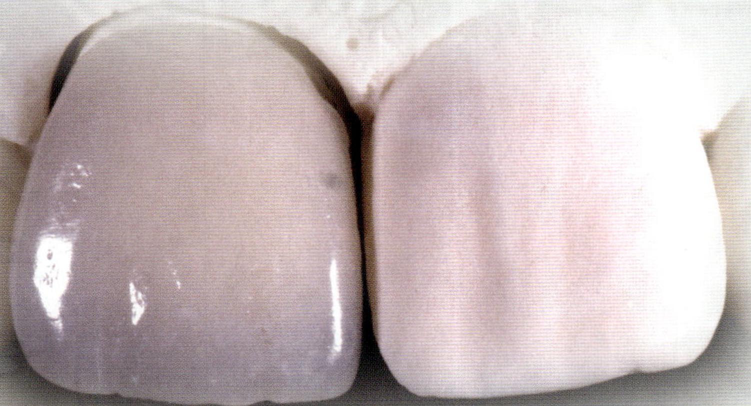

Fig 9-1d
Final result after firing the layers of ceramics and removing the platinum foil. The veneer is ready for cementation.

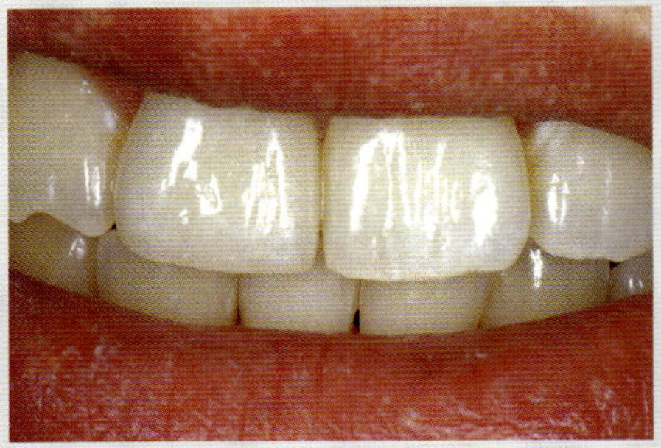

Fig 9-1e
Patient's smile after cementing the porcelain veneer.

Case 2

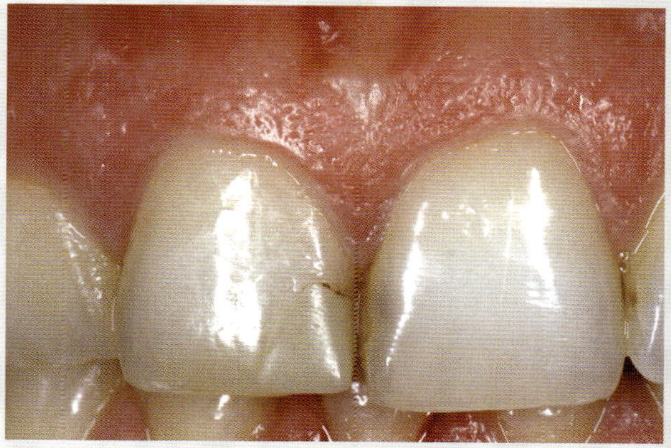

Fig 9-2a
The right central incisor has an old composite restoration of incorrect size and shape.

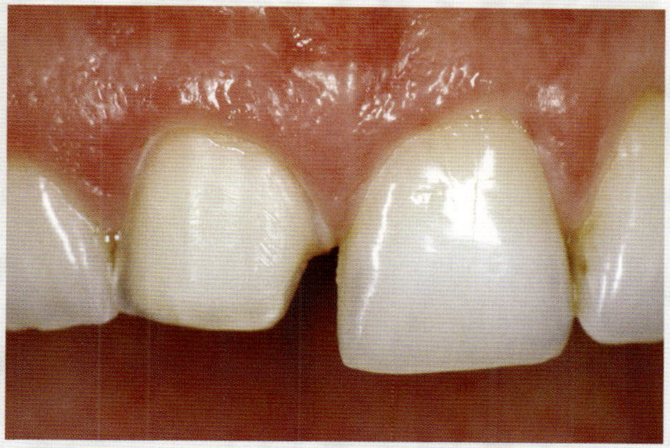

Fig 9-2b
Full-depth preparation, with a remaining thin layer of enamel.

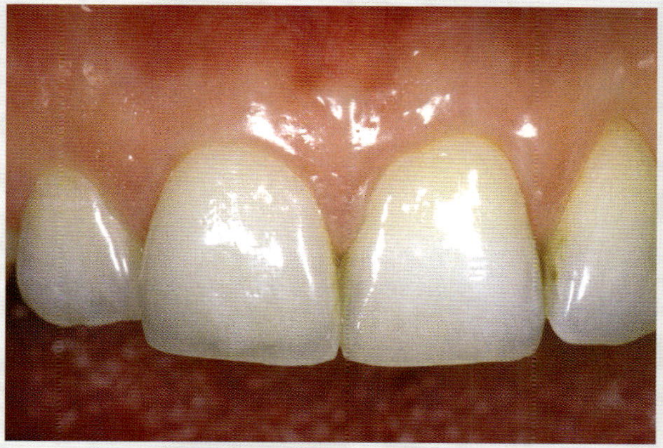

Fig 9-2c
By replacing the natural enamel with feldspathic ceramics, the proper contour and shape of the tooth can be created.

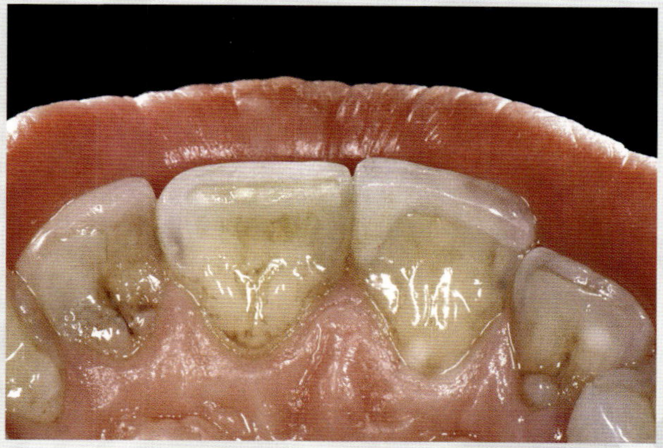

Fig 9-2d
Intraoral photograph after veneer cementation – palatal view.

PRACTITIONER'S ADVICE

Traditional preparation from the level of tooth structure, without mock-up, will be performed when we are absolutely sure that we want to make one veneer. It should be noted that any asymmetric prosthetic work is a difficult challenge for the dental technician!

Case 3

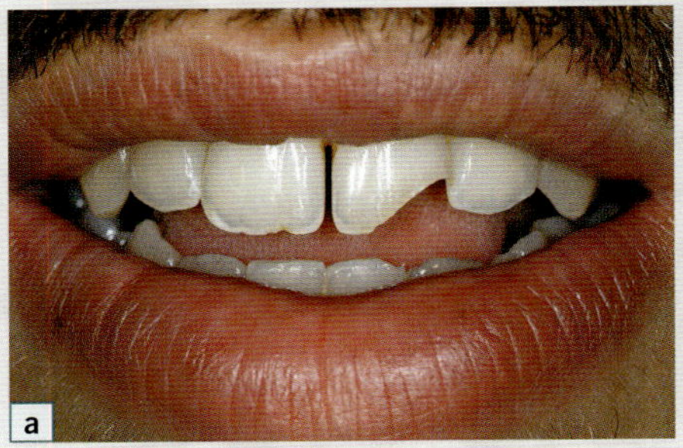
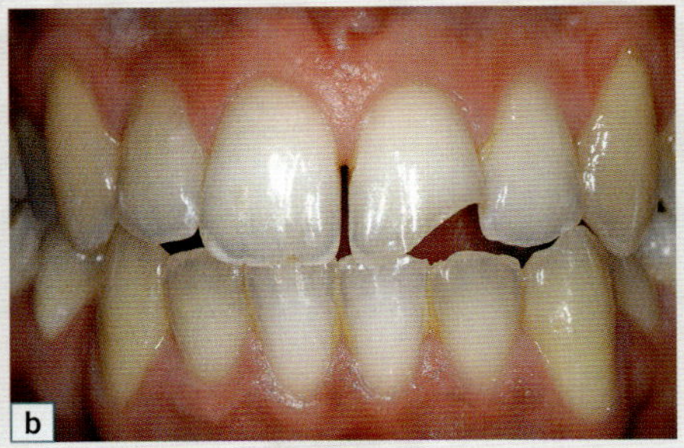

Figs 9-3a and 9-3b

(a) A patient presented to the dental office with a fractured tooth 21. (b) An intraoral photograph shows the size of the tooth defect.

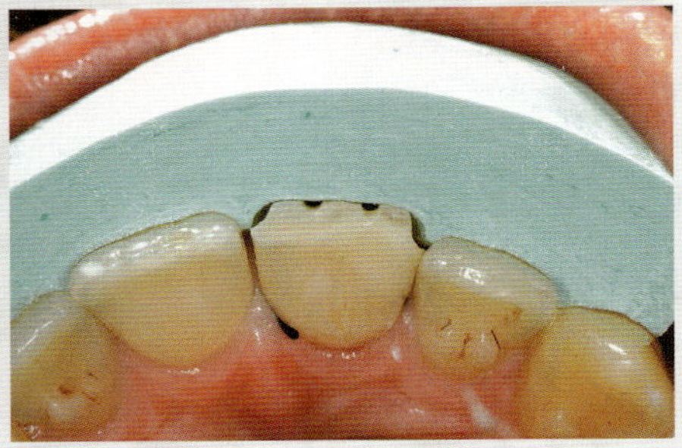

Fig 9-3c

Preparation was performed in the enamel, visible orientation grooves and applied silicone index as a "guidance" of the veneer preparation.

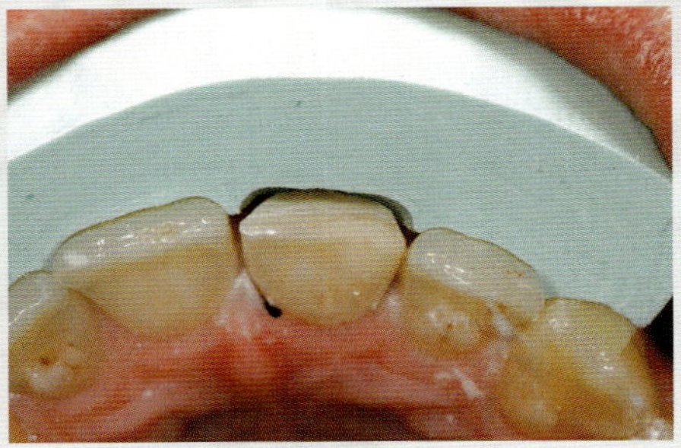

Fig 9-3d

It is clear how the presented veneer preparation technique allows you to obtain space for ceramic restoration that will not differ in shape from the adjacent teeth.

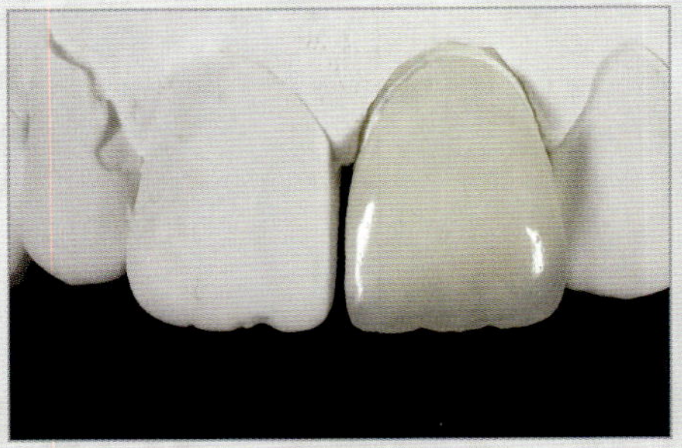

Fig 9-3e

Feldspathic ceramic fired on the refractory die. This is the first choice of material if a single veneer is made.

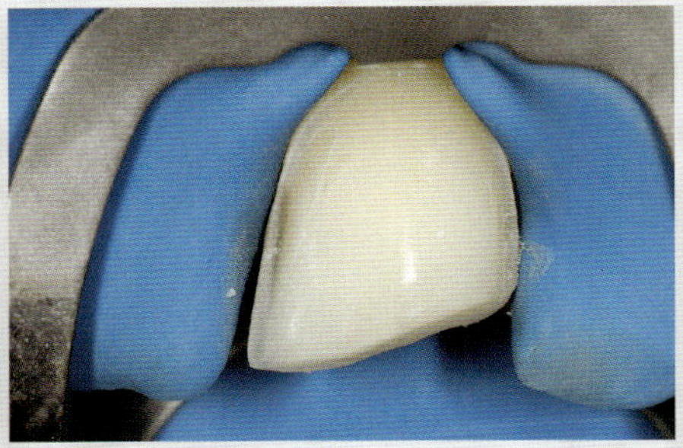

Fig 9-3f

Isolation with a rubber dam will allow adhesive cementation of the porcelain veneer.

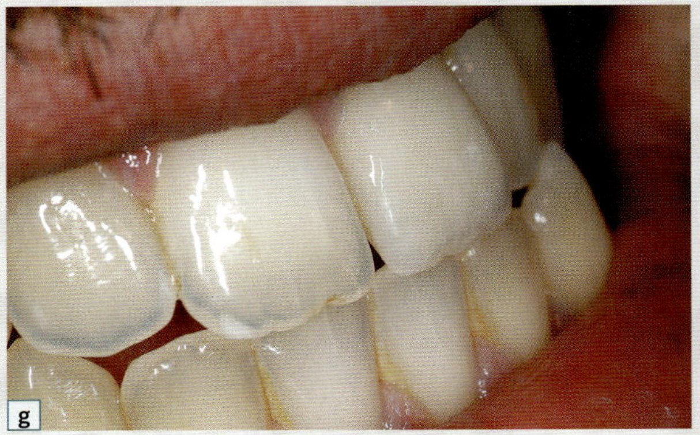
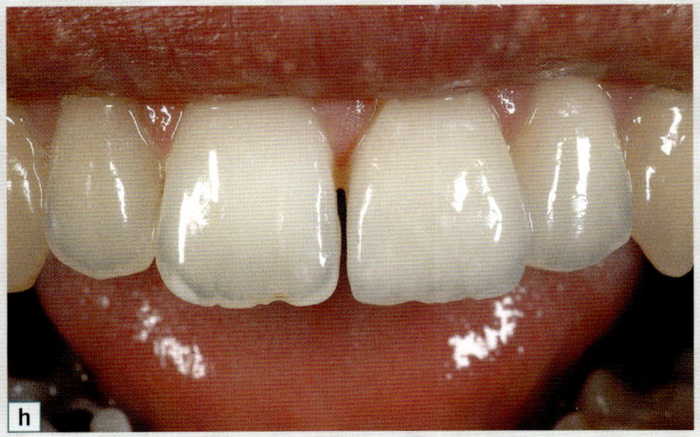

Figs 9-3g and 9-3h

The final esthetic result after veneer cementation. The patient accepted the compromise of performing only one asymmetric restoration (laboratory work was done individually in the patient's presence).

Case 4

Another clinical case illustrating a difficult esthetic restoration. The patient is very young, with healthy teeth which are an ideal model on the side unaffected by the trauma, and delicate periodontal tissues. In this kind of situation, it is very important to plan what type of ceramic material will be used before starting the tooth preparation, as the preparation must be performed according to the type of selected restorative material.

The treatment plan included the use of feldspathic ceramics made on a refractory die. A consequence of this choice is the necessity of performing a preparation that will be as deep as the future thickness of the restoration, in order to follow the contour of the adjacent teeth and to obtain a satisfying esthetic result.[7]

Feldspathic ceramic represents the best solution for restorations in the anterior segment, where we encounter different color saturation, variable brightness, and individual tooth characterization. The canine has very high color saturation, and the central incisor has very high brightness but low color saturation. The lateral incisor has characteristics between these two, so you need a material that can be layered and handled in various ways. An additional difficulty in this case is large tissue loss caused by the Class IV cavity. Therefore, it is very important to mask the surface of the lost dentin with more opaque material, which will not reflect light and will guarantee a natural final outcome.

Feldspathic ceramics are fragile, so for safety reasons, it must have an adequate thickness of 0.5–0.7 mm. Consequently, the tooth preparation has to be done at that depth to create a veneer, which does not extend beyond the contours of adjacent teeth.

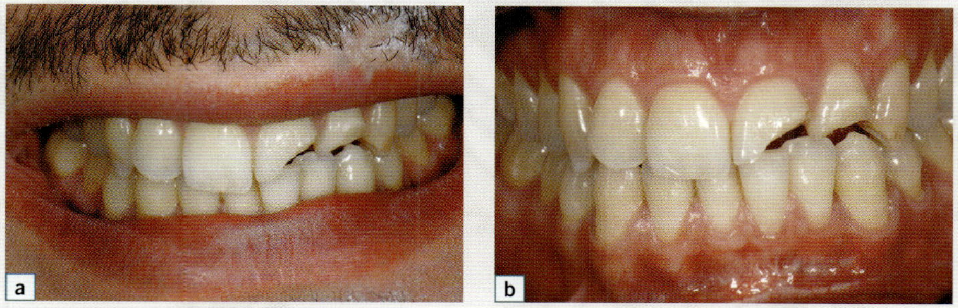

Figs 9-4a and 9-4b
A patient presented to the dental office due to a traffic accident, during which teeth 21, 22, and 23 were damaged.

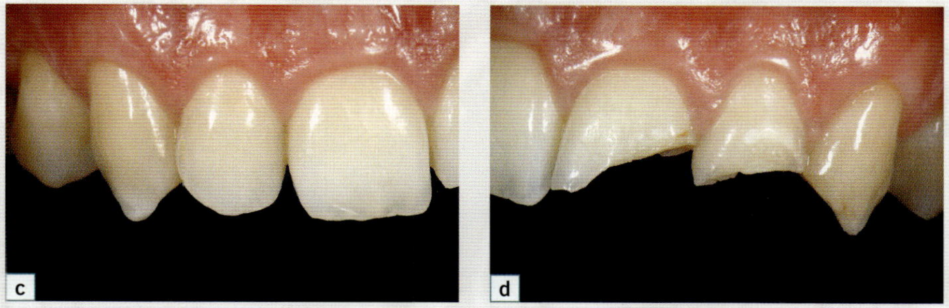

Figs 9-4c and 9-4d
(c) Differences in color saturation, brightness, tooth characteristics, and (d) extensive Class IV tissue loss involve more than half of the tooth.

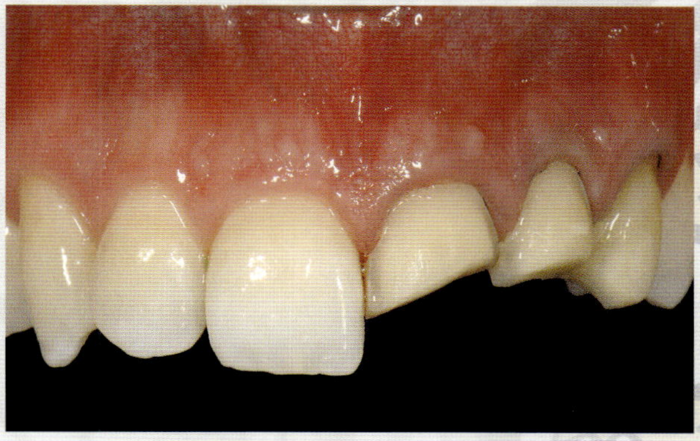

Fig 9-4e
When working on only half of the anterior dentition, we are forced to maintain the previous contour of asymmetrically located teeth. For this reason, a more invasive preparation is necessary, and this has to be compatible with the thickness of the future restoration.

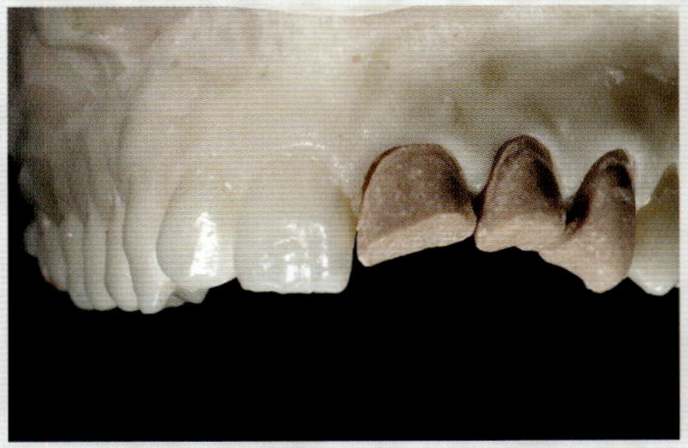

Fig 9-4f
From an esthetic point of view, the first choice of material in difficult cases is feldspathic ceramics made on a refractory die. Only this material enables direct layering when fabricating a reconstruction.

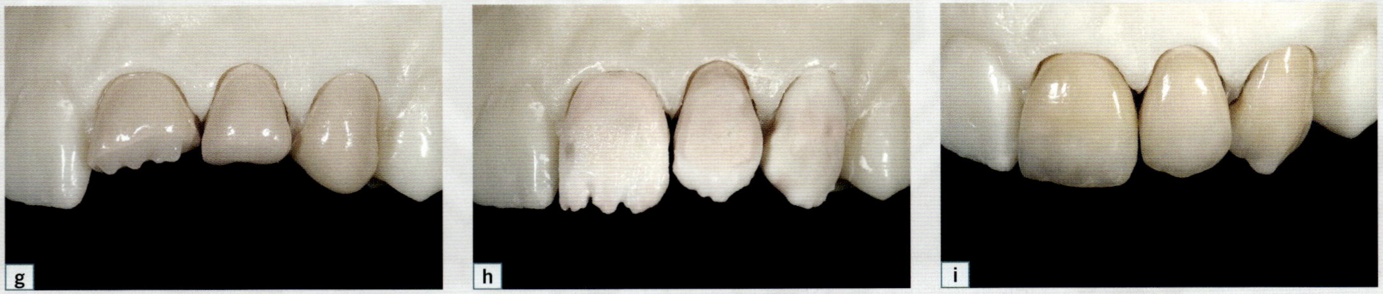

Figs 9-4g to 9-4i
Fabricating porcelain veneers 21, 22, and 23 in the dental laboratory.

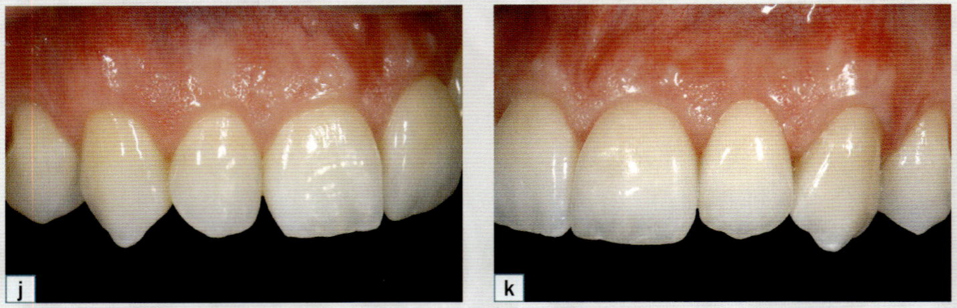

Figs 9-4j and 9-4k
Clinical situation after cementing veneers on teeth 21, 22, and 23 (j) from the right and (k) from the left semi-profile view.

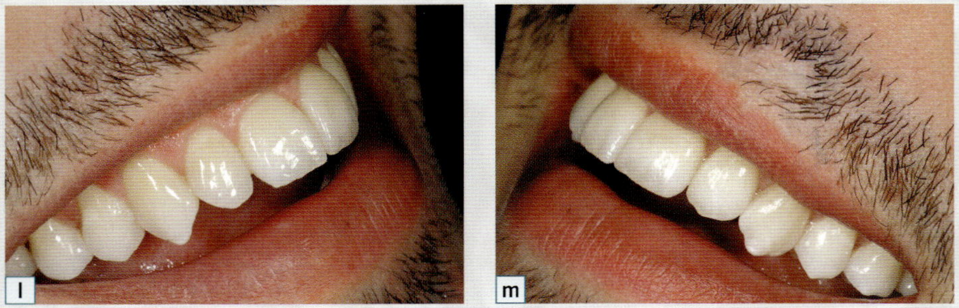

Figs 9-4l and 9-4m
Patient's smile after cementing veneers 21, 22, and 23 (l) from the right and (m) from the left semi-profile views.

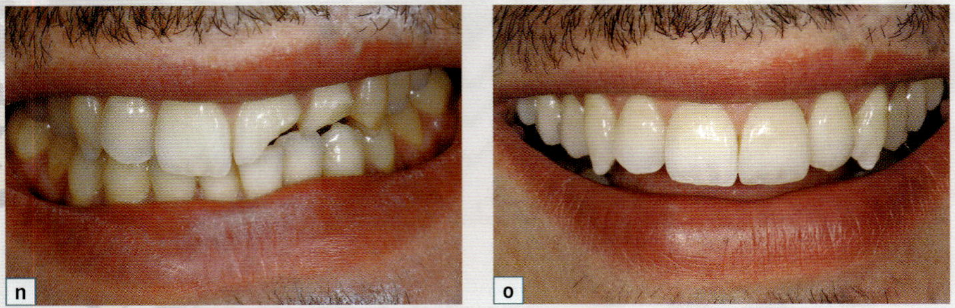

Figs 9-4n and 9-4o
Clinical situation (n) before and (o) after cementing veneers 21, 22, and 23.

B. FULL-DEPTH PREPARATION WITH ADDITIVE DIAGNOSTIC WAX-UP

Full-depth preparation with the use of a silicone index taken from the cast with additive diagnostic wax-up is certainly the most common today. It was introduced to the literature by Dr. Galip Gürel and Dr. Pascal Magne in 2003 and 2004. It allows excellent esthetic results to be obtained, while maintaining a large amount of enamel after tooth preparation.

This preparation technique is most often recommended when changing the esthetics of a larger group of teeth in the anterior segment when there is a possibility to modify the contour of the teeth in an additive way. It is described in detail in Chapter 6.

C. MINIMALLY INVASIVE PREPARATION

Minimally invasive preparation is a consequence of the development of the previous technique,[8] as well as a result of the availability of new ceramic materials on the market, which can be pressed to a very small thickness of 0.3 mm, for example, the Opal system (IPS e.max).

Such restorations are always additive to the tooth surface; they are rarely used for a single tooth reconstruction.[9] However, they can easily be used in a comprehensive anterior segment treatment. This technique is indicated when we do not want to change the shape and color of the tooth significantly or when these changes are minor, as well as when closing the diastema and gaps between the anterior teeth. Principles of material selection and of the dental technician's work are very similar to no-prep veneers. These restorations are characterized by minimal enamel preparation, involving tenths of a millimeter.

The author of this chapter prefers minimally invasive veneers over additive no-prep veneers because the advantage of minimal tooth preparation is a clearly marked preparation margin, which facilities the veneer positioning while cementing, which is not possible with no-prep veneers.

TIP

Covering the incisal edge with the veneer allows a more individual restoration to be created, reflecting all the characteristic features, which ensures an optimal esthetic restoration.

PREPARATION

The preparation technique begins with an additive diagnostic wax-up, then a silicone index is prepared on its basis, which helps control the preparation depth. Of course, the wax-up must be created to the full thickness of the future restoration. In this technique, if we start the preparation from the mock-up level, we should be very careful to keep the labial surface untouched or minimally affected by the bur and concentrate to clearly mark the outline of the restoration.

With such minimal preparation, it is necessary to use magnification, ie, dental loupes with four or fivefold magnification or, preferably, a microscope.

TIP

Although this approach is minimally invasive, certain rules from traditional preparations still apply.
These include:

- Reduction of the incisal edge to a depth of 1.5–2 mm in order to obtain sufficient space for the restoration
- Marked outline of the preparation margin with a minimal depth
- Minimal reduction of the labial surface

CEMENTATION

A well-marked border on the tooth circumference makes it possible to identify the preparation margin and easily apply rubber dam isolation, which is difficult to use in the no-prep technique where the preparation margin is not clearly marked.

Usually, dentists prefer to use a properly heated micro-hybrid composite when cementing veneers. However, in the case of very thin porcelain veneers, with a thickness of 0.2–0.3 mm, using a standard composite is difficult and may lead to cracking of the veneer during cementation.

For adhesive cementation of extremely delicate veneers, the author prefers to use a flowable **composite cement**. Due to its fluidity, this can be used as a thin layer and becomes the material of choice. When cementing thicker ceramic restorations, the color of the luting cement is not relevant, while **for very thin restorations, the choice of the right color is extremely important**.

Luting cement kits often include trial pastes based on water-soluble glycerin gel, and these correspond with the color of the composite cement (see Chapter 7).

CHOICE OF CERAMIC MATERIAL

Veneers can be fabricated with various types of ceramics, in particular:

- **Feldspathic ceramics** made on a refractory die or platinum foil (75–90 MPa)
- **Leucite-reinforced ceramics** (hot-pressed or fabricated in CAD/CAM technology) (120 MPa)
- **Lithium disilicate ceramics** (hot-pressed or fabricated in CAD/CAM technology) (400 MPa)

In everyday practice, the author prefers feldspathic or pressed ceramics due to the greatest experience in this range, instead of restorations fabricated using CAD/CAM technology.

Especially for ultrathin veneers, lithium disilicate pressed ceramics are preferred, as this can be fabricated to a thickness of only 0.3 mm while maintaining very high strength.

Fabricating such thin restorations by a dental technician, even though it may seem simple, is extremely complex and demands very high precision. Working with the veneers during the try-in and cementation stage is difficult because they are very fragile and therefore very susceptible to any damage.

Feldspathic ceramics provide very good precision and esthetics, but have a low elastic modulus of 75–90 MPa, making the material very fragile. Attention also should be paid to an interesting publication by Magne et al concerning the effects of luting composite shrinkage while cementing porcelain veneers and thermal loads on the stress distribution during variable thermal conditions.[10] The authors show through the finite element method the existence of a negative correlation between the thickness of the luting cement and porcelain veneer, and the distribution of stresses on the inner and outer surfaces.

Ceramic restorations underwent thermal shock testing, which showed a relationship between the thickness of the luting composite and the ceramics, and cracks in the porcelain veneers.

Thermal loads, in combination with stresses resulting from shrinkage of the composite material, are particularly dangerous for the veneers. Such loads lead to low compressive stresses, but they increase tensile stresses, which is very dangerous for porcelain veneers because this type of stress increases the risk of ceramic fracture.

The conclusions of this study are that the stress distribution is not related to the veneer's incisal edge length, but rather to the thickness of the ceramics on the labial surface, and the thickness of the luting cement layer.

Too thin veneers combined with their poor fit to the core surface (thick layer of the luting cement) have resulted in the appearance of higher stresses, as well as on the porcelain surface and between the junction of the tooth and the veneer.

In conclusion, the relationship between the thickness of the luting cement and the ceramics may have a significant impact on the stress distribution in the porcelain veneer. The labial and cervical areas are the most critical parts of the restoration if they are fabricated of a thin ceramic layer, due to insufficient space for the restoration.

TIP

Suppose the porcelain layer has to be very thin to maintain the natural contour of the tooth. In that case, only a perfect fit of the veneer in the tooth, with a gap in the range of up to 100 µm, can prevent a decrease of the CER/CPR ratio (the thickness of the ceramic layer in relation to the thickness of the luting cement layer) below the optimal value, which should always be greater than three.

Looking at the data from the literature, it can be concluded that the average size of the gap between the porcelain veneer and the tooth surface is over 100 µm (usually 100–140 µm) and exceeds the ideal CER/CPR ratio. For this reason, when fabricating thin veneers, it is recommended to use ceramics with higher flexural strength, such as lithium disilicate ceramics, which reach the strength of 400 MPa, even for thin restorations. This approach allows the risk of veneer fracture to be reduced significantly.

TIP

The choice of the ceramic material and the quality of the laboratory procedures has a significant impact on the durability of very thin porcelain veneers (the ability to achieve maximum tightness of the restoration).

In recent years, the author has used practically all types of ceramic materials available on the market. Based on experience, he is convinced that the most suitable material for thin porcelain veneers is lithium disilicate. Thanks to its high flexural strength, this is the most reliable material in the long term. Feldspathic ceramics offer the best esthetic results, but when very thin veneers are performed, they can turn out as fragile and unreliable over time.

Case 5: Lithium disilicate veneers

A female patient presented to the dental office in order to improve the esthetics of her smile. She complained about the discoloration of the two central incisors, which did not disappear after professional tooth whitening. She also wanted to improve the setting of the maxillary incisors but without orthodontic treatment. The dental tissues were healthy, so there was only an indication to change the superficial structure of the enamel. The treatment plan included correction of the midline, and changing the inclination of the central incisors. This was associated with minimal preparation because, in the absence of preparation, the labial contour of these two teeth would have to be significantly increased.

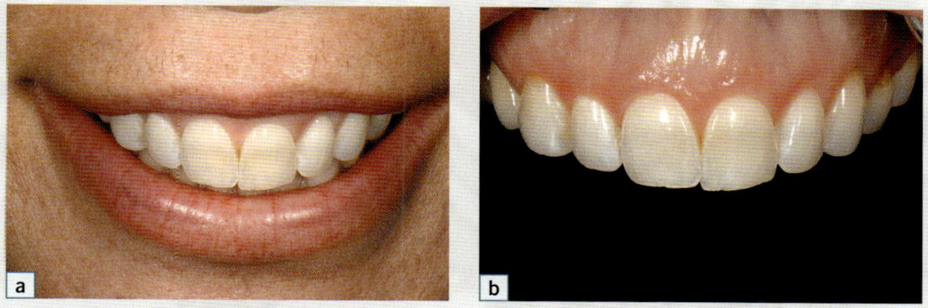

Figs 9-5a and 9-5b
Initial situation: discolored central incisors after whitening. The patient wished to improve the maxillary anterior teeth color and setting without orthodontic treatment.

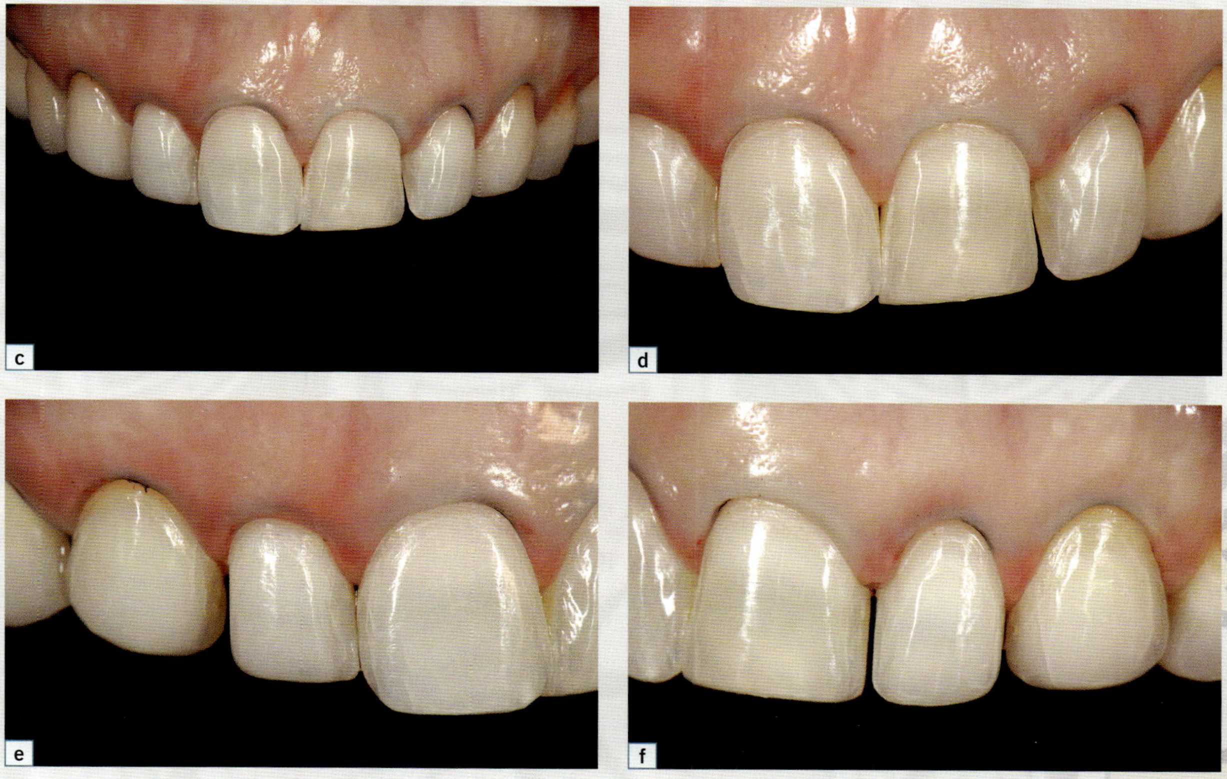

Figs 9-5c to 9-5f
Additive veneers were planned with minimal preparation (to facilitate the midline correction). Lithium disilicate from the Opal system (IPS e.max) was selected. It is an ideal material for such thin restorations because it has high bending strength – 400 MPa, which allows creation of very bright veneers pressed to a small thickness of 0.3 mm. This material is characterized by natural opalescence, even at minimum thickness, thanks to which the restoration has a very natural look under different lighting conditions.Moreover, lithium disilicate is a ceramic based on glass, so it can be cemented adhesively to the enamel surface.

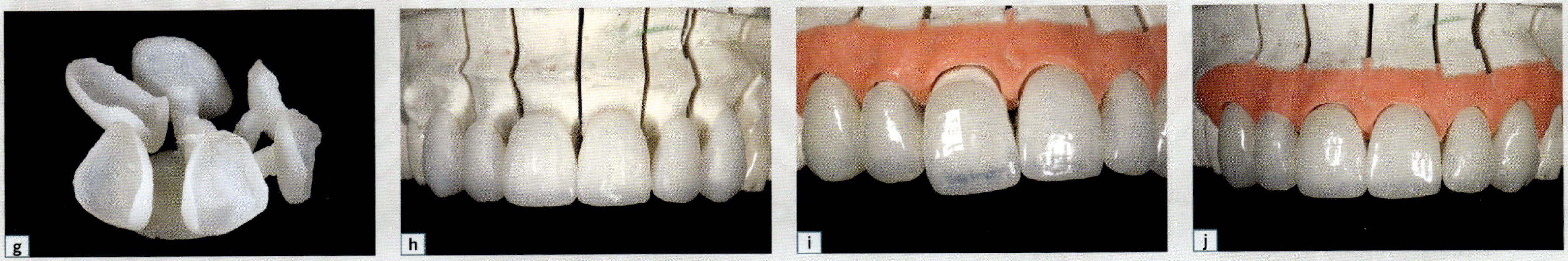

Figs 9-5g to 9-5j
The following laboratory procedures were performed: waxing-up the restoration on the working cast and, on its basis, preparing lithium disilicate veneers using the lost wax casting technique. In this way, veneers with a maximum thickness of 0.3 mm were fabricated. Such restorations can certainly be described as new artificial enamel, with which we replace the natural enamel (depending on the case, a staining or layering technique can be utilized, or a combination of both). It is very important to fabricate the veneer surface carefully, as it should have very precise micro and macrostructure.

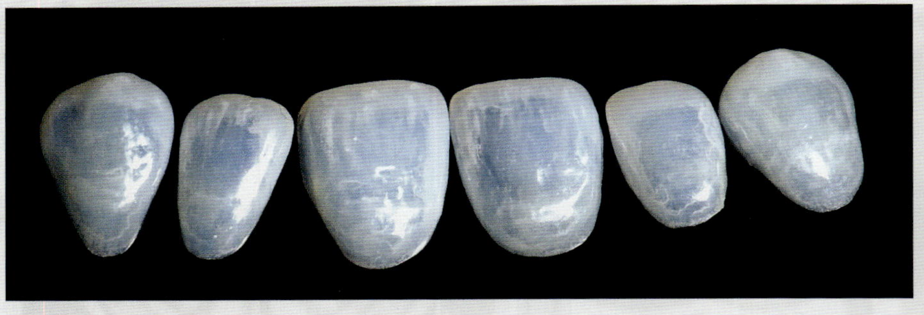

Fig 9-5k
Veneers fabricated in the dental laboratory are ready for adhesive cementation (laboratory work: DT Franco Feretti).

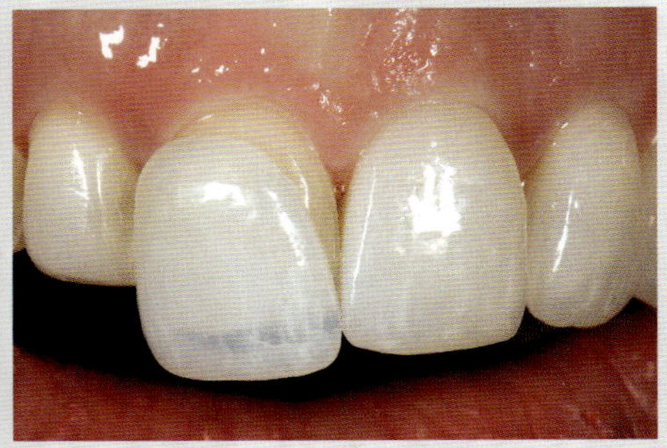

Fig 9-5l
Trying-in veneers before cementation.

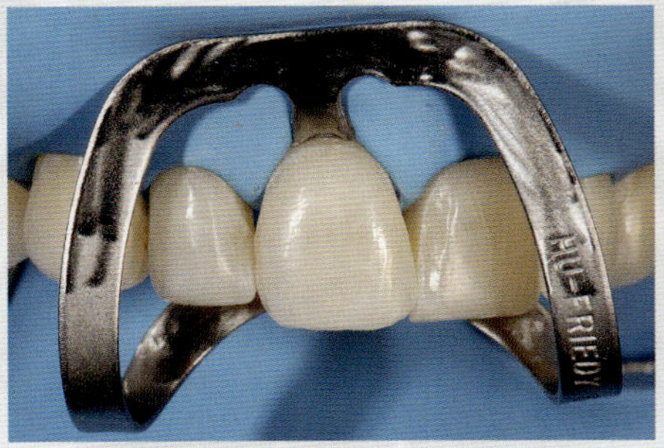

Fig 9-5m
Adhesive cementation in rubber dam isolation.

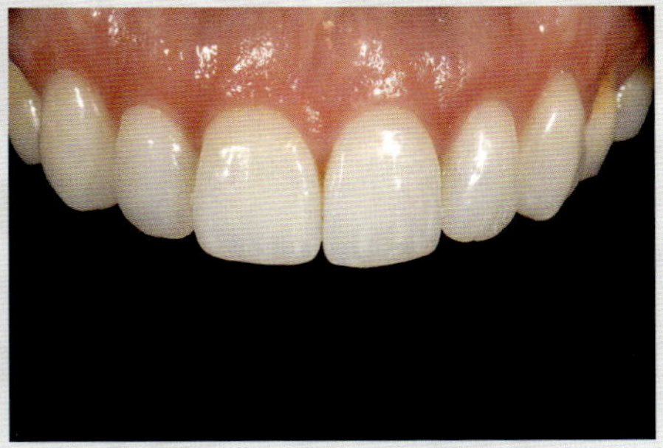

Fig 9-5n
Clinical situation after veneers cementation.

PRACTITIONER'S ADVICE

Micro and macrostructure of the porcelain veneers determine the natural and esthetic result of the treatment!

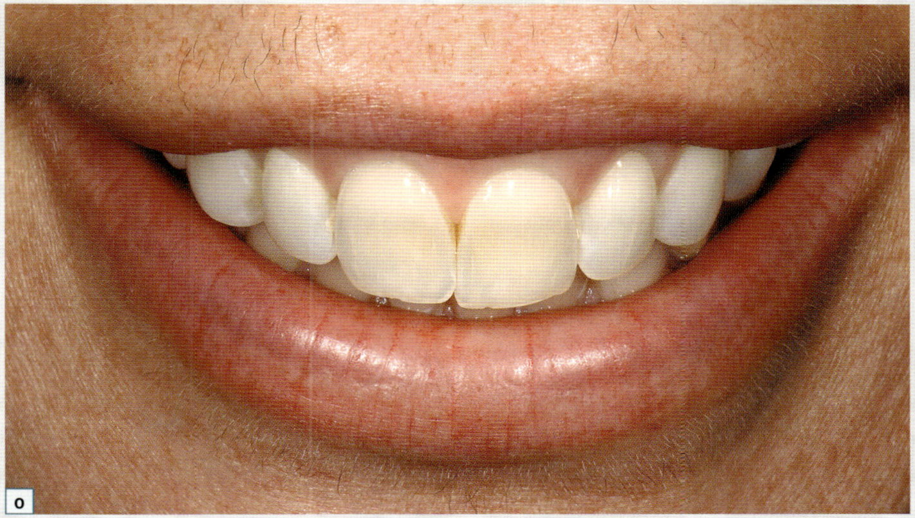

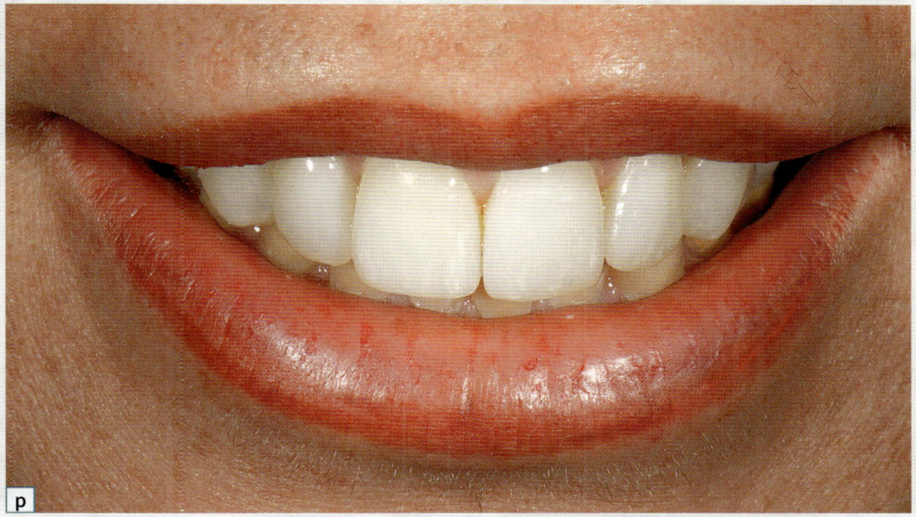

Figs 9-5o and 9-5p
Photographs of a satisfied patient (o) before and (p) after veneers cementation.

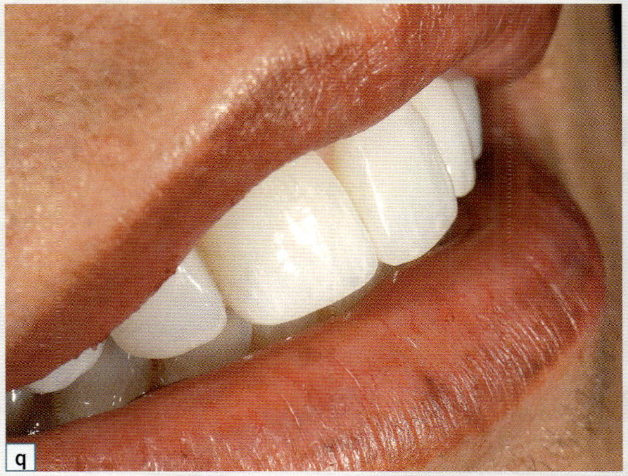

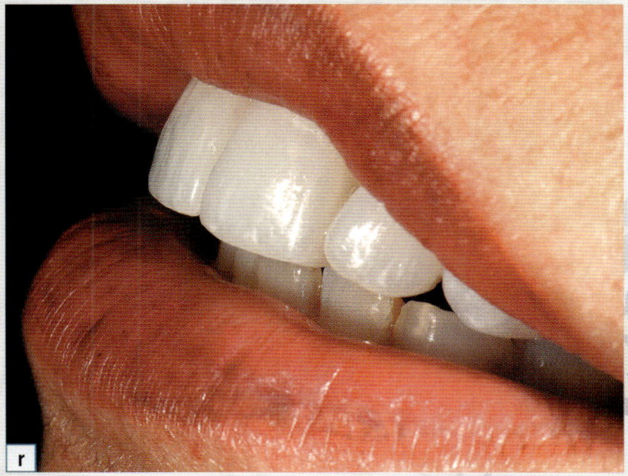

Figs 9-5q and 9-5r
Patient's smile from the semi-profile: perfect integration with the upper and lower lip.

Case 6: Feldspathic ceramics on a refractory die

This case presents a patient's treatment history after the first part of orthodontic therapy when severe gaps and diastema remained between the anterior teeth of the maxilla. Orthodontic treatment needed to be continued, which would be carried out using the Invisalign system after performing prosthetic restorations. Wide gaps between the anterior teeth allowed minimally invasive restorations with minimal tooth preparation and the use of feldspathic ceramics. **The patient had high esthetic expectations and wanted to achieve a natural effect.** This emphasis on improving esthetics resulted in the choice of feldspathic ceramics made on a refractory die. It must be emphasized that, although we currently have many good ceramic materials on the market, feldspathic porcelain undoubtedly remains the most suitable material from the esthetics point of view.

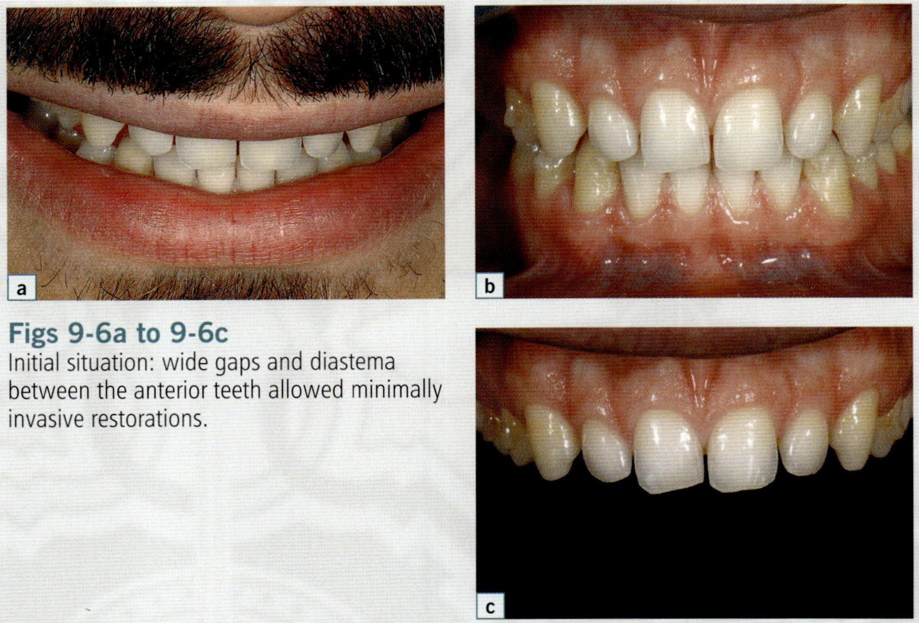

Figs 9-6a to 9-6c
Initial situation: wide gaps and diastema between the anterior teeth allowed minimally invasive restorations.

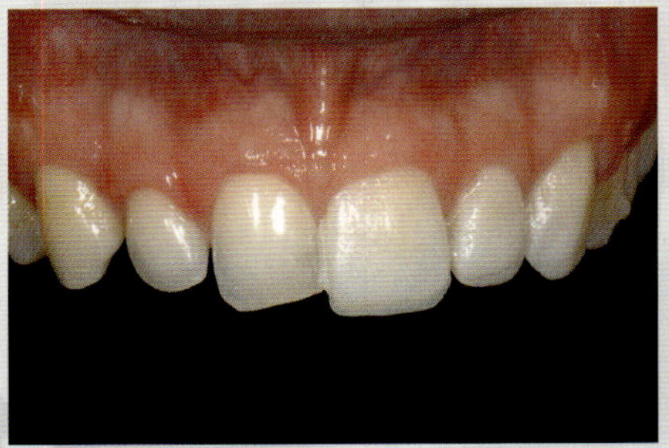

Fig 9-6d
Treatment was started with a diagnostic wax-up and by increasing the contour of the mock-up.

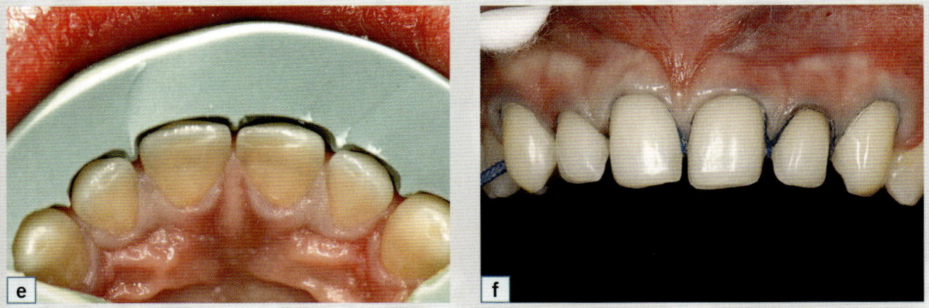

Figs 9-6e and 9-6f
The depth of the preparation is controlled with the silicone index. First, a small chamfer is created on the tooth circumference and the incisal edge is reduced to the depth provided during the wax-up. Next, the labial surface is minimally reduced, which is practically unnoticeable, to connect the preparation margins at the tooth circumference. The purpose of the minimally invasive preparation technique is to preserve the maximum amount of enamel substance, maintaining all the features characteristic for traditional preparation, but definitely reduced in depth.[11]

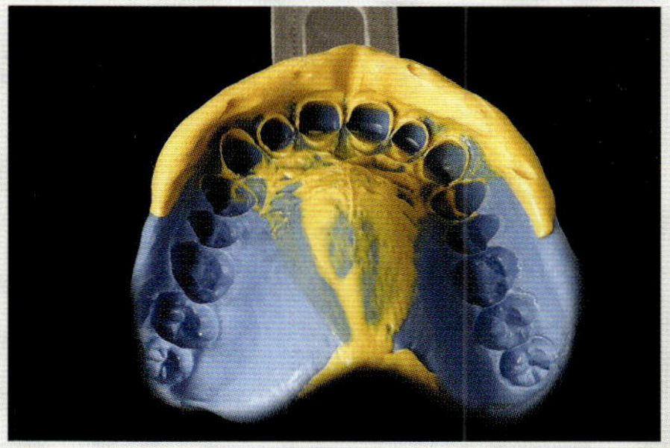

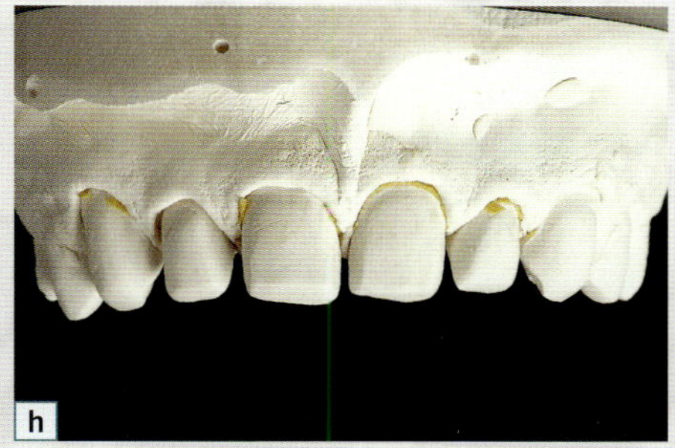

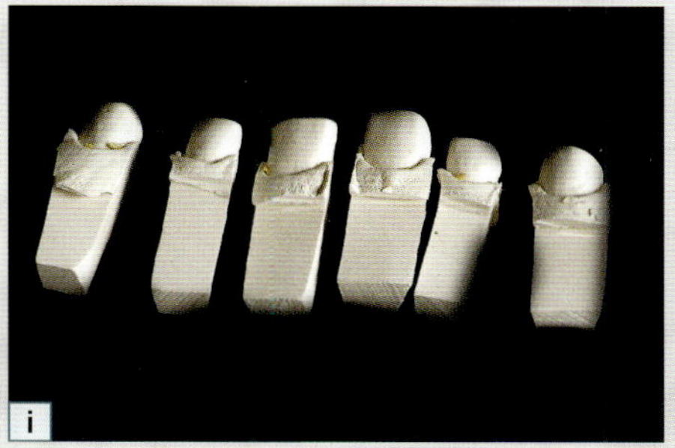

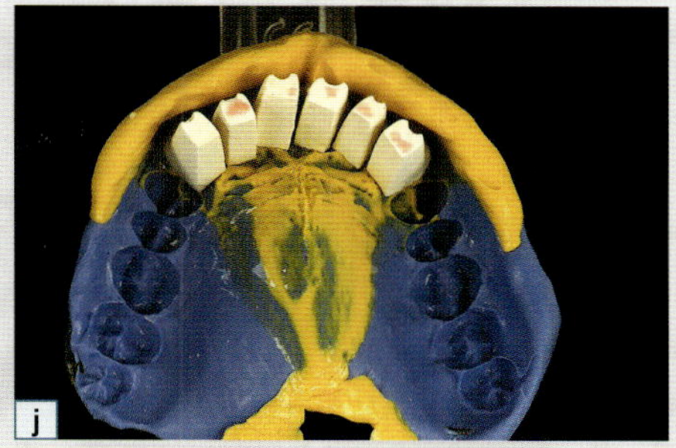

Fig 9-6g
Impressions taken with polyvinyl siloxane mass.

Figs 9-6h to 9-6s
Laboratory procedures while fabricating ultrathin veneers.

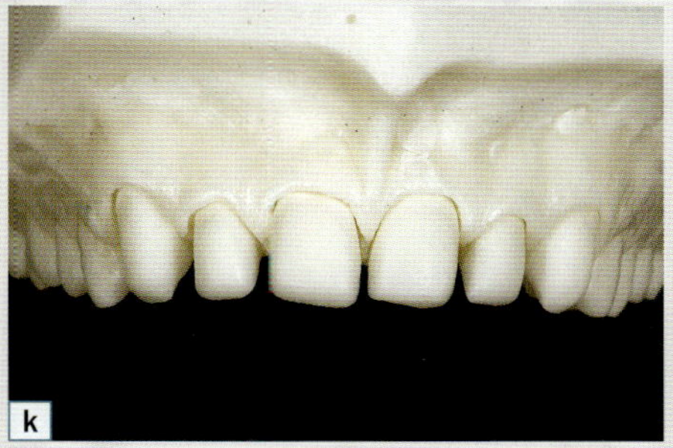

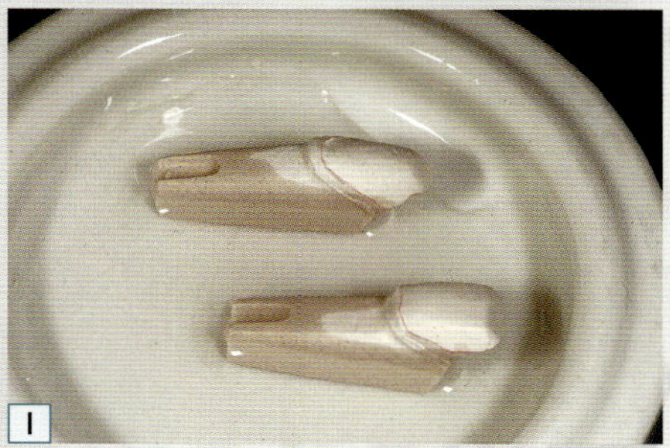

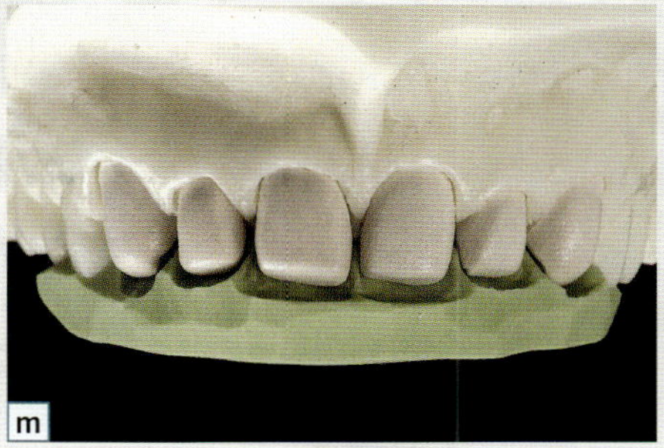

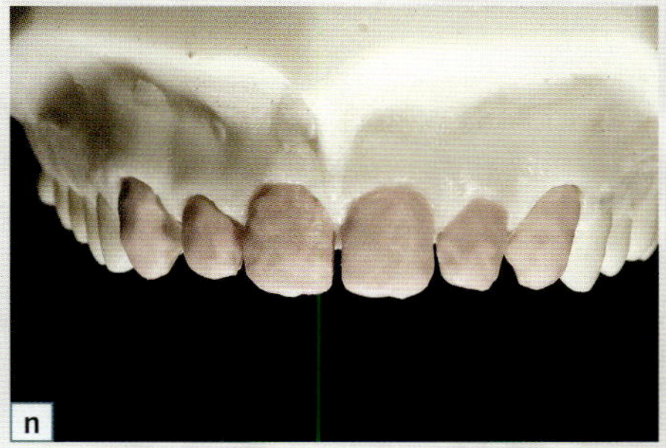

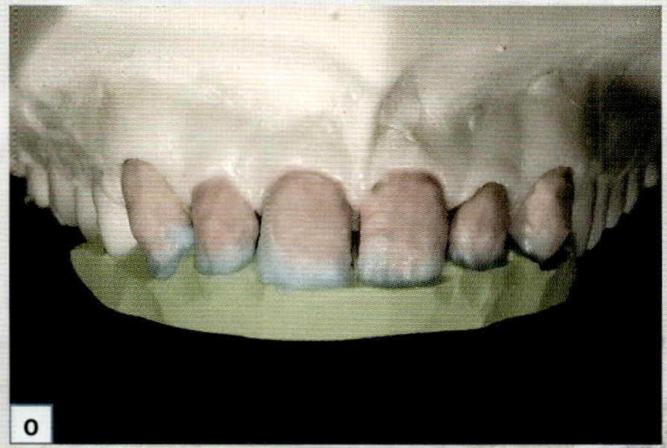

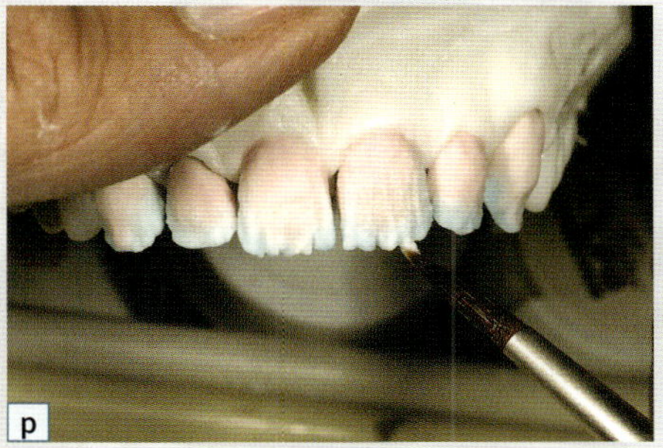

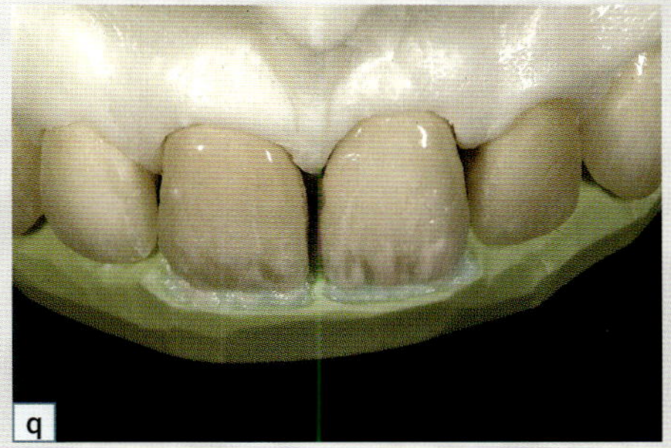

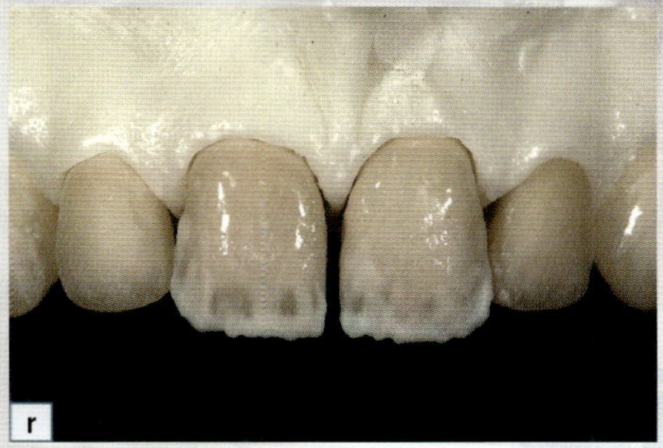

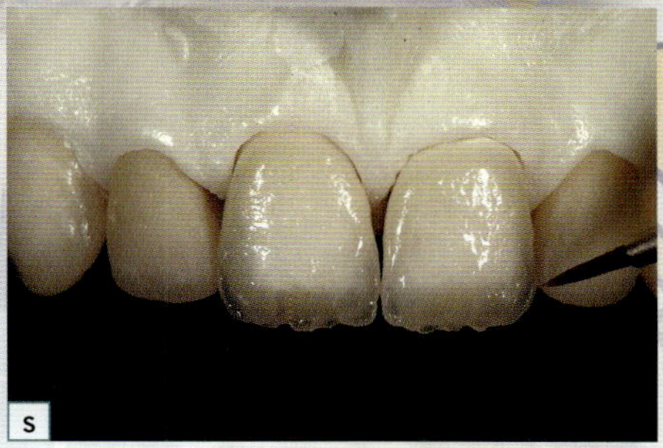

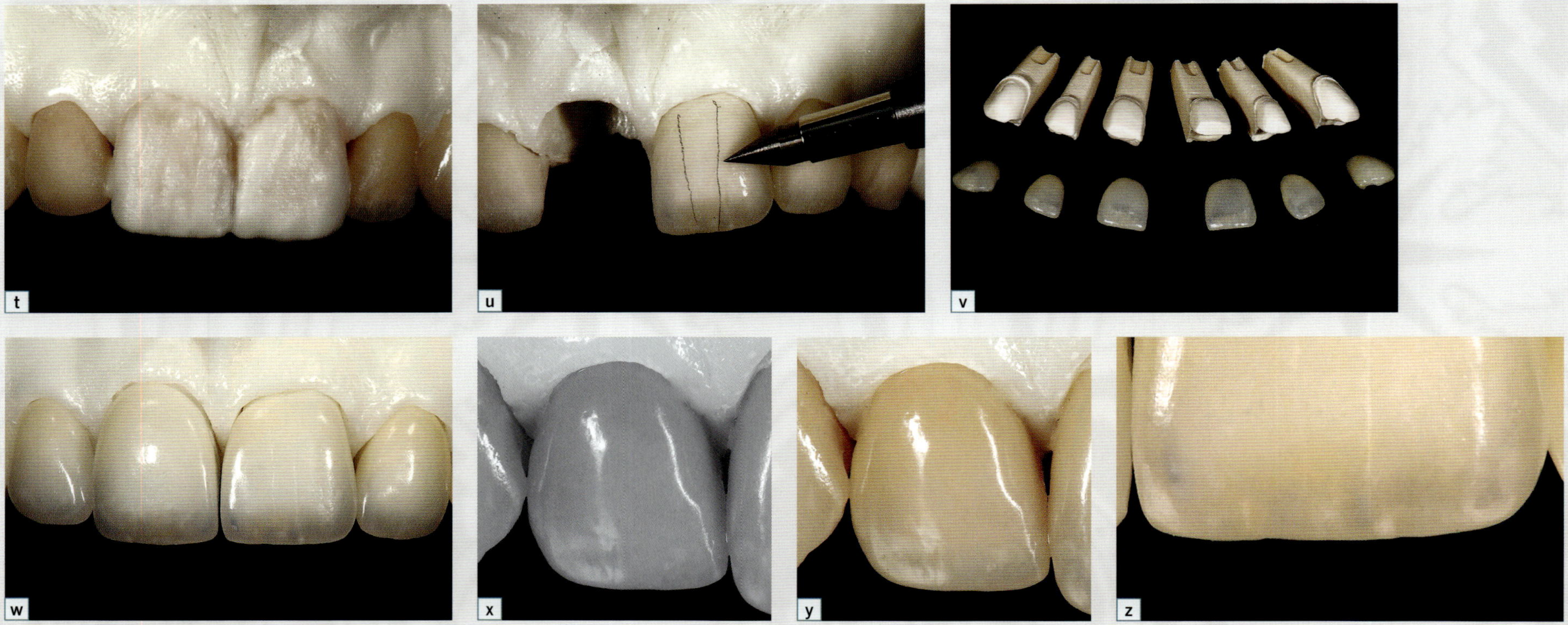

Figs 9-6t to 9-6z
Laboratory procedures while fabricating ultrathin veneers (laboratory work: DT Franco Feretti).

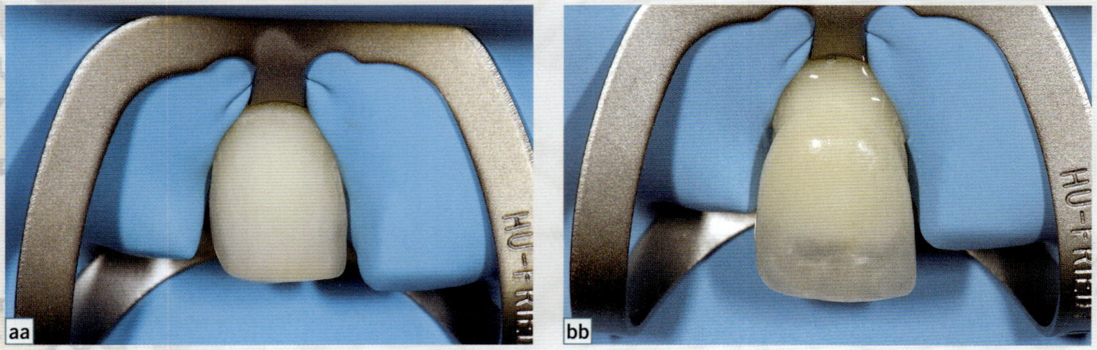

Figs 9-6aa and 9-6bb
When performing such thin restorations, we feel safer using sufficiently flowable luting cement and, for trial cementation, glycerin gels in shades corresponding to the luting cement. With such thin and translucent restorations, the color of the luting cement may have a crucial effect on the final esthetic result.[12]

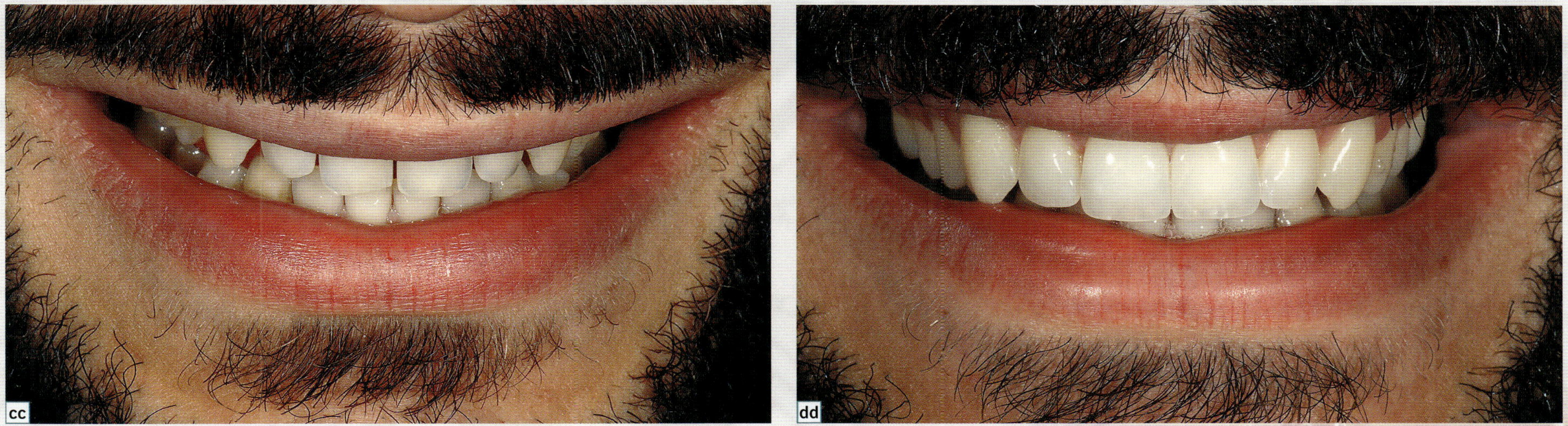

Figs 9-6cc and 9-6dd
(cc) Clinical situation before treatment and (dd) after porcelain veneers cementation.

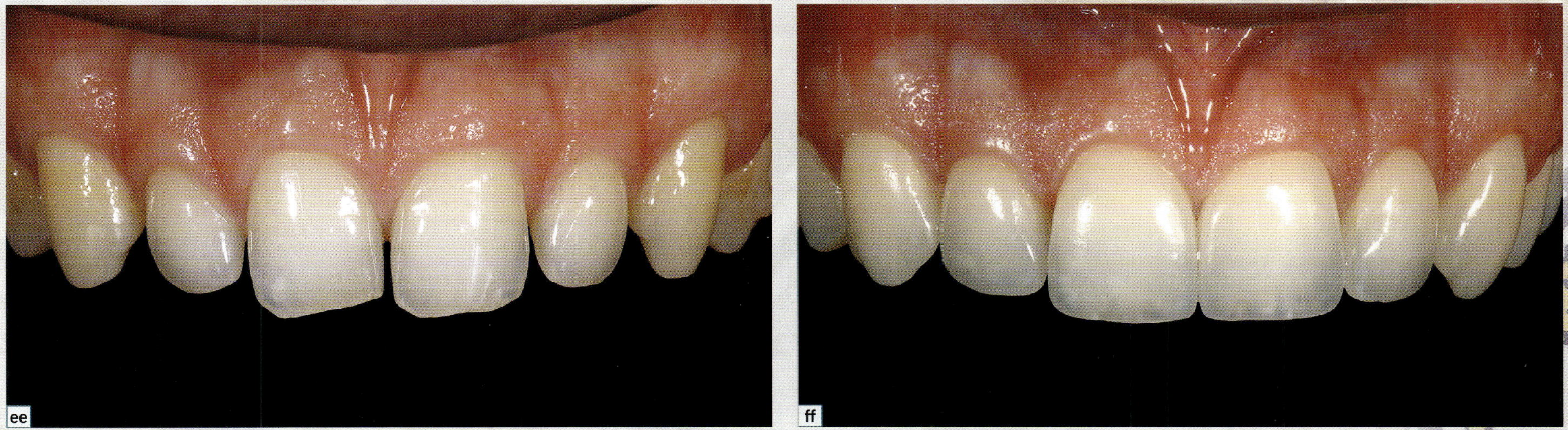

Figs 9-6ee and 9-6ff
Comparison of the photographs (ee) before and (ff) after treatment.

D. NO-PREP VENEERS

No-prep veneers are created without prior tooth preparation. This is by far the most conservative approach we can take when performing indirect restorations within the anterior teeth. As we know, this is not a novelty; this technique has advantages and disadvantages that should be carefully considered before offering a patient such a treatment solution.[13,14]

No-prep veneers appeared in the 1980s as an ultraconservative technique, easy to implement, minimally invasive for the patient and economical. Because it requires definitely less time and work at the dentist's chair than in the case of traditional veneers, no-prep veneers began to enjoy great popularity. In 1990–2000, the no-prep technique began to be replaced by more aggressive techniques due to the appearance of pressed ceramics, which required deeper tissue preparation. No-prep techniques returned to favor after 2000 in combination with new materials fabricated with the pressed technique, enabling the creation of thin restorations, which were a consequence of very aggressive and persuasive marketing.

Marketing presents no-prep veneers as very attractive for patients. The structural risk associated with the preparation drops to almost zero, which allows you to work without anesthesia and pain, which is the most common reason for most patients postponing visits until the last minute, especially those with dentophobia who often refrain from treatment even though they want to improve the esthetics of their smile.

Over the last 30 years, there has been a noticeable tendency to change the type of preparation and the most commonly used ceramic material. We went through minimally invasive restorations to more aggressive preparations, before returning to minimally invasive and no-prep restorations. However, **the veneer choice cannot dictate what is trendy or by marketing**. Over the years, our approach has become more conservative, and the preservation of the enamel and the vestibular dental structures became a priority. However, while no-prep restorations may seem easier to perform, they are associated with several clinical and laboratory problems.

> **TIP**
>
> There are clinical cases where the use of this method is contraindicated, or when thicker porcelain veneers are indicated. A typical example is major discoloration, where a thin restoration cannot mask the altered tooth color.

The purpose of this chapter is to evaluate this technique and discuss its advantages and disadvantages, so the reader can learn the appropriate indications for performing no-prep veneers and obtain predictable treatment results.

INDICATIONS

- Interdental gaps and incorrect Bolton index
- Moderate tooth discoloration resistant to whitening
- Abnormalities of tooth shape and size
- Closure of black triangles
- Lengthening the anterior teeth
- Correction of the teeth position (immediate prosthetic orthodontics)
- Patients with dentophobia

Optimal indications for this procedure are all cases where there is a place for correcting the incorrections, ie, everywhere that increasing the size and the shape of the tooth is esthetically beneficial and, for adults, when **open gaps and irregularities in the teeth shape** remain after orthodontic treatment.

A typical post-orthodontic indication is when we are dealing with an incorrect Bolton index, ie, the discrepancy between the width of the anterior teeth and the size of the dental arch, meaning that, after orthodontic treatment, despite the correct positioning of the canines, gaps remain between the anterior teeth. These are clinical cases that can be adequately corrected with the no-prep technique.

Another indication for this technique is the **closure of black triangles** in periodontal patients. A consequence of periodontal disease can be gingival recession, which also occurs in the interdental spaces (wide gaps between the teeth) and create a major esthetic problem that can be solved with no-prep additive veneers.

Another indication is **immediate prosthetic orthodontics**, ie, cases with incorrect positioning of the teeth in the anterior segment where instead of orthodontic treatment (the therapy of choice but often rejected by adult patients), malocclusion is corrected with additive ceramic restorations. In cases of moderate discoloration resistant to whitening, this method can be an attractive solution due to its excellent esthetics and low structural risk.

The next indication are patients with **dentophobia** for whom the possibility of treatment without anesthesia represents a more acceptable solution.

CONTRAINDICATIONS

- Major discolorations
- Tooth crowding
- Excessively rotated or slanted teeth
- Teeth with correct morphology and size

In all cases of anterior crowding with teeth rotations and inclinations, the no-prep technique is contraindicated because correcting such irregularities with these restorations would require a greater thickness of porcelain and would often be unesthetic. In such situations, the range of the tooth preparation has to be extended, allowing the fabrication of ceramic restorations of adequate thickness. In conclusion, the advantages of no-prep veneers are their small thickness (0.3 mm) and greater translucency while they are contraindicated when it is necessary to perform thicker restorations.

Sometimes, the fabricated veneer could be too thick as the dental technician needs to compensate for lack of appropriate preparation – in those cases, the no-prep restoration would cause marginal gingivitis in the place of contact with the soft tissues.

NO-PREP VENEERS: PROS AND CONS

Technically, the procedure is simple and has few following steps:

1. Initial assessment
2. Taking impressions and registering in the articulator
3. Fabricating no-prep veneers with the press ceramic technique
4. Try-in and cementing veneers

All these types of restorations are usually performed without anesthesia or rubber dam isolation. Undoubtedly, the simplicity of this procedure is what encourages dentists to use this technique, and it is also one of the reasons why it became popular again. However, from the clinical and laboratory point of view, this technique is associated with some difficulties, which makes the author of this chapter wary of this procedure and prompts the use of other solutions.

Let's start by analyzing the technical problems in the dental laboratory. Fabrication such thin restorations is not easy. It isn't easy to obtain adequate anatomical forms with the proper emergence profile without over-contouring. Moreover, the small thickness of the restorations requires enormous precision at every stage of fabrication.

Otherwise, the veneer can be damaged very easily. Performing a proper characterization of the surface, ie, the micro and macrostructure of the veneers, is technically a very difficult procedure, and the restoration can only be stained superficially.

Also, there are many critical steps from the clinical point of view. The small thickness of the veneers means that there is a small margin of manipulation, the try-in of the veneers must be performed with extreme caution, and adjustment of the contact points and the color is not without risk. The author has damaged veneers several times while try-in, to the point that he could not cement them during the scheduled appointment. This means a big loss because the time foreseen for this procedure is quite long.

Another important issue is the inability to place a rubber dam while cementing no-prep veneers, except in rare cases. This is because the preparation margin is not physically outlined. It is impossible to be sure that the rubber dam isolation is placed correctly and will not interfere in the proper positioning of the restoration during cementation.

Therefore, for cementation, a retraction cord is placed into the gingival sulcus, and the adjacent teeth are covered with Teflon tape. Light-curing cement with high fluidity is used for cementation to avoid the risk of veneer fracture.

NO-PREP VENEERS AND ORTHODONTIC TREATMENT

Figure 9-7 presents a female patient with ongoing adult orthodontic treatment. Before the end of this therapy, the patient decided to close the interdental gaps and to improve their incorrect shape. We often use this procedure in cooperation with orthodontists. Before the final phase of orthodontic treatment, the correct shape of the teeth is obtained. Treatment follows, and the final appearance is achieved with thin veneers.

The author has stated that this approach gives the best results in cases requiring interdisciplinary treatment. The interdental gaps and the tooth shape are corrected as precisely as possible, followed by the final stage of orthodontic treatment. Of course, this approach slightly increases the overall treatment time, but the achieved result is better and more predictable. In this particular case, the patient expected corrections without tooth preparation. She asked for the gaps to be closed in the most conservative way, so there were two possible treatment options: additive composite restorations or no-prep veneers.

After careful analysis of the advantages and disadvantages of each technique, no-prep ceramic restorations were selected.

REMEMBER

The no-prep technique only seems to be easier than the traditional one from the clinical and laboratory point of view. Given a choice, it is not a cementation technique that we would wish to propose to our patients. We recommend minimal preparation of the enamel, which will allow the avoidance of many mistakes related to the no-prep technique.

Case 7

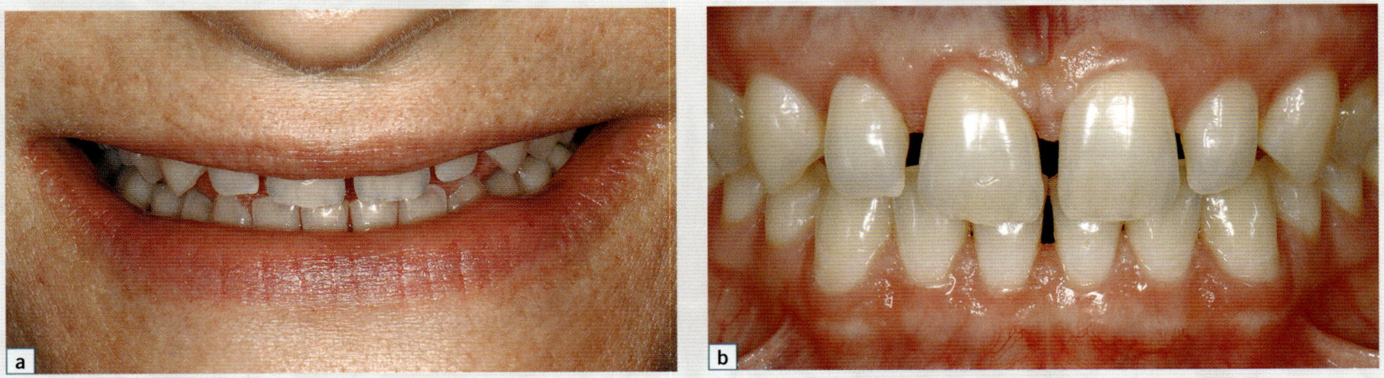

Figs 9-7a and 9-7b
A patient was referred to the dental office by the orthodontist before the end of orthodontic treatment.

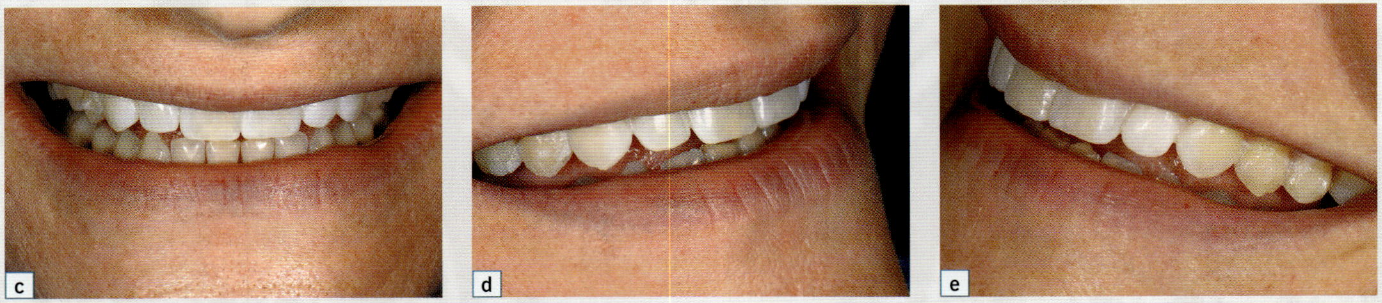

Figs 9-7c to 9-7e
Mock-up with temporary composite was created to allow the patient and the consultation team to evaluate the esthetics of restorations.

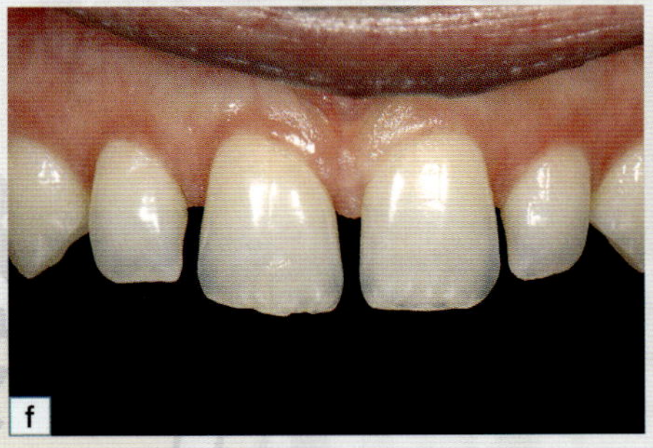

Fig 9-7f
Clinical situation before no-prep veneers cementation.

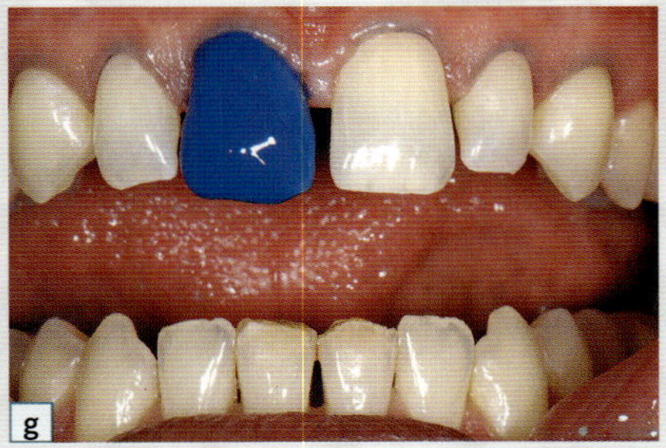

Fig 9-7g
Etching the tooth surface after placing the retraction cord into the gingival sulcus.

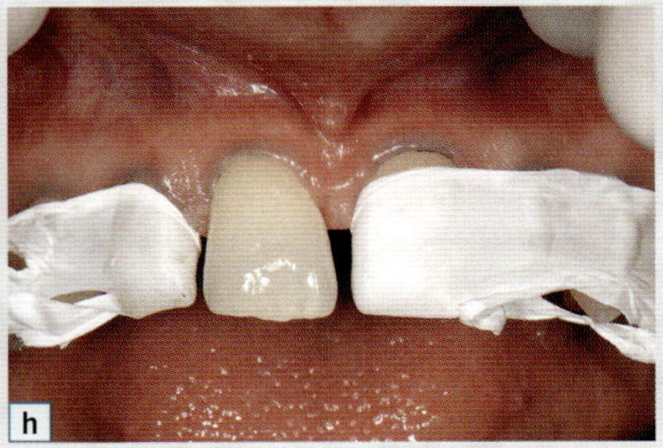

Fig 9-7h
Application of the bonding system.

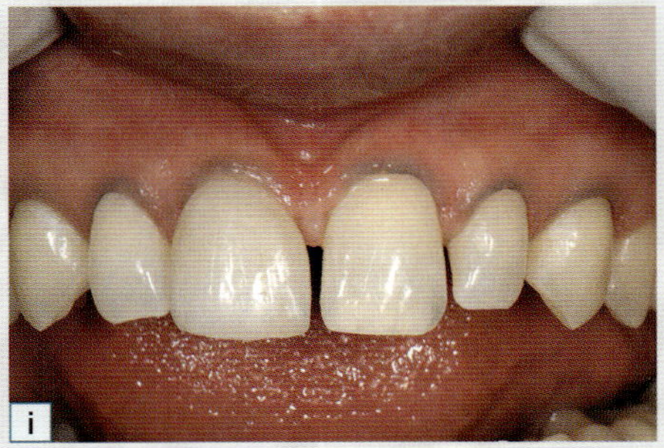

Fig 9-7i
Clinical situation after cementing no-prep veneer on tooth 11.

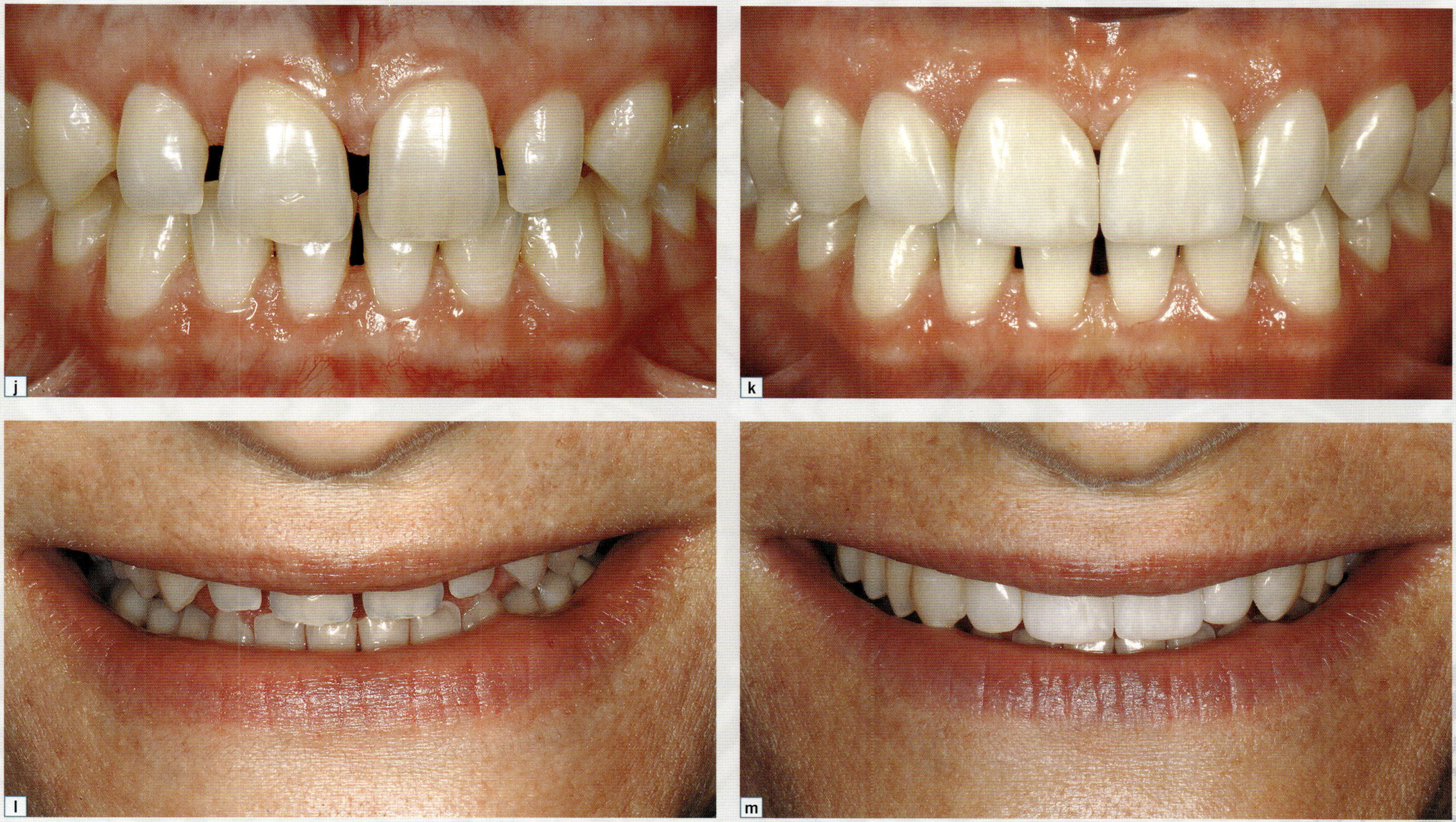

Figs 9-7j to 9-7m
Situation (j, l) before and (k, m) after cementing no-prep veneers on teeth 13, 12, 11, 21, 22, and 23.

Case 8

The presented clinical situation is very complex. A periodontal surgery intervention was necessary in order to restore the correct dento-gingival proportions. After 12 months (necessary for the soft tissues to heal), restorative treatment was started.

A female patient did not want to undergo orthodontic treatment, which in this case would have been the best option. Instead, she asked for her smile to be improved with porcelain veneers. This is a common case called instant orthodontics – you can solve esthetic problems during two appointments with adhesive restorations.

This case is an example of a perfect indication for porcelain veneers performed with the no-prep technique. The gaps between the teeth are wide and can remain closed by additive restorations while the canines are correctly positioned, and their color is acceptable for when fabricating very thin porcelain restorations of 0.2–0.3 mm thickness. Moreover, the patient herself asked for restorations without teeth preparation, fearing that such a procedure might damage her healthy dental tissue.

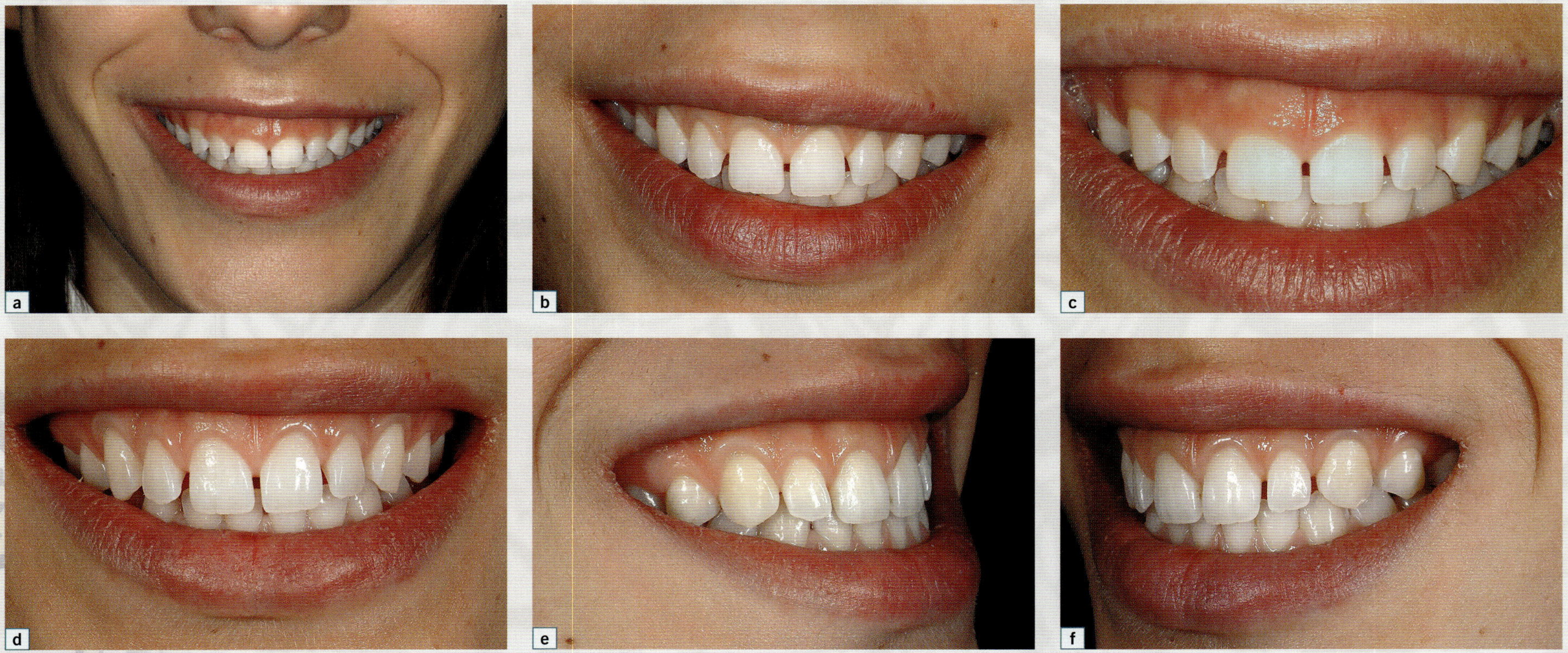

Figs 9-8a to 9-8f
A female patient presented to the dental office requesting esthetic treatment with no-prep porcelain veneers.

Step 1: **Prosthetic procedures (Figs 9-8a to 9-8j)**
The treatment plan in such cases is relatively simple. After the mock-up has been created and the patient has accepted it, silicone or polyether impressions are taken. Before taking the impressions, the author prefers to insert into the gingival sulcus a thin retraction cord soaked in a vasoconstrictor agent, in order to copy the subgingival area of the tooth and transfer the information to the dental laboratory. It is a very important stage of step 1, because the correct emergence profile of the veneers ensures adequate support for the soft tissues at the marginal gingival level and contributes to the extremely natural effect of the reconstruction.

Of course, this is all done without anesthesia and with minimal patient discomfort. Now, the impressions can be transferred to the dental laboratory to pour a working cast and fabricate the final restorations. It should be noted that the functional occlusal registration was performed at the previous appointment, ie, in protrusion and eccentric movements. Additionally, a facebow registration was taken, which will enable the casts to be mounted in a partially adjustable articulator. It is a very important stage of the procedure because when performing non-invasive restorations, we are forced to change the shape and length of the anterior teeth, which functionally affects the mandible and condylar movements. In addition, mounting in an articulator is essential for the dental technician because it means they can achieve the correct equilibrium between the function of the anterior segment and the esthetics of the patient's smile.

Step 2: **Laboratory procedures (Figs 9-8k to 9-8t)**
Laboratory procedures are definitely more complicated than clinical management. Fabricating such thin veneers is a big challenge. Achieving all necessary anatomical effects, applying complex layers, and finishing the veneers is especially difficult and can lead to damage to the restorations. The working cast was poured with removable dies according to Geller (this is also known as an anatomical cast). The advantage of this procedure is that, on the main cast, we can maintain the shape and volume of the soft tissues while also being able to remove the gypsum die of one single tooth, which simplifies veneer fabrication.

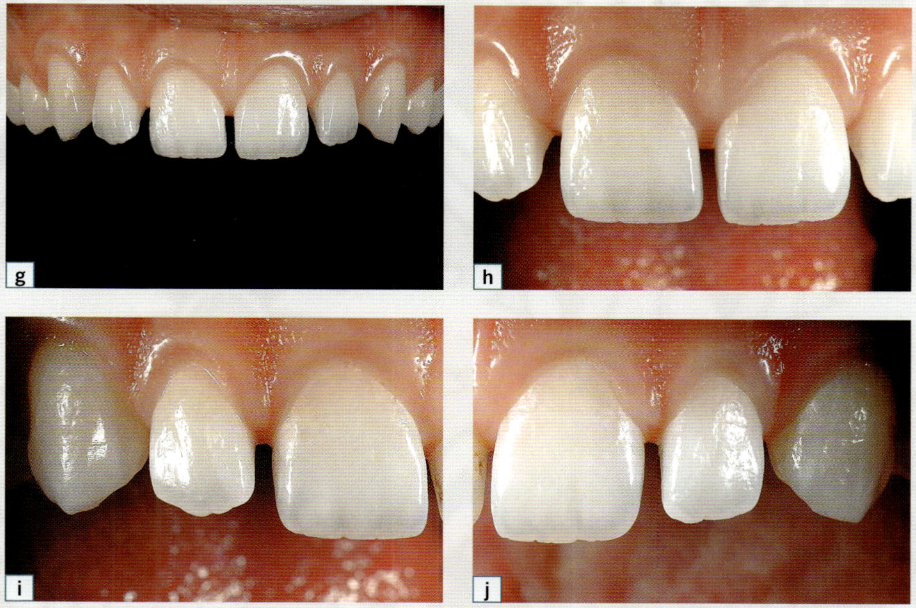

Figs 9-8g to 9-8j
Clinical situation after the gingiva has healed and before taking an impression.

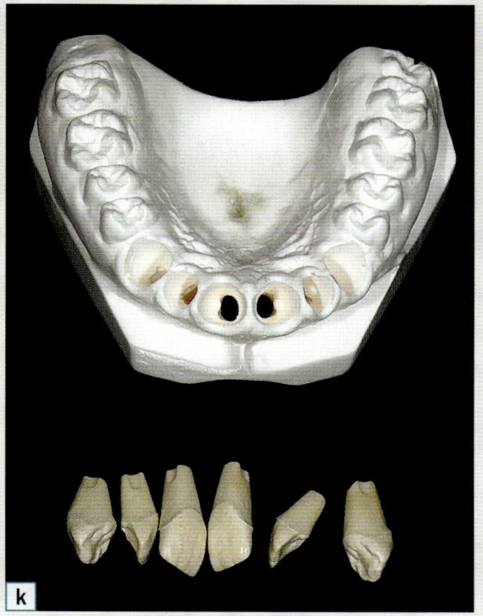

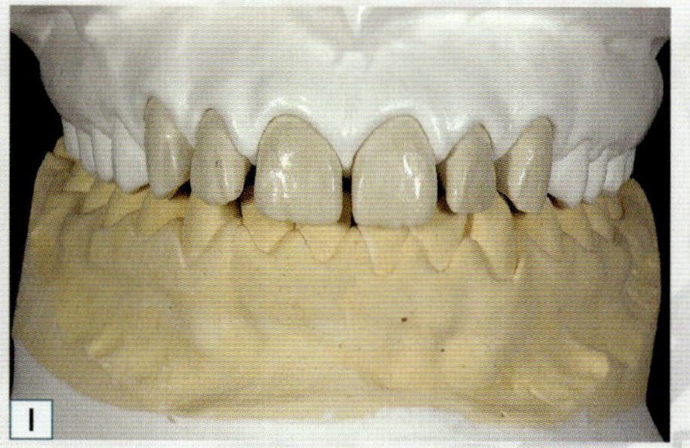

Figs 9-8k and 9-8l
Laboratory procedures when fabricating no-prep veneers of thermoplastic feldspathic ceramics.

For pouring the cast, we can use a hard gypsum Class IV or special resins designed for casts that are more durable. In this case, Class IV plaster was used, with a special resin to create the dies. The resin is harder than the plaster and guarantees a better preparation margin of the restorations. Thermoplastic feldspathic ceramics were chosen for the veneers (heat-pressed feldspathic), which can be pressed to a small thickness of 0.3 mm. An alternative material is lithium disilicate.

After waxing-up and pressing the ceramics, the light staining and finishing phases are performed. Steps such as staining or the possible application of the outer layer of ceramics are performed on the pressed restoration surface. The final phase, ie, creating macro and microstructure, and polishing is performed with great care.

Then, the restorations are ready to be tried in and cemented.

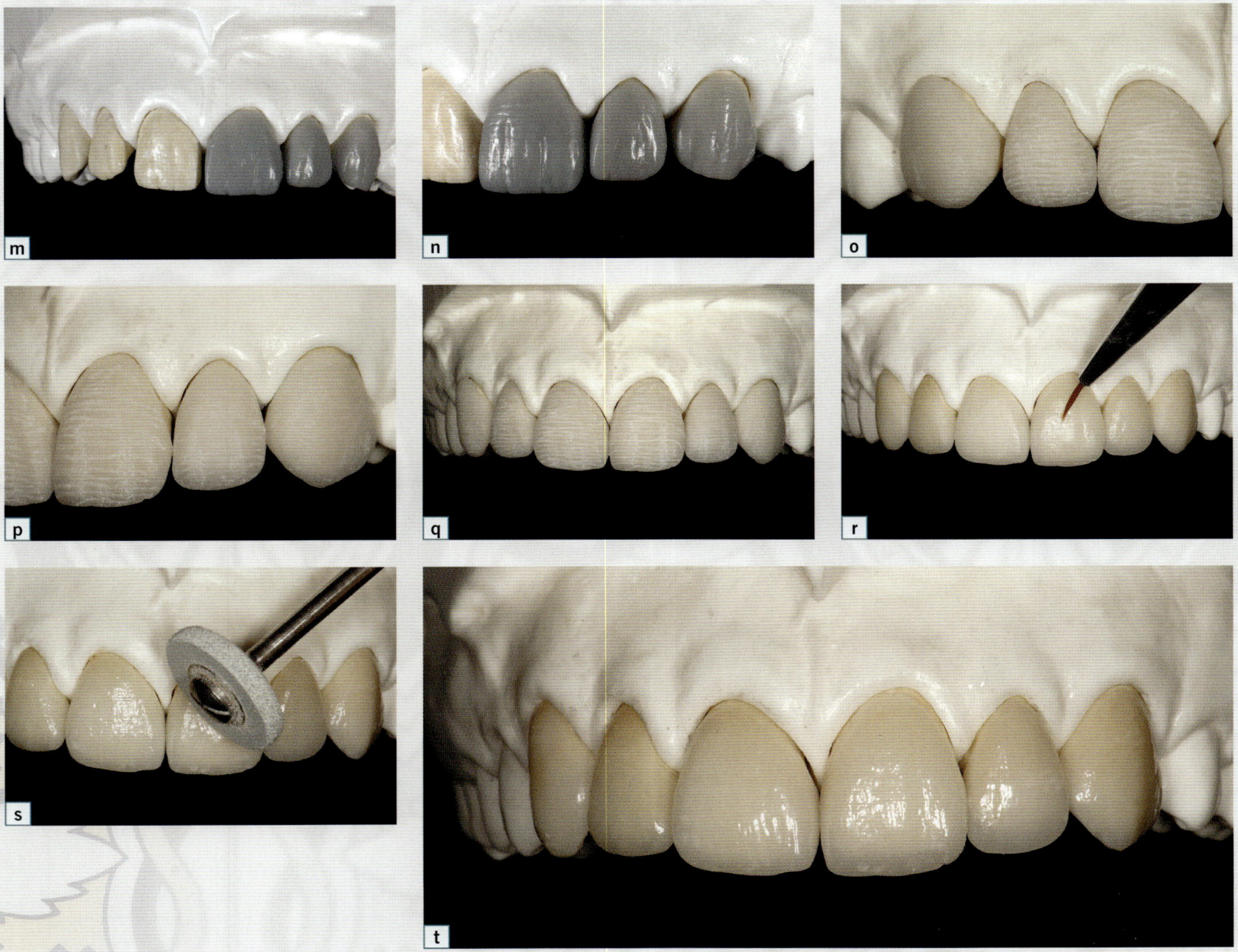

Figs 9-8m to 9-8t
Laboratory procedures for no-prep veneers fabricated of thermoplastic feldspathic ceramics (laboratory work: DT Franco Ferretti).

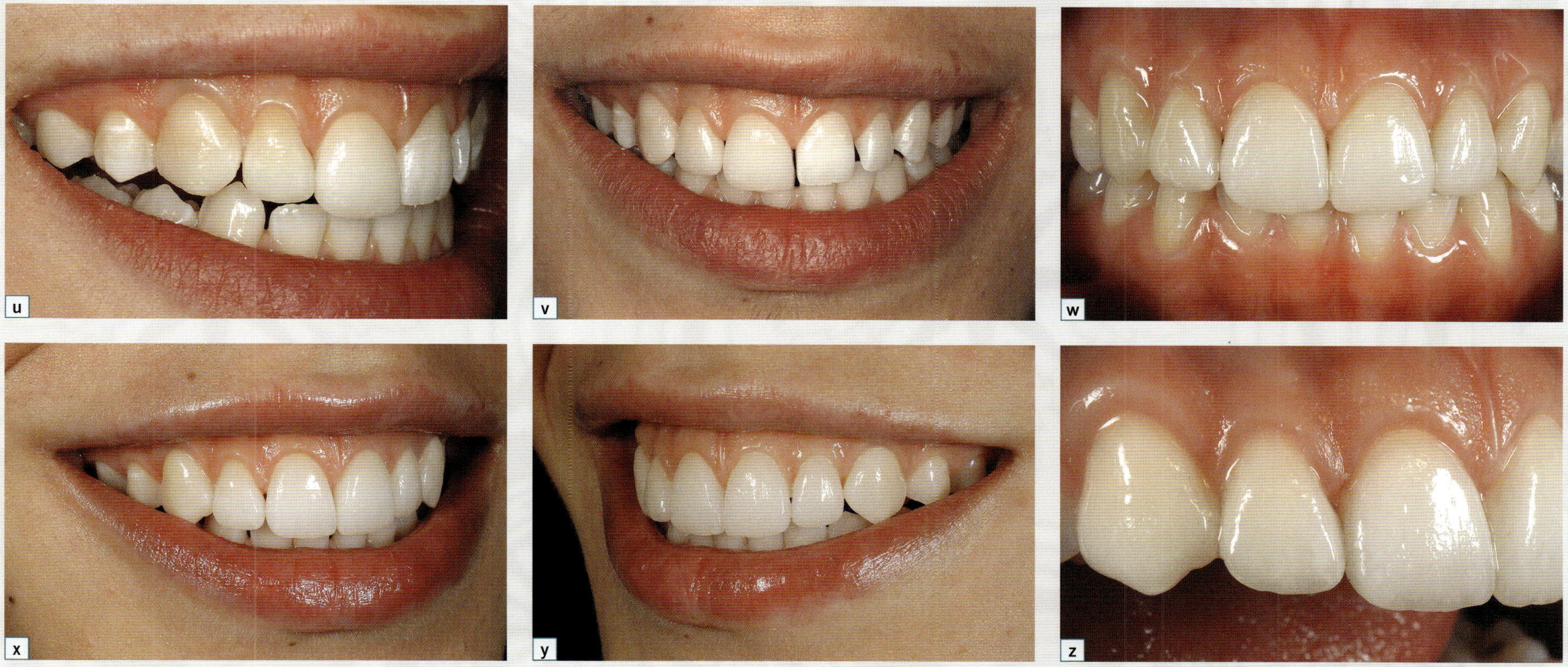

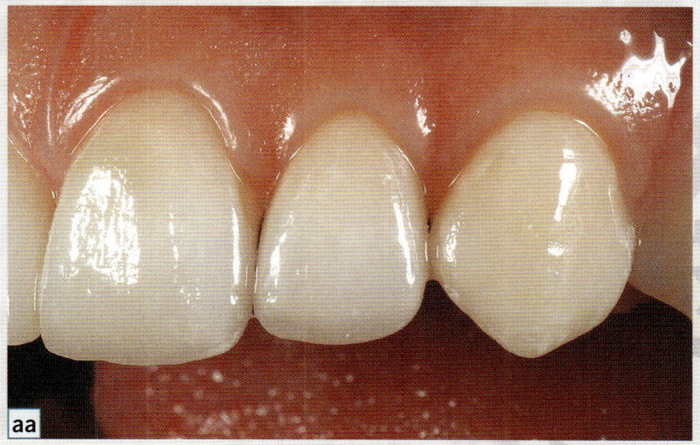

PRACTITIONER'S ADVICE

At the try-in stage, evaluate:

- Marginal integrity
- Contact points
- Color and shape
- Smile composition

Plan a suitable amount of time for this!

Figs 9-8u to 9-8aa
(u, v) Try-in and test cementation stage of no-prep veneers are carried out to assess marginal adaptation, fitting of the proximal surfaces, color, shape, and smile composition.
(w to aa) Clinical situation 7 days after veneers cementation.

Step 3: Veneer try-in and cementation (Figs 9-8u to 9-8cc)

The appointment when the veneers are to be placed is a special challenge. Before the final cementation, several test procedures must be performed. In the first phase, we try-in the veneers individually and check the marginal adaptation's quality.

In the case of an incorrect fit, we perform a test using a silicone mass that allows detection and correction of any places with increased friction on the surface of the internal restoration. Then, we initially try in all the veneers, starting with the canines, and checking the contact points' accuracy. If there is too much friction within the contact points, it will be difficult to place the veneers perfectly on the tooth surface, which can lead to fracture. This stage is extremely important, and we perform it with great thoroughness until we obtain optimal adaptation of all the restorations. Next, we need to evaluate the esthetics and the color. We need to remember that, when cementing veneers with greater thickness, the color of luting cement is not that important. Still, in situations involving very thin restorations, the color of the luting cement may significantly impact the final appearance of the restoration. When cementing thicker veneers, we usually use micro-hybrid composites, and for thin restorations, flowable light-cured composite cement, which gives us much time to adequately remove excess. Application of luting cement with such properties facilitates the correct placement of thin veneers and reduces fracture risk during the cementation phase (see Chapter 7).

Most of the composite luting cement systems available on the market veneer include try-in pastes based on water-soluble glycerin and of the same color and translucency as the final cement. It is a very important component of the system because it allows you to reliably assess the final esthetic result of the restoration.

Light curing is performed after the complete removal of excess. Personally, the author prefers not to remove flowable light-cured composite cement excess after initial polymerization because it may cause a marginal leak and lead to visible discoloration over time. Thorough removal of excess luting cement in the flowable phase provides better closure of possible micro-leaks.

In the final stage, veneers are polished with appropriate rubbers. Using milling cutters to finish the restoration's margin is inadvisable because it would be impossible to polish it perfectly. Rough surfaces will contribute to plaque colonization and inevitably lead to marginal gingival inflammation.

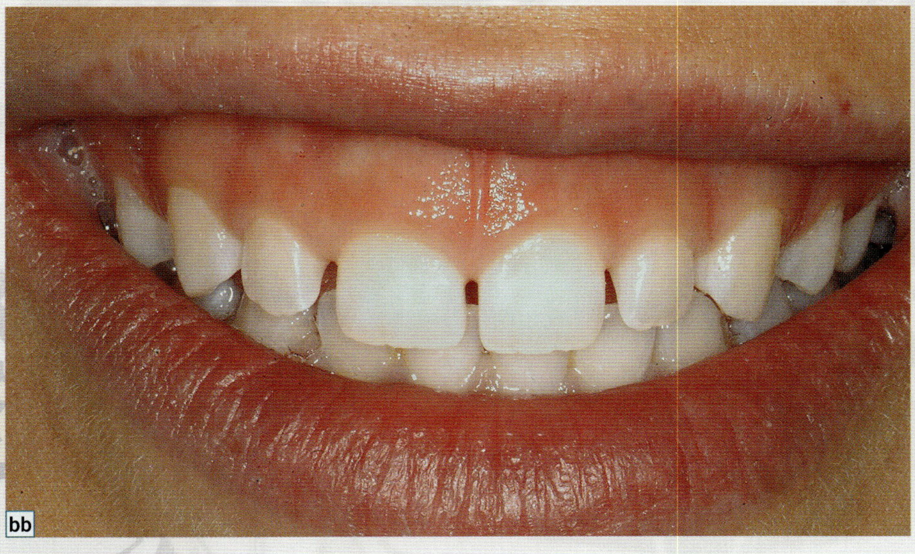

bb

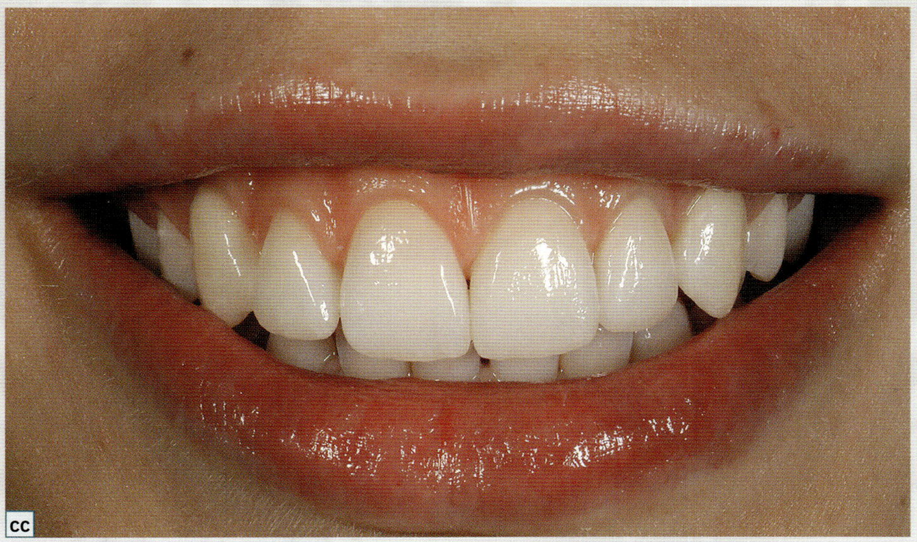

cc

Figs 9-8bb and 9-8cc

Clinical situation (bb) before treatment and (cc) after no-prep veneers cementation.

SUMMARY

After performing a certain number of clinical cases using the no-prep technique, the author came to conclusions, which differ from the opinion of many fellow dentists and of many patients:

1. The "simplicity" of performing no-prep veneers is a myth. It is more a marketing opinion used in relation to the patients for whom conservative therapy, without the need of anesthesia and tooth preparation, is very attractive.
2. The no-prep technique is not simple, and neither are the associated clinical and laboratory procedures. It also has many limitations in terms of clinical use.
3. From a clinical point of view, the most critical point in the no-prep technique is the cementation phase, if you want to do it perfectly. Handling no-prep veneers must be done extremely gently due to their small thickness, as these restorations are fabricated of fragile material, and they can be easily damaged during the try-in stage in the patient's mouth.
4. Lack of preparation margin results in making mistakes while positioning the veneers, which may obstruct the placement of other restorations. This can be prevented by using a positioning key made of resin or silicone mass, but it only solves part of the problem.
5. From the point of view of the dental laboratory, there are many difficulties. Creating such thin, anatomical, and beautiful veneers is extremely difficult, regardless of the type of ceramics used. The small amount of available space does not facilitate the work. It is a time-consuming procedure and more complex than with other traditional veneers.
6. No-prep veneers do not have many indications. Remembering about all the aforementioned limitations, we can perform them in carefully selected patients, for example, in people with dentophobia, as well as in situations of wide interdental gaps in the anterior segment, in the case of lateral incisors in the shape of icicles, or in situations of significant abrasion or erosion where it is not necessary to mask discoloration.
7. Minimal preparation of the tooth surface and creating thin veneers is conservative enough for the hard dental tissues. It provides equilibrium between perfect esthetics and minimal invasiveness. It guarantees stability and durability, as well as high predictability of successful long-term maintenance results, as confirmed by the scientific literature.[15–18]

REFERENCES

1. Magne P, Hanna J, Magne M. The case for moderate "guided prep" indirect porcelain veneers in the anterior dentition. The pendulum of porcelain veneer preparations: from almost no-prep to over-prep to no-prep. Eur J Esthet Dent 2013;8:376–388.
2. Garber DA, Goldstein RE, Feinman RA. Porcelain Laminate Veneers. Chicago, IL: Quintessence, 1998.
3. Strub JR, Türp JC. Esthetics in dental prosthetics. In: Fischer J. Esthetics and Prosthetics. Chicago, IL: Quintessence, 1999.
4. Magne P, Magne M. Use of additive wax-up and direct intraoral mock-up for enamel preservation with porcelain laminate veneers. Eur J Esthet Dent 2006;1:10–19.
5. Gürel G. Predictable, precise, and repeatable tooth preparation for porcelain laminate veneers. Pract Proced Aesthet Dent 2003;15:17–24.
6. Gürel G, Morimoto S, Calamita MA, Coachman C, Sesma N. Clinical performance of porcelain laminate veneers: outcomes of the aesthetic pre-evaluative temporary (APT) technique. Int J Periodontics Restorative Dent 2012;32:625–635.
7. Gracis S, Thompson VP, Ferencz JL, Silva NR, Bonfante EA. A new classification system for all-ceramic and ceramic-like restorative materials. Int J Prosthodont 2015;28:227–235.
8. Thomas MS, Pralhad S, Basaiwala AK. Concept of minimally invasive indirect veneers. N Y State Dent J 2017;83:32–36.
9. Sisler ZS. No-preparation veneers: a minimally invasive approach for a naturally esthetic smile. Compend Contin Educ Dent 2018;39:714–720.
10. Magne P, Versluis A, Douglas WH. Effect of luting composite shrinkage and thermal loads on the stress distribution in porcelain laminate veneers. J Prosthet Dent 1999;81:335–344.
11. Da Cunha LF, Reis R, Santana L, Romanini JC, Carvalho RM, Furuse AY. Ceramic veneers with minimum preparation. Eur J Dent 2013;7:492–496.
12. Coachman C, Gürel G, Calamita M, Morimoto S, Paolucci B, Sesma N. The influence of tooth color on preparation design for laminate veneers from a minimally invasive perspective: case report. Int J Periodontics Restorative Dent 2014;34:453–459.
13. D'Arcangelo C, Vadini M, D'Amario M, Chiavaroli Z, De Angelis F. Protocol for a new concept of no-prep ultrathin ceramic veneers. J Esthet Restor Dent 2018;30:173–179.
14. Wells D. Low-risk dentistry using additive-only ("no-prep") porcelain veneers. Compend Contin Educ Dent 2011;32:50–55.
15. Friedman MJ. A 15-year review of porcelain veneer failure: a clinician's observations. Compend Contin Educ Dent 1998;19:625–636.
16. Calamia JR, Calamia CS. Porcelain laminate veneers: reasons for 25 years of success. Dent Clin North Am 2007;51:399–417.
17. Beier US, Kapferer I, Burtscher D, Dumfahrt H. Clinical performance of porcelain laminate veneers for up to 20 years. Int J Prosthodont 2012;25:79–85.
18. Layton D, Walton T. An up to 16-year prospective study of 304 porcelain veneers. Int J Prosthodont 2007;20:389–396.

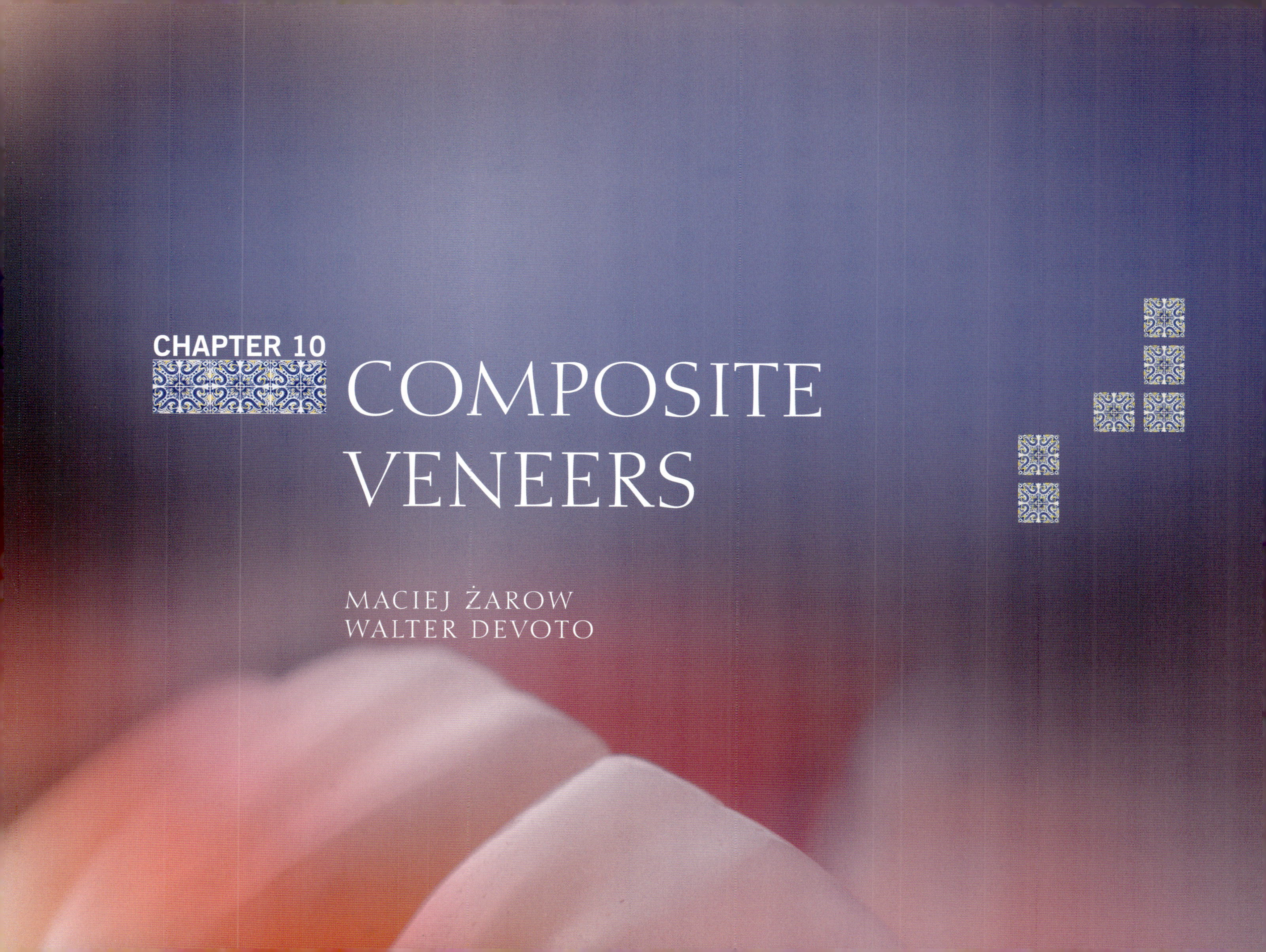

CHAPTER 10

COMPOSITE VENEERS

MACIEJ ŻAROW
WALTER DEVOTO

In the past, creating composite veneers required artistic craftsmanship from the dentist, and the final treatment result depended mostly on their manual skills. Can such veneers be performed repeatedly, and how can their risk of failure be reduced?

Composite veneers

There are many alternative methods of solving esthetic problems rather than porcelain veneers. However, composite restorations have become the most popular and developing trend in recent years. When and in what kind of clinical cases are they a good treatment indication for the patient?

COMPOSITE VENEERS: ADVANTAGES AND LIMITATIONS

ADVANTAGES

- **Minimally invasive**: Minimal or no preparation
- **Repairable:** Can be easily repaired in the event of chipped veneer/restoration
  Corrections: It is possible to make corrections after performing the restorations (unlike with cemented porcelain veneers)
- **Time:** Reduction in the number of appointments necessary to implement the esthetic treatment plan: in most cases – up to only one visit required
- **Restorations are performed in the dental office:** No need for complex collaboration with the dental laboratory[1–17]
- **Economics:** The restorations are definitely cheaper for the patient

Unlike in the case of porcelain veneers, asymmetrical restorations (the possibility of performing one veneer) are an indication for composite veneers. While working with the porcelain, it is recommended to carry out at least two symmetrical veneers simultaneously to achieve a predictable result.

LIMITATIONS

Limitations in performing composite veneers are as follows:

- **Discolorations:** Difficulty in masking the dark color in the event of discoloration
- **Comprehensive treatment:** Difficult when performing complex esthetic treatment (controlling the shape and the color of multiple anterior teeth)

Composite veneers require much attention when it comes to gingival profile and reducing the risk of composite resin excess in the cervical zone, as well as the patient's awareness about the daily oral hygiene, the use of appropriate toothpaste (with reduced abrasion), and professional repolishing.

TOOTH DISCOLORATION AFTER ROOT CANAL TREATMENT AND COMPOSITE VENEERS

Discolored teeth after root canal treatment can be properly bleached internally, thanks to which the reconstruction will be much easier and will not require external masking. It is obvious that discoloration can have a negative impact on the final esthetic result of the restoration.[18–21] Internal whitening can be performed using the walking bleach technique, successfully implemented for several decades all over the world, in accordance with the following procedures:

- **Endo assessment:** Condition assessment of the root canal treatment and the periapical tissues; retreatment should be considered in case of an underfilled root canal or periapical lesions
- **Assessment of tooth structure:** Condition assessment of the hard dental tissues, especially the quantity and quality at the cervical level. Lack of appropriate thickness in this part of the tooth and possible cracks with subgingival direction will be a contraindication for internal bleaching
- **Cleaning the tooth surface from inside the chamber:** The labial surface has to be perfectly clean to allow the whitening agent to diffuse effectively toward the labial surface of the tooth (it is recommended to use microabrasion with 27 μm aluminum oxide particles for this purpose, working with appropriate magnification under a microscope)

- **Make sure that the horns of the tooth chamber do not contain pulp residues:** Remains of the pulp often cause the discoloration to reoccur sometime after internal bleaching, so it is extremely important to clean this part of the tooth chamber
- **Creating the barrier:** Measure the height of the tooth crown from the labial surface and transfer this length (taking the incisal edge as a reference point) to the tooth chamber; create a barrier within the root canal opening 1 mm below the gingival margin (Fig 10-1a). The barrier should protect the alveolar bone and the gingival attachment from the proximal surfaces, which is why the material should be arch-shaped with more material creating the barrier approximately (Figs 10-1b and 10-1c). What is the best material for the barrier? Unfortunately, it cannot be a composite resin due to the bonding system that would block the dentinal tubules and the diffusion of the whitening agent. Glass-ionomer or traditional phosphate cement remains the best material as they are easy to shape and set rapidly. If it is necessary to use a bur or ultrasonic tip to make adjustments, these two materials are easy to correct.

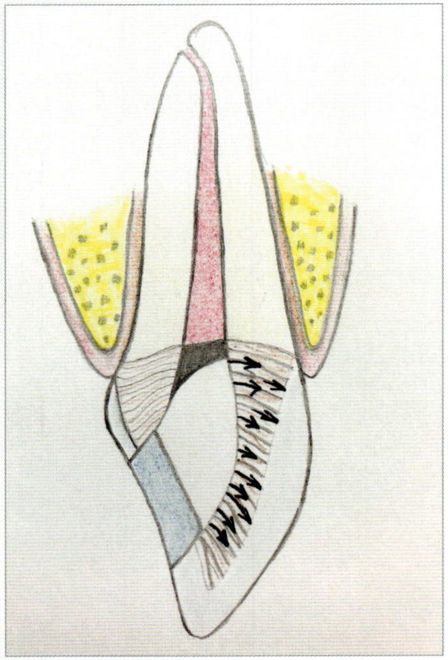

Fig 10-1a
Barrier design for internal bleaching – the sagittal section shows how the material should be positioned so as not to block the penetration of the whitening agent in the labial direction, along the dentinal tubules.

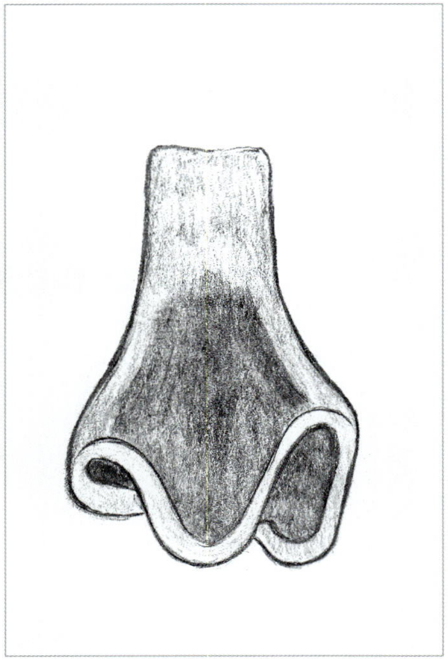

Fig 10-1b
The arch-shaped barrier protects the alveolar bone and the gingival attachment in the interdental space.

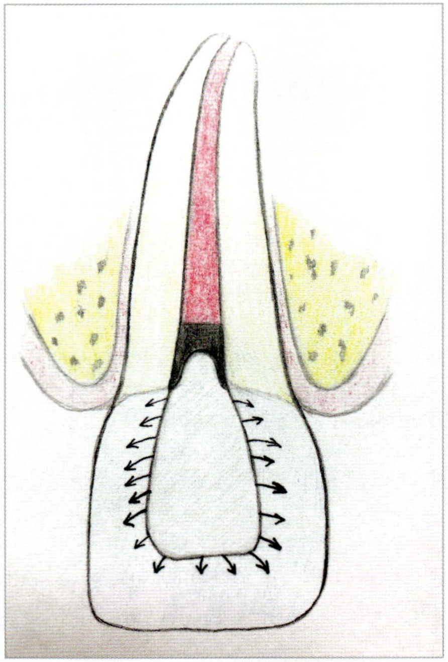

Fig 10-1c
Design of the barrier – frontal section.

> **TIP**
> Make sure that the barrier does not block the dentinal tubules on the labial surface of the tooth crown. If blocking occurs, bleaching will not be effective!

- **Application of the bleaching agent:** The material of choice (when it comes to bleaching after root canal treatment) is 10% sodium perborate mixed with distilled water or 3% hydrogen peroxide. This material can be used only outside the European Union as it is prohibited within the bloc (Annex III of the cosmetics directive 76/768/EEC).[22] In the European Union, the material of choice is 10% carbamide peroxide, which is routinely used for vital teeth whitening. The problem in this case is the proper application of the carbamide peroxide in the consistency of the gel, so it remains in contact with the labial surface and allows diffusion of the whitening agent along the dentinal tubules.
- **Closing the whitening agent in the tooth chamber:** After cleaning the whitening agent from the edges of the cavity, a small cotton ball is inserted into the chamber, leaving space for 0.5–1 mm of restorative material, such as RelyX Unicem (3M), which is a self-adhesive cement and shows good retention in such cases. The whitening agent should be left in the tooth chamber for a period of 3–7 days.

> **TIP**
>
> Always make sure that the root canal-treated tooth during the bleaching process is eased from the occlusion as a measure to prevent tooth fracture!

- **Replacing the bleaching agent:** Depending on the need, the bleaching agent can be replaced once or twice (in total, the bleaching agent can be maximally inserted into the tooth chamber up to three times). The faster the whitening is performed and the fewer consecutive visits to replace the whitening agent, the lower the risk of any possible fracture or cracking. Apart from the effect of the whitening agent itself, a possible weakening of the hard dental tissues may occur during functions such as biting or chewing since the tooth during bleaching is a kind of empty tube susceptible to fractures. Decreasing this risk by reducing the bleaching time and providing the patient with accurate information about the precautions to be taken in connection with the bleaching process are indicated
- **Application of calcium hydroxide paste for the next 14 days:** This raises the pH level that was disturbed during internal bleaching. In addition, the hard dental tissues need at least 2 weeks after whitening to be able to bond adhesively
- Tooth reconstruction with a composite resin: 14–21 days after teeth whitening[18–26]

Case 1: Discolored non-vital teeth

A female patient presented to the dental office in order to improve the esthetics of discolored teeth 11 and 12 (Figs 10-2a and 10-2b). The placement of four porcelain veneers improved the symmetry of the entire smile, along with diastema closure between the central incisors and resolution of the discoloration problem. However, the patient expected a less invasive solution and an attempt was performed to whiten discolored teeth 11 and 12 internally and obtain composite veneers without preparation.

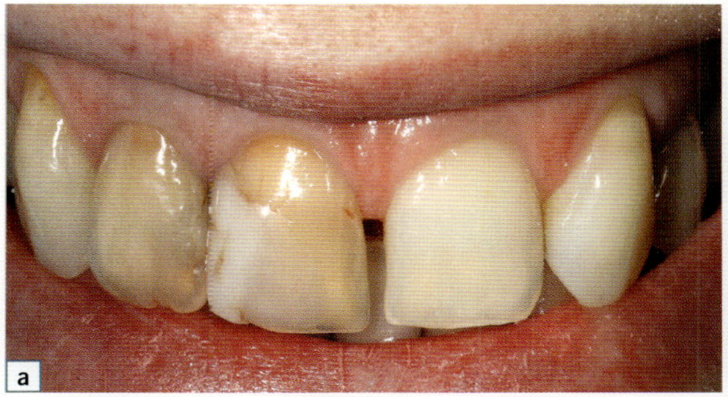

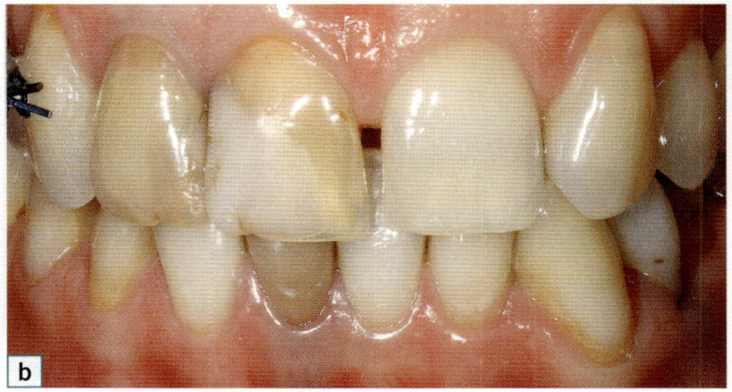

Figs 10-2a and 10-2b
Intraoral photographs of the patient who presented to the dental office in order to improve the esthetics of teeth 11 and 12.

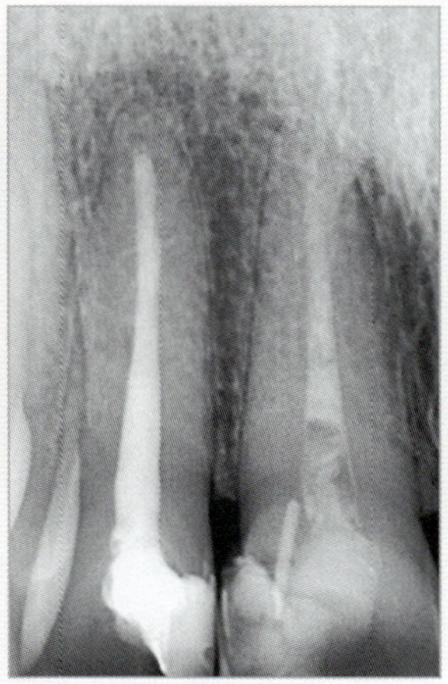

Fig 10-2c
Radiograph of teeth 11 and 12 after root canal treatment shows that the root canals are probably filled with pastes, and the filling material is not reaching the apex – so endodontic retreatment should be performed.

Step 1: Root canal retreatment

The quality of root canal fillings in teeth 11 and 12 was assessed (Fig 10-2c), and a decision was taken to perform endodontic retreatment. During the treatment, attention was paid to the remnants of the pulp horns of the tooth chamber (a common cause of discoloration) (Fig 10-2d). Retreatment was performed by filling the root canals with thermoplastic condensable gutta-percha (System B, Obtura) (Figs 10-2e and 10-2f).

Step 2: Bleaching the discolored teeth

A glass-ionomer cement barrier was created (Fig 10-2g), and a bleaching agent (Fig 10-2h) – sodium perborate mixed with 3% hydrogen peroxide (other bleaching agents must currently be used in the European Union) – was applied into the tooth chamber.

The clinical situation after the first whitening session is shown in Fig 10-2i, and after the second one in Fig 10-2j. Next, impressions were taken for the whitening splint (Fig 10-2k). At the following appointment, while keeping the barrier (Fig 10-2l) and with an open pulp chamber from the palatal surface, "inside-outside" bleaching was performed involving the simultaneous use of the bleaching agent (10% carbamide peroxide) inside and outside for 3 days (Fig 10-2m). The modified whitening splint had special openings on the adjacent teeth (Fig 10-2n) to facilitate the removal of excess bleaching agent (Fig 10-2p), so they would not be whitened accidentally. The final result after whitening is shown in Fig 10-2o.

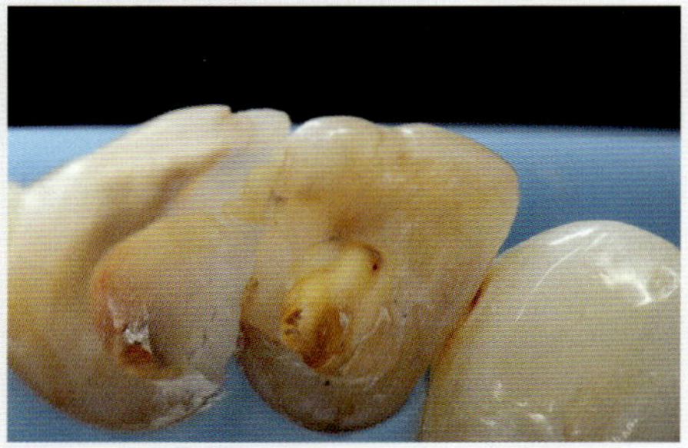

Fig 10-2d
In tooth 12, visible pulp remnants are located in the horn of the tooth chamber.

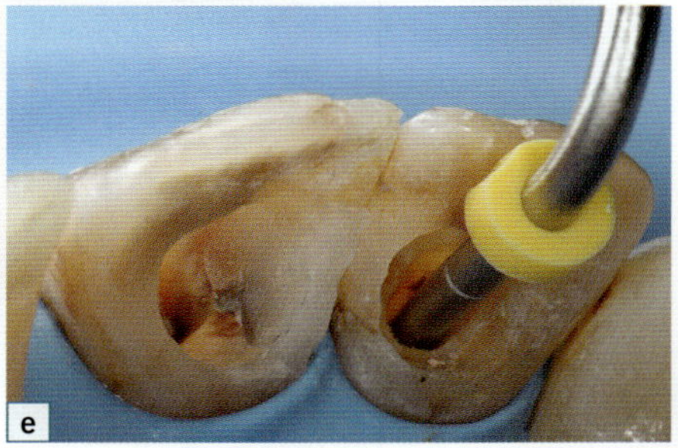

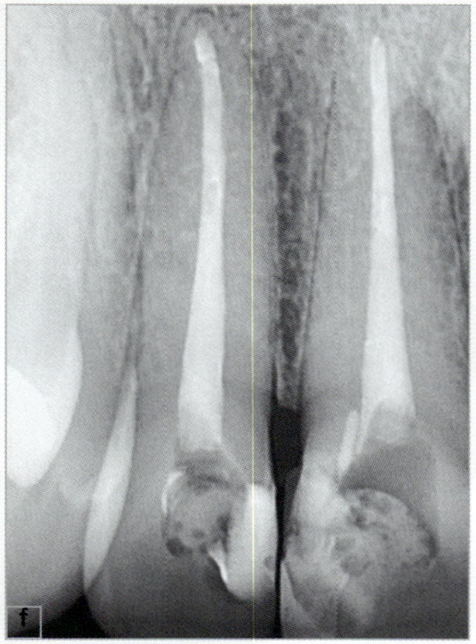

Figs 10-2e and 10-f
(e) Retreatment: filling the root canals with thermoplastic condensable gutta-percha (System B). (f) Radiograph of teeth 11 and 12 taken after endodontic retreatment.

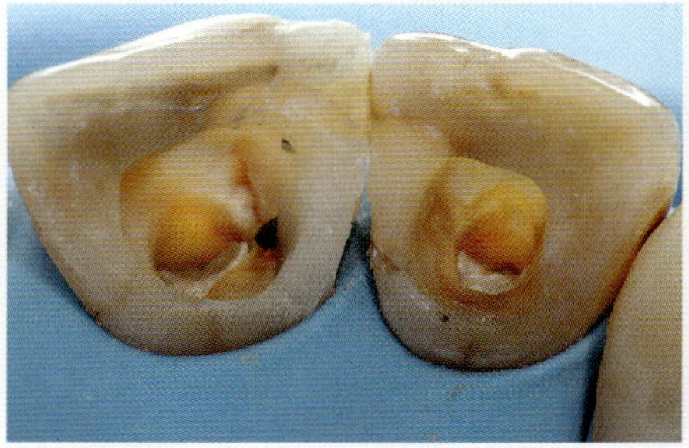

Fig 10-2g
Clinical situation after applying the barrier in teeth 11 and 12.

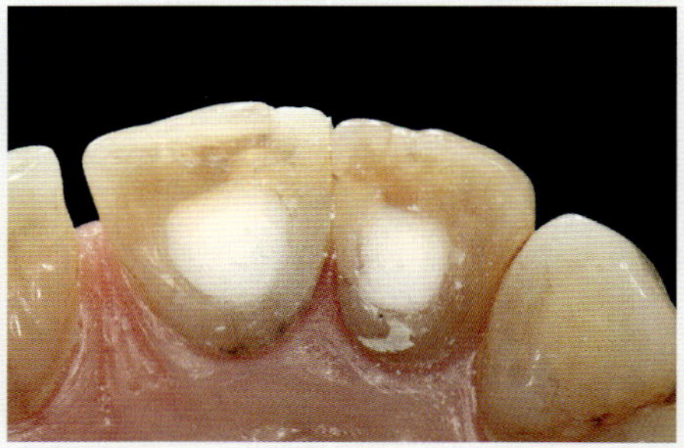

Fig 10-2h
Bleaching agent applied in the chamber of teeth 11 and 12.

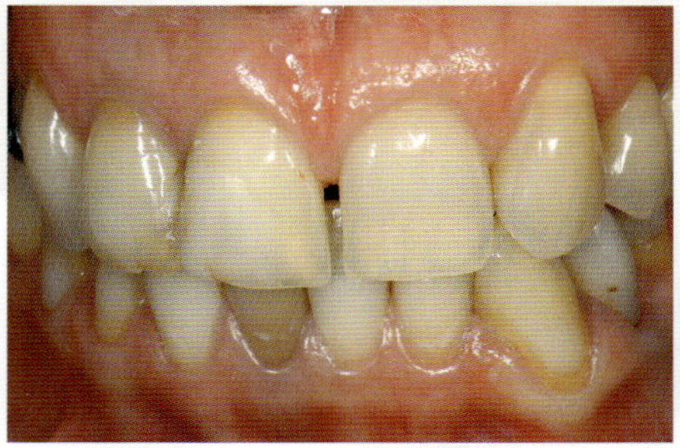

Fig 10-2i
Clinical situation after the first bleaching session – visibly brightening teeth, compared to the initial situation.

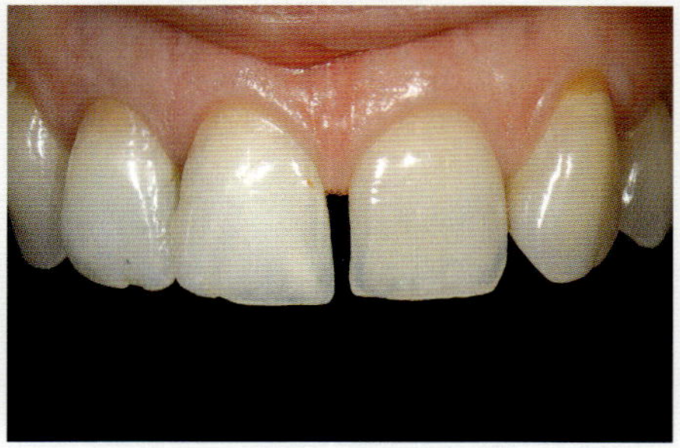

Fig 10-2j
Clinical situation after second bleaching session – evident brightening of teeth 11 and 12 compared to the initial situation.

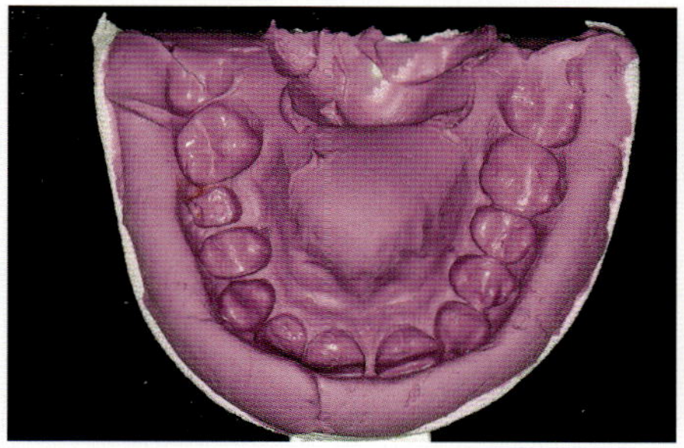

Fig 10-2k
Alginate impression was taken to create a splint and carry out the "inside-outside" bleaching technique.

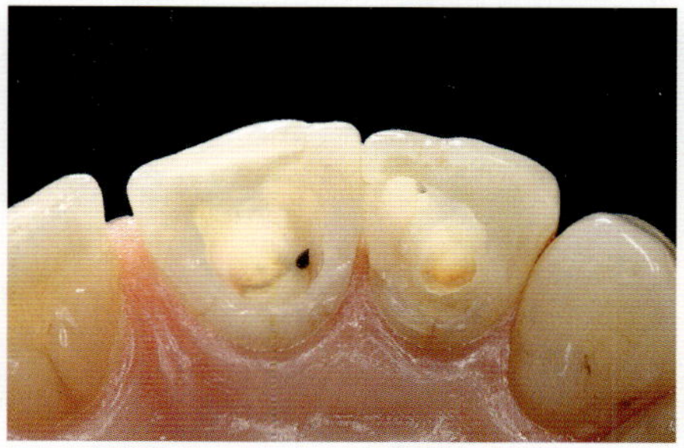

Fig 10-2l
The barrier was sealed to ensure perfect tightness of the root canals.

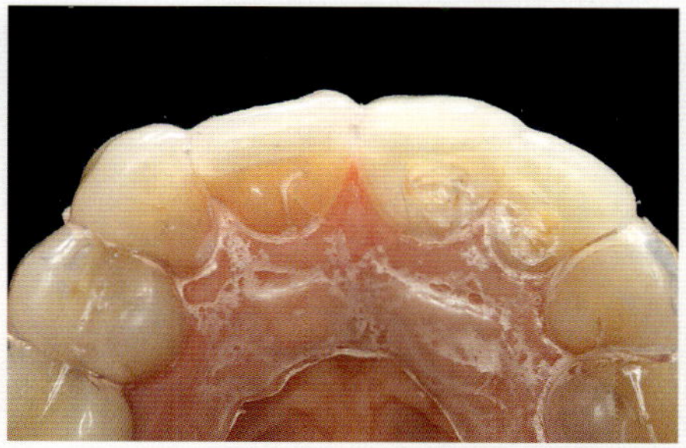

Fig 10-2m
The patient was informed how to apply the bleaching gel (10% carbamide peroxide) into the tooth chamber …

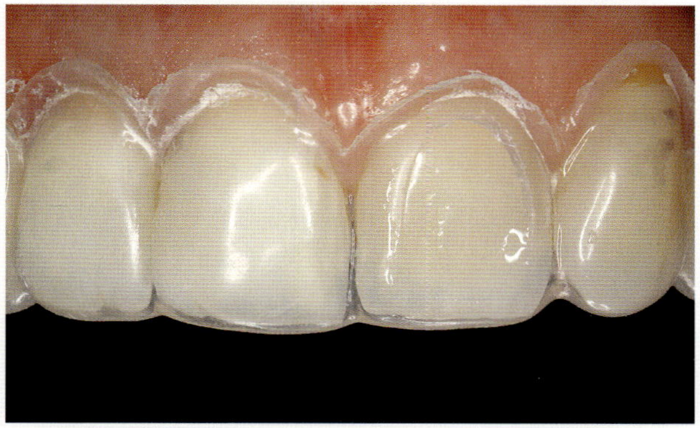

Fig 10-2n
… and externally into the whitening splint. Whitening was recommended for the next 3 days with the recommendation of great caution when consuming foods.

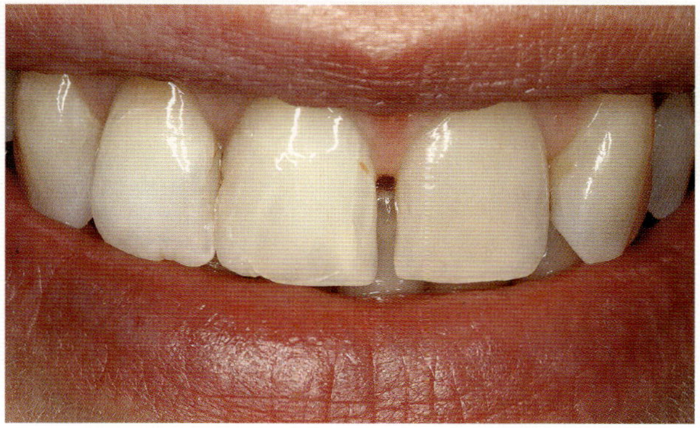

Fig 10-2o
Clinical situation after completing bleaching of the teeth with root canal treatment.

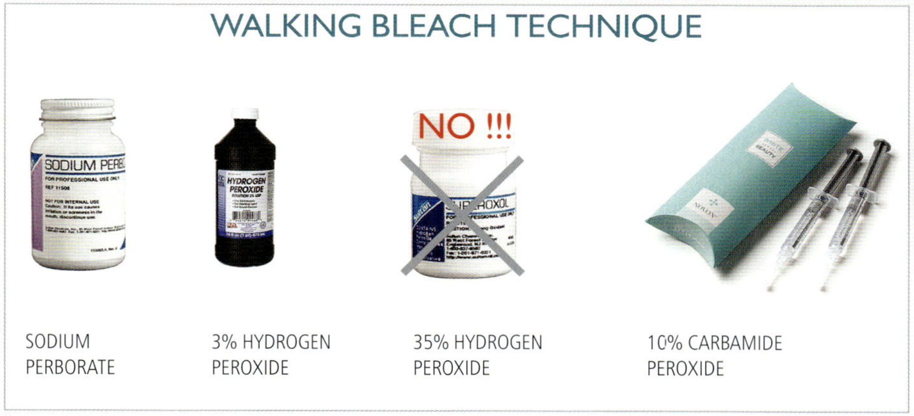

Fig 10-2p
Agents used in the walking bleach technique: (from left) sodium perborate, which should be mixed with 3% hydrogen peroxide or with distilled water; 35% hydrogen peroxide is not recommended in any situation (due to risk of external cervical resorption); 10% carbamide peroxide, which at the moment remains as the material of choice in European Union under the new regulations.

Step 3: Removal of the old composite restorations and obtaining new restorations

Two weeks after the whitening procedure was completed (for this period, calcium hydroxide was placed into the tooth chamber), the restorative phase could be completed. The teeth were isolated with a rubber dam, and the old composite resin restorations were removed (the rubber dam certainly made this easier) with diamond burs, microabrasion, and a scalpel (Figs 10-2q to 10-2t). The clinical situation immediately before the final restorative phase is presented in Figs 10-2u and 10-2v. After thorough air abrasion and etching with orthophosphoric acid (Fig 10-2w), the bonding system was applied. The inside of the tooth chamber was filled with a very bright opaque flowable composite (Essentia ML, GC) (Fig 10-2x) and a layer of a bright dentin composite (UD1 Micerium) (Fig 10-2y).

Using an enamel layer of composite resin (BF2, Micerium) and the silicone index, the palatal wall was formed (Fig 10-2z) and then, with the matrix bands for premolars (Quickmat Sectional Matrix, Polydentia) placed perpendicularly, the proximal surfaces were created (Fig 10-2aa). In tooth 11, a Class 4 cavity was restored with dentin composite (UD3, Micerium). After that, a veneer matrix was fixed (Unica Anterior, Polydentia) (Figs 10-2bb and 10-2cc), and the inverted U-shaped "frame" was carried out with a flowable composite (G-aenial Universal Flo, GC), and final enamel layer (BF2, Micerium) was applied inside the "frame" (Fig 10-2dd). The shaping of the veneer was performed with the Profin contra-angle handpiece (Figs 10-2ee and 10-2ff) and a diamond bur no. 832-204-012 (Komet Brasseler) in order to achieve symmetry with the adjacent central incisor (Figs 10-2gg and 10-2hh).

When the shape was similar to the symmetrically located tooth, characterization was performed. Vertical lines were drawn with a pencil, corresponding to the vertical grooves of the adjacent tooth, and recreated on the composite veneer using a bur no. 832-204-012 (Figs 10-2ii and 10-2jj). Then, the horizontal lines were drawn and appropriate characterization was performed with the same bur (Figs 10-2kk and 10-2ll). The final result is shown in Fig 10-2mm. Photographs taken on a follow-up visit show the natural integration of composite resin restorations into the patient's smile and the surrounding hard and soft tissues (Figs 10-2nn to 10-2pp). In the meantime, in order to further improve the esthetics, the diastema was reduced through a composite microrestoration of tooth 21 and internal bleaching of discolored tooth 42.

In conclusion, it is worth emphasizing that the bleaching effect can be extremely beneficial, facilitating the composite as a restorative material. This, in turn, allows simpler and faster implementation of an esthetic restoration, which can also be less invasive.

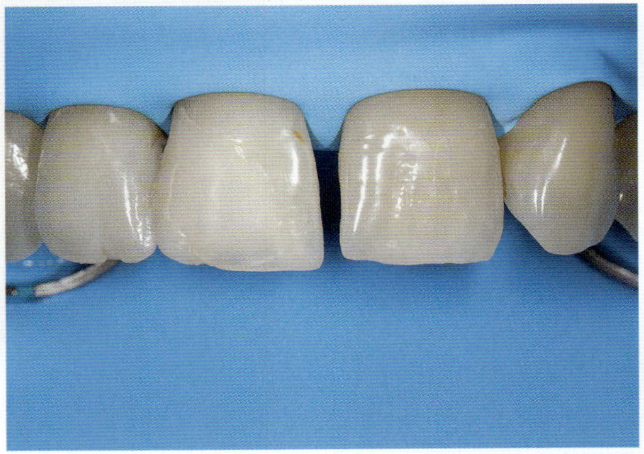

Fig 10-2q
Rubber dam isolation was placed to better recognize the old restoration margin while removing the fillings.

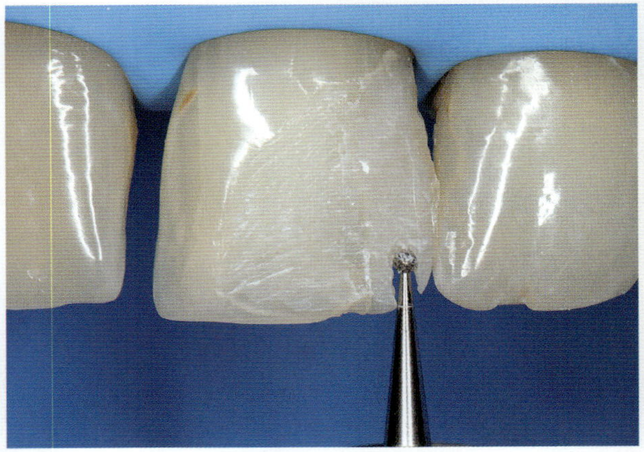

Fig 10-2r
Removal of the old restorations with a small ball-shaped diamond bur with increasing speed red band 1:5 contra-angle handpiece.

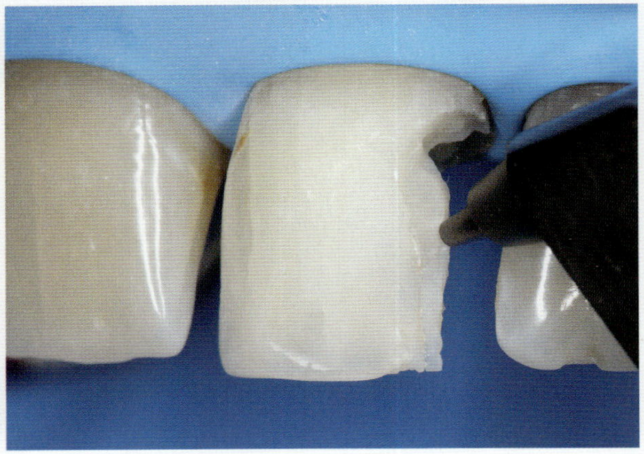

Fig 10-2s
Microabrasion with 27 μm particles of aluminum oxide.

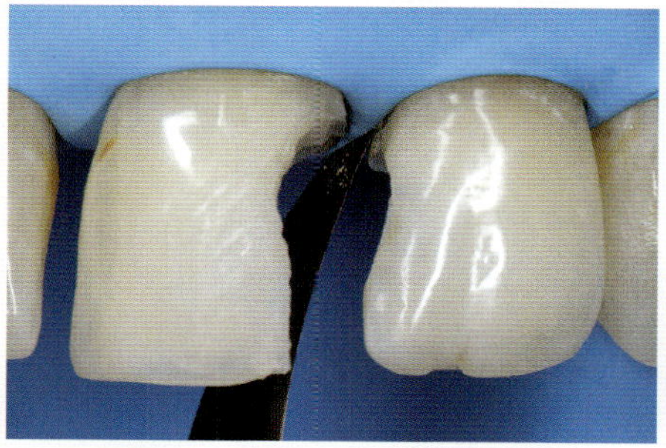

Fig 10-2t
Removal of the remaining subgingival excess material by a scalpel no. 12.

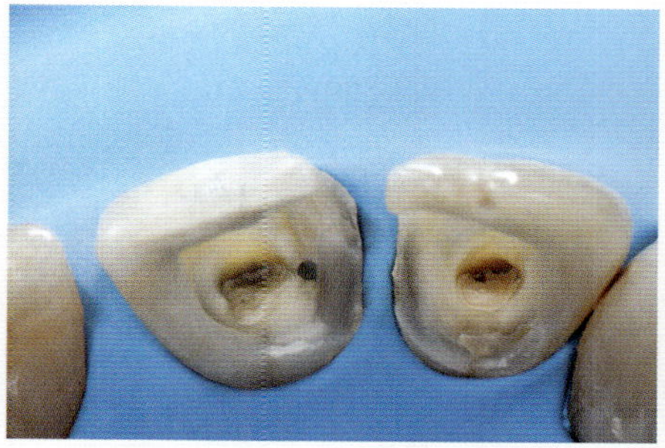

Fig 10-2u
Clinical situation after removing the majority of the old composite resin.

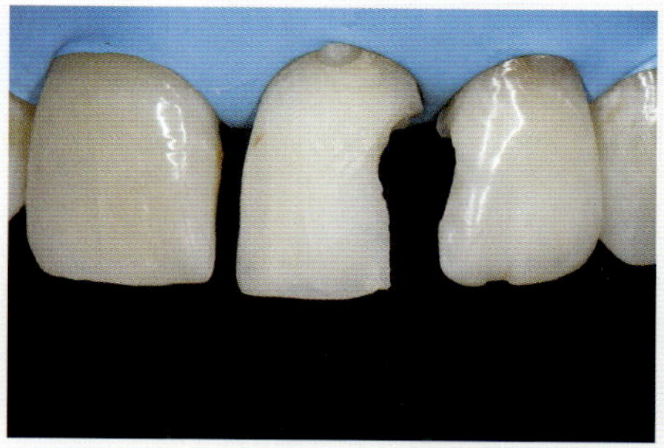

Fig 10-2v
A visible chamfer in tooth 11 – the clinical situation after air abrasion of the labial surface.

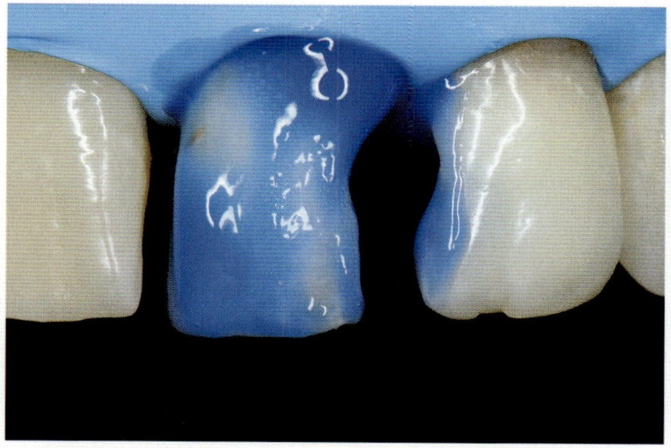

Fig 10-2w
Etching the labial surface of the teeth with orthophosphoric acid.

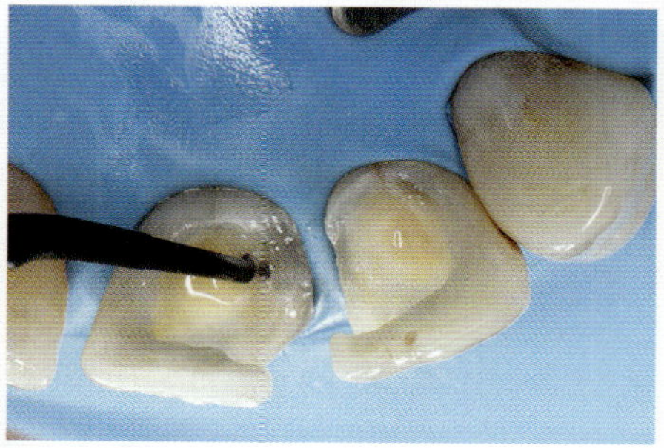

Fig 10-2x
Filling cervical part of the tooth chamber with very bright opaque flowable composite resin.

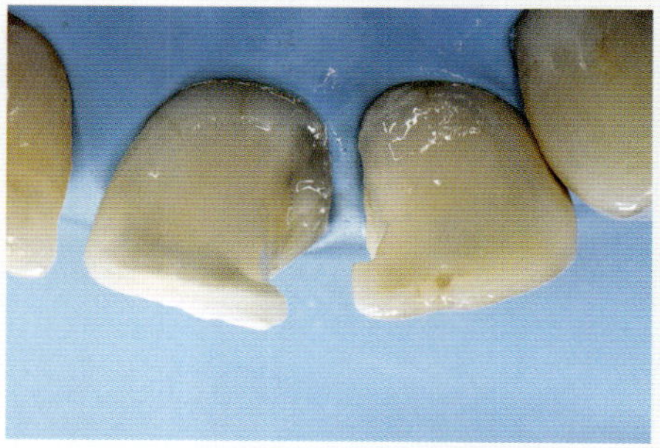

Fig 10-2y
Placing a very bright dentin layer.

PRACTITIONER'S ADVICE

Application of a very bright composite resin in the pulp chamber is important for the future esthetics of the root-filled tooth!

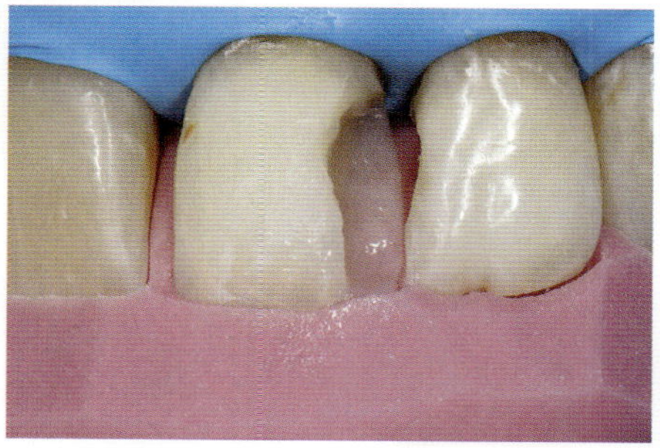

Fig 10-2z
Reconstruction of the palatal surface with enamel composite and silicone index.

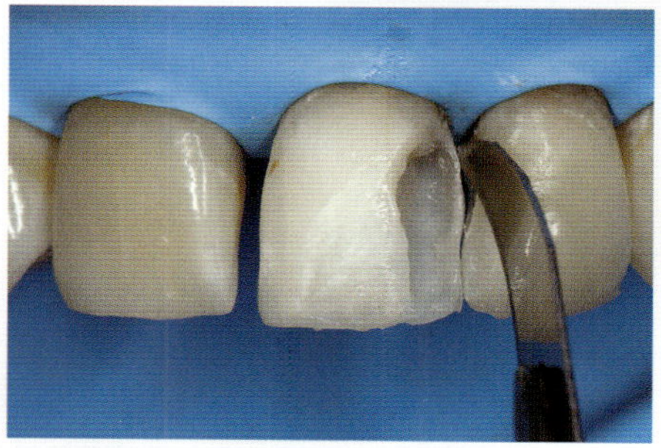

Fig 10-2aa
Clinical situation after reconstructing the proximal surface with the enamel composite.

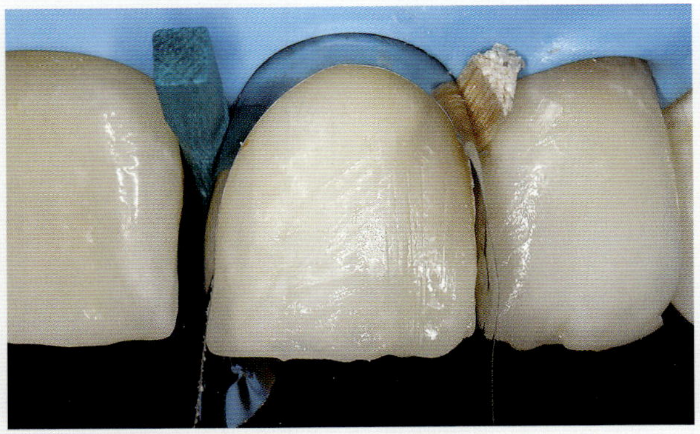

Fig 10-2bb
Unica Anterior Matrix (Polydentia) was adapted with wooden wedges ...

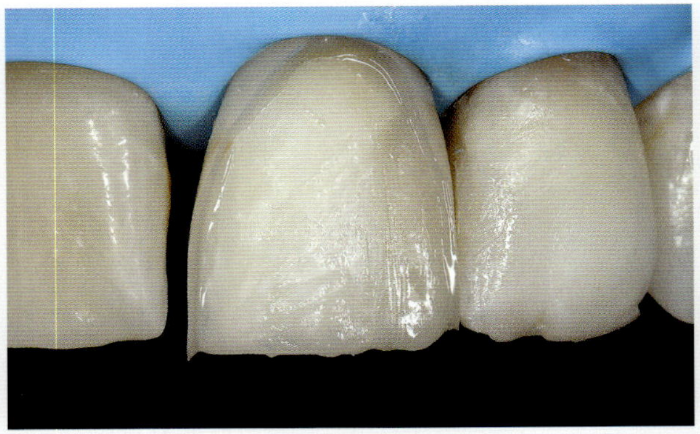

Fig 10-2cc
... and, after applying a flowable composite (G-aenial Universal Flo, GC), it was polymerized, and the matrix band was removed. This is how the "frame" was created to facilitate the application of the final layers.

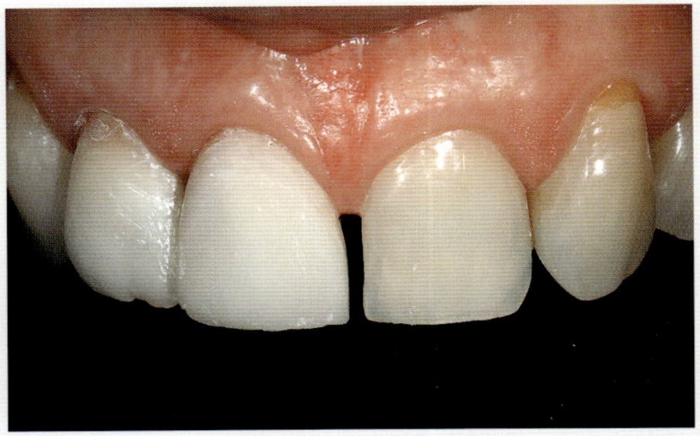

Fig 10-2dd
Situation after applying the external enamel layer on tooth 11 and after restoring tooth 12.

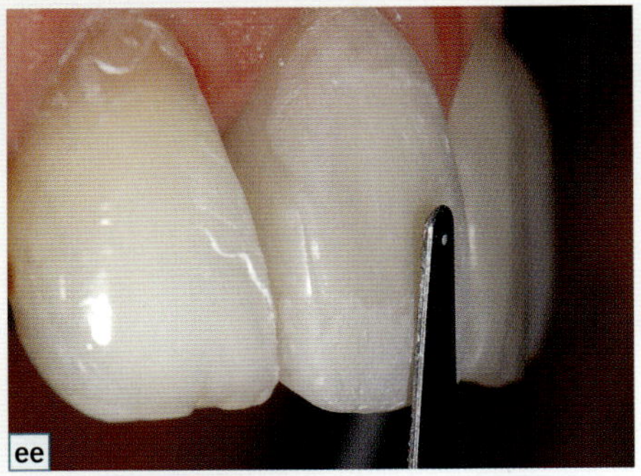

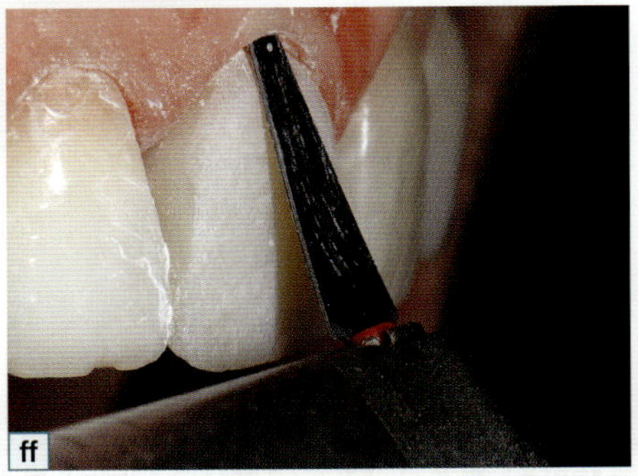

Figs 10-2ee and 10-ff
The veneers were shaped appropriately with a Profin contra-angle handpiece.

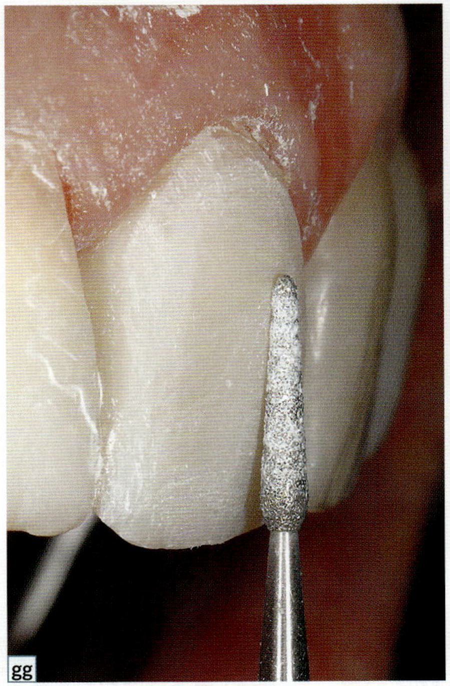

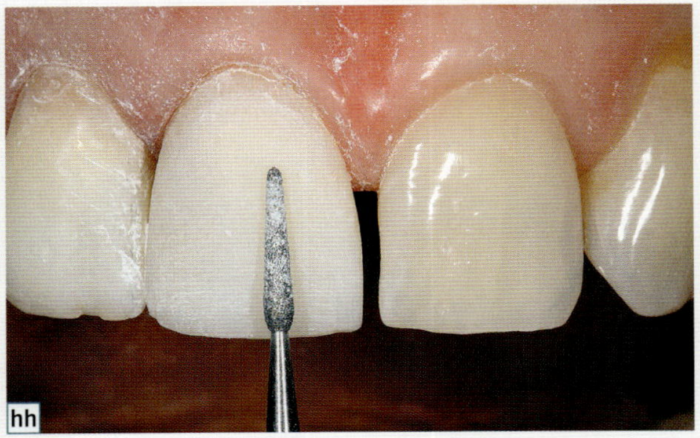

Figs 10-2gg and 10-2hh
The shape was performed with a diamond bur no. 832-204-012 (Komet Brasseler).

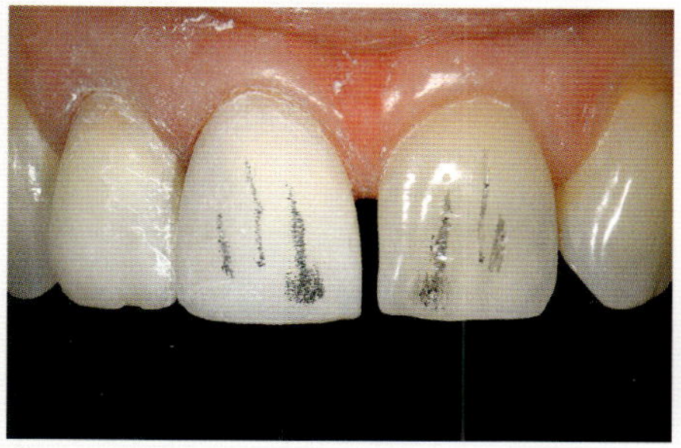

Fig 10-2ii
In order to perform an appropriate characterization, vertical lines were drawn with a pencil, corresponding to vertical grooves …

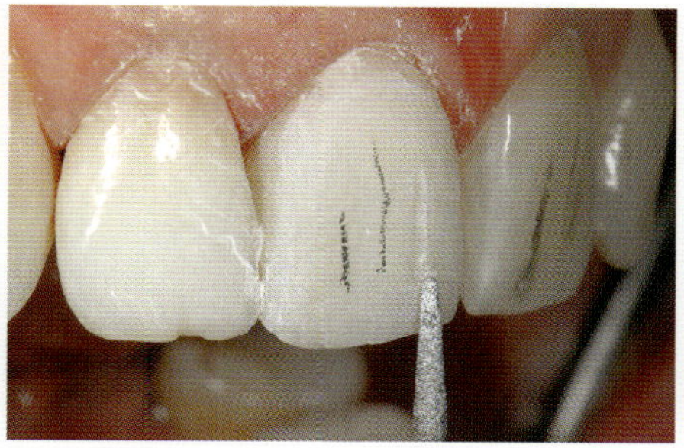

Fig 10-2jj
… next, the characterization of the vertical grooves of the adjacent central incisor was transferred on the veneer.

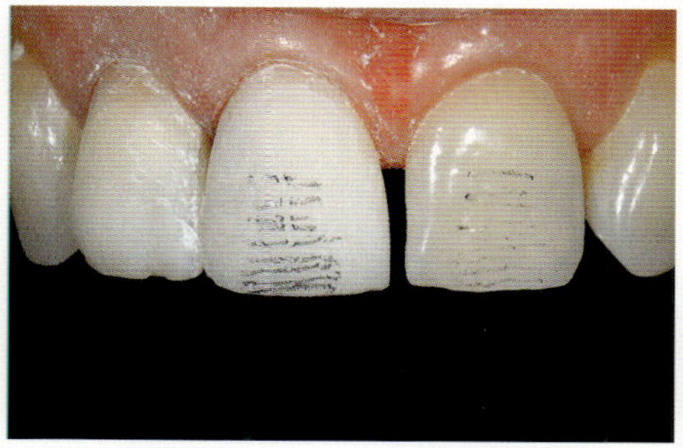

Fig 10-2kk
Then, with a pencil, the horizontal characterizations were drawn corresponding to the adjacent central incisor …

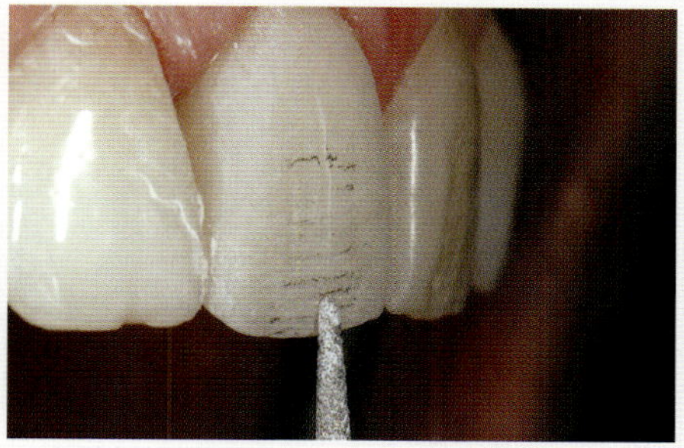

Fig 10-2ll
… and adequately delicate horizontal grooves were performed with a diamond bur no. 832-204-012 (Komet Brasseler).

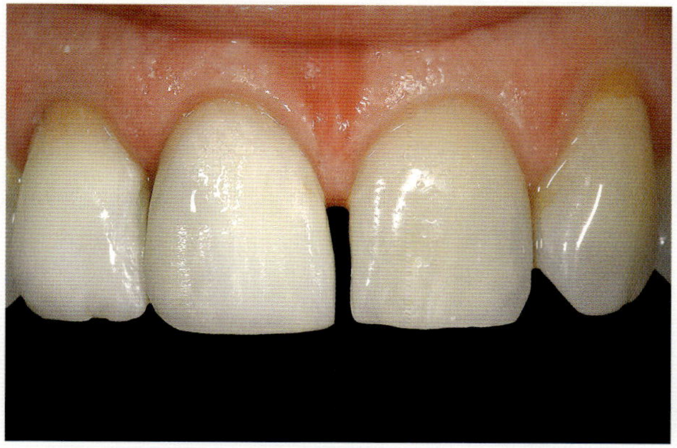

Fig 10-2mm
The final result of reconstructing teeth 11 and 12 after internal bleaching and endodontic retreatment.

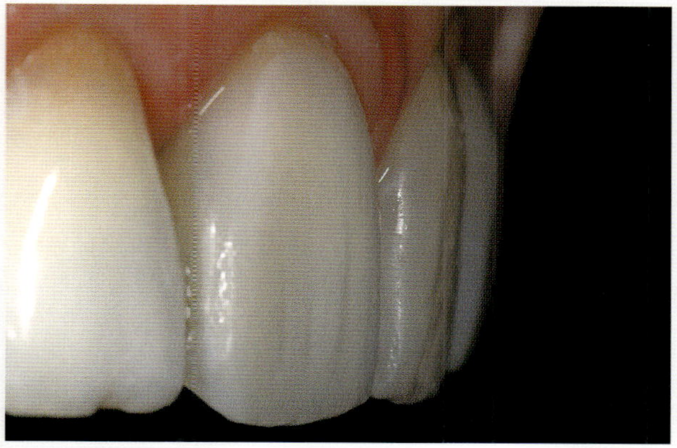

Fig 10-2nn
Intraoral photograph of composite restorations 11 and 12 taken from a semi-profile.

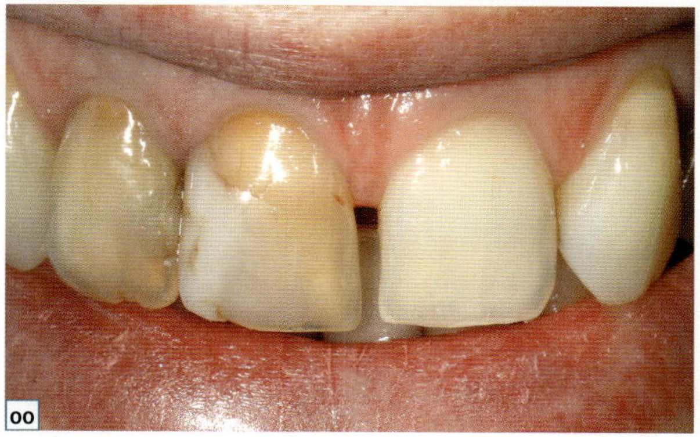

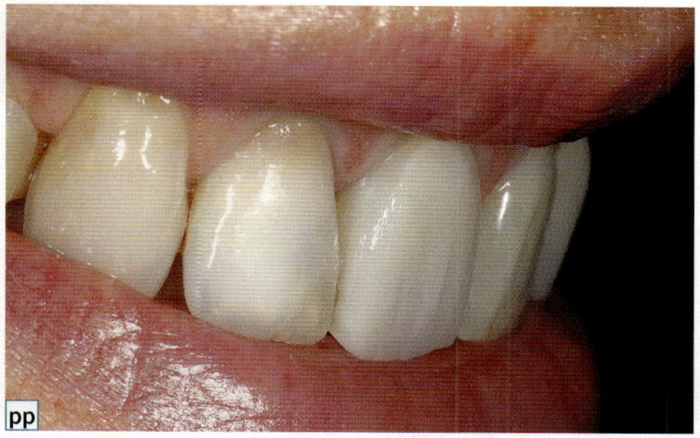

Figs 10-2oo and 10-pp
(oo) Intraoral photograph before starting the treatment and (pp) the patient's smile from semi-profile view (restored teeth after internal bleaching and endodontic retreatment).

Case 2: Discolored non-vital teeth

A female patient presented to the dental office to improve the shape and the color of tooth 21 (Figs 10-3a to 10-3c). She expected that the tooth's esthetics would be improved with an all-ceramic crown. A radiograph was taken, revealing that discolored tooth 21 had undergone root canal treatment. A less invasive procedure was planned in the form of internal bleaching and, in the case of a positive result of bleaching, a direct composite restoration was planned.

Step 1: Root canal retreatment

Endodontic retreatment was carried out due to the old root canal endodontic paste (Figs 10-3d and 10-3e), which was not favorable to maintain the bleached color of the tooth in the future (one of the reasons for recurrence of the discoloration are the old endodontic pastes containing dyes).

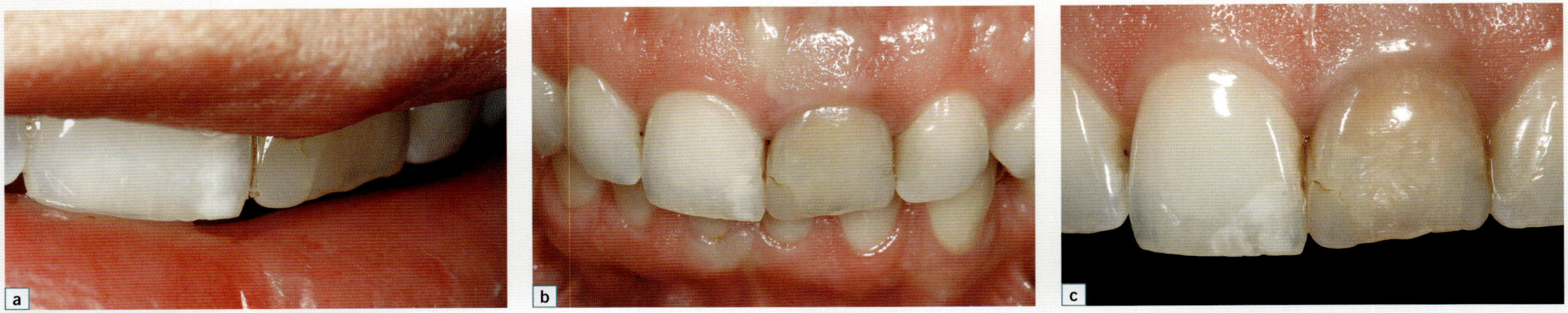

Figs 10-3a to 10-3c
Extraoral and intraoral photographs of the patient who presented to the dental office to improve the esthetics of discolored tooth 21.

Fig 10-3d
Radiograph of the discolored tooth. The root canal is filled properly, but the filling material is a paste, which may pose a risk of discoloration reoccurrence after bleaching.

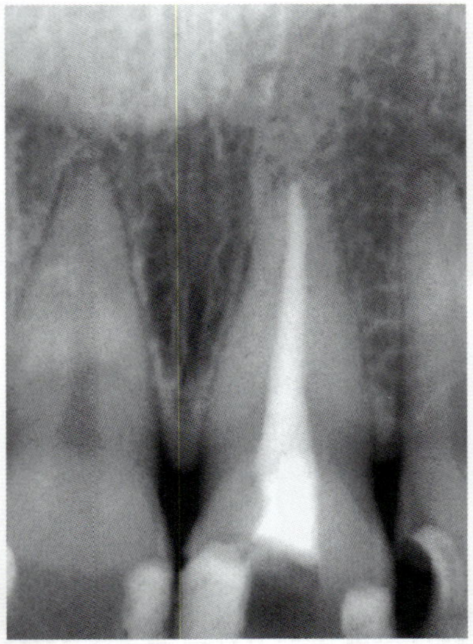

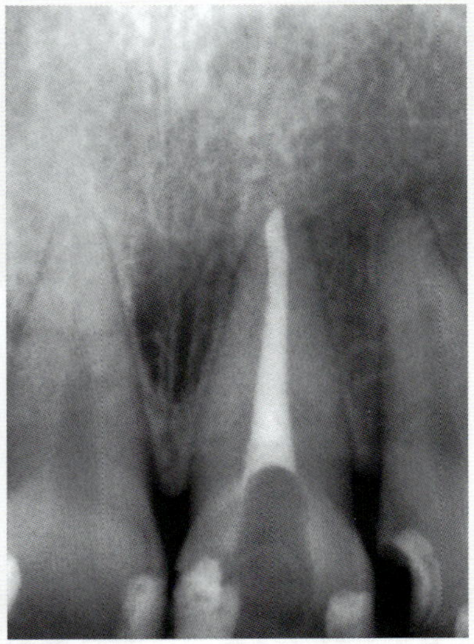

Fig 10-3e
Radiograph of tooth 21 after root canal retreatment. Root canal filled with thermoplastic gutta-percha.

Step 2: Bleaching the discolored tooth

In the next stage, internal bleaching was performed under the procedures described in Case 1, making a barrier (Fig 10-3f), and applying the sodium perborate in three following appointments into the pulp chamber (Fig10-3g). A direct composite resin veneer could be planned since the bleaching gave a positive result (Fig 10-3h). If the whitening procedure had been unsuccessful, the patient should have been offered two indirect veneers on the maxillary central incisors.

Step 3: Replacing the old fillings and a fiberglass post cementation

Two weeks after the bleaching, restorative treatment was carried out. A provisional restoration was performed to simulate the tooth's final shape, and a silicone index was taken (Fig 10-3i). The teeth were isolated with a rubber dam, all old restorations were removed (Fig 10-3j), and a white fiberglass post was cemented (Ena Post, Micerium) (Figs 10-3k to 10-3o). The reason to cement a fiberglass post was the unstable occlusion in the posterior segment (risk of future anterior overloading) and to enhance the fluorescence effect of the final composite restoration.[23]

PRACTITIONER'S ADVICE

If you have any structural or functional doubts about the anterior root treated tooth and internal bleaching, then cement a fiberglass post.[23]

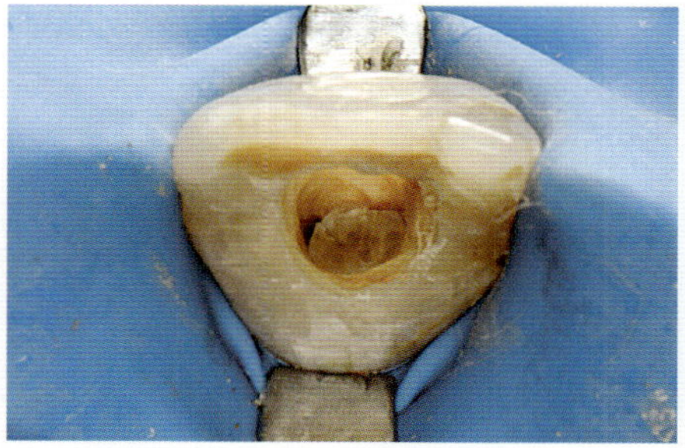

Fig 10-3f
A barrier was obtained in the root canal opening before starting the internal bleaching of tooth 21.

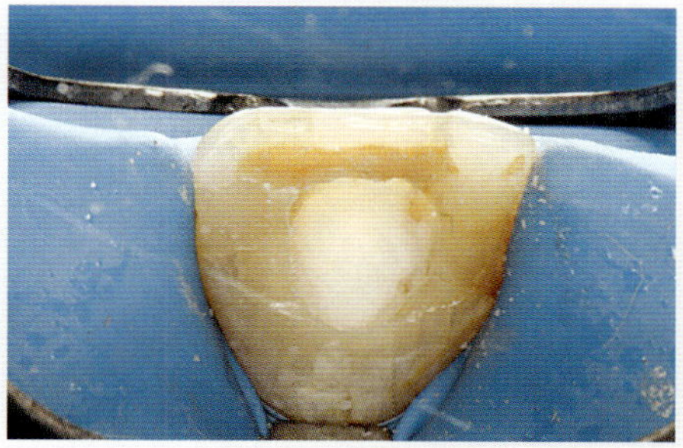

Fig 10-3g
After applying the bleaching agent (sodium perborate mixed with 3% hydrogen peroxide) into the pulp chamber – palatal view.

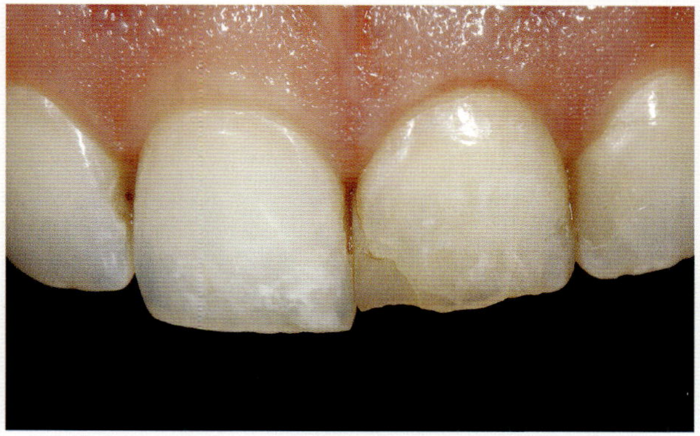

Fig 10-3h
Clinical situation after completing the bleaching (three sessions).

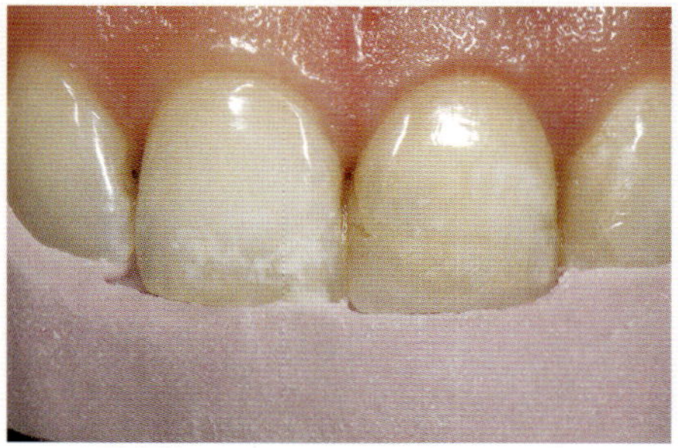

Fig 10-3i
A provisional composite restoration was performed in order to take a silicone index for further tooth reconstruction.

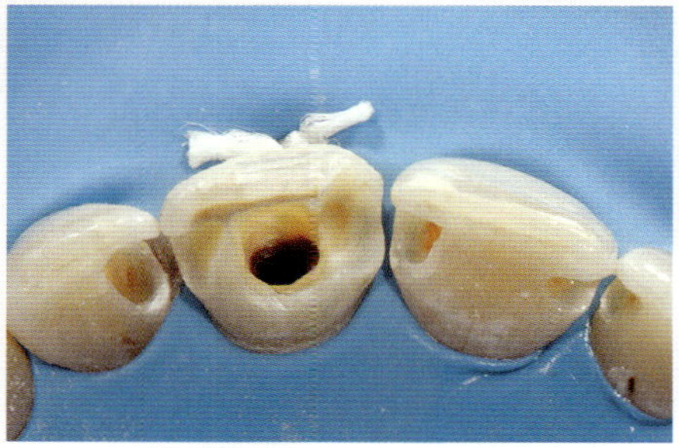

Fig 10-3j
Two weeks after completing the bleaching, the restorative phase was started. The teeth were isolated with a rubber dam, and the old restorations were removed.

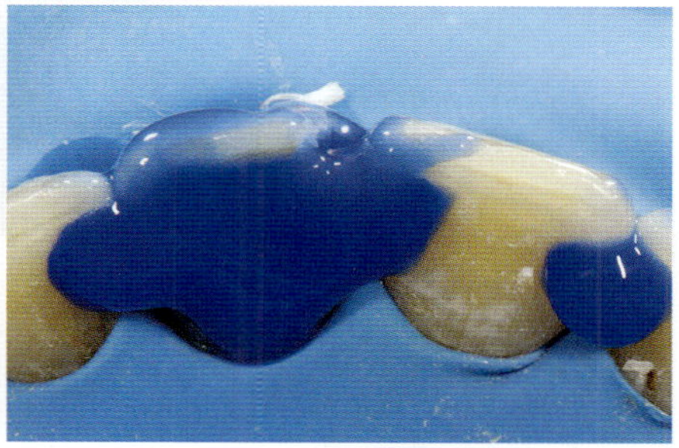

Fig 10-3k
The appropriate space for the fiberglass post was prepared, with the root canal dentin being airborne-particle abraded with aluminum oxide 27 μm, and etched with orthophosphoric acid.

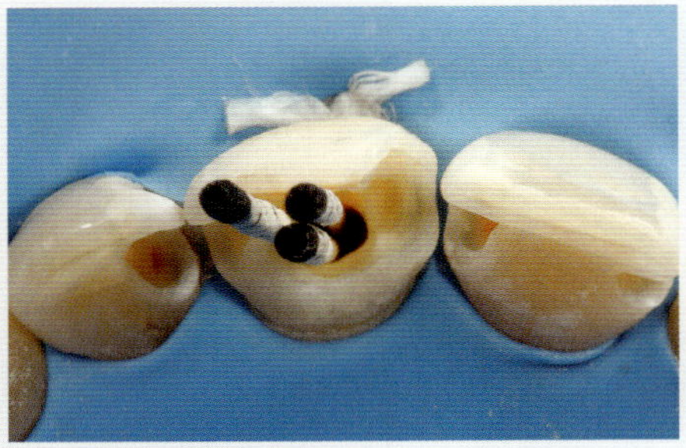

Fig 10-3l
… after rinsing thoroughly, the root canal was dried with paper points …

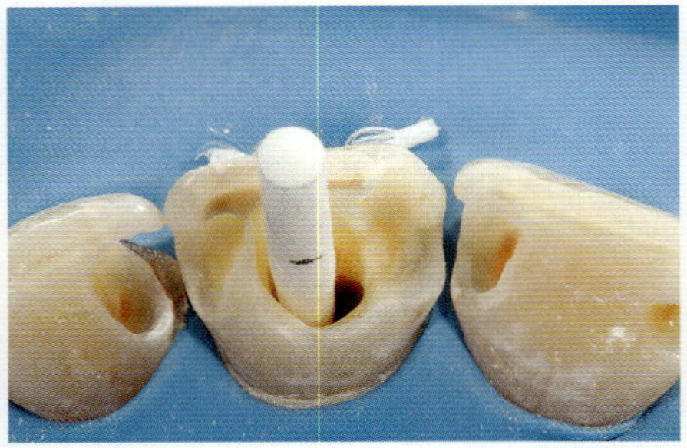

Fig 10-3m
… the appropriate size of fiberglass post was selected …

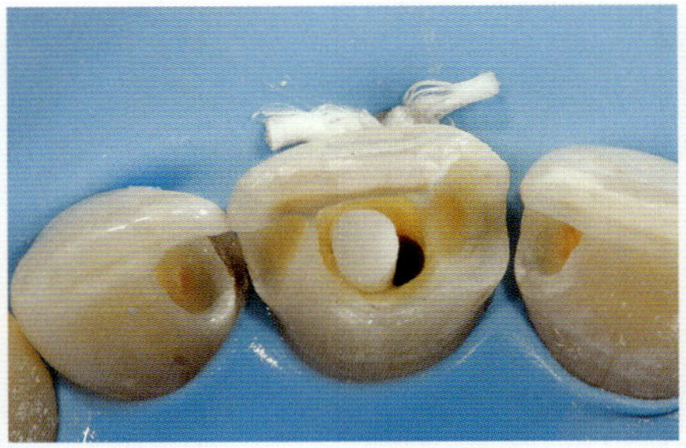

Fig 10-3n
… and the post was adjusted, so it does not extend beyond the volume of the final reconstruction …

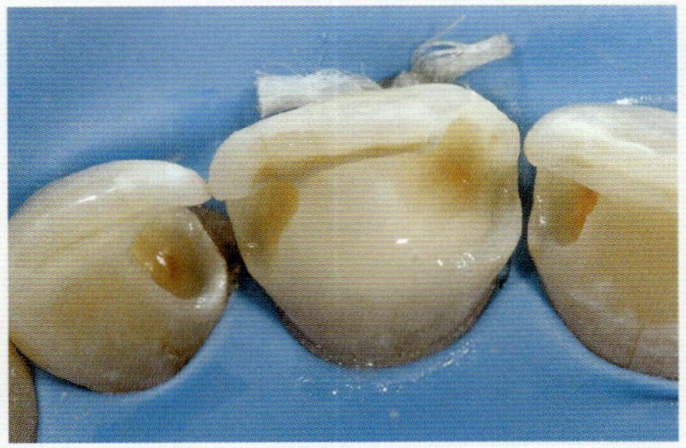

Fig 10-3o
… next, the bonding system was applied, and the fiberglass post was cemented.

Step 4: Composite veneer

Thanks to the silicone index the palatal surface was formed, and then a minimally invasive veneer preparation was performed (Fig 10-3p). After preparing the labial surface for adhesive restoration, the proximal surfaces were created using an enamel layer of composite resin (Figs 10-3q and 10-3r). Then, mamelons were shaped using a dentin layer (Fig 10-3s). Before the polymerization of the mamelons, the Misura instrument (LM-Arte) was used in order to check if there would be enough space for the final enamel layer. Next, the Intensive White dye was applied, imitating the white stains (Fig 10-3t), which were found on the adjacent central incisor (the patient wanted the veneer to be as similar as possible to the adjacent tooth), and the final enamel layer was applied (Fig 10-3u). Final shaping and characterization were carried out with a bur no. 832-204-012 (Komet Brasseler). Polishing was carried out using brushes (Goat-Hair Brush Wheel RA, SHINY S, Micerium) with a SHINY Finishing Pastes (Micerium, A – 3 μm diamond paste, B – 1 μm diamond paste and C – aluminum oxide). The patient's smile after completing the treatment is shown in Fig 10-3v.

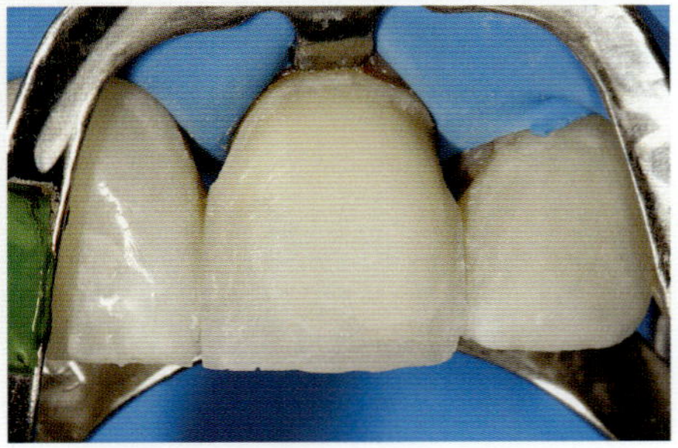

Fig 10-3p
After creating the entire palatal surface, the minimally invasive preparation on tooth 21 was performed (the preparation was needed as the restoration of tooth 21 could not be performed as more convex than the natural tooth 11. Moreover, external veneer was intended to block future discoloration reoccurrence).

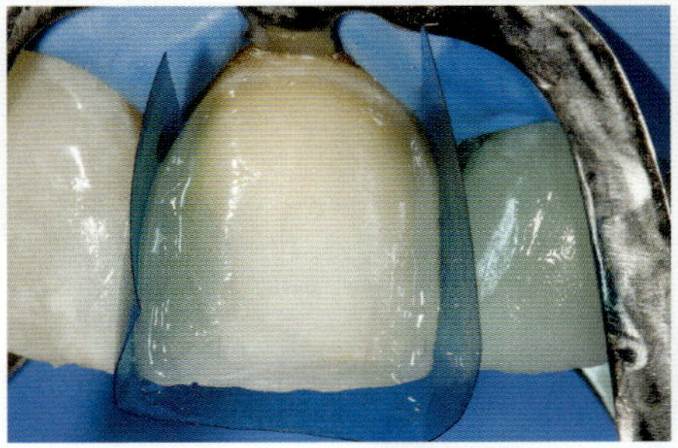

Fig 10-3q
A transparent VariStrip matrix (Blue View VariStrip, Garrison Dental) was placed on the proximal surfaces to form the veneer's proximal surfaces.

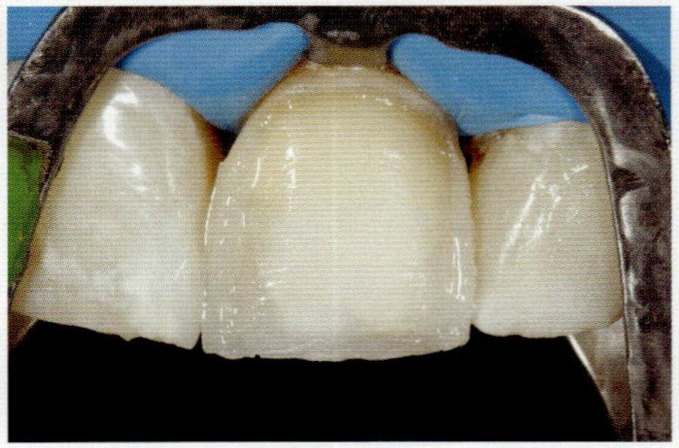

Fig 10-3r
After polymerization, the matrix was removed; the restoration of proximal surfaces will facilitate direct veneer fabrication.

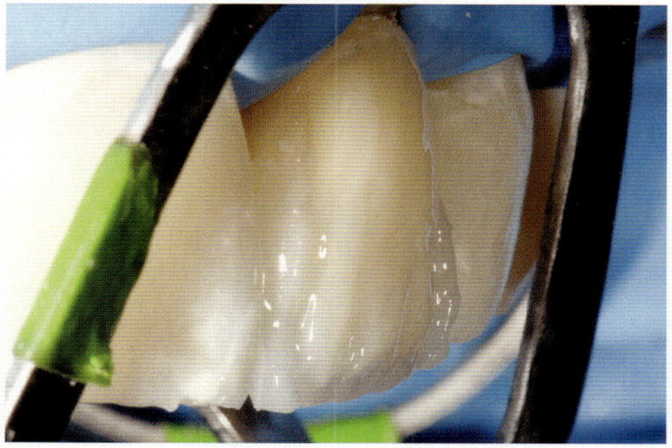

Fig 10-3s
Shaping mamelons with dentin composite resin (UD3, Micerium).

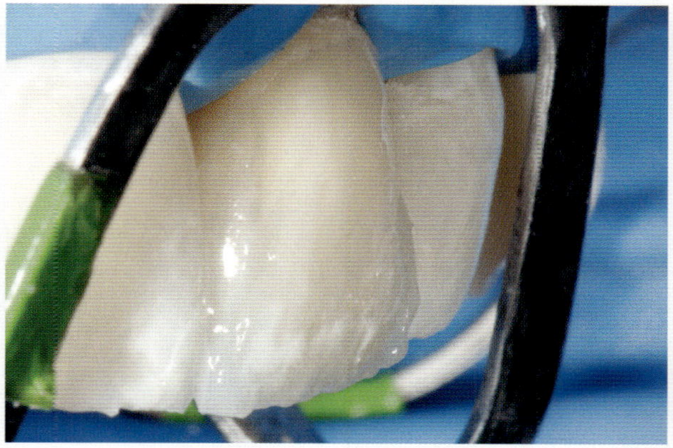

Fig 10-3t
After polymerizing the dentin layer, imitation of a white spot was applied similarly to the symmetrical central incisor …

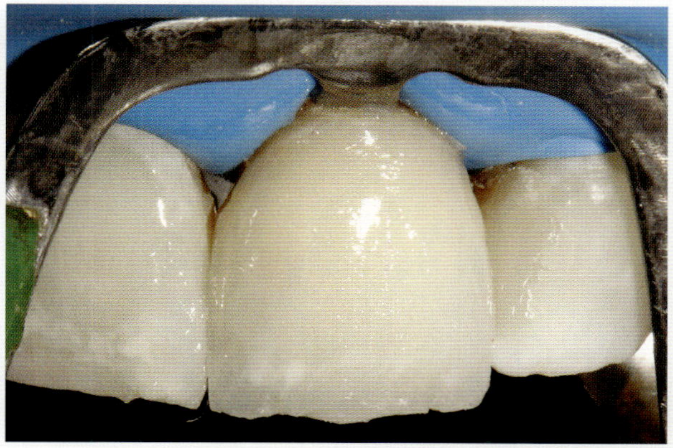

Fig 10-3u
… next, the final enamel layer was applied.

REMEMBER

Important factors determining the choice of therapy for the discolored tooth after root canal treatment:

- If there is a possibility of bleaching the tooth, restoring them with a direct composite resin is relatively easy. In case of severe discoloration and contraindication for internal bleaching, it is difficult and not predictable to block the discoloration using only direct composite.
- If the discoloration is asymmetrical and it can be bleached, the direct composite restoration is more predictable to perform. If we decide to perform porcelain veneers, it is safer to make them symmetrically on both central incisors.[18,21]

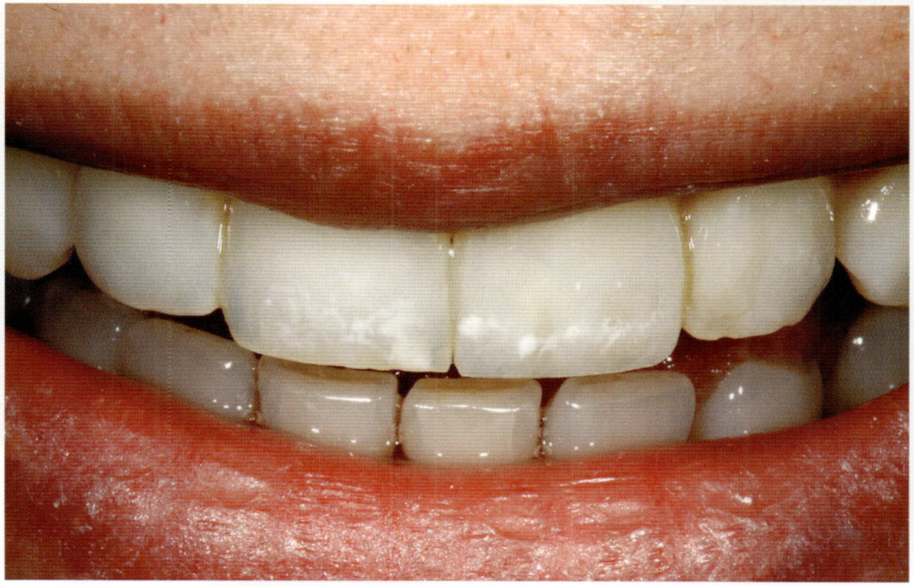

Fig 10-3v
Patient's smile after treatment.

SIMPLIFIED COMPOSITE VENEERS PERFORMED WITH THE STYLE ITALIANO TECHNIQUE

In the past, creating composite veneers required artistic craftsmanship from the dentist, and the final result depended on their manual skills. How can the risk of failure be reduced? How can the unpredictability be limited and young dentists be taught to carry out composite restorations repeatedly? These questions impacted the work of the Style Italiano dentists who undertook the responsibility of creating a technique and instruments that would increase the predictability of treatment in the oral cavity. One of the improvements was the introduction of the Unica Anterior Matrix into clinical practice. This thin matrix is designed to create outlines for direct composite resin veneer. Creating this contour was always the most difficult part and posed the risk of composite excess in the cervical area or margin gaps in the proximal surfaces area. How to perform direct composite veneers today?[27–29]

Preliminary stage

In this stage, we prepare a silicone index based on the mock-up or the wax-up (the length and shape of the teeth should always be verified after the initial application of the temporary composite, taking photographs, and engaging in a thorough discussion with the patient about the expected outcome and all details of which are presented in the previous chapters). When increasing the length of the anteriors, the incisal edge (its palatal part) should be extended with an enamel layer of composite resin using the silicone index – this is how we determine the future length of the tooth and, at the same time, the esthetics of the incisal edge (Fig 10-4a).

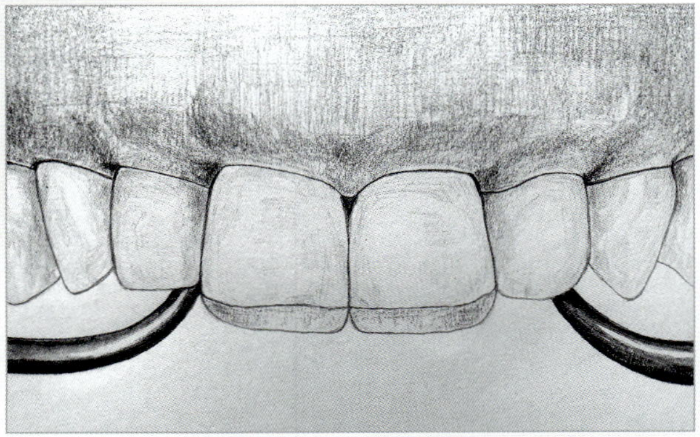

Fig 10-4a
The preliminary stage of performing composite veneers: the incisal edge was formed (with the palatal index) …

Step 1: Unica Anterior

After stabilizing a thin Unica Anterior Matrix in an appropriate position, the flowable composite resin can be easily applied along the matrix. After light-curing the "frames," the restoration is almost ready (Figs 10-4b and 10-4c).

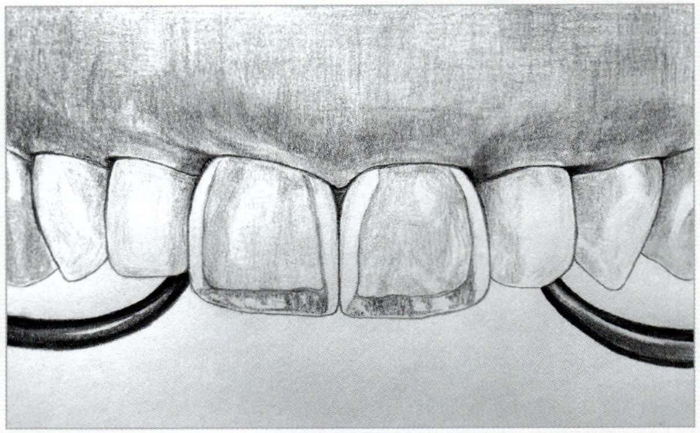

Fig 10-4b
… next, on the anterior teeth, a special veneer matrix called Unica Anterior was situated.

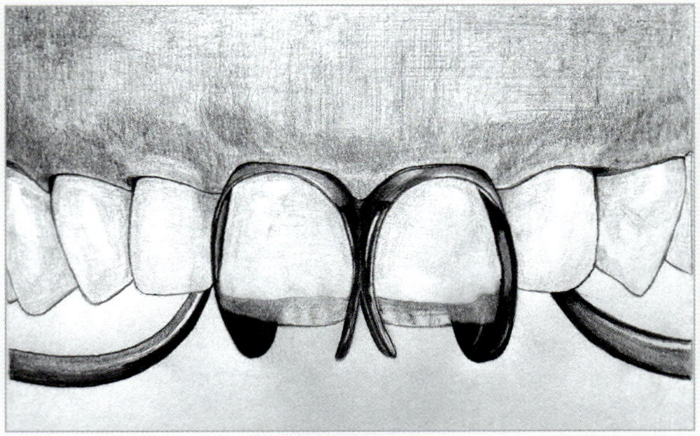

Fig 10-4c
"Frames" of the veneers were created by light-curing the flowable composite along the Unica Anterior Matrix – situation after removing the matrices.

Step 2: Dentin

The dentin composite layer was applied between the "frames," and mamelons were formed with a Fissura instrument (LM-Arte) before light-curing (Fig 10-4d). Ensure that an appropriate space of 0.5 mm is left for the outer layer of the enamel composite. For this purpose, we use a Misura instrument (LM-Arte). Next, the dentin mamelons should be light cured.

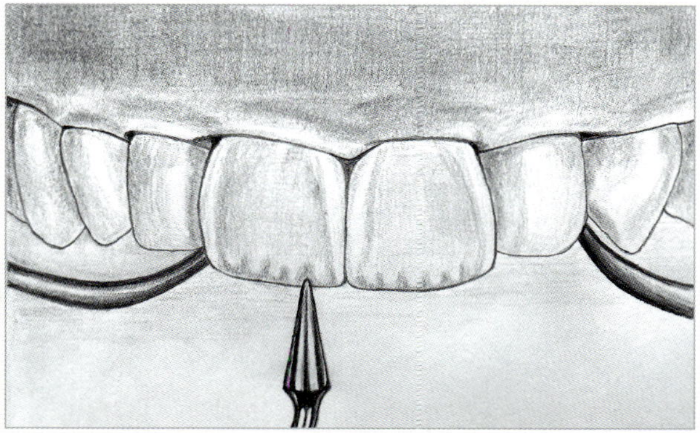

Fig 10-4d
Step 2 of performing composite veneers: shaping the mamelons with a Fissura instrument in the dentin composite layer.

Step 3: Enamel

In the next step, the enamel layer is applied and spread on the entire outer surface with the flexible spatula (Applica LM-Arte) or with a composite resin brush (Fig 10-4e).

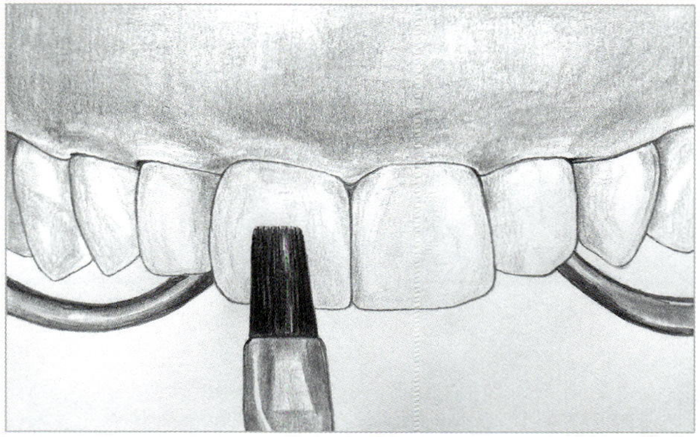

Fig 10-4e
Step 3: spreading the enamel layer (you can perform this with a flexible spatula, eg, Applica or a composite brush).

Step 4: Characterization of the surface

The formed and polymerized surface is a starting point for further characterization to match the shape of adjacent. This can be performed with a Profin contra-angle handpiece or a bur no. 832-204-012 (Fig 10-4f) after marking on the labial surface of the tooth the transition line between the labial, proximal and cervical surfaces.

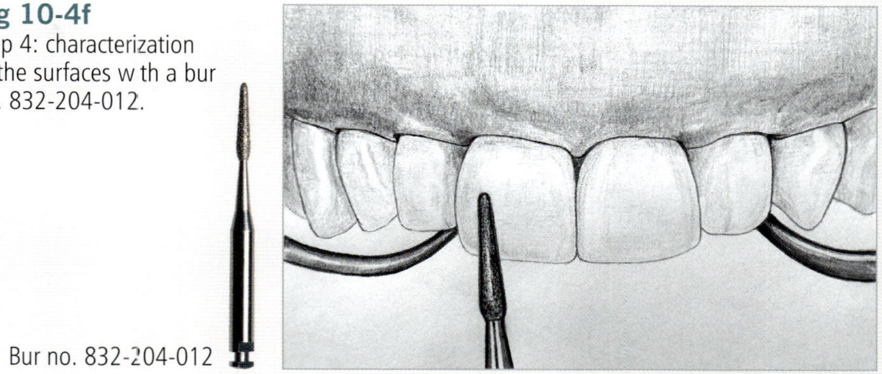

Fig 10-4f
Step 4: characterization of the surfaces with a bur no. 832-204-012.

Step 5: Final polishing

Polishing should not be done at high speed to avoid overheating the composite resin (ideally 5,000-10,000 rpm). In this chapter, the polishing system introduced by Dr. Lorenzo Vanini is proposed, which contains three pastes: A – 3 μm diamond paste, B – 1 μm diamond paste, and C – aluminum oxide. The first two pastes are dedicated for initial polishing with a Goat-Hair Brush (Fig 10-4g) and the last one for final polishing with a felt polishing wheel.

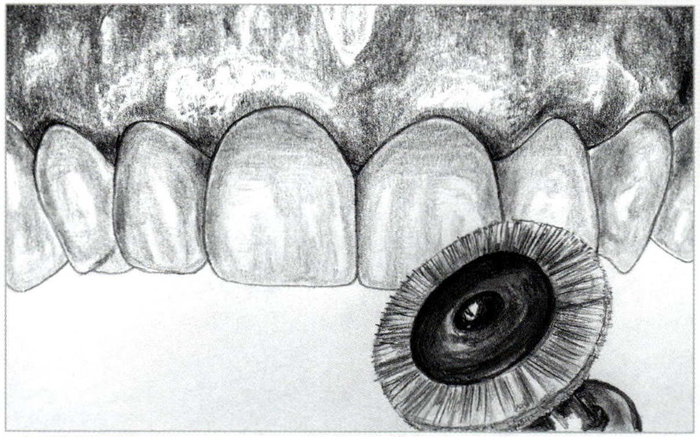

Fig 10-4g
Step 5: polishing with a Goat-Hair Brush Shiny S.

Case 3: Simplified direct composite veneers

A 61-year-old female patient presented to the dental office to improve the esthetics of her anterior incisors (Fig 10-5a). The patient was analyzed for tooth structure loss and in terms of function. The occlusal conditions were improved, making it possible to extend the anterior teeth adequately to the upper and lower lip position. This chapter describes only the technique of performing no-prep composite veneers. The mock-up analysis indicated that the tooth enlargement both incisally and labially would be esthetically beneficial for the patient smile. In addition, the patient insisted on a more economical solution, which would not affect the remaining dental structures of the anterior teeth. Direct composite veneers without preparation on teeth 12–22 seemed to be the best solution, taking into account the patient's expectations.

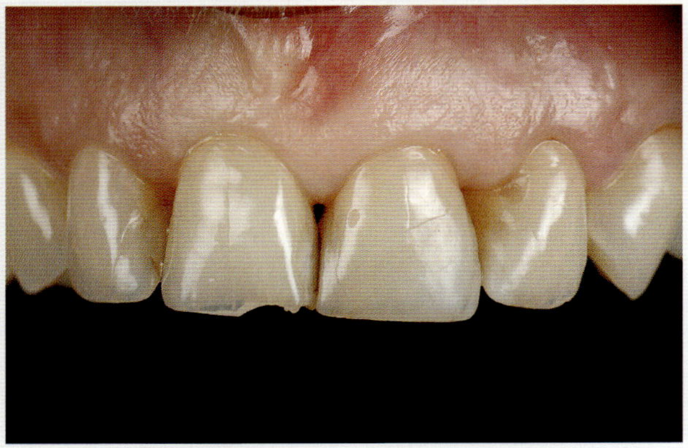

Fig 10-5a
A female patient presented to the dental office with a wish to improve the esthetics of the anterior teeth: four direct composite veneers were planned.

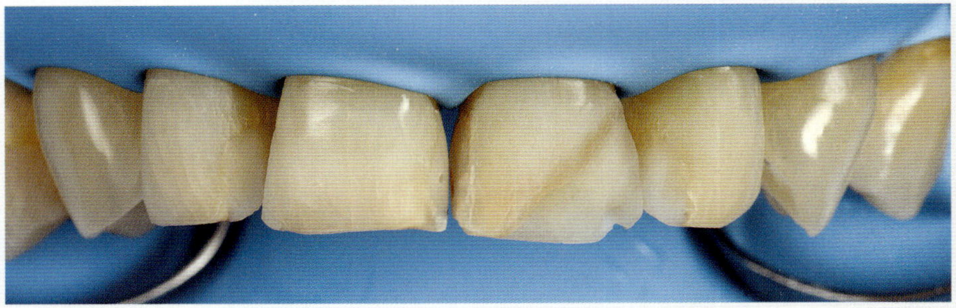

Fig 10-5b
Rubber dam isolation was performed, teeth 21 and 22 had old composite materials removed from the labial surface. Then, the tooth structure was airborne-particle abraded.

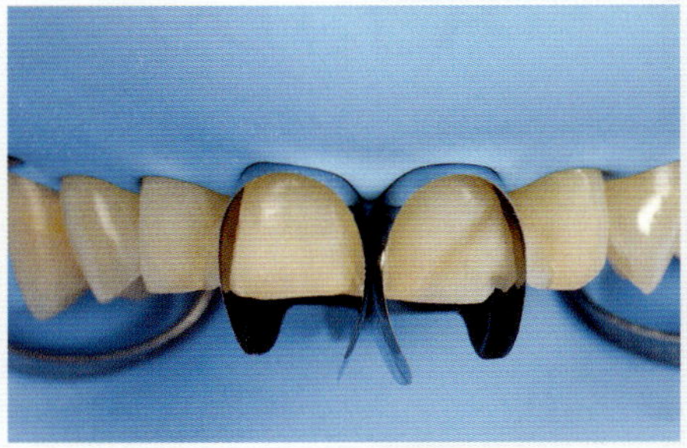

Fig 10-5c
Two Unica Anterior Matrices were placed ...

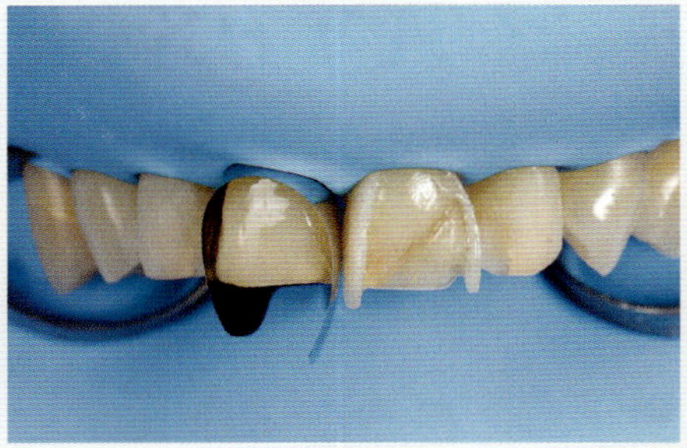

Fig 10-5d
... and a flowable composite resin was injected along each matrix and light cured.

Step 1: Unica Anterior

The anterior teeth were isolated with a rubber dam (Fig 10-5b), and restorative procedures were carried out: the outer part of the old composite was removed (the palatal part was maintained due to the good marginal seal of the restoration), the tooth surface was airborne-particle abraded and etched, and the bonding system was applied. The Unica Anterior Matrices were placed on both central incisors followed by a flowable resin application (Fig 10-5c) along the matrix, thus forming the "frames" of the restoration (Fig 10-5d). The planned length of the tooth from the palatal side was formed with enamel composite applied previously on a prepared silicone index (Fig 10-5e).

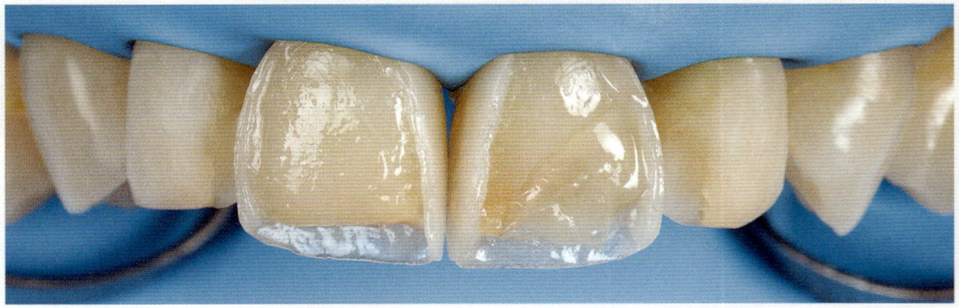

Fig 10-5e
Intraoral photograph after creating the direct composite veneer frames with the Unica Anterior Matrix. Palatal surfaces of the incisors were formed using the silicone index.

Step 2: Dentin

A dentin layer of composite resin was applied between the previously polymerized "frames" of the tooth, and the mamelons were shaped (Fig 10-5f) with a Fissura instrument. After making sure that enough space was left for the outer layer, the dentin mamelons were polymerized.

Step 3: Enamel

Next, the enamel layer was spread with a flexible spatula (Applica, LM-Arte). The pre-shaped enamel layer was polymerized (Fig 10-5g). The same procedures were repeated when performing direct composite resin veneers on teeth 12 and 22 (Figs 10-5h to 10-5j).

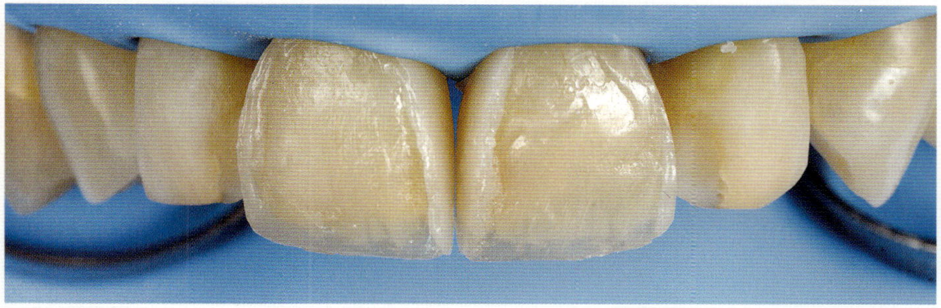

Fig 10-5f
After the dentin layer was applied, the mamelons were shaped with the Fissura instrument.

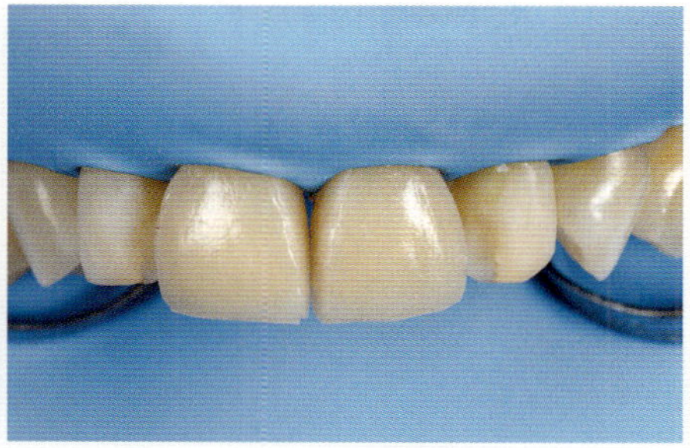

Fig 10-5g
Clinical situation after applying and modeling the enamel layer of the composite veneers on teeth 11 and 21.

> **PRACTITIONER'S ADVICE**
>
> When performing a veneer "frame," use a flowable composite. Control the extrusion from the syringe to avoid any unnecessary excess!

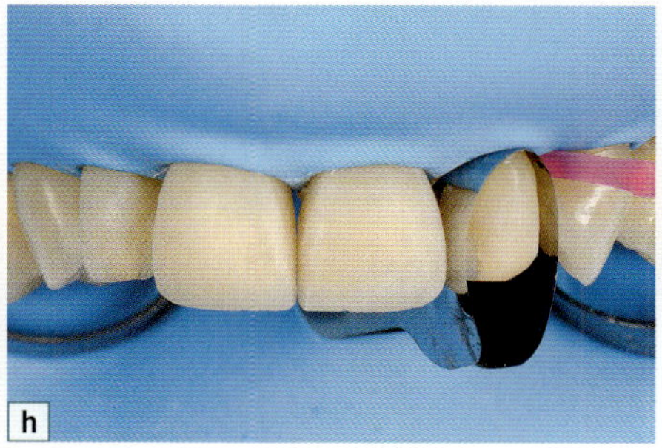

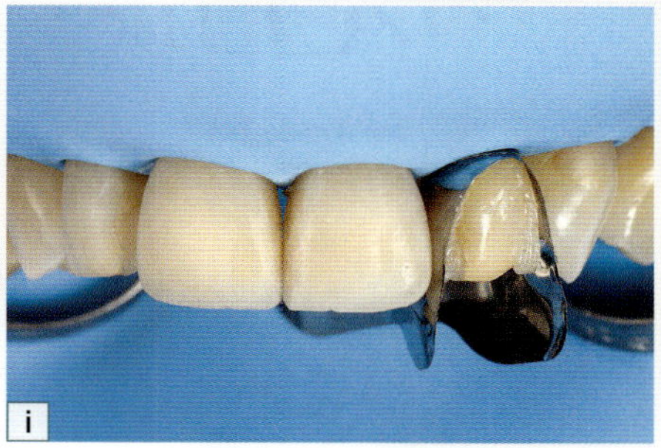

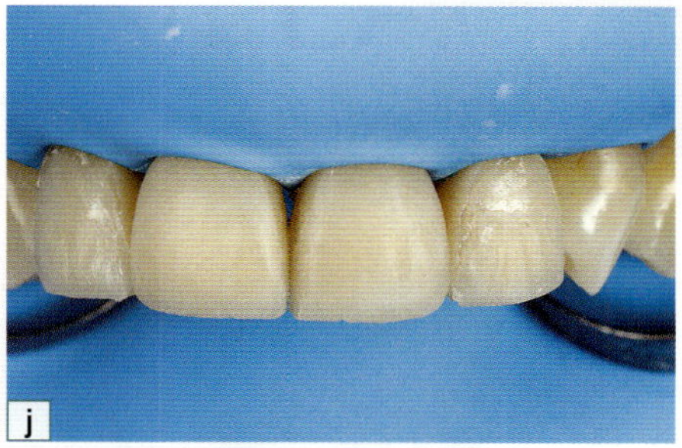

Figs 10-5h to 10-5j
Steps of performing direct composite veneers on the maxillary lateral incisors.

Steps 4 & 5: Characterization and polishing

The characterization and polishing were performed in accordance with the procedures described in the previous section, achieving the effect presented in Figs 10-5k to 10-5n.

Figs 10-5k and 10-5l
Photographs of direct veneers taken from the semi-profile.

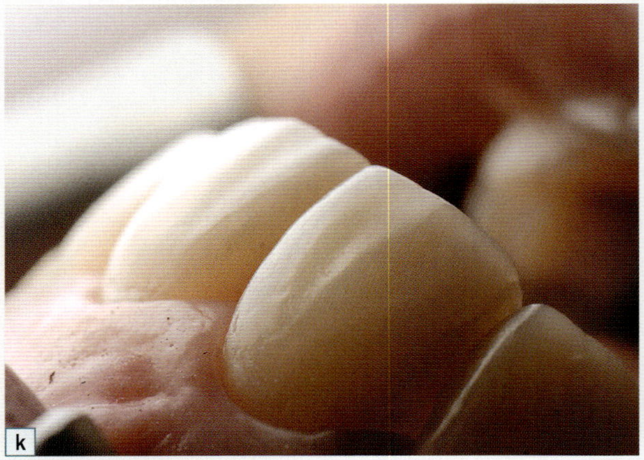

k

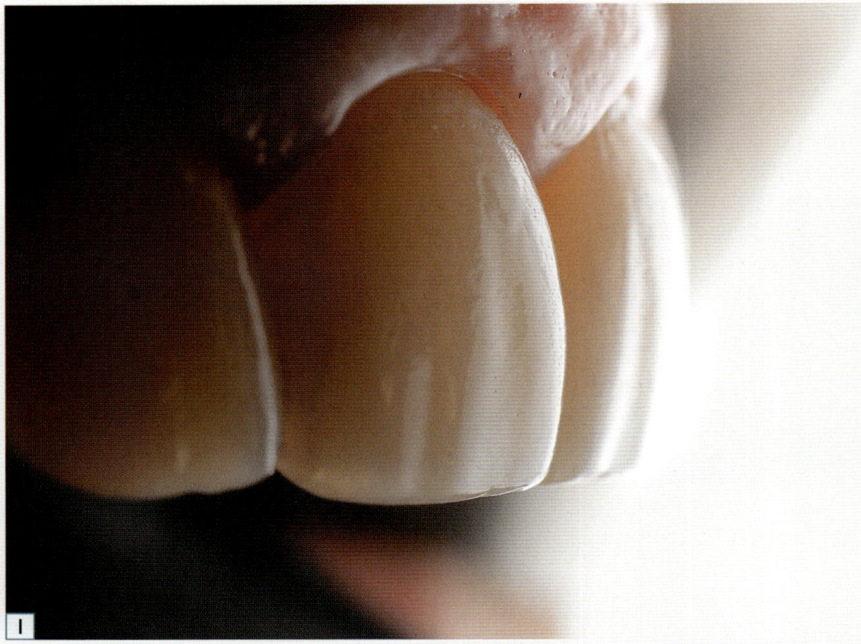

l

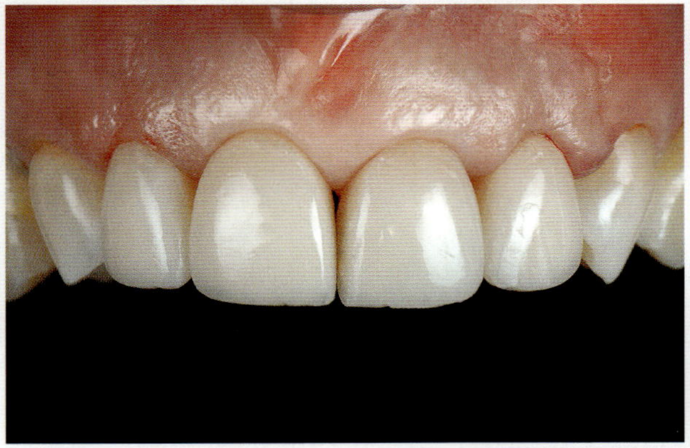

Fig 10-5m
Intraoral photograph of direct composite veneers.

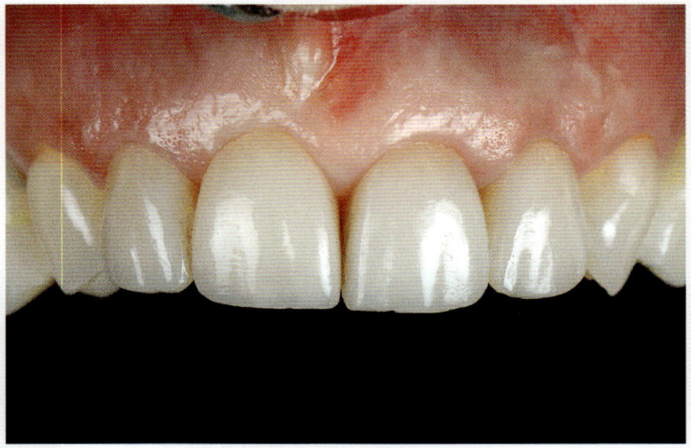

Fig 10-5n
Follow-up visit 12 months after performing veneers.

PRACTITIONER'S ADVICE

Spend enough time when characterizing and polishing. Rushing at this stage can ruin the final effect of direct composite veneer.

INDIRECT COMPOSITE VENEERS

Composite veneers can also be performed in an indirect way. It is not a very popular treatment technique because it is much cheaper and faster (during one visit) to perform direct veneers. The indications for such veneers are generally similar to porcelain veneers. However, it is worth paying attention to specific indications for indirect composite veneers:

- Young patients before the end of the growth period
- Patients before or during orthodontic treatment (as a provisional or a final stage, if the treatment meets the patient's and dentist's expectations)
- Clinical situations where direct composite veneers could be too difficult to execute for the dentist due to the inability to create the proper shape and color (for example, if there are several veneers to perform, or existing discoloration is difficult to mask with direct composite)

Two cases of indirect composite veneers are presented in the following subsections, one of which concerns a juvenile patient and the other an adult who avoided tooth preparation thanks to direct veneers.

Case 4: Adolescent patient

A 17-year-old female patient presented to the dental office with a fractured tooth 21 (Fig 10-6a), which had been root canal-treated in the past. The fracture of the tooth was juxtagingival on the palatal surface (Fig 10-6b), the tooth was restored with a fiberglass post, and in the radiograph, there was a lesion in the periapical tissues (Fig 10-6c).

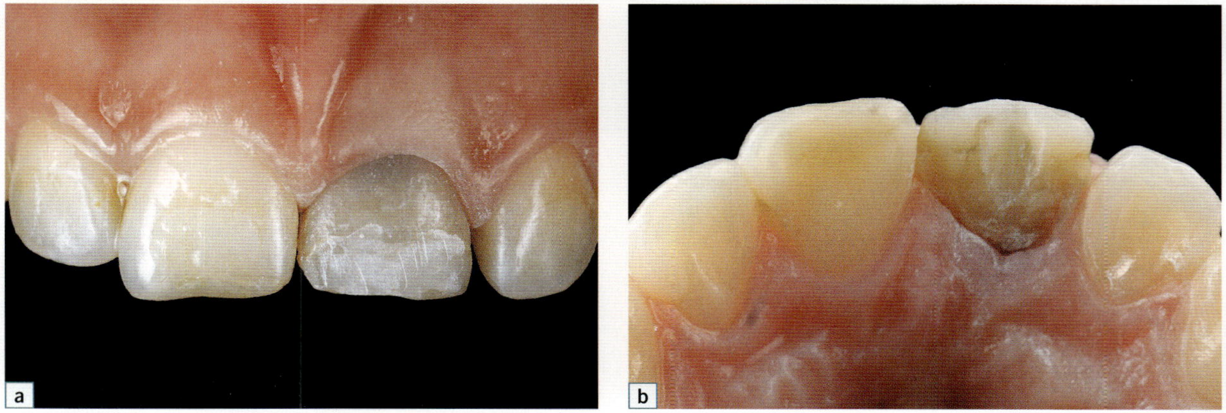

Figs 10-6a and 10-6b
(a) A 17-year-old female patient presented to the dental office with a fractured tooth 21. (b) The tooth was juxtagingivally fractured from the palatal surface.

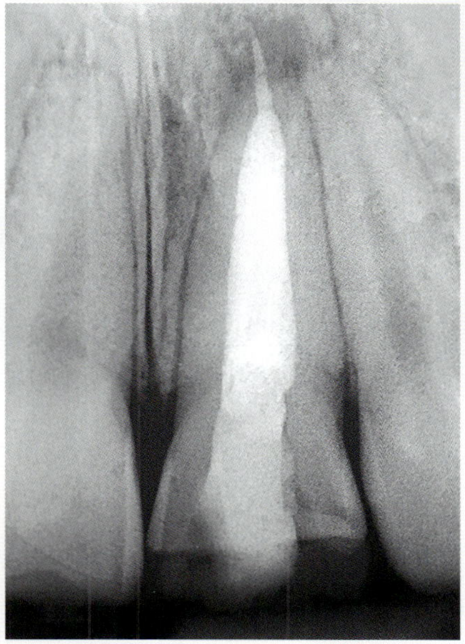

Fig 10-6c
Radiograph of the lesion in the periapical tissues.

Step 1: Root canal retreatment

During the endodontic retreatment, perforation on the labial surface was identified (Fig 10-6d). Since it was situated within the gingival sulcus, this problem was solved by gingivectomy followed by restoring the perforation from the labial surface (Fig 10-6e). Root canal treatment ended with thermoplastic gutta-percha filling, and a fiber post was cemented in the wide root canal. The palatal part of the tooth crown was restored with composite resin.

Step 2: Wax-up, mock-up, and impressions

A wax-up was fabricated in the dental laboratory, and a transparent silicone index was made (Figs 10-6f and 10-6g). The mock-up was carried out in the patient's oral cavity with a flowable composite (Fig 10-6h) polymerized through the transparent index (Fig 10-6i). Once the esthetic concept had been accepted (Figs 10-6j and 10-6k), the mock-up through preparation was performed (Figs 10-6l to 10-6n) under control of adjusted silicone index (Fig 10-6o). The excess composite was removed with an Eccesso (LM-Arte) instrument (Fig 10-6p), and the preparation was finished in such a way that the margins were clearly visible for the dental technician (Fig 10-6q). After that, two retraction cords were placed (Figs 10-6r and 10-6s). A metal strip was placed between a strong contact point of teeth 11 and 12 in order to separate adjacent surfaces. Then, the thicker retraction cords were removed, and impressions were taken (Figs 10-6t to 10-6x). Impressions were sent to the dental laboratory, and the teeth were provided with the provisional veneers (Fig 10-6y).

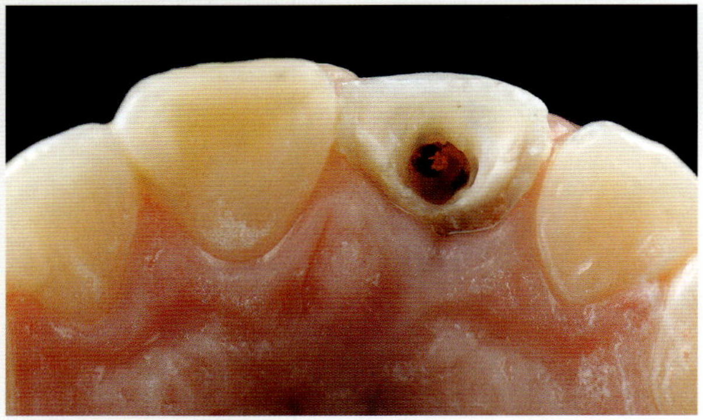

Fig 10-6d Perforation is visible on the labial surface.

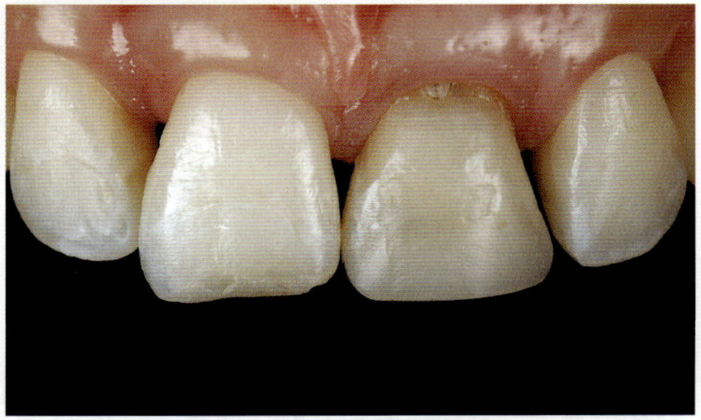

Fig 10-6e Clinical situation after gingivectomy.

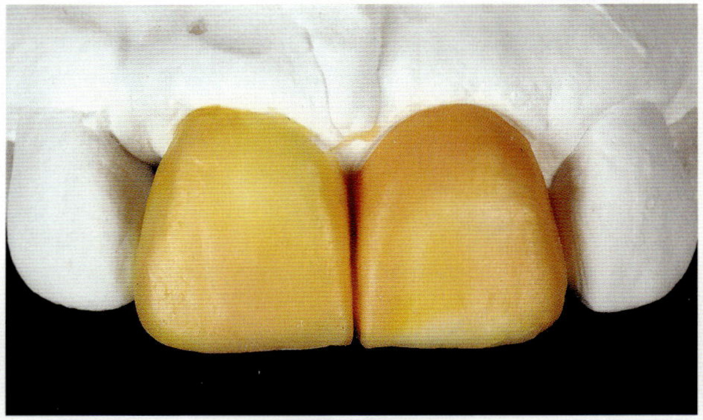

Fig 10-6f Diagnostic wax-up of teeth 11 and 21, in accordance with the planned indirect composite veneers.

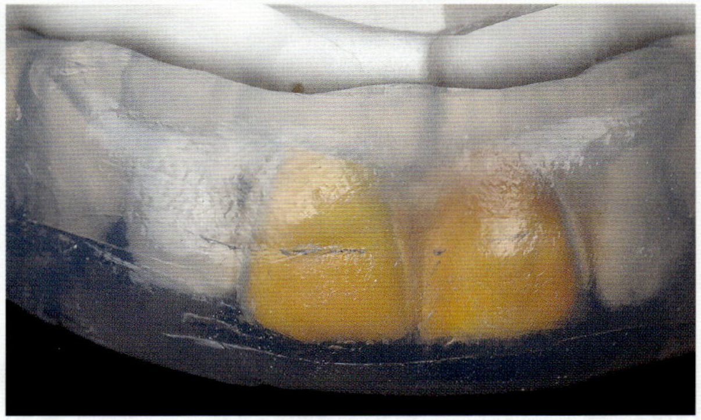

Fig 10-6g Taking a transparent silicone index from the diagnostic wax-up.

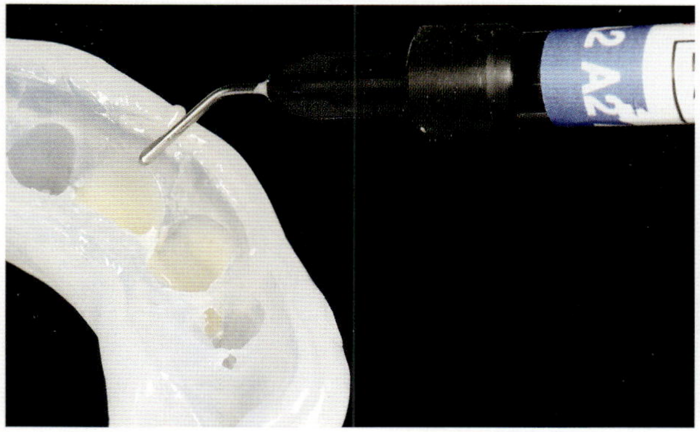

Fig 10-6h
A flowable composite was applied to the silicone index.

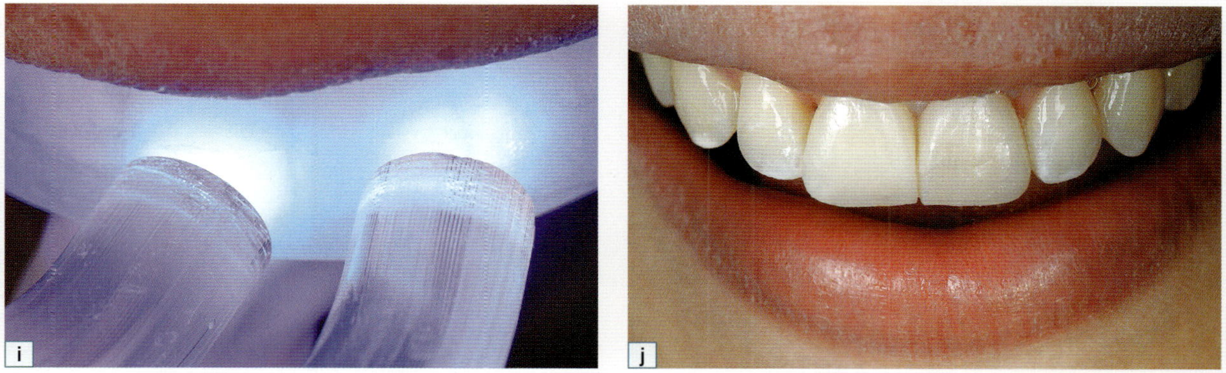

Figs 10-6i and 10-6j
(i) Silicone index was placed on the maxillary arch and light-cured, (j) obtaining a direct mock-up on teeth 11 and 21, which was assessed, in the presence of the patient, in the photographs.

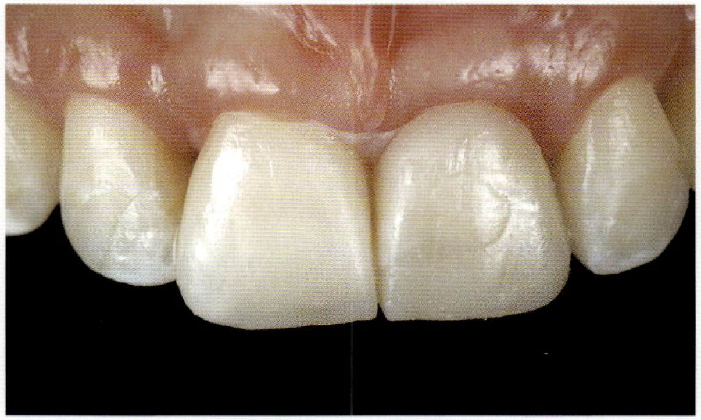

Fig 10-6k
Composite resin mock-up on teeth 11 and 21.

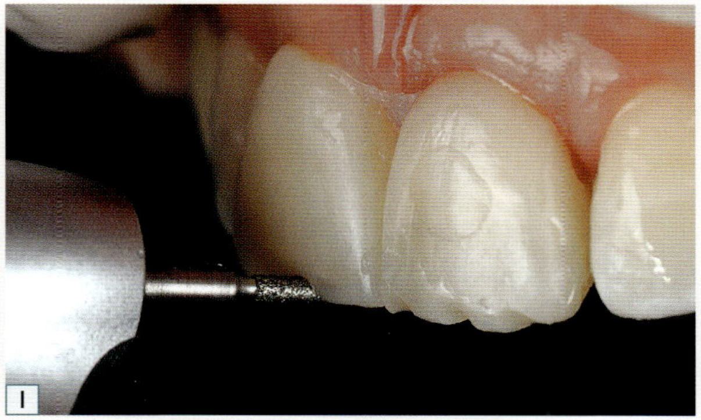

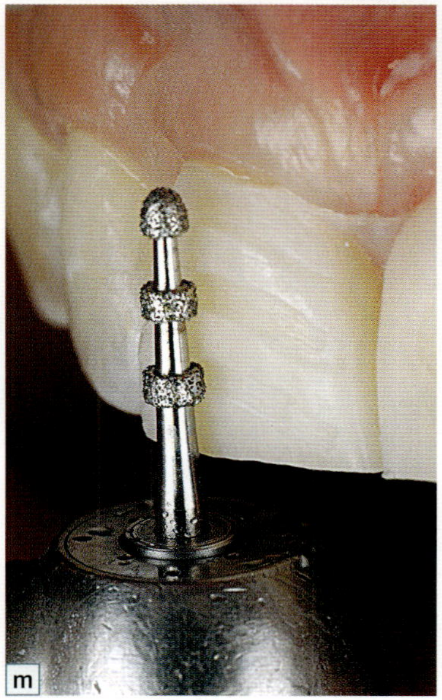

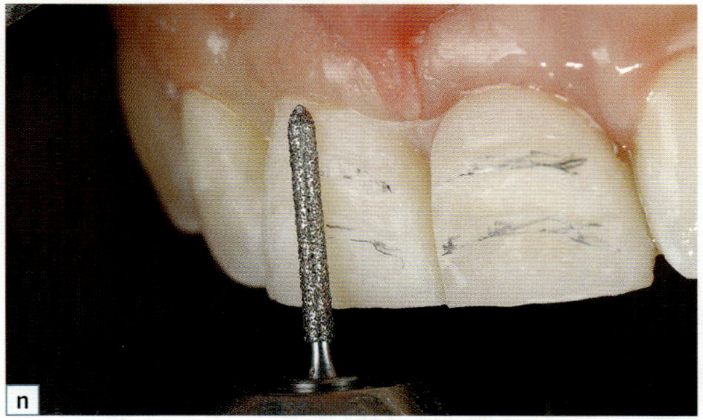

Figs 10-6l to 10-6n
Mock-up through preparation for indirect composite veneers.

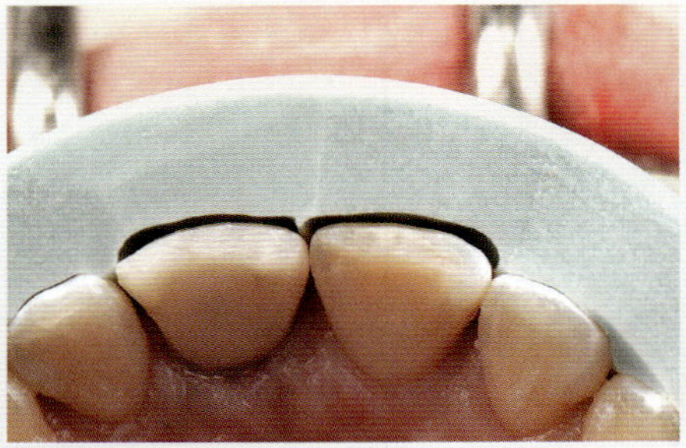

Fig 10-6o
Controlling the veneer preparation with the adjusted silicone index placed on teeth 11 and 21.

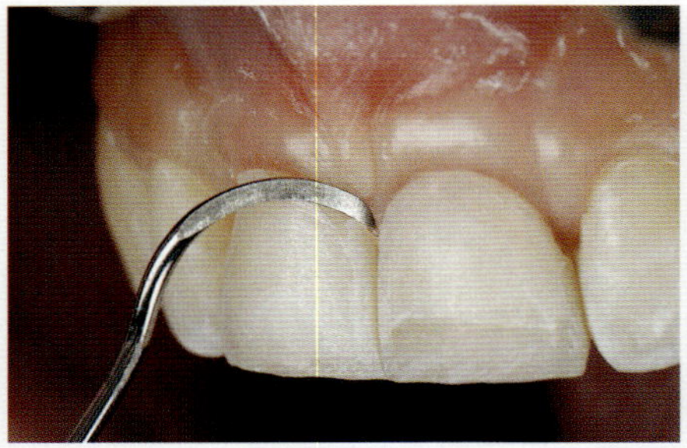

Fig 10-6p
Removing the excess composite mock-up from the proximal surfaces with the Eccesso instrument.

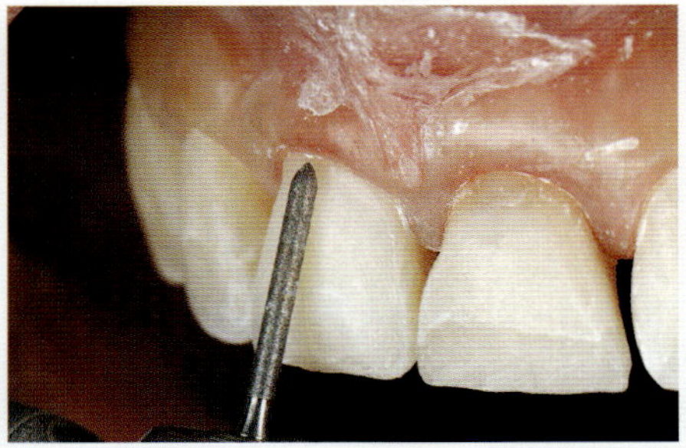

Fig 10-6q
Finishing the preparation margin for indirect composite veneers.

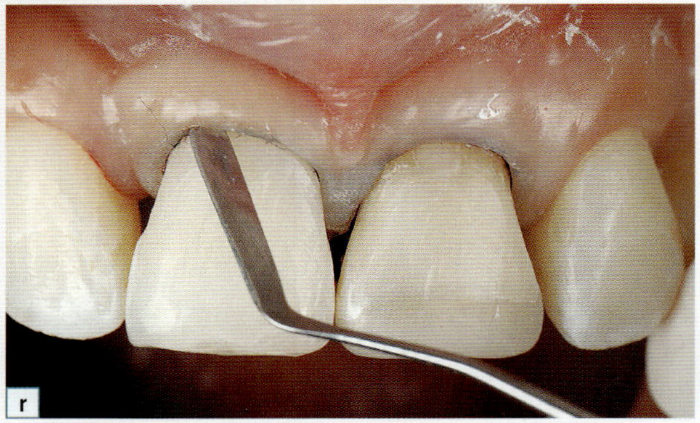

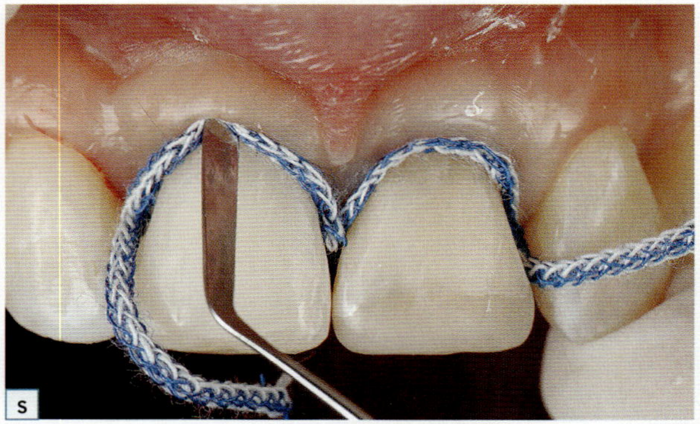

PRACTITIONER'S ADVICE

In the case of a tight contact point, you can place a metal strip between proximal surfaces immediately before taking an impression!

Figs 10-6r and 10-6s
(r) Placing the first and (s) the second retraction cord.

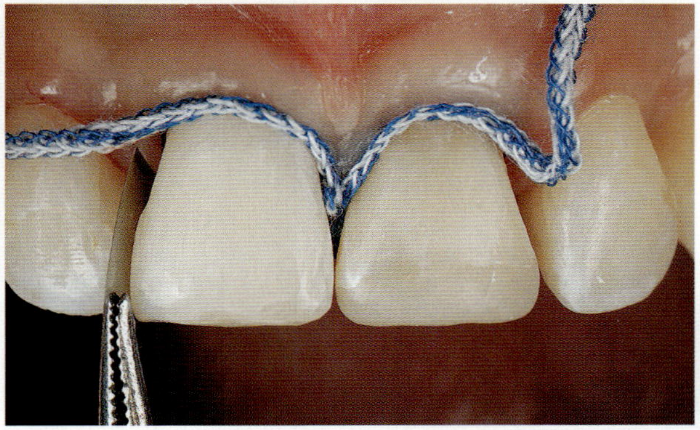

Fig 10-6t
Placing a metal strip between a tight contact point of teeth 11 and 12.

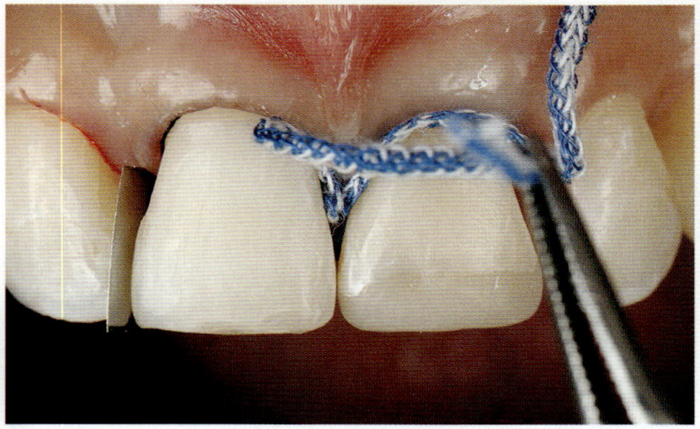

Fig 10-6u
Right before the injection of the impression material, the dental assistant removes the thicker retraction cord …

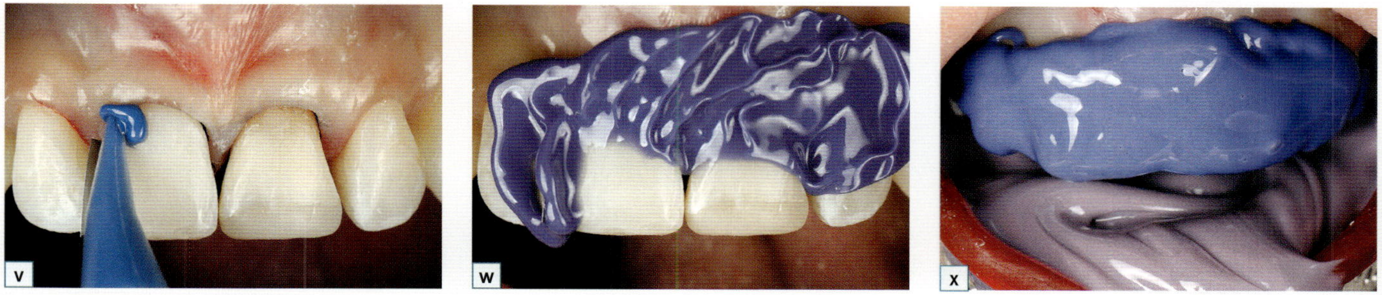

Figs 10-6v to 10-6x
... (v and w) next, the dentist injects the medium body impression paste along the gingival margin of teeth 11 and 21, and (x) along the proximal, labial, and palatal surfaces, followed by insertion of impression tray, filled with heavy body mass on the entire maxillary arch.

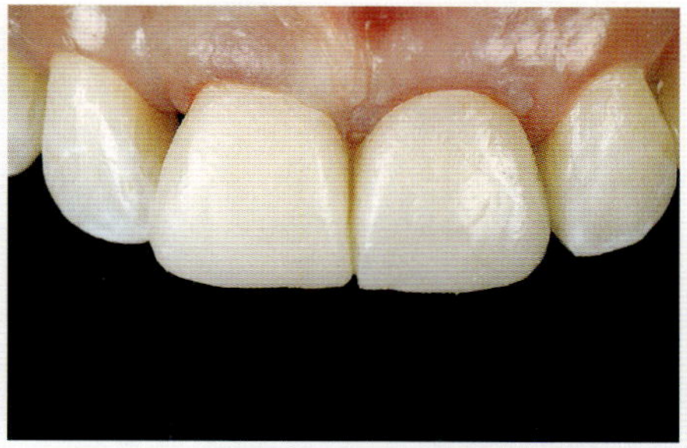

Fig 10-6y
Provisional veneers were placed on teeth 11 and 21.

Step 3: Cementing and control

At the next appointment, two indirect composite veneers were cemented in rubber dam isolation. The final esthetic result, a few days after cementing the veneers, is presented in Fig 10-6z. The 12-month follow-up is shown in Fig 10-6aa and the follow-up after 36 months in Fig 10-6bb. It should be emphasized that, in the case of composite veneers, repolishing is recommended to restore the original esthetic effect. The good thing about composite restoration, also the indirect one, is the possibility of small corrections with the direct resin if needed.

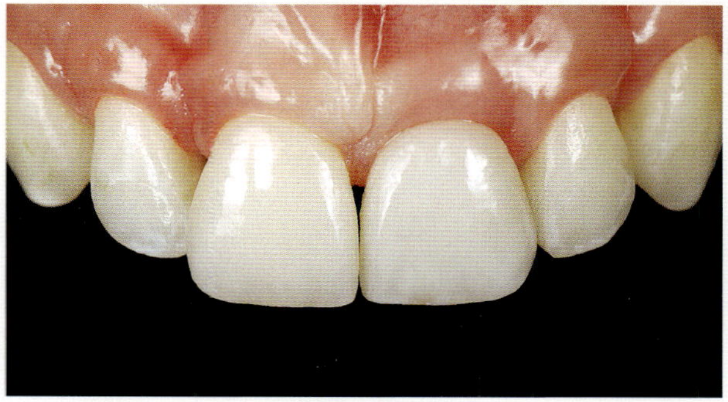

Fig 10-6z
Indirect composite veneers a few days after cementation.

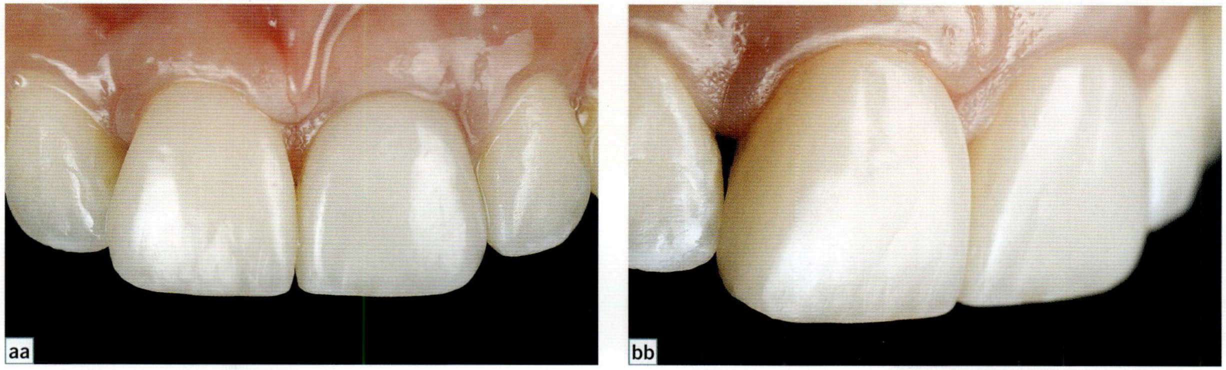

Figs 10-6aa and 10-6bb
Follow-up of the indirect composite veneers: (aa) 12 months and (bb) 36 months after cementation.

Case 5: No-prep composite veneers

Veneers without preparation are not easy to perform using the indirect method with porcelain or composite material. However, in some clinical situations, when maxillary teeth are in retrusion or in case of tooth structure vestibular deficiency, modifying the shape by adding the material will positively impact the esthetic result. Additionally, when the indirect material is a composite, the dentist has more options and the possibility of merging the direct and indirect methods using the same material (as in the case of undercuts to avoid preparation).

A patient presented to the dental office seeking comprehensive dental treatment (Figs 10-7a to 10-7e). Generalized tooth wear with a horizontal wear pattern was diagnosed with numerous erosions. He was also missing several molar teeth. After dental prophylaxis appointments, needed endodontic retreatments and replacement of defective restorations, the patient was offered comprehensive implant-prosthetic treatment. The esthetic treatment plan was visualized through the wax-up (Fig 10-7f) and mock-up, and the patient was enthusiastic about it. Unfortunately, he had to postpone the treatment plan for financial reasons and asked for an alternative therapy method. Thanks to deprogramming (with KD), the occlusion was registered in the centric relation (CR) (Fig 10-7g), and a functional wax-up with occlusal vertical dimension (OVD) alteration was fabricated, in accordance with the esthetic needs (Fig 10-7h).

PRACTITIONER'S ADVICE

Taking photographs of our patients with lips in repose is the key element of esthetic treatment planning.

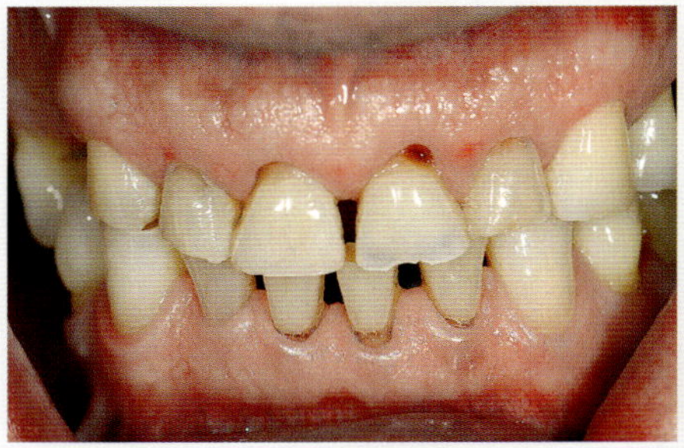

Fig 10-7b
Intraoral photograph in the position of maximum intercuspation.

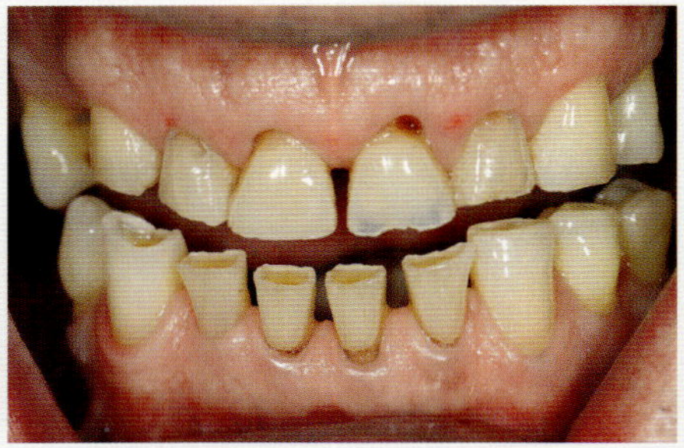

Fig 10-7c
Photograph of gentle tooth disclusion (visible horizontal wear pattern).

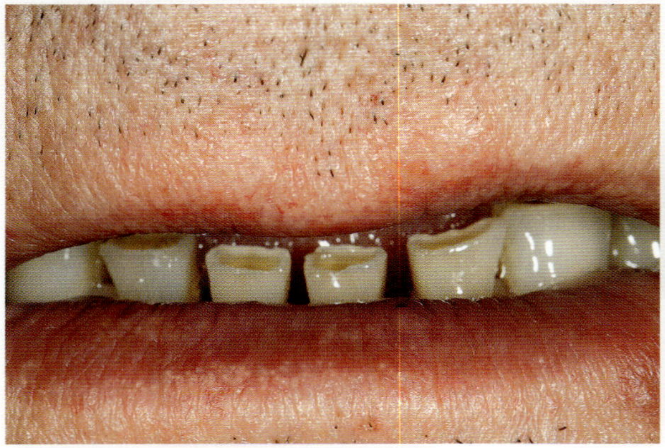

Fig 10-7a
Photograph of the patient with the lips in repose.

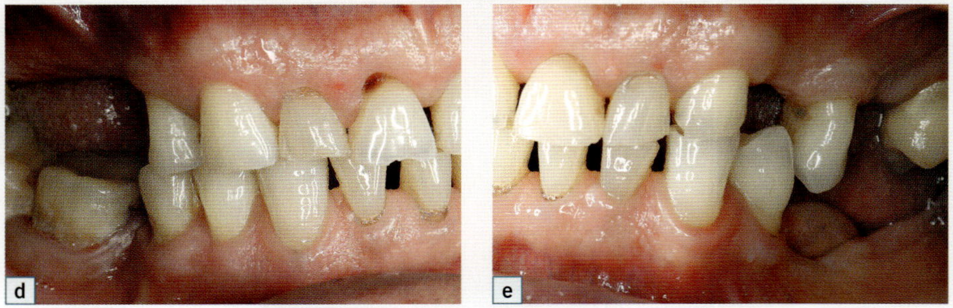

Figs 10-7d and 10-7e
Maximum intercuspation (d) from the right and (e) from the left semi-profile.

It was proposed to implement the treatment plan through direct composite restorations in the mandibular arch, indirect composite restorations in the maxillary arch, and skeletal dentures as a temporary solution to rehabilitate the missing posteriors. Based on the lower wax-up, a transparent silicone index was performed, which was adjusted individually to each tooth (Fig 10-7i) in order to copy the occlusal surface designed in the lab.

The entire mandibular arch was restored with direct composite resin without any tooth preparation (Fig 10-7j). In the next stage, the maxillary teeth were restored with the objective of avoiding additional tooth preparation. Impressions were taken and, in the dental laboratory, six no-prep indirect composite restorations were fabricated (Figs 10-7k and 10-7l).

By increasing the OVD, there was a significant space for the restorative material between the mandibular and maxillary arches, and it was convenient to select the no-prep technique.[30]

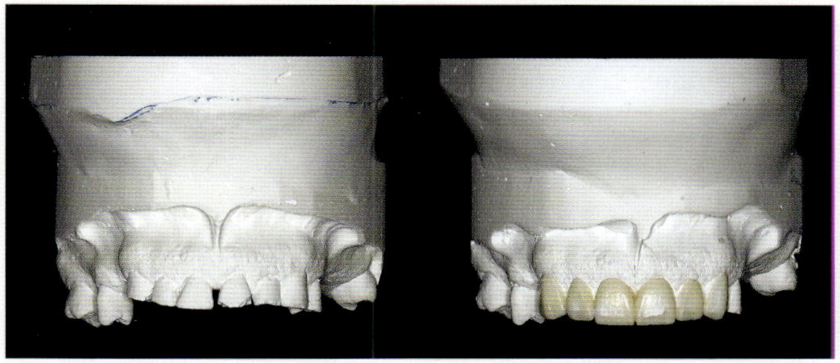

Fig 10-7f
Upper diagnostic casts: situation before (left side) and after waxing-up the upper model (right side) (wax-up: DT Iwona Domagała).

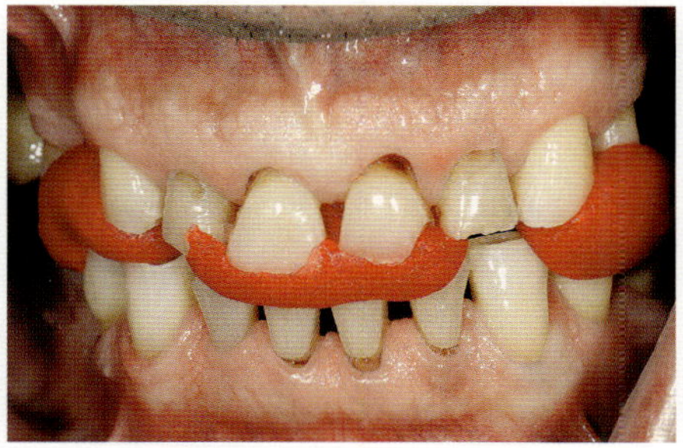

Fig 10-7g
CR registration with Pattern Resin.

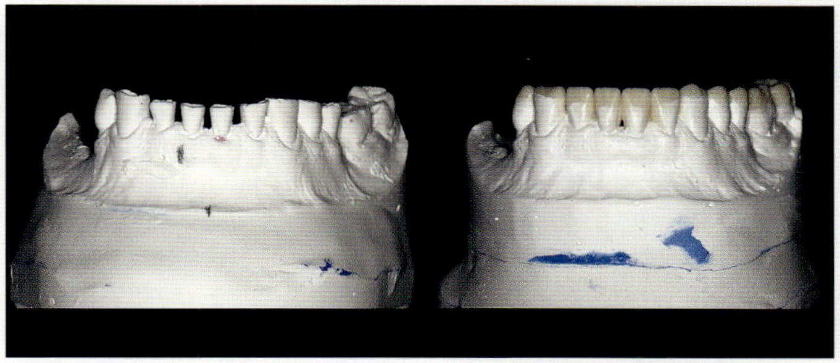

Fig 10-7h
Lower diagnostic casts: situation before (left side) and (right side) after waxing-up the mandibular model (wax-up: DT Iwona Domagała).

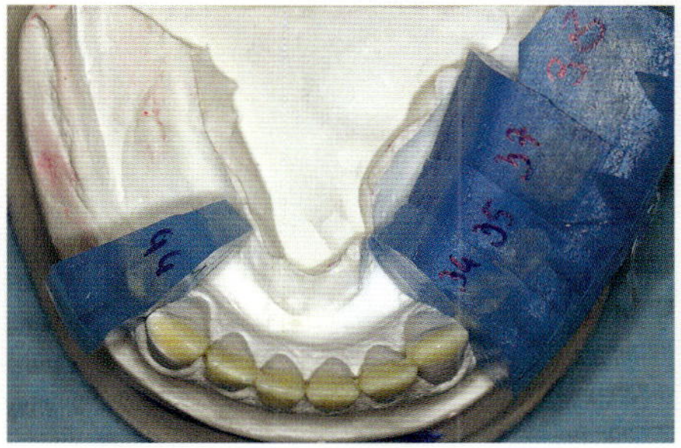

Fig 10-7i
The transparent silicone index, cut into segments to restore the worn mandibular arch with the index technique.

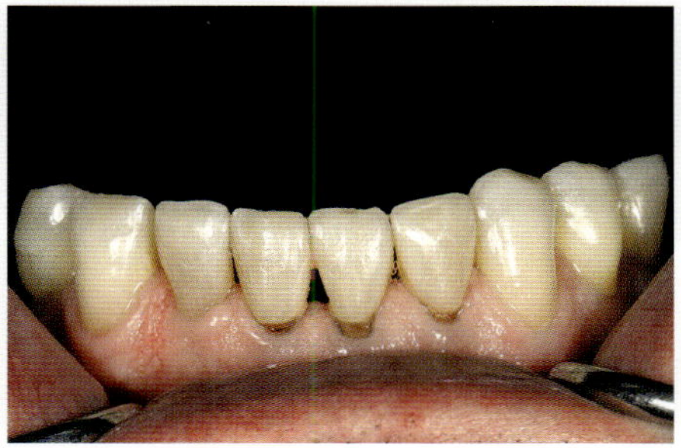

Fig 10-7j
Clinical situation after restoring the mandibular arch with direct additive composite restoration (reconstruction of the mandibular arch: Dr. Teresa Szupiany-Janeczek).

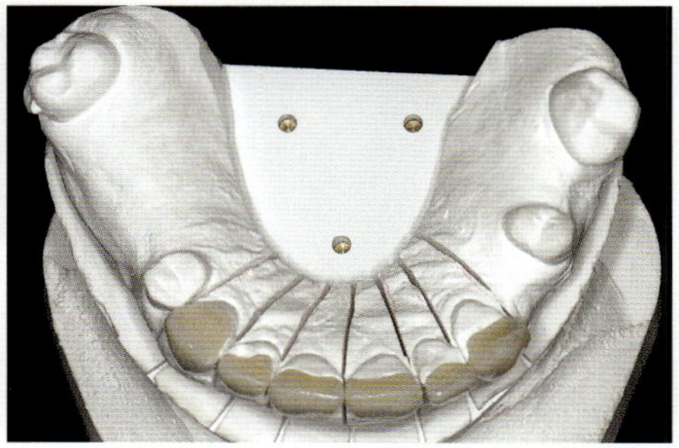

Fig 10-7k
No-prep indirect composite restorations on the cast.

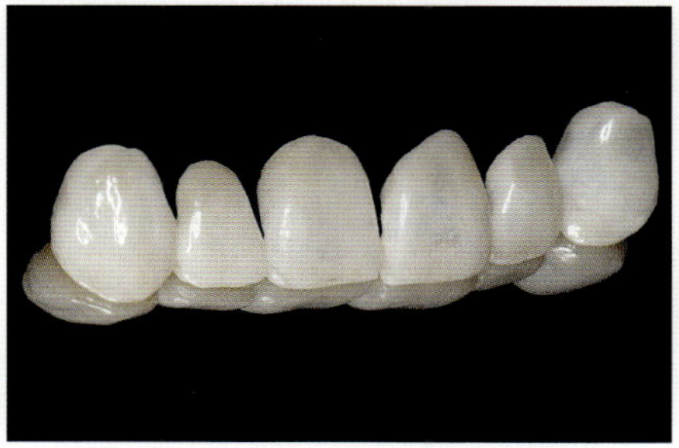

Fig 10-7l
No-prep indirect composite restorations (Enamel Plus) ready for cementation (laboratory work: DT Roman Frączek).

The dental technician was asked not to pay attention to existing undercuts (Fig 10-7m) as these would be filled with direct composite resin. The restorations were tried in, checked for esthetics, followed by cementation. Teeth were isolated with a rubber dam, airborne-particle abraded with an air abrasion unit (27 μm aluminum oxide), etched, rinsed, dried, and the bonding system was applied (Figs 10-7n to 10-7q). The cementing composite resin (Enamel Plus, Micerium) was heated in the same way as for porcelain veneer cementation and then applied to the inner surface of the restoration before the veneers were placed in the correct position (Figs 10-7r and 10-7s). Any marginal gaps resulting from the worn teeth anatomy (abfractions, erosions, abrasions) were filled with the direct composite resin – the same one used in the lab while fabricating the indirect restorations (Fig 10-7t).

Veneers on the two central incisors were light-cured only after ensuring they were in the correct position (Figs 10-7u and 10-7 v). After complete polymerization of each side (60 seconds), the excess material was removed with a scalpel no. 12 (Fig 10-7w). Then, the restoration margins were finished with a Profin contra-angle handpiece (Figs 10-7x and 10-7y). In the next phase, the veneers were cemented on the lateral incisors (Figs 10-7z to 10-7bb) and the canines (Fig 10-7cc). The result after the no-prep veneers cementation is shown in Fig 10-7dd.

Because the patient had problems with precise mandible closure and determining the occlusal contact points following cementation, a quick deprogramming was performed (30 minutes) using a small amount of direct composite resin light-cured on the palatal surface of the central incisors (Figs 10-7ee and 10-7ff). Then, reducing step by step the composite resin from the surface of the "fast deprogrammer" (Fig 10-7gg), the patient's occlusion was equilibrated until bilateral, multiple, and simultaneous contact points between the opposing teeth were achieved. The final result of treatment a few months after cementation is presented in Figs 10-7hh and 10-7ii. The clinical situation after delivering the skeletal dentures is shown in Fig 10-7jj. The 12-month follow-up is presented in Figs 10-7kk and 10-7ll.

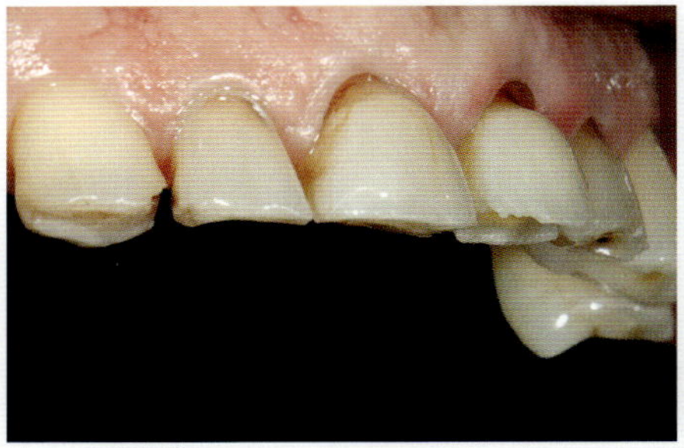

Fig 10-7m
The photograph shows the extent of tooth structure loss due to many factors, such as attrition, erosion, abfraction or abrasions.

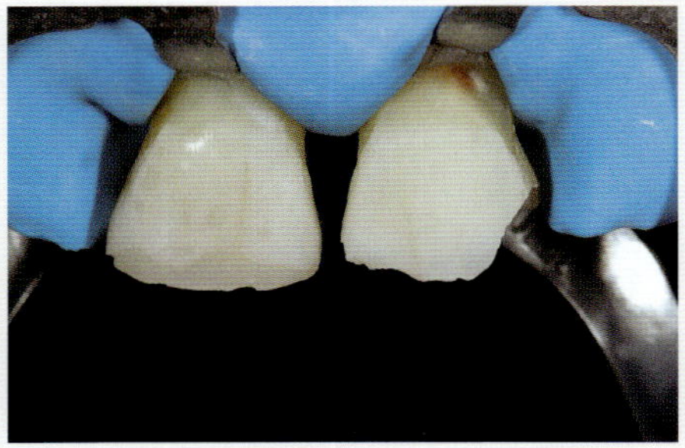

Fig 10-7n
Rubber dam isolation of the maxillary central incisors: the situation after airborne-particle abrasion with aluminum oxide particles.

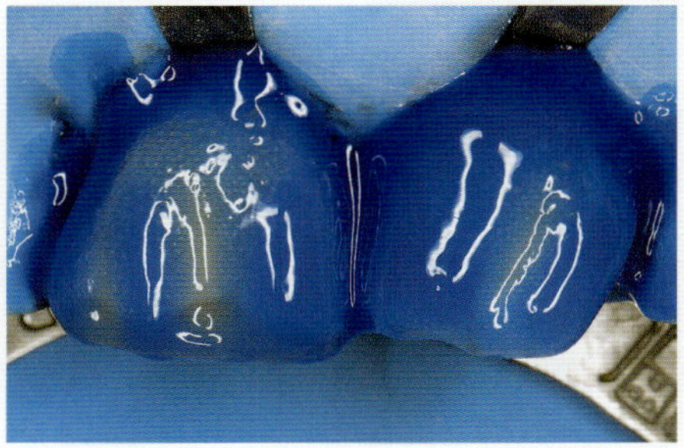

Fig 10-7o
Etching with orthophosphoric acid.

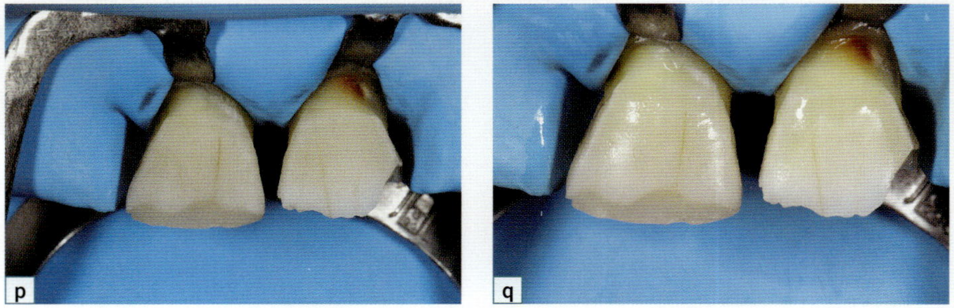

Figs 10-7p and 10-7q
Situation after (p) etching, rinsing, and drying, (q) followed by bonding system application.

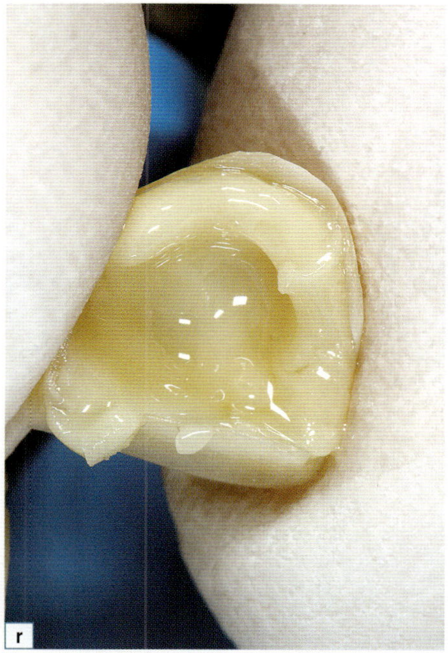

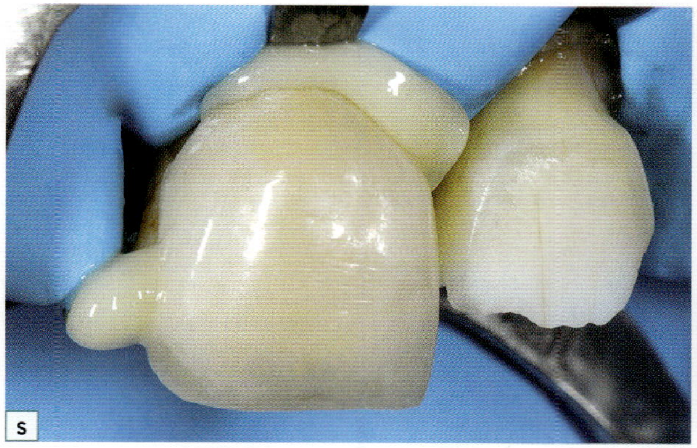

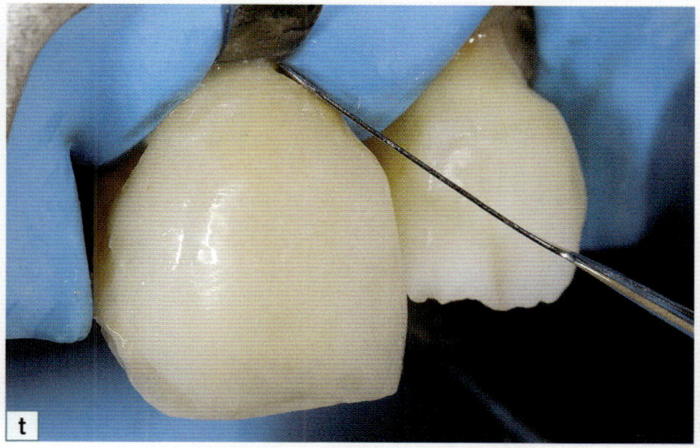

Figs 10-7r to 10-7t
(r) A heated composite (Enamel Plus UD3) was applied to the inner surfaces of the indirect restoration; (s) cementation on tooth 11. (t) The excess material had been thoroughly removed, and the margin gaps (caused by numerous undercuts and lack of preparation) had been filled directly with the composite resin.

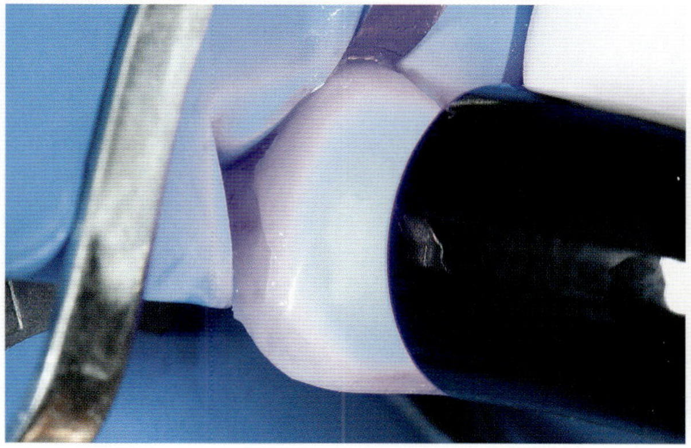

Fig 10-7u
After inserting the second restoration on the maxillary left central incisor and ensuring it was correctly positioned, the luting cement was polymerized.

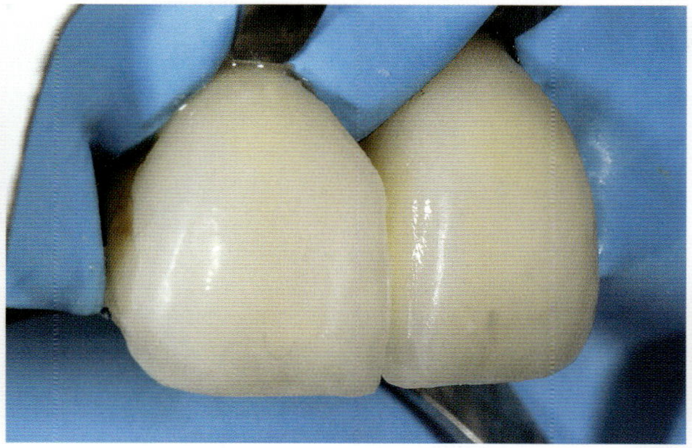

Fig 10-7v
Situation after light-curing two maxillary central incisors.

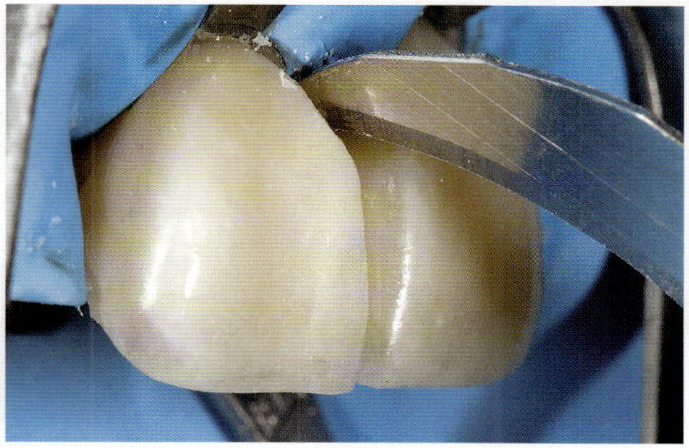

Fig 10-7w
Removal of the polymerized composite resin excess with a scalpel no. 12.

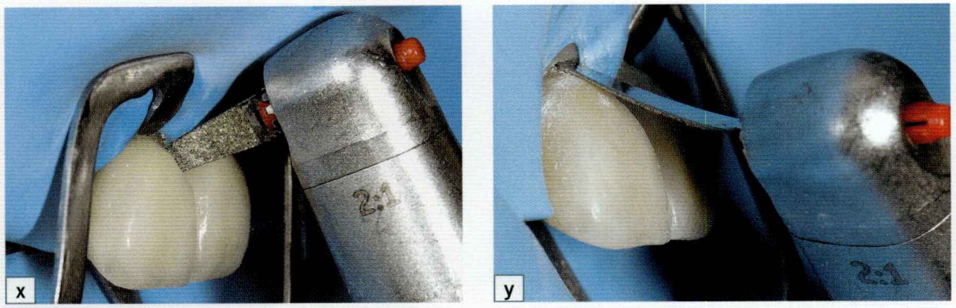

Figs 10-7x and 10-7y
Removal of polymerized excess material with a Profin contra-angle handpiece.

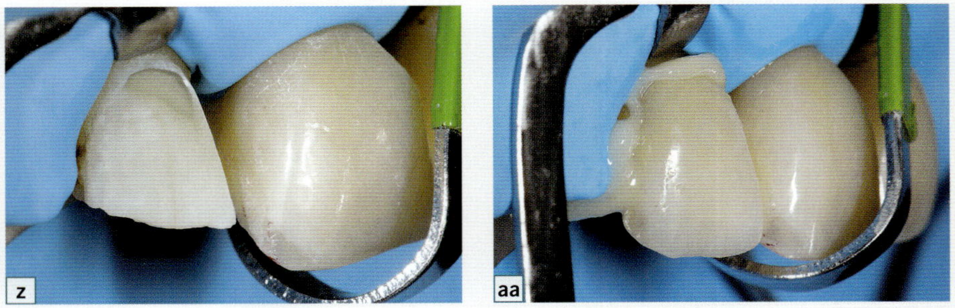

Figs 10-7z and 10-7aa
(z) Situation after isolating the maxillary lateral incisors with a rubber dam and (aa) after the indirect restorations cementation with the heated composite.

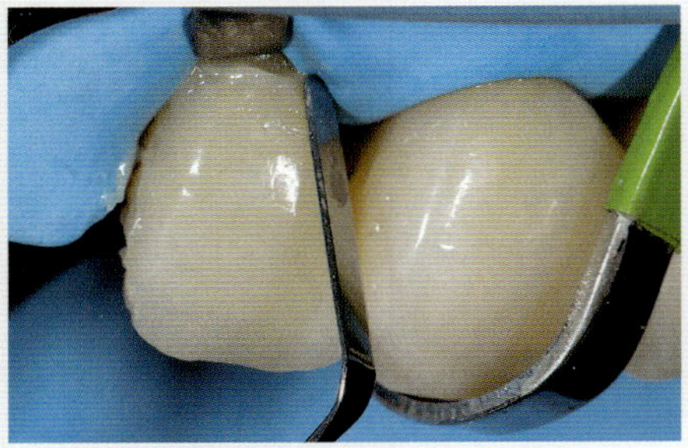

Fig 10-7bb
Marginal sealing with the same composite resin that was used for cementation.

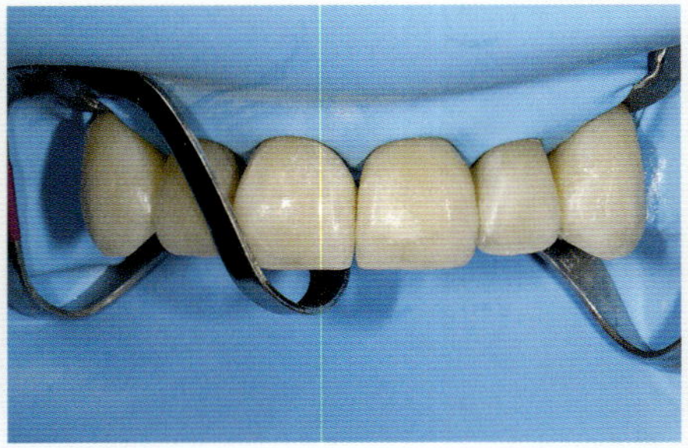

Fig 10-7cc
Clinical situation after cementation of six composite indirect restorations.

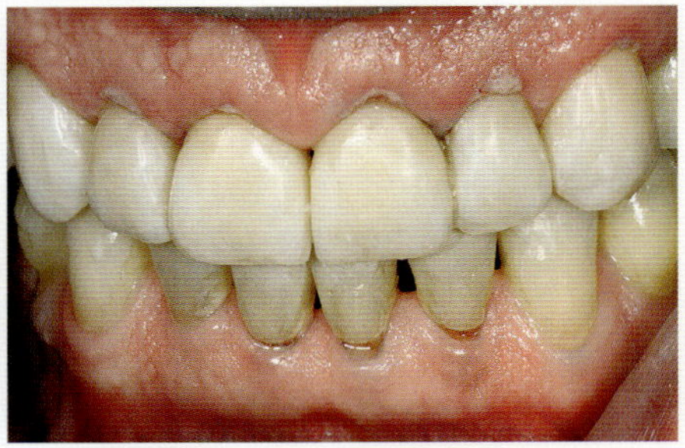

Fig 10-7dd
Situation after removing the rubber dam.

PRACTITIONER'S ADVICE

If you have difficulties identifying the premature contacts, perform the "quick deprogramming" with composite resin material light-cured on the palatal surfaces of the maxillary incisors!

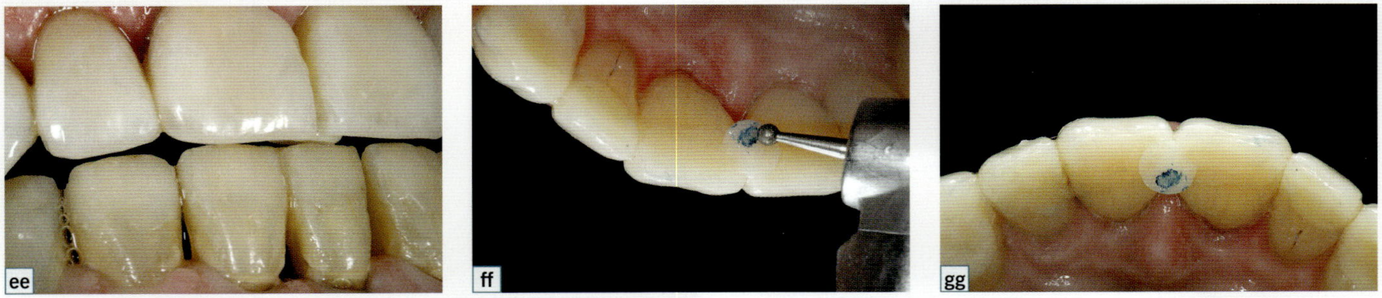

Figs 10-7ee to 10-7gg
Quick deprogramming enables muscle relaxation of the temporomandibular joint (TMJ) and facilitates proper occlusal equilibration.

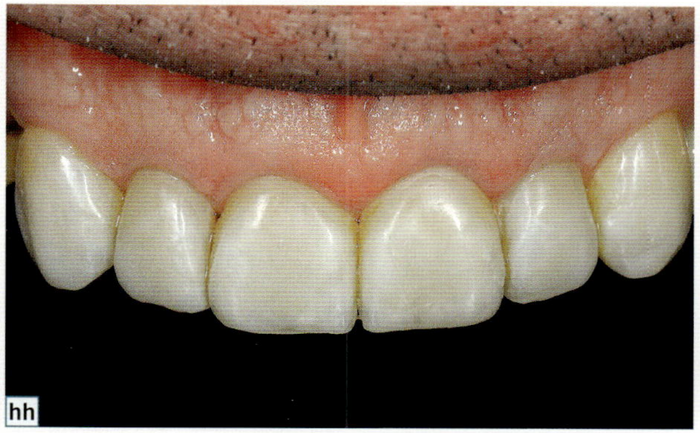

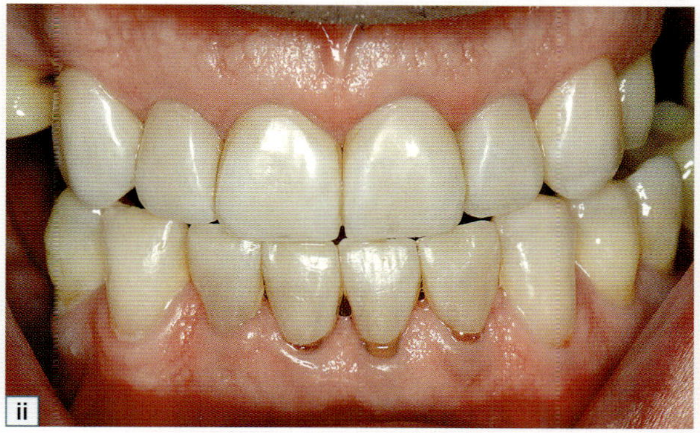

Figs 10-7hh and 10-7ii
Final result a few months after final cementation.

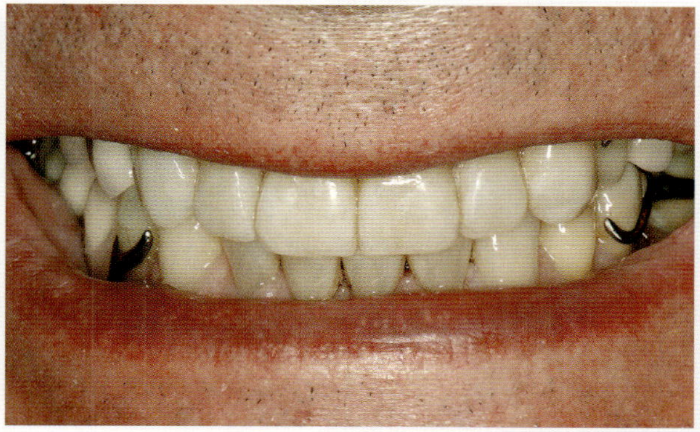

Fig 10-7jj
Clinical situation after delivering the skeletal dentures restoring missing teeth (as an alternative solution before implant placement can be performed).

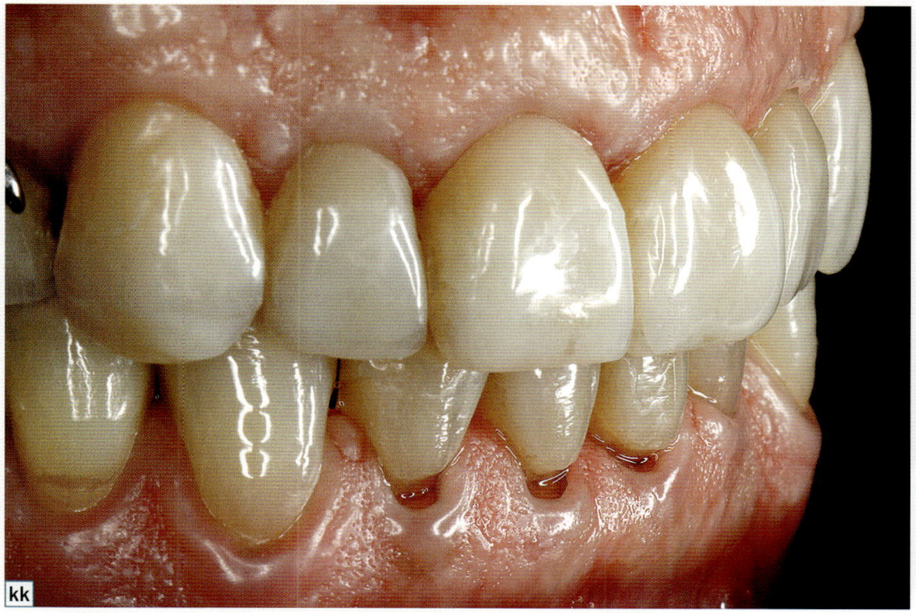

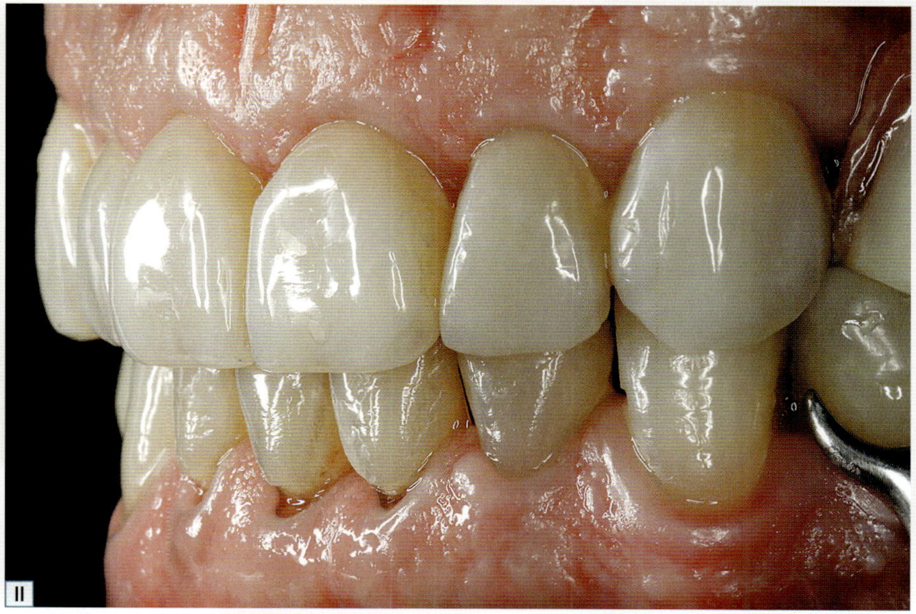

Figs 10-7kk and 10-7ll
Clinical follow-up after 12 months.

OTHER SOLUTIONS FOR ESTHETIC PROBLEMS

In the past decades, we have often seen restorative treatments involving extensive tooth preparation, even in controversial situations.[31] This was related to the trend of covering the teeth with ceramics or composites.

One such controversial indication was enamel hypoplasia in a clinical form of white spots. Today, many of these problems can be solved by the resin infiltration technique. This method was developed in the 1970s with the intention of treating initial caries, but only a decade ago it was commercialized as the Icon product (DMG). In this technique, after appropriate white spots etching (multiple etching of the lesion with 15% hydrochloric acid and dehydration with ethanol), the resin infiltrates it, replacing the demineralization areas. As a result of the histological similarity of initial carious spots and white spots caused by fluorosis, resin infiltration also has excellent results in these kinds of cases. It is due to the alteration of the refractive index, which is similar in value to the changes observed in healthy enamel.

Before infiltrating the anterior teeth with resin, it is recommended to whiten them, which is especially beneficial in case of amber or brownish spots, which can be turned by the bleaching agent into white spots, more susceptible to acid action and infiltration. Bleaching also reduces the contrast between the white spots and the surrounding tissues. The resin infiltration brings a better final esthetic outcome.[31–35] For deep lesions, which can be confirmed with the illumination technique, the acid action and the resin penetration can be insufficient. Therefore, microabrasion is recommended in order to remove the outer layer of the discolored enamel and allow easier penetration of resin monomers. It is important to eliminate the water from the micropores caused by the erosive acid action!

Case 6: White spots on the teeth

A 19-year-old female patient presented to the dental office because of white and amber-brownish spots on teeth 11, 33, and 42 (Fig 10-8a). The patient had already visited the dental office 5 years ago, but at that time it was decided not to perform the whitening procedure due to her young age, and the resin infiltration technique was not at that time widespread (Figs 10-8b and 10-8c). A thorough analysis of photographs was performed (Figs 10-8d to 10-8f), and the patient was qualified for teeth whitening. For this, 10% carbamide peroxide was utilized using splints for 2 weeks during nighttime. The post-bleach inspection confirmed the transformation of the brown spots into white spots (Figs 10-8g and 10-8h). At the next appointment, 3 weeks after bleaching, the resin infiltration was tested on the white spots of mandibular teeth (Fig 10-8i). A gentle microabrasion was performed with 27 μm aluminum oxide, and hydrochloric acid was applied to the white spots for 120 seconds (Icon-Etch, DMG), and rubbed in with a microbrush (Fig 10-8j). Next, the acid was rinsed with water spray for 30 seconds and dried thoroughly.

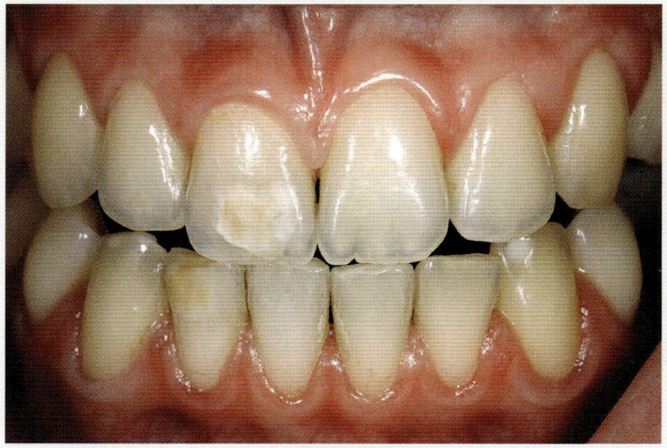

Fig 10-8a Intraoral photograph of the patient who presented to the dental office to improve the esthetics of teeth 11, 33, and 42.

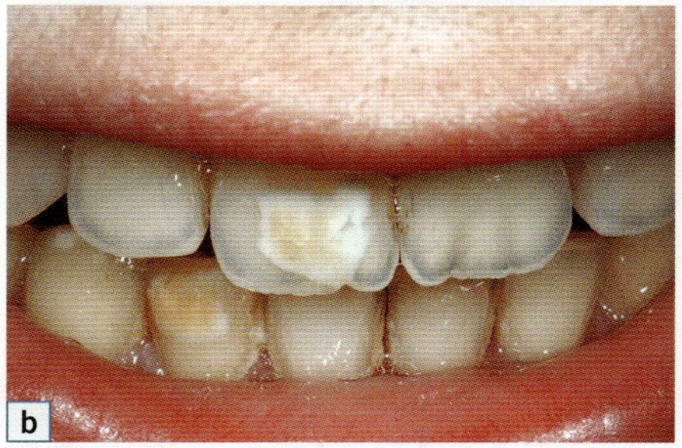

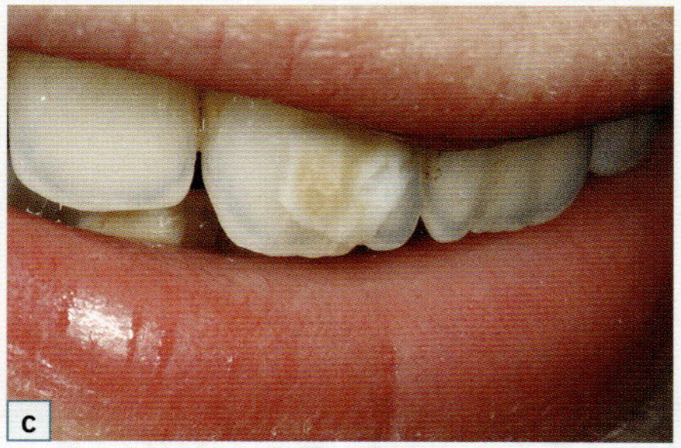

Figs 10-8b and 10-8c Photographs of the patient's smile taken 5 years ago, she presented for the first appointment in our dental office.

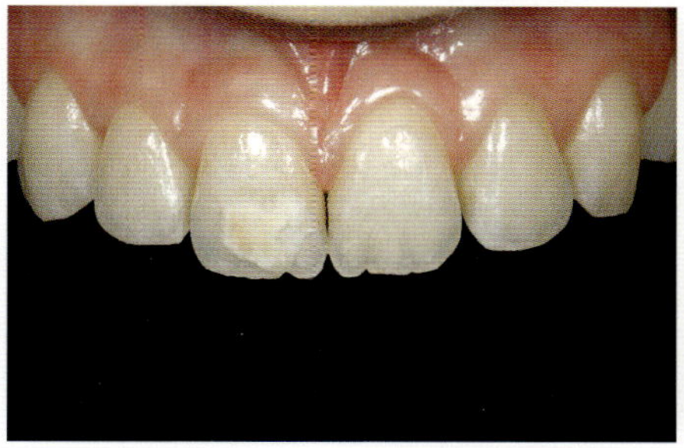

Fig 10-8d
Maxillary anterior teeth with white spots.

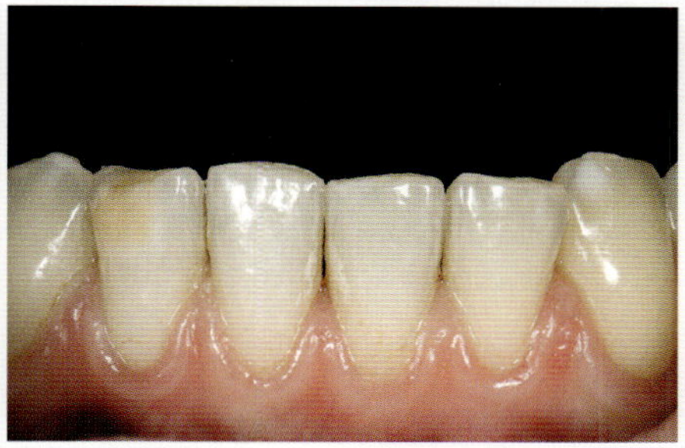

Fig 10-8e
Mandibular anterior teeth with white spots.

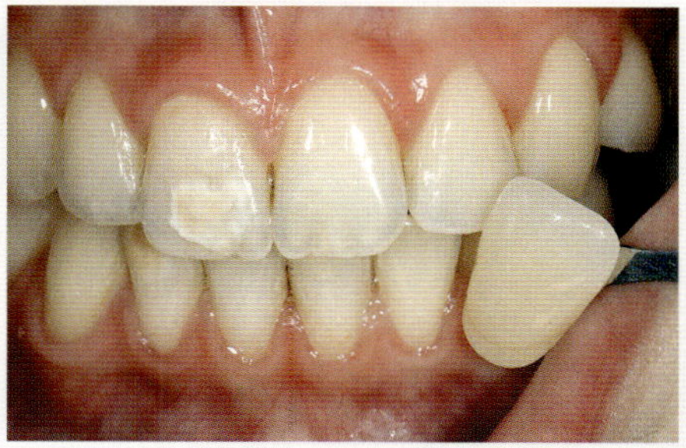

Fig 10-8f
Color of the teeth compared to the Vita shade guide before whitening.

PRACTITIONER'S ADVICE

Before performing resin infiltration, it is highly recommended that the patient undergoes teeth whitening!

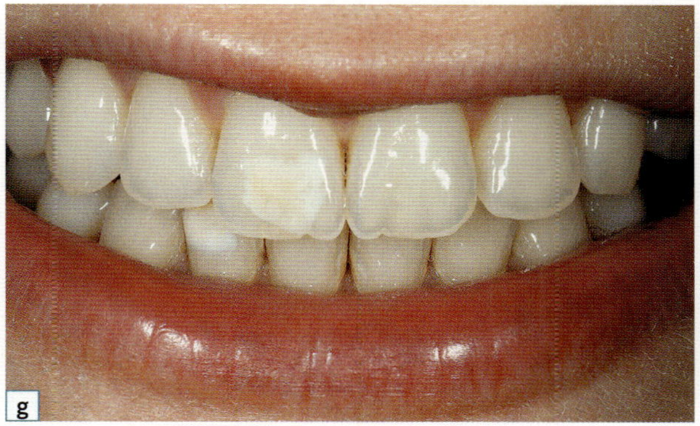

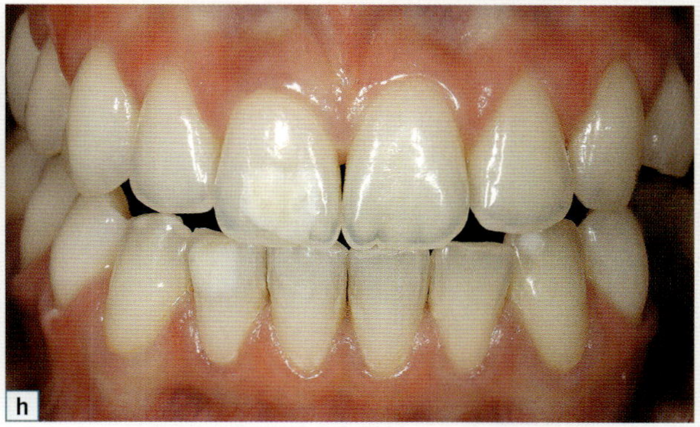

Figs 10-8g and 10-8h
Clinical situation after tooth whitening with 10% carbamide peroxide: (g) photograph of the patient's smile and (h) intraoral photograph.

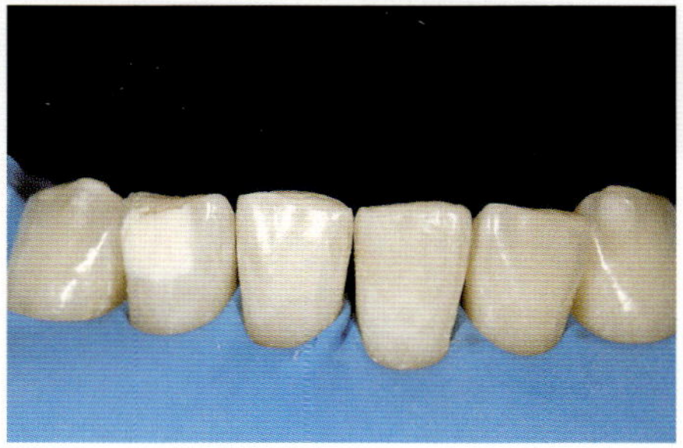

Fig 10-8i
Rubber dam isolation of the mandibular anterior teeth.

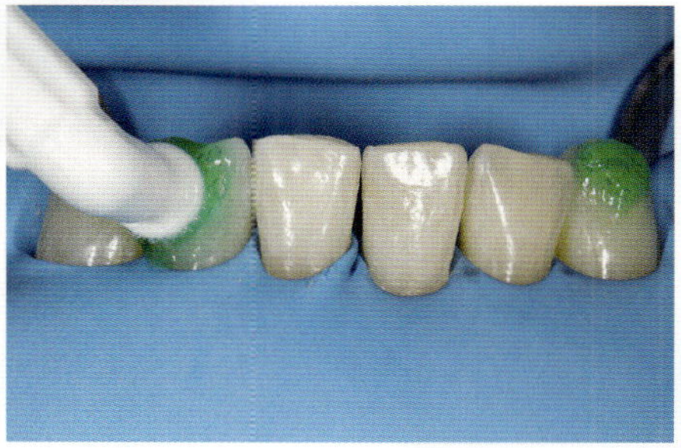

Fig 10-8j
15% hydrochloric acid was applied to the white spots and rubbed into the tooth surface.

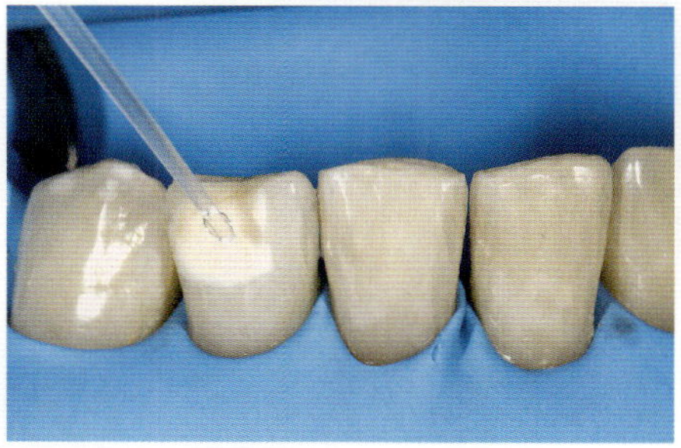

Fig 10-8k
Dehydration through a 30-second application of 99% ethanol (Icon Dry).

Dehydration occurs through a 30-second application of 99% ethanol (Icon Dry) (Fig 10-8k), but some authors recommend keeping ethanol on the tooth surface for up to 120 seconds. The hydrochloric acid, then ethanol sequence should be repeated up to four times in the same way (Figs 10-8l and 10-8m). After several repetitions of the sequence, the white spot appears to be a lot less opaque and almost disappears. At this moment, the tooth surface should be dried in order to evaporate the ethanol.

In the next step, the proper infiltration with TEGDMA resin is obtained. This resin is more liquid and resistant to the water environment. After applying it on the tooth surface, it is recommended to leave it for three minutes and then light-cured for 40 seconds (Fig10-8n). The infiltration process should be repeated – leaving the resin for one minute and light-curing after applying a layer of glycerin to minimize the oxygen inhibition layer (Fig 10-8o). After polymerization, gentle polishing can proceed (Fig 10-8p) using a Goat-Hair Brush (Shiny S) and 1 μm diamond paste (Enamel Plus Shiny B).

Teeth 42 and 33 were infiltrated according to the described procedure (Fig 10-8q). At the next appointment, an identical procedure was performed for the right central incisor of the maxilla. By testing the technique on the less "esthetically sensitive" mandibular arch, it was possible to discuss the treatment effect with the patient and proceed with the treatment on the tooth in the maxillary arch. The procedures were repeated according to principles described earlier (Figs 10-8r to 10-8x).

The final effect of transforming white spots using the resin infiltration technique is presented in Figs 10-8y to 10-8aa.

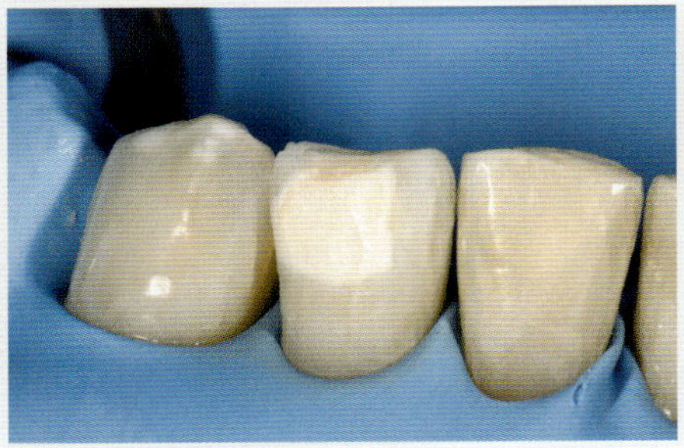

Fig 10-8l
Situation after subsequent etching with the hydrochloric acid ...

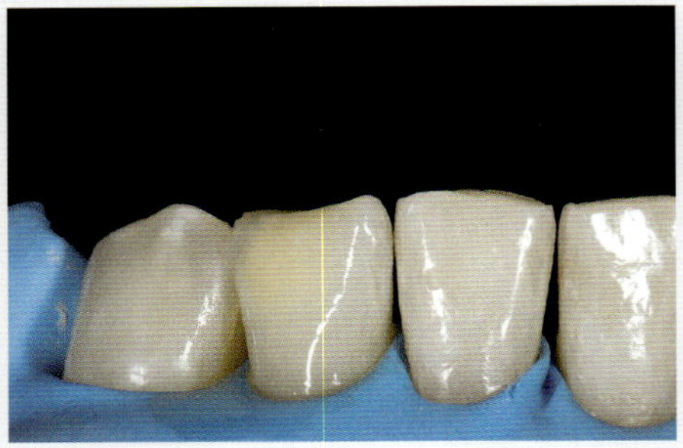

Fig 10-8m
... and after the final application of ethanol.

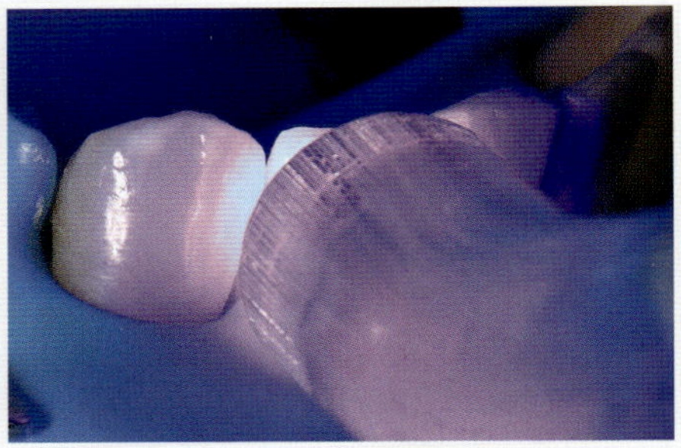

Fig 10-8n
Now, when the matte and white dental tissues have become more translucent, the resin with high fluidity was applied. Three minutes later, it was light-cured for 40 seconds.

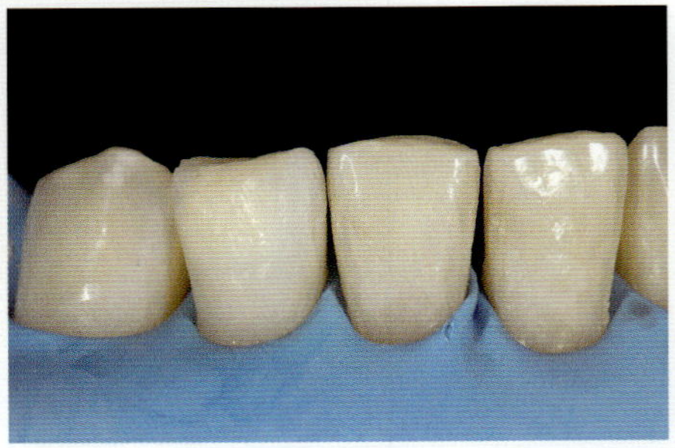

Fig 10-8o
Clinical situation after final polymerization of the resin.

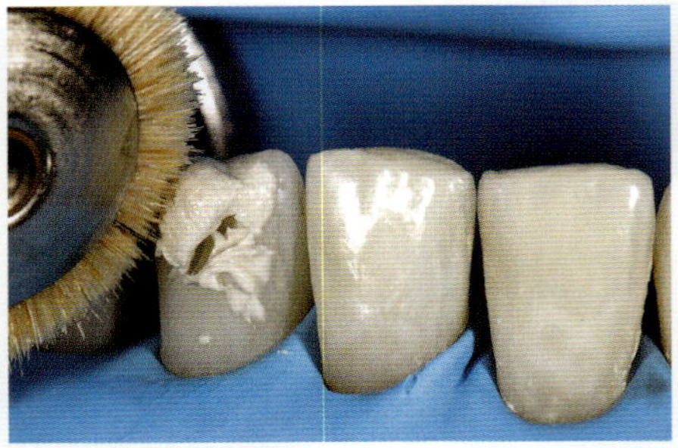

Fig 10-8p
Polishing with a Goat-Hair Brush and 1 μm diamond paste.

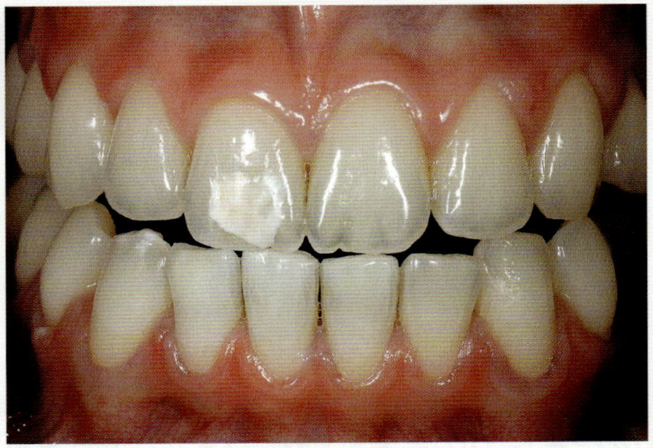

Fig 10-8q
Clinical situation after the alteration of the white spots' translucency, thanks to resin infiltration.

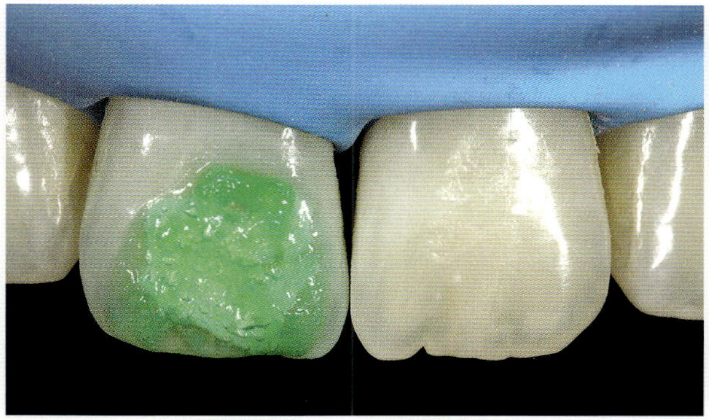

Fig 10-8r
Isolation with rubber dam and application of hydrochloric acid on the white spot on tooth 11.

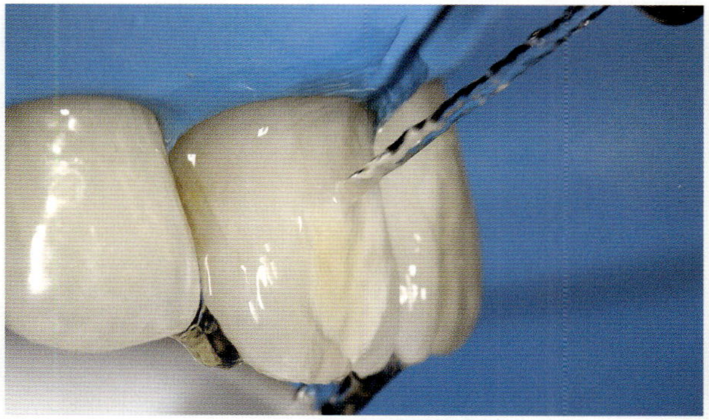

Fig 10-8s
Thorough rinsing of hydrochloric acid.

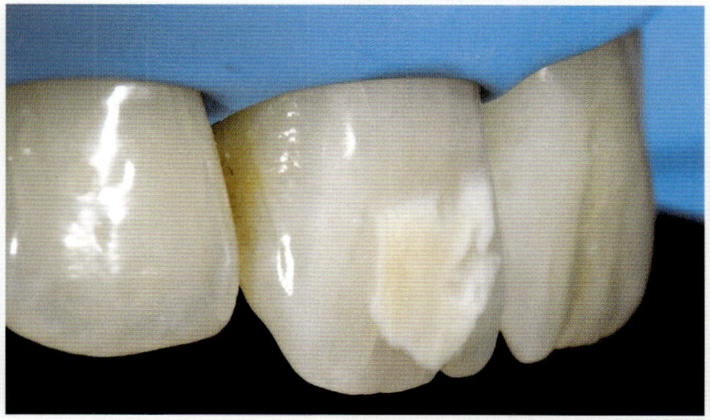

Fig 10-8t
Situation before the application of ethanol.

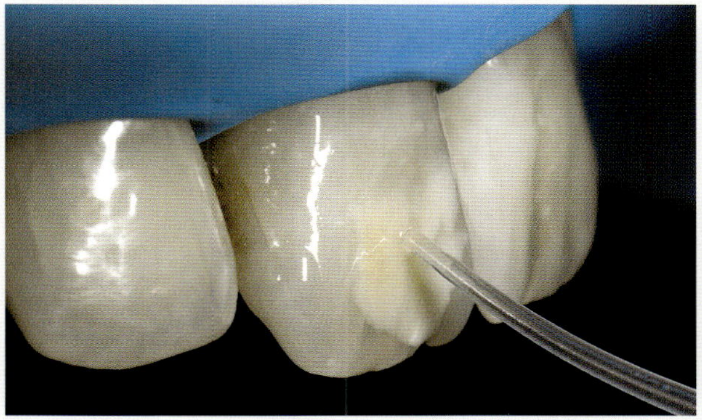

Fig 10-8u
Ethanol is applied on the matte and white spots.

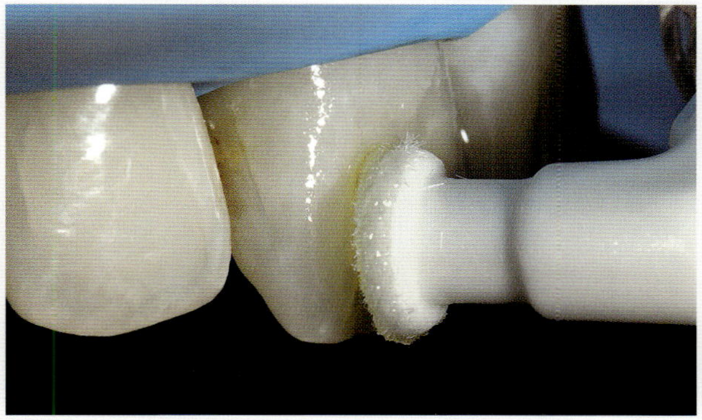

Fig 10-8v
Rubbing the resin into the tooth surface.

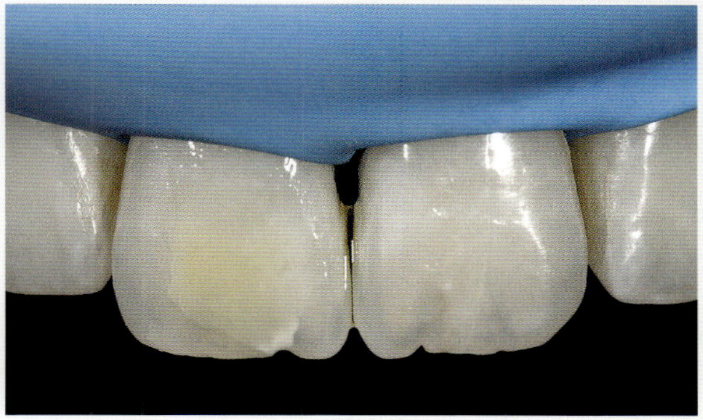

Fig 10-8w
Situation after resin application.

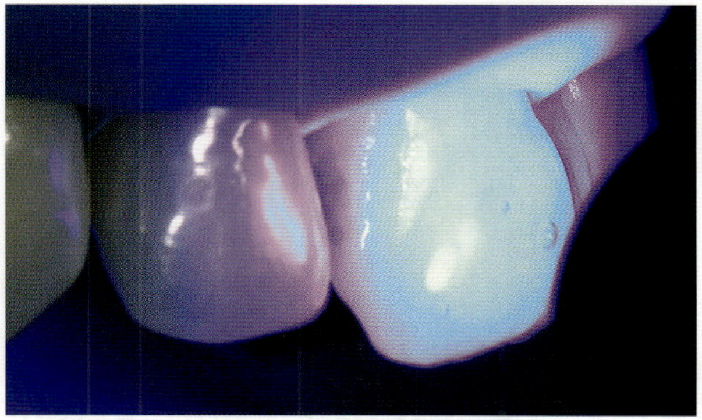

Fig 10-8x
Polymerization of the resin with a light-curing lamp.

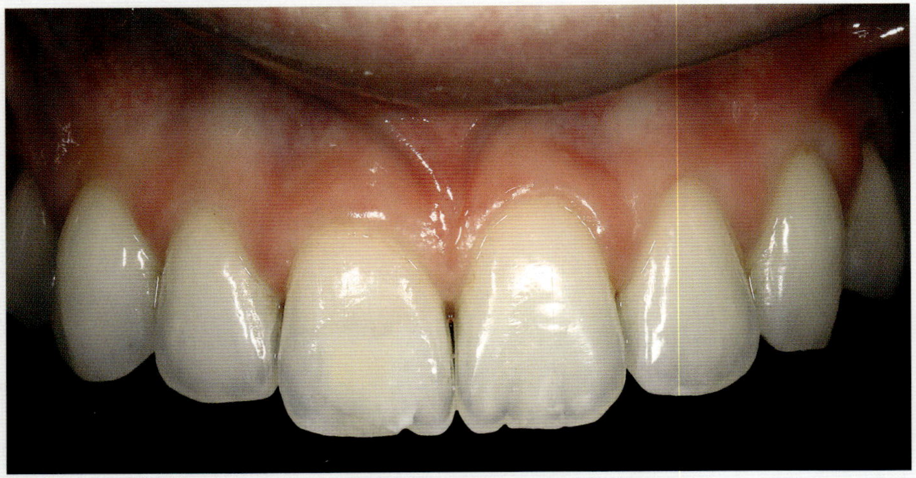

Fig 10-8y
Clinical situation after completing the treatment of white spots on tooth 11.

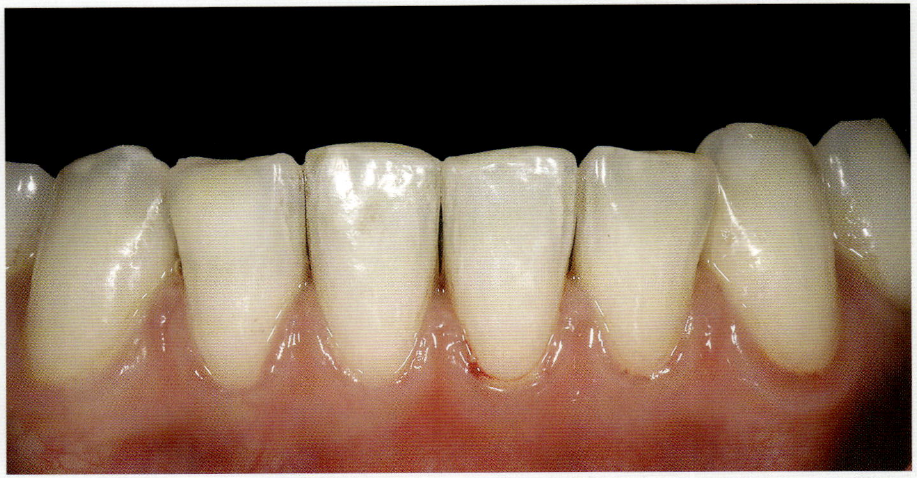

Fig 10-8z
Clinical situation after treatment of white spots on teeth 42 and 33.

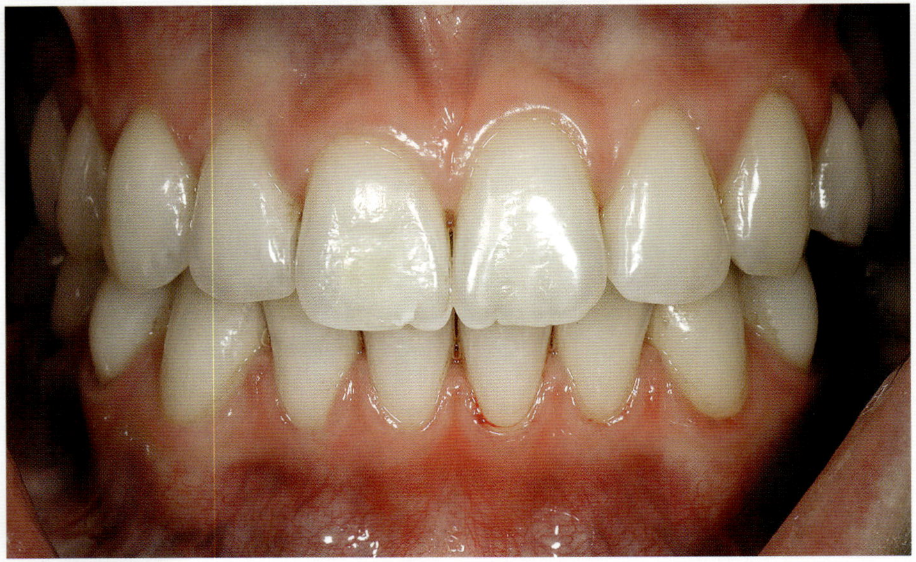

Fig 10-8aa
Clinical follow-up several months after treatment with resin infiltration.

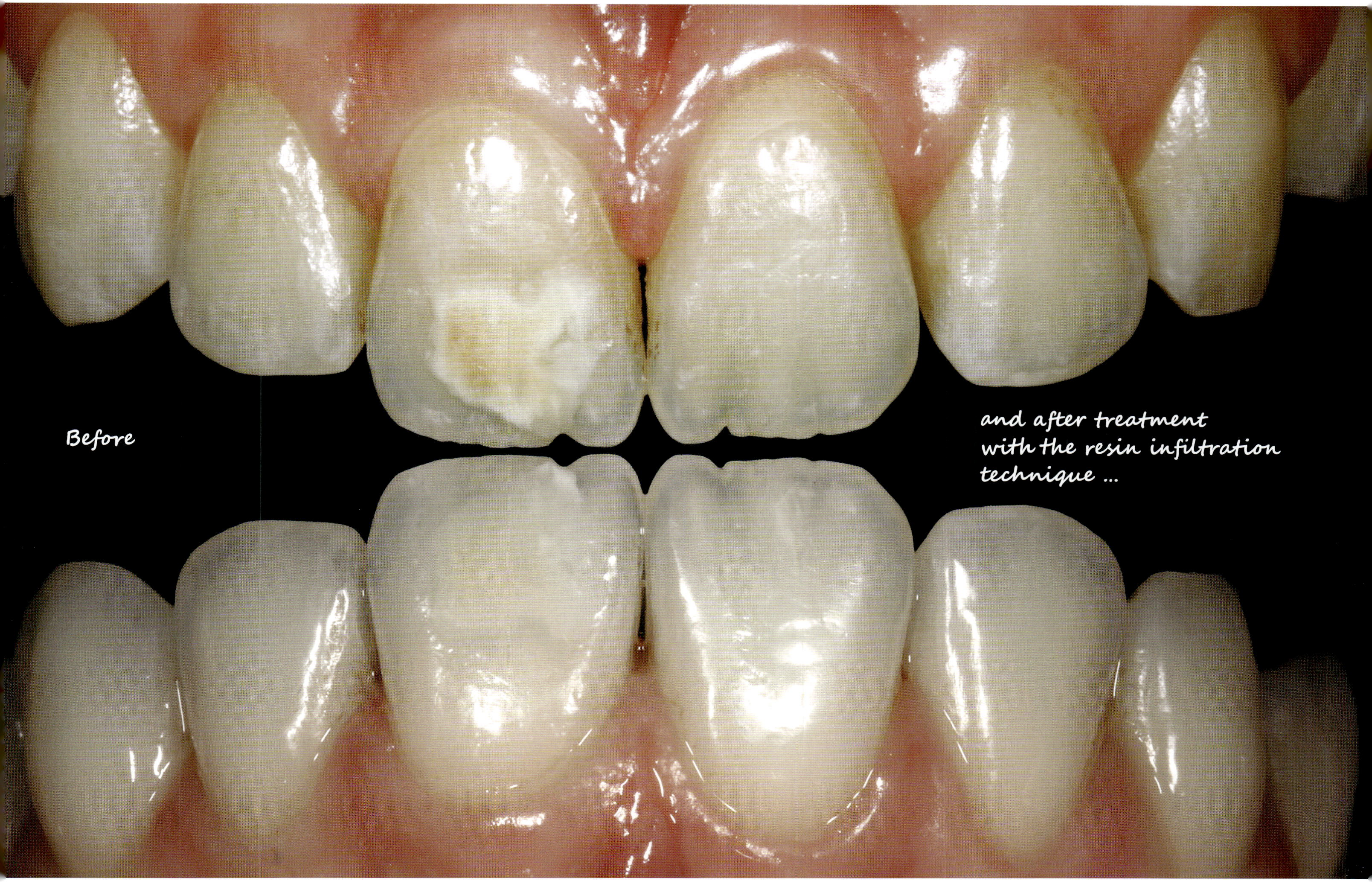
Before
and after treatment
with the resin infiltration
technique ...

REFERENCES

1. Zarow M, D'Arcangelo C, D'Amario M, Marzo G. Conservative approach for the management of congenital bilateral agenesis of permanent mandibular incisors: case report and literature review. Eur J Paediatr Dent 2015;16:154–158.
2. Devoto W, Saracinelli M, Manauta J. Composite in everyday practice: how to choose the right material and simplify application techniques in the anterior teeth. Eur J Esthet Dent 2010;5:102–124.
3. Devoto W, Pansecchi D. Composite restorations in the anterior region: clinical and aesthetic performances. Pract Proced Aesthet Dent 2007;19:465–470.
4. Yanikian C, Yanikian F, Sundfeld D, Lins R, Martins L. Direct composite resin veneers in nonvital teeth: a still viable alternative to mask dark substrates. Oper Dent 2019;44: 159–166.
5. Van de Sande FH, Moraes RR, Elias RV, Montagner AF, Rodolpho PA, Demarco FF, Cenci MS. Is composite repair suitable for anterior restorations? A long-term practice-based clinical study. Clin Oral Investig 2019;23:2795–2803.
6. Collares K, Opdam NJM, Laske M, Bronkhorst EM, Demarco FF, Correa MB, Huysmans MCDNJM. Longevity of anterior composite restorations in a general dental practice-based network. J Dent Res 2017;96:1092–1099.
7. Casagrande L, Laske M, Bronkhorst EM, Huysmans MCDNJM, Opdam NJM. Repair may increase survival of direct posterior restorations – a practice-based study. J Dent 2017;64:30–36.
8. Paolone G, Orsini G, Manauta J, Devoto W, Putignano A. Composite shade guides and color matching. Int J Esthet Dent 2014;9:164–182.
9. Villarroel M, Fahl N, De Sousa AM, De Oliveira OB Jr. Direct esthetic restorations based on translucency and opacity of composite resins. J Esthet Restor Dent 2011;23:73–87.
10. Terry DA. Dimensions of color: creating high-diffusion layers with composite resin. Compend Contin Educ Dent 2003;24(Suppl 2):3–13.
11. Terry DA. Direct applications of a nanocomposite resin system: Part 2 – Procedures for anterior restorations. Pract Proced Aesthet Dent 2004;16:677–684.
12. Terry DA. Developing natural aesthetics with direct composite restorations. Pract Proced Aesthet Dent 2004;16:45–52.
13. Terry DA. Restoring the incisal edge. N Y State Dent J 2005;71:30–35.
14. Vanini L, Mangani FM. Determination and communication of color using the five color dimensions of teeth. Pract Proced Aesthet Dent 2001;13:19–26.
15. Vanini L, De Simone F, Tammaro S. Indirect composite restorations in the anterior region: a predictable technique for complex cases. Pract Periodontics Aesthet Dent 1997;9: 795–802.
16. Fahl Júnior N. The direct/indirect composite resin veneers: a case report. Pract Periodontics Aesthet Dent 1996;8:627–638.
17. Baratieri LN, Araujo E, Monteiro S Jr. Color in natural teeth and direct resin composite restorations: essential aspects. Eur J Esthet Dent 2007;2:172–186.
18. Zarow M. Nonvital tooth bleaching: a case discussion for the clinical practice. Compend Contin Educ Dent 2016;37:268–276.
19. Baratieri LN, Ritter AV, Monteiro S Jr, Caldeira de Andrada MA, Cardoso Vieira LC. Nonvital tooth bleaching: guidelines for the clinician. Quintessence Int 1995;26:597–608.
20. Plotino G, Buono L, Grande NM, Pameijer CH, Somma F. Nonvital tooth bleaching: a review of the literature and clinical procedures. J Endod 2008;34:394–407.
21. Zarow M, Szczeklik K. Faccette dirette in composito come prevenzione della discolorazione dopo lo sbiancamento di denti non vitali. Case report. Il Dentista Moderno 2015;9: 126–134.
22. Greenwall L. Tooth Whitening Techniques. Boca Raton, FL: CRC Press, 2017.
23. Zarow M, Ramírez-Sebastià A, Paolone G, et al. A new classification system for the restoration of root filled teeth. Int Endod J 2018;51:318–334.
24. Dietschi D. Nonvital bleaching: general considerations and report of two failure cases. Eur J Esthet Dent 2006;1:52–61.
25. Garcia-Godoy F, Dodge WW, Donohue M, O'Quinn JA. Composite resin bond strength after enamel bleaching. Oper Dent 1993;18:144–147.
26. Lai SC, Mak YF, Cheung GS, et al. Reversal of compromised bonding to oxidized etched dentin. J Dent Res. 2001;80:1919–1924.
27. Villares CF. Shape modification with Unica anterior. Available at: www.styleitaliano.org/shape-modification-with-unica-anterior/
28. Ottoboni T. Direct veneers, the single incisor challenge. Available at: www.styleitaliano.org/direct-veneers-the-single-incisor-challenge/
29. Saracinelli M. Direct composite for no-prep aesthetics & function. Available at: www. styleitaliano.org/aesthetics-function-a-no-prep-direct-composite-case/
30. Kois JC. Occlusal vertical dimension: what is the controversy? Compend Contin Educ Dent 1997;18:1164.
31. Bamashmous MS. Veneer or Interproximal Enamel Reduction? J Contemp Dent Pract 2018;19:749–751.
32. Meyer-Lueckel H, Chatzidakis A, Naumann M, Dörfer CE, Paris S. Influence of application time on penetration of an infiltrant into natural enamel caries. J Dent 2011;39:465–469.
33. Tirlet G, Chabouis HF, Attal JP. Infiltration, a new therapy for masking enamel white spots: a 19-month follow-up case series. Eur J Esthet Dent 2013;8:180–190.
34. Borges AB, Caneppele TM, Masterson D, Maia LC. Is resin infiltration an effective esthetic treatment for enamel development defects and white spot lesions? A systematic review. J Dent 2017;56:11–18.
35. Kim S, Kim EY, Jeong TS, Kim JW. The evaluation of resin infiltration for masking labial enamel white spot lesions. Int J Paediatr Dent 2011;21:241–248.
36. Zarow M. Brown and white spots on teeth: micro-invasive treatment. Available at: www.styleitaliano.org/brown-white-spots-teeth-micro-invasive-treatment/

CHAPTER 10+

DIGITAL VENEERS

DANIELE RONDONI

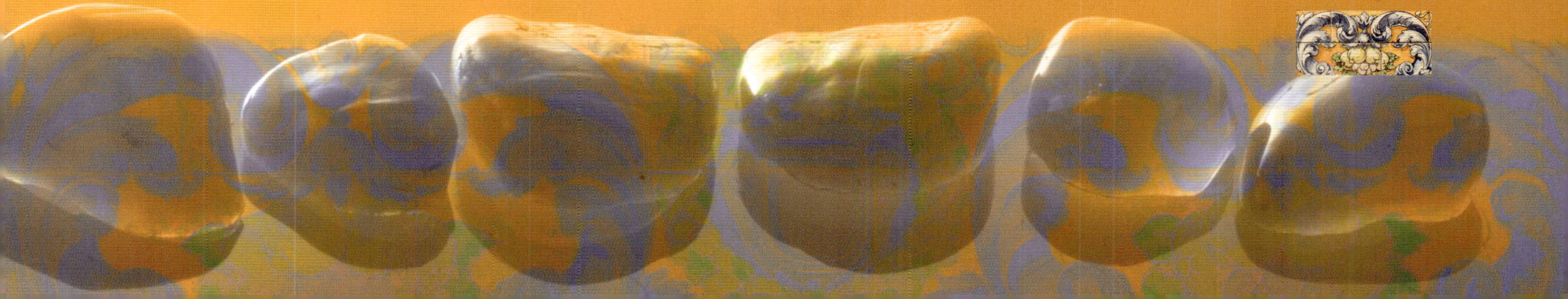

Traditional laboratory
procedures can now be
simplified and accelerated
through digital workflow.
The variety of material
solutions available
with the digital option
allows you to choose
the appropriate technique
for a given treatment plan,
which may affect
the final quality
of the prosthetic work ...

Digital veneers

Digital protocols, which have become widely implemented in dentistry in recent years, have brought revolutionary change in work organization due to the new generation of materials and greater possibilities offered by work based on the concept of a "design" in clinical management.

PORCELAIN VENEERS: A DIGITAL PLATFORM

This chapter presents the practical aspects of work organization between the dental office and the dental laboratory, necessary for digital planning and digital fabrication of porcelain veneers. Three clinical cases are discussed, showing the possibility of using various new materials. The possibility to use a material adequate for the planned treatment is a fundamental advantage now offered by digital laboratories. An additional advantage of digitization is the ability to work remotely. A dentist may work in the UK, and a dental technician, for example, in Italy, or vice versa. The power of today's technology and the reduced time of transferring digital impressions and other data means faster and more efficient work![1–4]

BENEFITS FOR THE DENTIST

- Control and predictability of the results
- Possibility to use all-new generation materials
- More options offered to the patients
- Improved quality with a reduced number of visits, which will be of shorter duration
- Ability to better understand patients' needs (communication via visualization)
- Improvement of communication with the dental laboratory and elimination of misunderstandings

BENEFITS FOR THE PATIENT

- Possibility to visualize the final result before starting treatment
- Higher level of trust in the dentist and the whole dental team
- Possibility to provide the dentist with all information about expectations and doubts
- Shorter treatment time

BENEFITS FOR THE DENTAL TECHNICIAN

- Possibility to use all-new generation materials
- All the possible prosthetic solutions can be shown to the dentist quickly and easily
- Preparation of the reconstruction project and presenting it to the dentist and the patient
- Possibility to predict potential problems and eliminate ineffective procedures
- Possibility to proceed simply by following established protocol
- Ability to spend more time on precise finishing of the restorations requiring manual work
- Obtaining synergy in cooperation with the dentist
- Shorter treatment time

PROCEDURE PROTOCOL

A 2D digital project is a preliminary template for an analog project, and can be checked in the patient's oral cavity through a mock-up – created with a silicone index and a polymerized composite resin.

Using a 3D program, a virtual reconstruction project is performed, along with the prototype model, which can be used to prepare the mock-up and to mill the final restoration immediately using digital methods.

Case 1: Esthetic treatment in the anterior segment (Figs 10-9a to 10-9i)

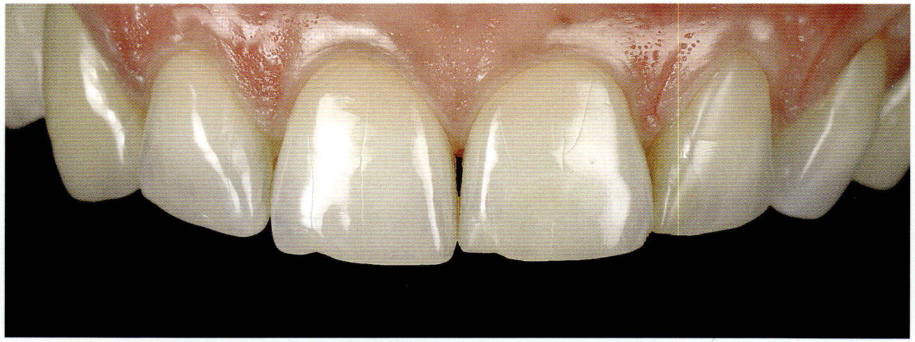

Fig 10-9a
The patient was initially qualified for esthetic improvement of the maxillary arch.

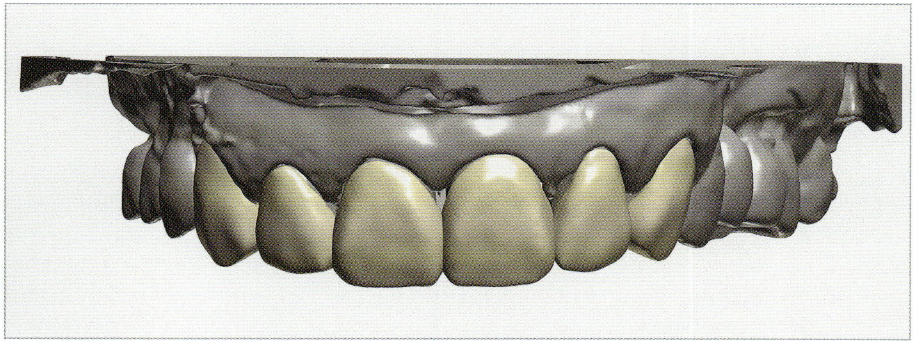

Fig 10-9b
3D digital design presenting the treatment plan.

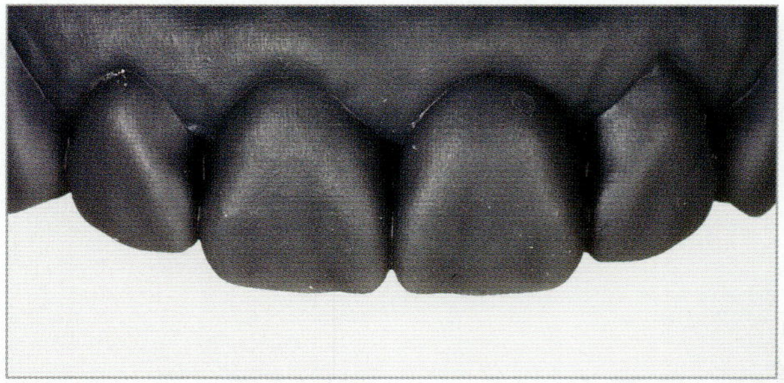

Fig 10-9c
Printed wax-up model.

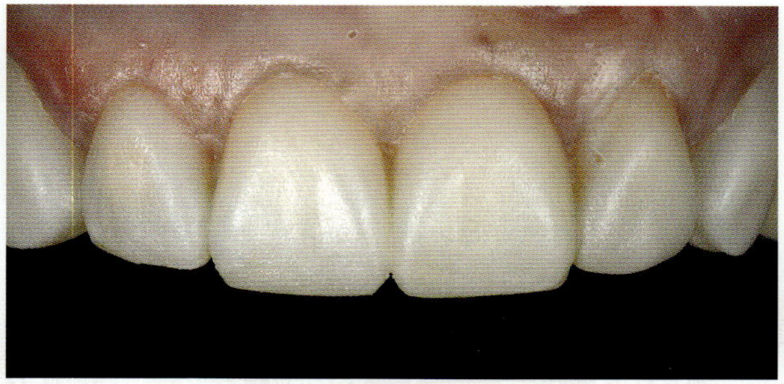

Fig 10-9d
Mock-up performed with a flowable composite.

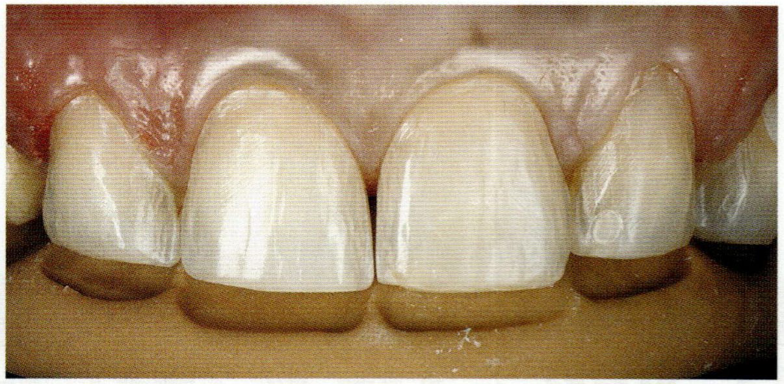

Fig 10-9e
Minimally invasive preparation controlled with the silicone index.

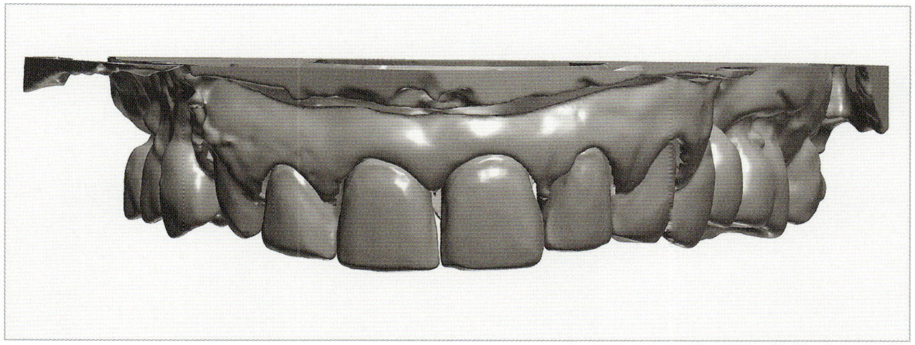

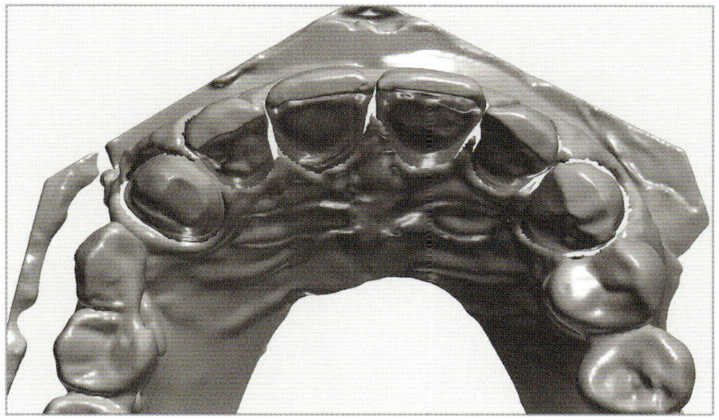

Fig 10-9f
3D digital image after minimally invasive tooth preparation.

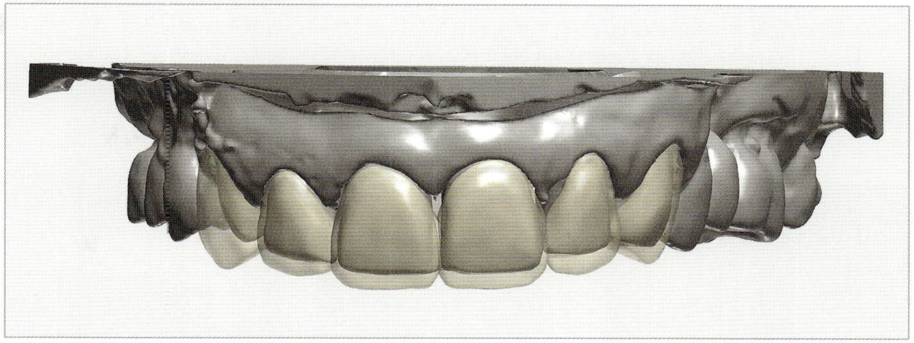

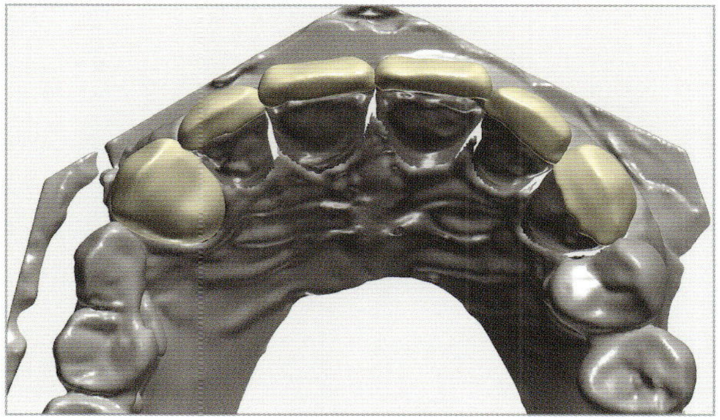

Fig 10-9g
Checking the digital design after applying it on the model with teeth after preparation.

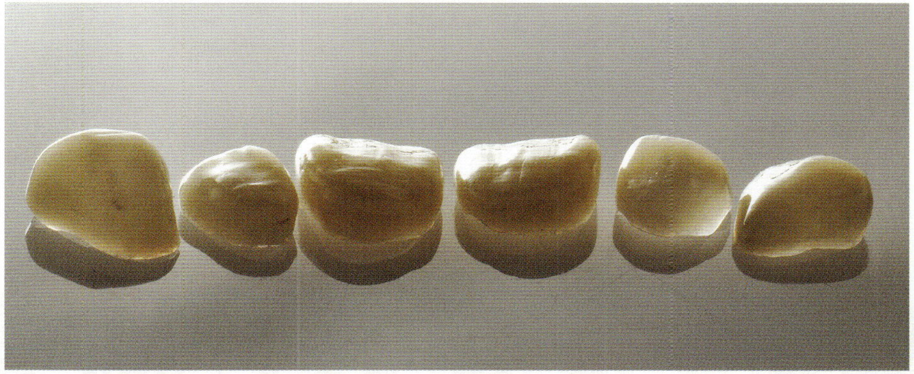

Fig 10-9h
Six lithium disilicate veneers without the need for cutting back, thanks to the new liquid ceramic technology.

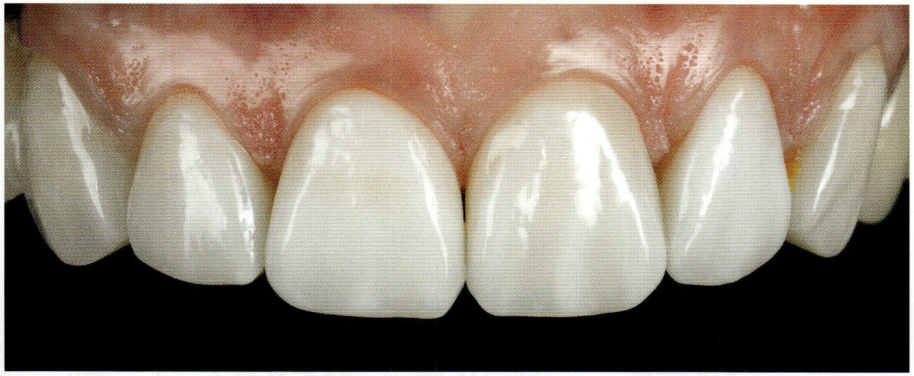

Fig 10-9i
Final result after veneers cementation.

Case 2: Comprehensive treatment with esthetic and functional reconstruction (Figs 10-10a to 10-10s)

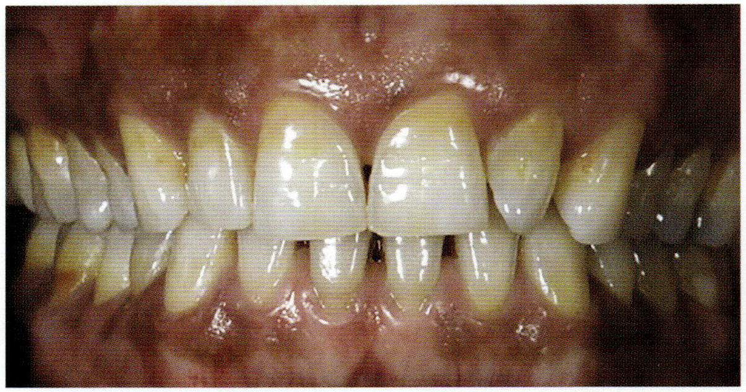

Fig 10-10a
Preliminary situation: initial plan combined esthetic and functional treatment.

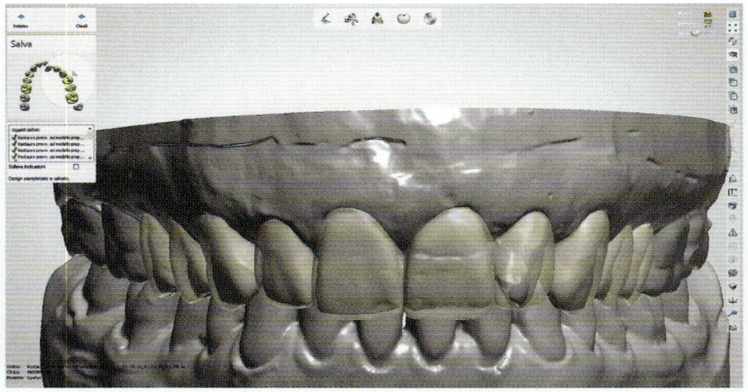

Fig 10-10b
Digital smile design in the anterior segment.

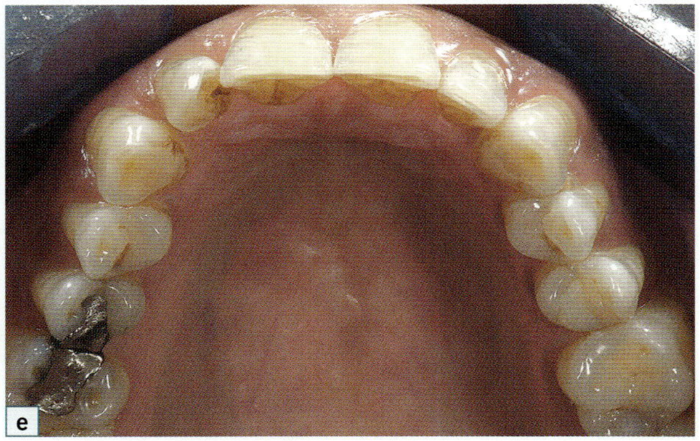

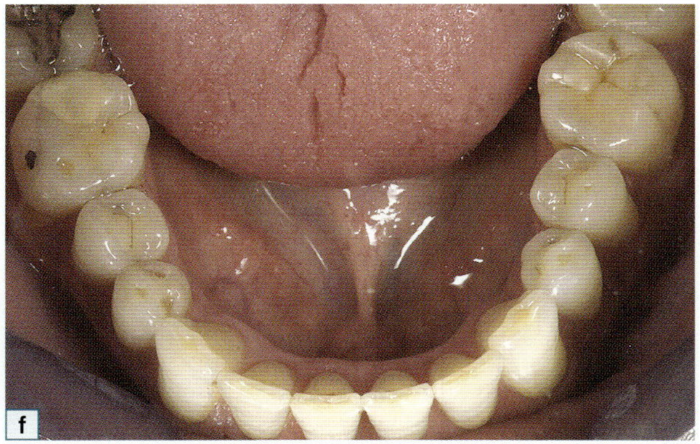

Figs 10-10e and 10-10f
Initial situation: view of the occlusal surfaces of the maxillary and mandibular arches.

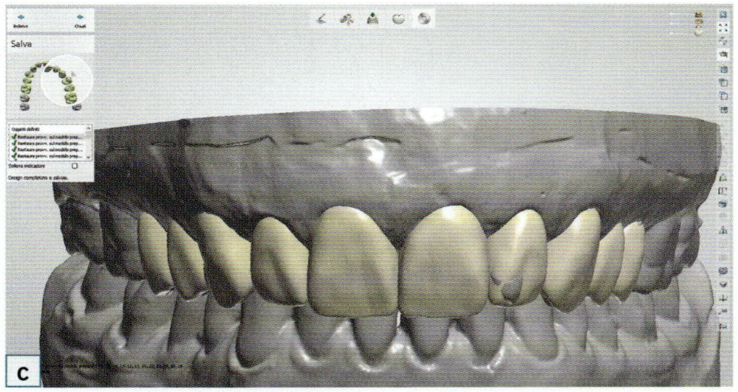

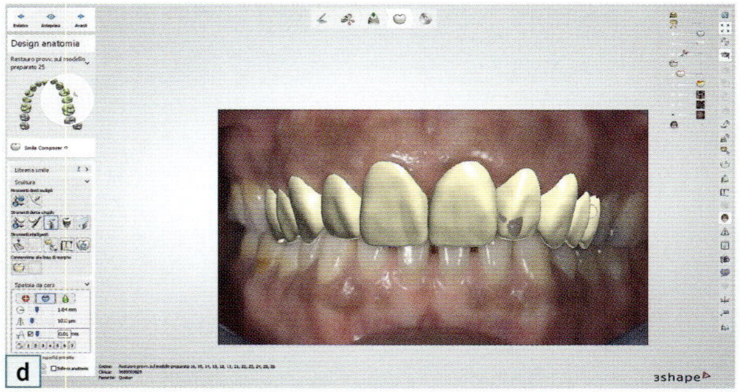

Figs 10-10c and 10-10d
3D digital design of the new esthetics.

REMEMBER

Regardless of the treatment method (analog or digital), always remember to verify the treatment plan with the mock-up. Thanks to that, you will know more about the patient's expectations!

Figs 10-10g and 10-10h
Digital models.

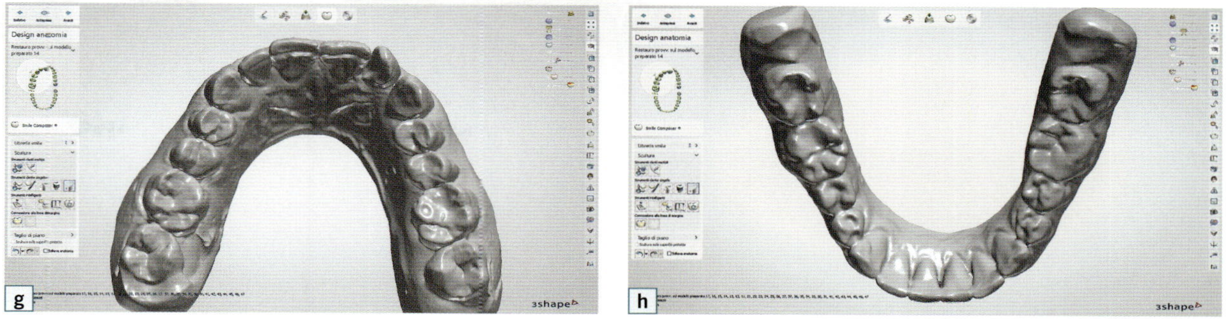

Figs 10-10i and 10-10j
Control of the digital design in the maximum intercuspation.

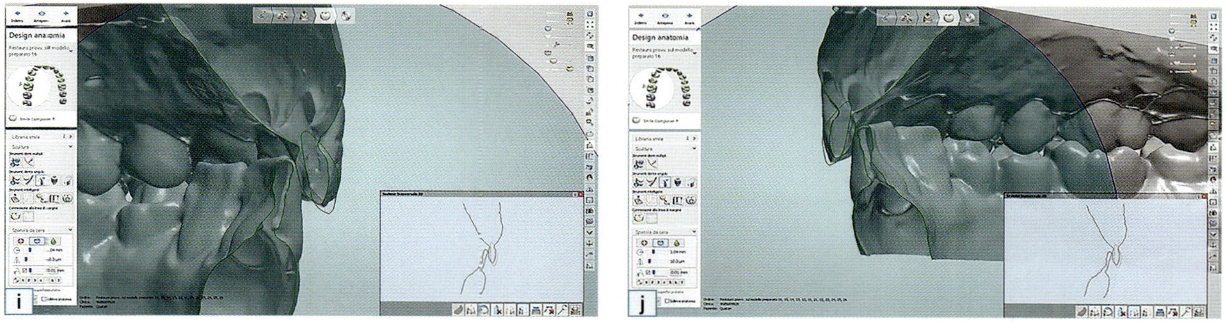

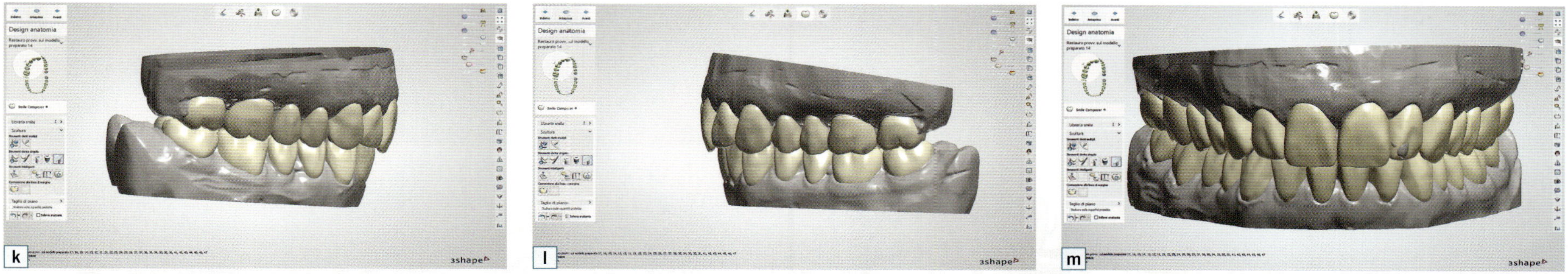

Figs 10-10k to 10-10m
Full 3D digital design.

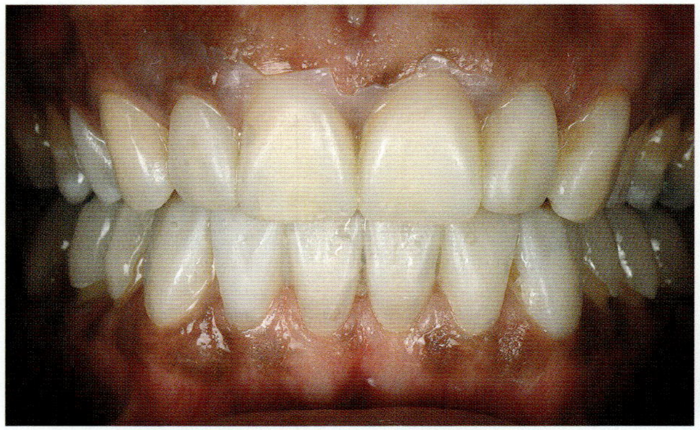

Fig 10-10n
Mock-up performed with flowable composite.

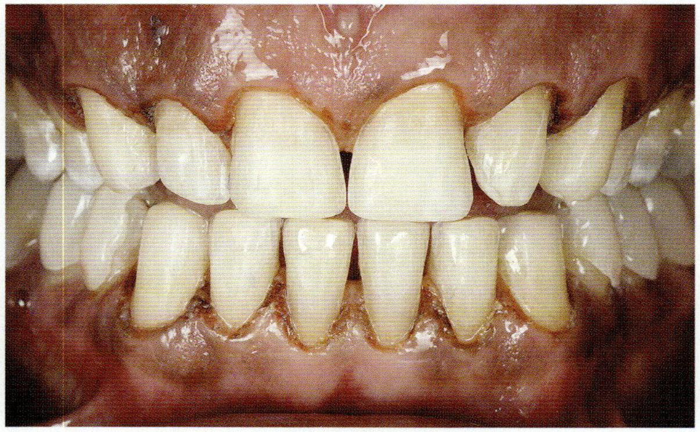

Fig 10-10o
Minimally invasive veneer preparation in the anterior segment.

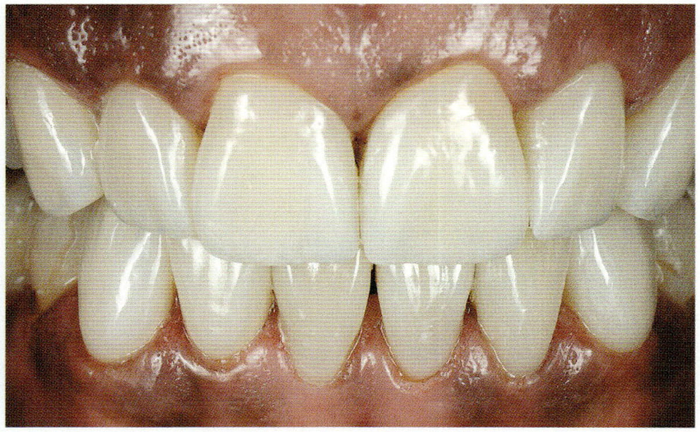

Fig 10-10p
Post-treatment situation: twelve lithium disilicate veneers without cutting back fabricated liquid ceramics.

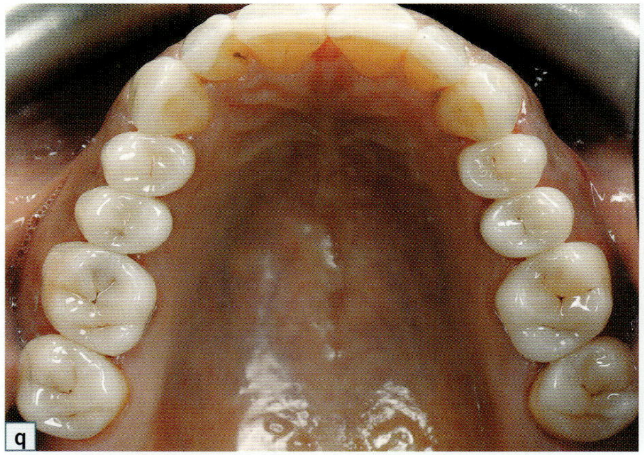

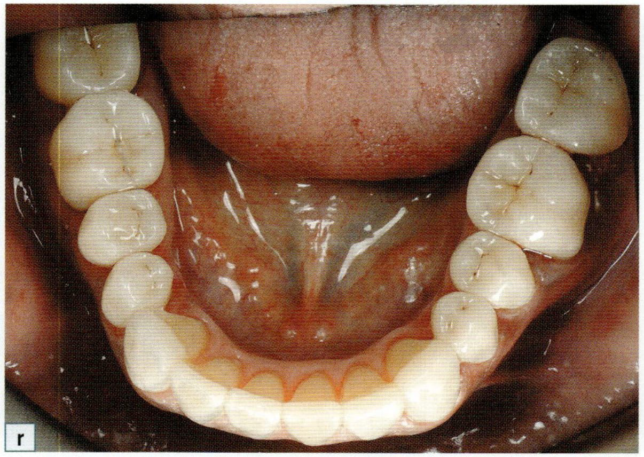

Figs 10-10q and 10-10r
Restored (q) maxillary and (r) mandibular arches: 16 veneers/onlays milled from lithium disilicate without cutting back the ceramics.

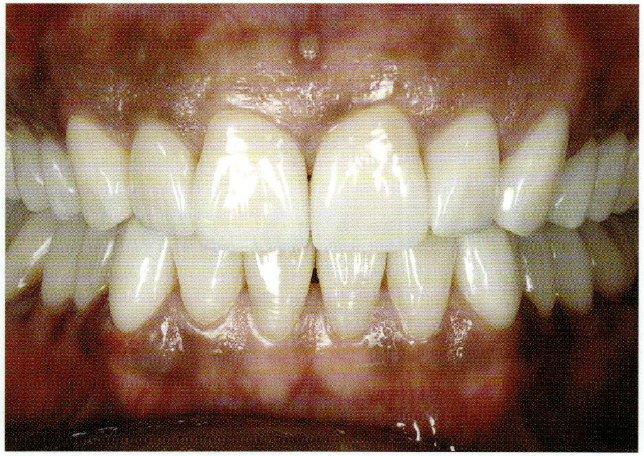

Fig 10-10s
The esthetic and functional result after 7 days.

Case 3: Hybrid solution: zirconium oxide combined with lithium disilicate (Figs 10-11a to 10-11o)

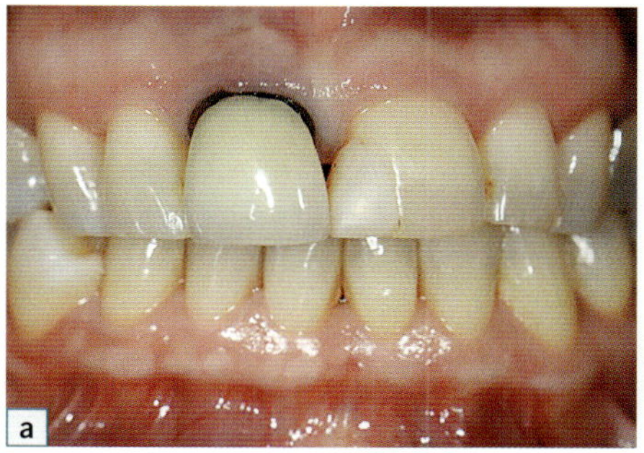

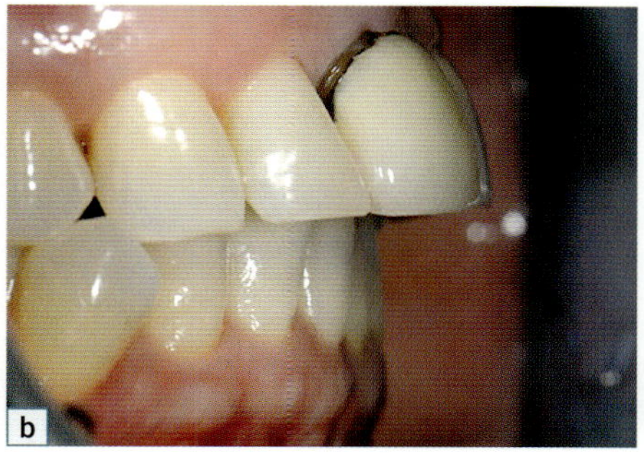

Figs 10-11a and 10-11b
Initial situation: a prosthetic crown on tooth 11 and a veneer on tooth 21 were planned.

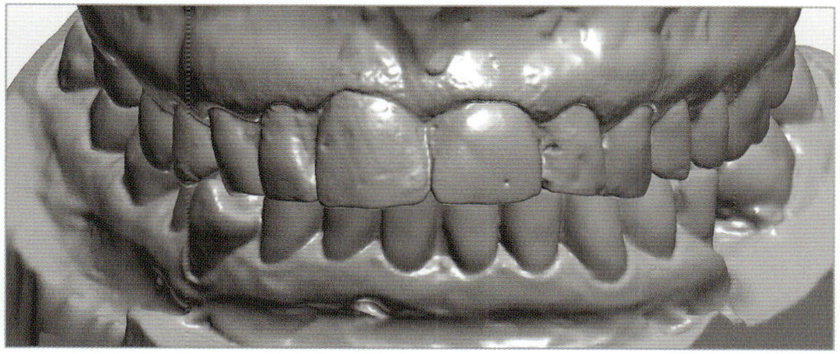

Fig 10-11c
The digital model presents the initial situation.

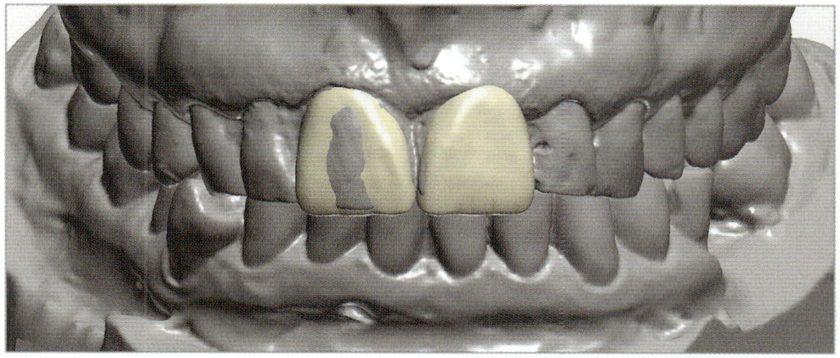

Fig 10-11d
3D digital project.

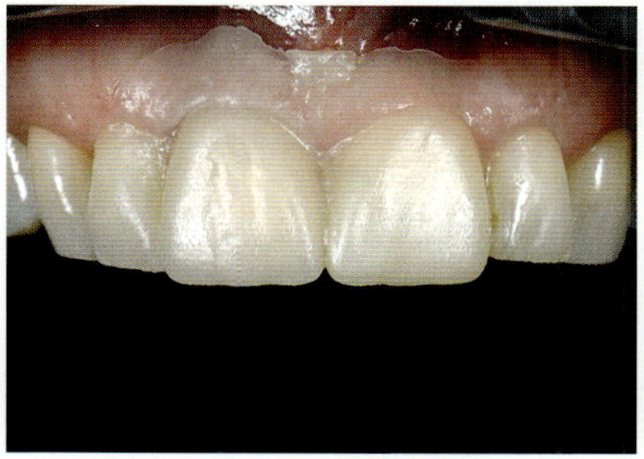

Fig 10-11e
Mock-up was performed with the indirect technique.

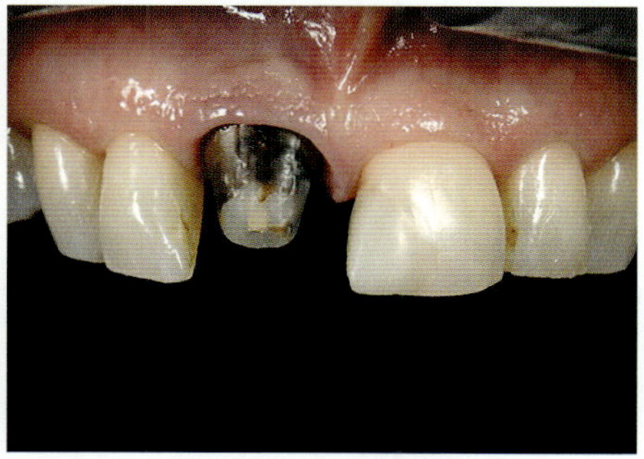

Fig 10-11f
Tooth 11 after prosthetic crown preparation.

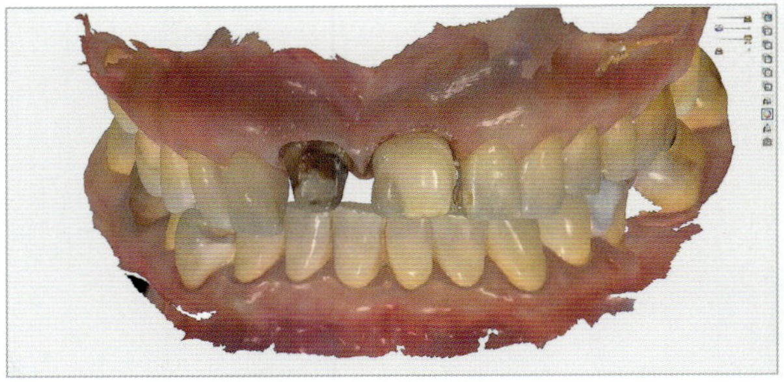

Fig 10-11g
Digital impression taken with an intraoral scanner.

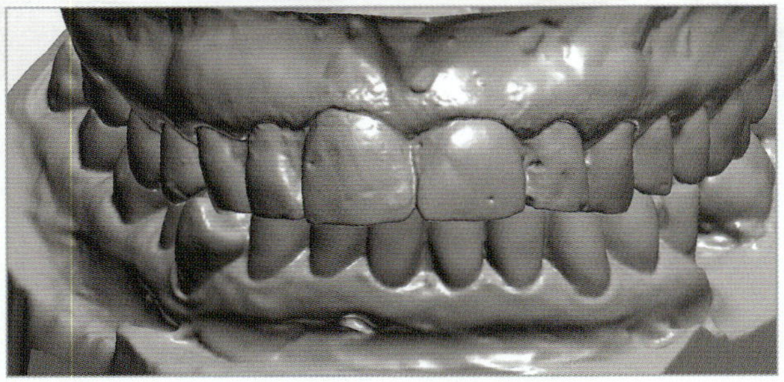

Fig 10-11h
Digital impression obtained with the use of laboratory software.

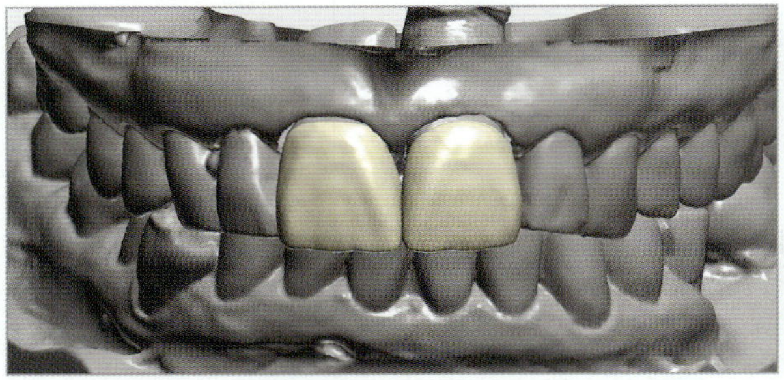

Fig 10-11i
Step 1: 3D design of a zirconium oxide crown and a veneer (teeth 11 and 21).

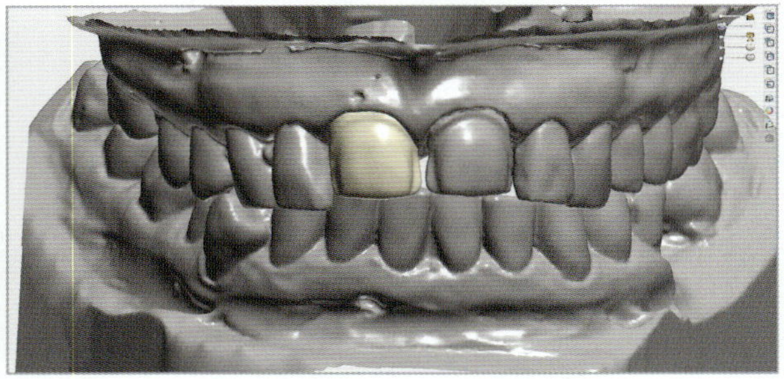

Fig 10-11j
Step 2: partial design of the hybrid crown fabricated of zirconium oxide.

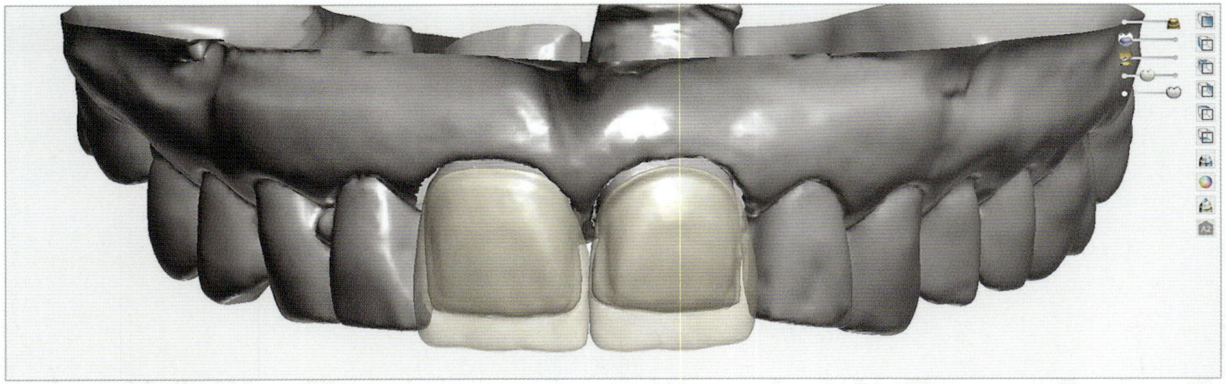

Fig 10-11k
Step 3: digital design of lithium disilicate restorations. (In the case of tooth 11, a hybrid crown was planned: zirconium oxide as the base and lithium disilicate as the outer layer of the restoration).

In summary, it can be concluded that the new possibilities created by digital dentistry allow more dynamic, synchronized work (workflow) between the dental office and the dental laboratory. Today's dental technicians can actively participate in recording each patient's additional parameters (intraoral scanners) and enjoy more freedom to create restorative solutions regarding the morphology and the functional treatment.[5–9]

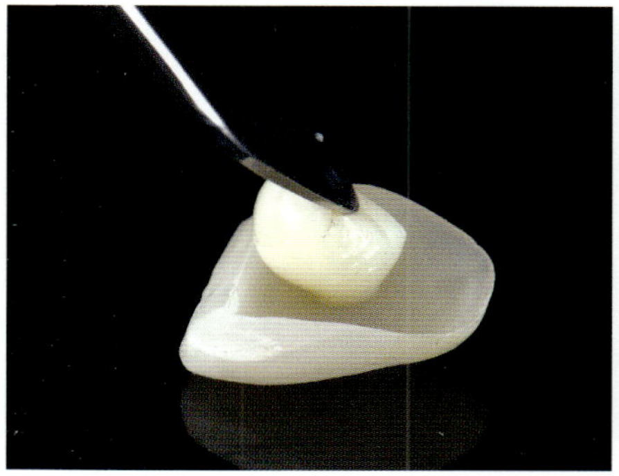

Fig 10-11l
The porcelain veneer cementation.

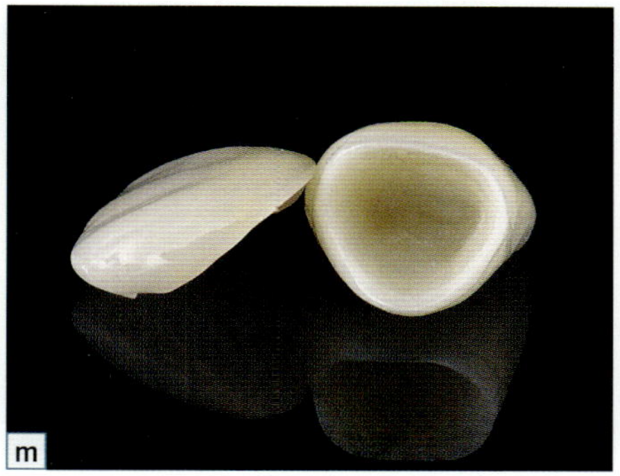

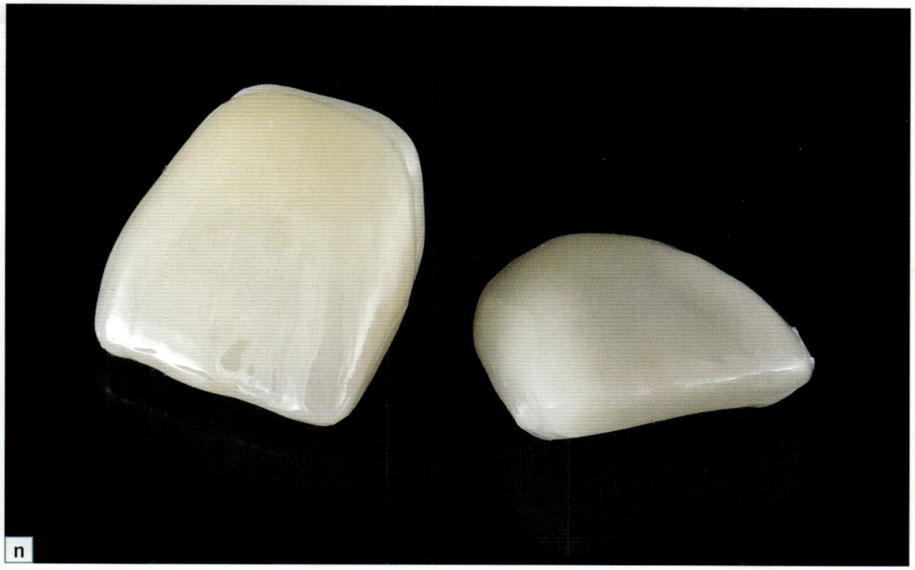

Figs 10-11m and 10-11n
Lithium disilicate veneer fabricated without cutting back (tooth 21), and a hybrid prosthetic crown with the palatal part fabricated from mechanically polished multilayer zirconium oxide and the labial surfaces created of lithium disilicate, bonded adhesively in the laboratory. As a result, the same material was used in the labial part of teeth 11 and 21.

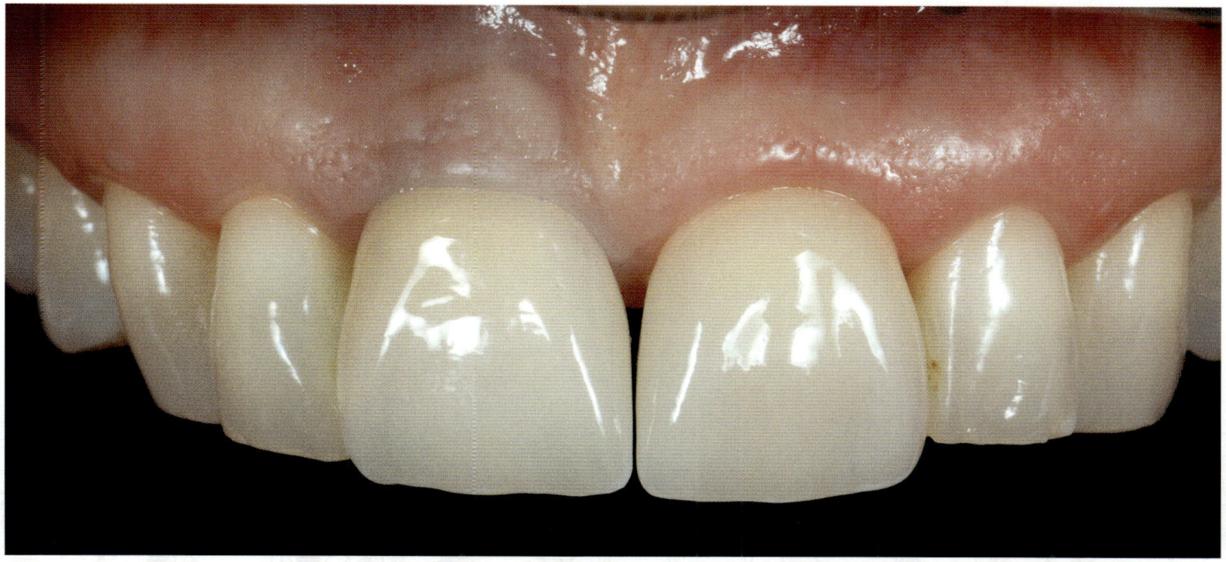

Fig 10-11o
Situation after completing the digitized treatment, without printing any models.

REFERENCES

1. De Freitas BN, Tonin BSH, Macedo AP, et al. Adaptation accuracy of milled lithium disilicate crowns: a 2D and 3D microCT analysis. J Esthet Restor Dent 2020;32:403–409.
2. Anadioti E, Aquilino SA, Gratton DG, Holloway JA, Denry I, Thomas GW, Qian F. 3D and 2D marginal fit of pressed and CAD/CAM lithium disilicate crowns made from digital and conventional impressions. J Prosthodont 2014;23:610–617.
3. Gold SA, Ferracane JL, da Costa J. Effect of crystallization firing on marginal gap of CAD/CAM fabricated lithium disilicate crowns. J Prosthodont 2018;27:63–66.
4. Zimmermann M, Valcanaia A, Neiva G, Mehl A, Fasbinder D. Digital evaluation of the fit of zirconia-reinforced lithium silicate crowns with a new three-dimensional approach. Quintessence Int 2018;49:9–15.
5. Ting-Shu S, Jian S. Intraoral digital impression technique: a review. J Prosthodont 2015;24:313–321.
6. Aswani K, Wankhade S, Khalikar A, Deogade S. Accuracy of an intraoral digital impression: a review. J Indian Prosthodont Soc 2020;20:27–37.
7. Ahlholm P, Sipilä K, Vallittu P, Jakonen M, Kotiranta U. Digital versus conventional impressions in fixed prosthodontics: a review. J Prosthodont 2018;27:35–41.
8. Shamseddine L, Majzoub Z. Relative translucency of a multilayered ultratranslucent zirconia material. J Contemp Dent Pract 2017;18:1099–1106.
9. Yu NK, Park MG. Effect of different coloring liquids on the flexural strength of multilayered zirconia. J Adv Prosthodont 2019;11:209–214.

SUMMARY

This textbook presents many clinical
cases of indirect veneers – fabricated
from porcelain and composite,
as well as direct composite veneers.
Each of these techniques has its own
indications, but also limitations.
Here, a summary of the most
important advantages of both
techniques is presented
to help the dentist
make an optimal decision
in everyday practice.

ADVANTAGES OF DIRECT COMPOSITE VENEERS

- They do not require a dental laboratory
- They allow faster execution of esthetic restorations
- They are more economical
- Their repairs are much easier, and a chip or a defect can be modified quickly and without significant financial expense for the dental office
- They allow for color or shape corrections when necessary (for example, when the patient is not satisfied with the final result)
- In many clinical situations, tooth preparation is not required (no-prep composite veneers)
- When performing composite veneers in the mandibular teeth, they perfectly fulfill the functional tasks related to the envelope of function (the composite material can be easily adjusted to avoid the constricted chewing pattern after treatment)

ADVANTAGES OF INDIRECT PORCELAIN VENEERS

- When performing comprehensive treatment including multiple teeth, it is easier to control the overall smile esthetic (inclination of the axis of individual teeth, the relationship of the central incisors to the lateral incisors, etc.)
- Covering discoloration is more predictable, as the dental technician has more options to achieve this
- More durable due to the extraoral fabrication process and easier finishing of the material
- Their esthetics do not depend profoundly on the manual and esthetic skills of the dentist, but more on the initial planning, cooperation with the dental laboratory, and know-how of the dental technician fabricating the final restorations

The table on the following page is helpful for practitioners as it includes the parameters for discussion while selecting the type of restoration, ie, between a direct composite veneer and an indirect porcelain veneer.

Table 10-1 Parameters for selecting veneers

Parameter for discussion	Direct composite veneers	Indirect porcelain veneers
Patient's age	Adolescent patients are also an indication due to the minimal invasiveness and ease of performing corrections at the patient's growth stage	Adolescent patients are contraindicated due to the tooth preparation for veneers and the incomplete growth of the patient's masticatory complex
Discolorations	Less predictable result of masking of discoloration	Easier masking of discoloration
Location in the dental arch	It is possible to perform both symmetrically and asymmetrically positioned restorations	Difficult and unpredictable in the case of fabrication single indirect veneer on the central incisor (asymmetrically positioned restorations)
Number of restorations to be performed	Difficult to control when performing comprehensive treatment (on many teeth)	Ideal for comprehensive treatment (six, eight, or more teeth in the maxillary arch)
Maxillary or mandibular arch	Maxillary or mandibular arch	It is difficult to perform in the mandibular arch: small teeth, appropriate space in the occlusion is necessary, risk to create the constricted chewing pattern
Durability	The composite resin material is polymerized intraorally	Veneer surface guarantees adequate durability due to the laboratory fabrication
Economy	Less expensive for the dentist and the patient	Much more expensive due to the work done in the dental laboratory and multiple appointments
Repair	Easy to fix/adjust (color, shape, chipping)	After cementation, the color cannot be modified, and if chipping occurs, it usually requires replacement of the veneer
Esthetics	Depends more on the manual and esthetic skills of the dentist	Mainly depends on the know-how of the dental technician

Video list

Title	Page	QR code	URL address
Alternative treatment of an adolescent	31		https://books.dentist.com.pl/venners/1
Correction no-prep with the composite	33		https://books.dentist.com.pl/venners/2
Whitening and shape correction with the composite	34		https://books.dentist.com.pl/venners/3
How to avoid preparation – shape correction with composite	37		https://books.dentist.com.pl/venners/4
Preparation through the mock-up*	116		https://books.dentist.com.pl/venners/5
The 45 degrees preparation*	118		https://books.dentist.com.pl/venners/6
Index check*	119		https://books.dentist.com.pl/venners/7
Impression for porcelain veneers*	123		https://books.dentist.com.pl/venners/8
Provisional veneers*	127		https://books.dentist.com.pl/venners/9
Etching the veneers with hydrofluoric acid**	148		https://books.dentist.com.pl/venners/10
Filling the veneerME with alcohol**	148		https://books.dentist.com.pl/venners/12
Ultrasonic bath**	148		https://books.dentist.com.pl/venners/13
Initial veneer rinsing**	149		https://books.dentist.com.pl/venners/11
Final veneer rinsing**	149		https://books.dentist.com.pl/venners/14
Final veneer drying**	149		https://books.dentist.com.pl/venners/15
Veneers cementation – preparation of the tooth hard tissues*	151		https://books.dentist.com.pl/venners/16
Placing veneers – cementation procedure*	154		https://books.dentist.com.pl/venners/17
Performing mock-up	175		https://books.dentist.com.pl/venners/18
Preparation through the mock-up	176		https://books.dentist.com.pl/venners/19

* Film editing: Dr. Maja Stępień
** With the consent of Style Italiano and Dr. Galip Gürel